2009
YEAR BOOK OF
MEDICINE®

The 2009 Year Book Series

Year Book of Anesthesiology and Pain Management™: Drs Chestnut, Abram, Black, Gravlee, Lee, Mathru, and Roizen

Year Book of Cardiology®: Drs Gersh, Cheitlin, Elliott, Graham, Sundt, and Waldo

Year Book of Critical Care Medicine®: Drs Dellinger, Parrillo, Balk, Bekes, Dorman, and Dries

Year Book of Dermatology and Dermatologic Surgery™: Drs Thiers and Lang

Year Book of Diagnostic Radiology®: Drs Osborn, Abbara, Birdwell, Elster, Levy, Manaster, Oestreich, Offiah, Rosado de Christenson, and Walker

Year Book of Emergency Medicine®: Drs Hamilton, Bruno, Handly, Quintana, and Werner

Year Book of Endocrinology®: Drs Schott, Apovian, Clarke, Eugster, Ludlam, Meikle, Ovalle, Schinner, and Schteingart

Year Book of Gastroenterology™: Drs Talley, Dempsey, Harnois, Lange, Pearson, Picco, Rombeau, and Scolapio

Year Book of Hand and Upper Limb Surgery®: Drs Yao and Steinmann

Year Book of Medicine®: Drs Barker, Berney, Garrick, Gersh, Khardori, LeRoith, Talley, and Thigpen

Year Book of Neonatal and Perinatal Medicine®: Drs Fanaroff, Benitz, Neu, and Papile

Year Book of Neurology and Neurosurgery®: Drs Klimo and Rabinstein

Year Book of Obstetrics, Gynecology, and Women's Health®: Drs Dungan and Shulman

Year Book of Oncology®: Drs Thigpen, Arceci, Bauer, Byhardt, Gordon, and Lawton

Year Book of Ophthalmology®: Drs Rapuano, Cohen, Eagle, Flanders, Hammersmith, Myers, Nelson, Penne, Sergott, Shields, Tipperman, and Vander

Year Book of Orthopedics®: Drs Morrey, Beauchamp, Huddleston, Swiontkowski, and Trigg

Year Book of Otolaryngology-Head and Neck Surgery®: Drs Sindwani, Balough, Franco, Gapany, and Mitchell

Year Book of Pathology and Laboratory Medicine®: Drs Raab, Parwani, Bejarano, and Bissell

Year Book of Pediatrics®: Dr Stockman

Year Book of Plastic and Aesthetic Surgery™: Drs Miller, Bartlett, Garner, McKinney, Ruberg, Salisbury, and Smith

Year Book of Psychiatry and Applied Mental Health®: Drs Talbott, Ballenger, Buckley, Frances, Krupnick, Mack, and Markowitz

Year Book of Pulmonary Disease®: Drs Barker, Jones, Maurer, Raza, Tanoue, and Willsie

Year Book of Sports Medicine®: Drs Shephard, Cantu, Feldman, Jankowski, Khan, Nieman, Pierrynowski, and Rowland

Year Book of Surgery®: Drs Copeland, Bland, Daly, Eberlein, Fahey, Jones, Mozingo, Pruett, and Seeger

Year Book of Urology®: Drs Andriole and Coplen

Year Book of Vascular Surgery®: Drs Moneta, Gillespie, Starnes, and Watkins

2009

The Year Book of
MEDICINE®

Editors

James A. Barker
Seth M. Berney
Renee Garrick
Bernard J. Gersh
Nancy M. Khardori
Derek LeRoith
Nicholas J. Talley
J. Tate Thigpen

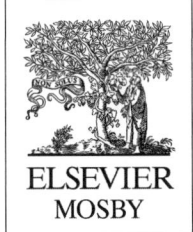

ELSEVIER
MOSBY

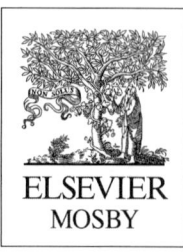

ELSEVIER
MOSBY

Vice President, Continuity: John A. Schrefer
Developmental Editor: Rachel A. Glover
Production Supervisor: Donna M. Skelton
Electronic Article Manager: Travis L. Ross
Illustrations and Permissions Coordinator: Linda S. Jones

Printed in the United States of America
Composition by TnQ Books and Journals Pvt Ltd, India
Printing/binding by Sheridan Books, Inc.

Editorial Office:
Elsevier
Suite 1800
1600 John F. Kennedy Blvd
Philadelphia, PA 19103-2899

International Standard Serial Number: 0084-3873
International Standard Book Number: 978-1-4160-5745-1

Editorial Board

Editors
James A. Barker, MD
Professor of Medicine and Chief, Pulmonary and Critical Care Medicine, University of South Carolina; Medical Director, MICU, PCU, and Respiratory Therapy, Palmetto Richland Hospital, Columbia, South Carolina

Seth Mark Berney, MD
Professor of Medicine, Chief, Section of Rheumatology; Director, Center of Excellence for Arthritis and Rheumatology, Louisiana State University Health Sciences Center School of Medicine, Shreveport, Louisiana

Renee Garrick, MD
Nephrology Associates, Valhalla, New York

Bernard J. Gersh, MB, ChB, DPhil, FRCP
Professor of Medicine, Mayo Clinic College of Medicine; Consultant, Division of Cardiovascular Diseases, Mayo Clinic, Rochester, Minnesota

Nancy M. Khardori, MD
Professor of Medicine and Microbiology/Immunology; Chief, Division of Infectious Diseases, Southern Illinois University School of Medicine, Springfield, Illinois

Derek LeRoith, MD, PhD
Chief, Division of Endocrinology and Diabetes, Mount Sinai School of Medicine, New York, New York

Nicholas J. Talley, MD, PhD
Chair, Department of Internal Medicine, Mayo Clinic Florida, Jacksonville, Florida

James Tate Thigpen, MD
Professor of Medicine and Director, Division of Oncology, University of Mississippi Medical Center, Jackson, Mississippi

Contributors

Rheumatology
Molly Boyd, MD
Fellow, Section of Hematology/Oncology, Feist-Weiller Cancer Center, Louisiana State University Health Sciences Center School of Medicine, Shreveport, Louisiana

Nicole Cotter, MD
Fellow, Section of Rheumatology, Center of Excellence for Arthritis and Rheumatology, Louisiana State University Health Sciences Center School of Medicine, Shreveport, Louisiana

Richa Dhawan, MD
Assistant Professor, Section of Rheumatology, Center of Excellence for Arthritis and Rheumatology, Louisiana State University Health Sciences Center School of Medicine, Shreveport, Louisiana

Table of Contents

Journals Represented

Journals represented in this YEAR BOOK are listed below.

Academic Emergency Medicine
Acta Obstetricia et Gynecologica Scandinavica
American Heart Journal
American Journal of Cardiology
American Journal of Clinical Nutrition
American Journal of Emergency Medicine
American Journal of Epidemiology
American Journal of Gastroenterology
American Journal of Infection Control
American Journal of Kidney Diseases
American Journal of Medicine
American Journal of Ophthalmology
American Journal of Respiratory and Critical Care Medicine
American Surgeon
Annals of Emergency Medicine
Annals of Internal Medicine
Annals of the Rheumatic Diseases
Annals of Thoracic Surgery
Archives of Internal Medicine
Archives of Surgery
Arthritis & Rheumatism
British Journal of Dermatology
British Journal of Surgery
British Medical Journal
Burns
Cancer
Cancer Research
Chest
Circulation
Clinical Endocrinology
Clinical Infectious Diseases
Digestive Diseases and Sciences
Europace
European Journal of Echocardiography
European Heart Journal
Fertility and Sterility
Gastroenterology
Gastrointestinal Endoscopy
Gut
Gynecologic Oncology
Heart Rhythm
Hepatology
Intensive Care Medicine
International Journal of Cardiology
International Journal of Obesity
International Journal of Obesity (London)
International Journal of Radiation Oncology Biology Physics

Journal of Bone Mineral Research
Journal of Cardiac failure
Journal of Cardiovascular Electrophysiology
Journal of Clinical Endocrinology & Metabolism Journal of Clinical Microbiology
Journal of Clinical Oncology
Journal of Clinical Rheumatology
Journal of General Internal Medicine
Journal of Heart and Lung Transplantation
Journal of Infectious Diseases
Journal of Pediatrics
Journal of Rheumatology
Journal of the American Board of Family Medicine
Journal of the American College of Cardiology
Journal of the American College of Cardiology: Cardiovascular Interventions
Journal of the American College of Radiology
Journal of the American College of Surgeons
Journal of the American Medical Association
Journal of the American Society of Nephrology
Journal of the National Cancer Institute
Journal of Thoracic and Cardiovascular Surgery
Journal of Urology
Kidney International
Lancet
Lancet Oncology
Lupus
Medicine
Metabolism
Metabolism Clinical and Experimental
Molecular Cancer Therapeutics
Nature
Nature Genetics
Nephrology Dialysis Transplantation
New England Journal of Medicine
Obstetrics & Gynecology
Pediatric Infectious Disease Journal
Pediatrics
Proceedings of the National Academy of Sciences of the United States of America
Respiratory Medicine
Scandinavian Journal of Rheumatology
Seminars in Radiation Oncology
Surgery
Thorax
Transplantation
Transplantation Proceedings
Tuberculosis

Standard Abbreviations

The following terms are abbreviated in this edition: acquired immunodeficiency syndrome (AIDS), cardiopulmonary resuscitation (CPR), central nervous system (CNS), cerebrospinal fluid (CSF), computed tomography (CT), deoxyribonucleic acid (DNA), electrocardiography (ECG), health maintenance organization

(HMO), human immunodeficiency virus (HIV), intensive care unit (ICU), intramuscular (IM), intravenous (IV), magnetic resonance (MR) imaging (MRI), ribonucleic acid (RNA), and ultrasound (US).

NOTE

The YEAR BOOK OF MEDICINE is a literature survey service providing abstracts of articles published in the professional literature. Every effort is made to assure the accuracy of the information presented in these pages. Neither the editors nor the publisher of the YEAR BOOK OF MEDICINE can be responsible for errors in the original materials. The editors' comments are their own opinions. Mention of specific products within this publication does not constitute endorsement.

To facilitate the use of the YEAR BOOK OF MEDICINE as a reference tool, all illustrations and tables included in this publication are now identified as they appear in the original article. This change is meant to help the reader recognize that any illustration or table appearing in the YEAR BOOK OF MEDICINE may be only one of many in the original article. For this reason, figure and table numbers will often appear to be out of sequence within the YEAR BOOK OF MEDICINE.

PART ONE

RHEUMATOLOGY

SETH MARK BERNEY, MD

Introduction

What has happened since the closing months of 2008? My daughter earned her driver's license; Barack Obama won the presidential election and vowed to repair the economy, bring home the troops, and fix the health care system; my beloved Phillies won the World Series; and both General Motors and Chrysler filed for Chapter 11 bankruptcy.

My contributors and I have diligently reviewed many papers and selected those that represent the most interesting or important findings from the past year and grouped them into 9 chapters for the Rheumatology section: Rheumatoid Arthritis, Systemic Lupus Erythematosus, Vasculitis, Fibromyalgia, Scleroderma, Juvenile Idiopathic Arthritis, Osteoporosis, Spondyloarthropathy, and Miscellaneous. Because of space constraints, we unfortunately could not include other deserving articles.

While this book's purpose is to review the literature from the prior year, questions that we should consider in the coming year include: 1) Will the tyrosine kinase inhibitor GLEEVEC® (imatinib mesylate) benefit patients with scleroderma? 2) Will the two new tumor necrosis factor (TNF) inhibitors become "me-too" drugs or provide an improvement over the currently available anti-TNF medications? 3) When will the American College of Rheumatology formally incorporate musculoskeletal ultrasound training into rheumatology fellowship programs? 4) Will the new voluntary Pharmaceutical Research and Manufacturers of America (PhRMA) marketing and ethical conduct recommendations change the perceived or actual physician conflict of interest, and will it affect the cost of medications? Or is it a farce and just for show? 5) How prevalent will progressive multifocal leukoencephalopathy (PML) become, and will it limit the use of certain cell-depleting therapies and other biologics? 6) What health care delivery and availability changes will occur under President Obama, and how will it affect providers, suppliers, and patients? Or will everybody refuse to cooperate because of the fear that they will lose money, leaving the underinsured to fend for themselves again?

Seth Mark Berney, MD

1 Rheumatoid Arthritis

Introduction

This chapter contains 9 articles arranged in 2 groups. The first group consists of 6 articles that analyze the effectiveness of several medications. The remainder of the Rheumatoid Arthritis articles discuss the dissociation between clinical remission and continued joint destruction, the association of biologics and malignancy, and the recognition that pulmonary tuberculosis patients have serum anti-CCP antibodies.

Seth Mark Berney, MD

Comparison of methotrexate monotherapy with a combination of methotrexate and etanercept in active, early, moderate to severe rheumatoid arthritis (COMET): a randomised, double-blind, parallel treatment trial

Emery P, Breedveld FC, Hall S, et al (Univ of Leeds, UK; Leiden Univ Med Centre, Netherlands; Cabrini Health Hospital, Malvern, VIC, Australia; et al)
Lancet 372:375-382, 2008

Background.—Remission and radiographic non-progression are goals in the treatment of early rheumatoid arthritis. The aim of the combination of methotrexate and etanercept in active early rheumatoid arthritis (COMET) trial is to compare remission and radiographic non-progression in patients treated with methotrexate monotherapy or with methotrexate plus etanercept.

Methods.—542 outpatients who were methotrexate-naive and had had early moderate-to-severe rheumatoid arthritis for 3–24 months were randomly assigned to receive either methotrexate alone titrated up from 7·5 mg a week to a maximum of 20 mg a week by week 8 or methotrexate (same titration) plus etanercept 50 mg a week. Coprimary endpoints at 52 weeks were remission measured with the disease activity score in 28 joints (DAS28) and radiographic nonprogression measured with modified total Sharp score. Treatment was allocated with a computerised randomisation and enrolment system, which masked both participants and carers. Analysis was done by modified intention to treat with last

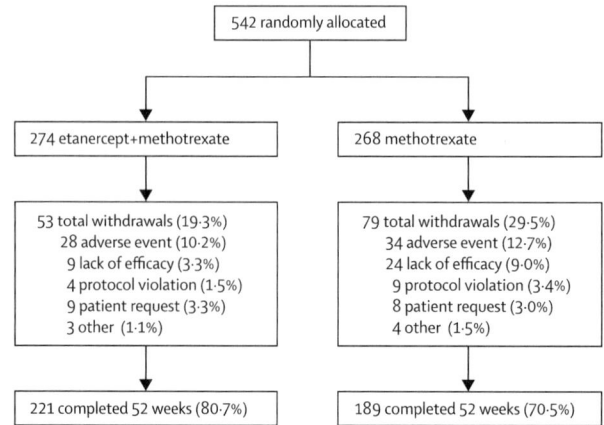

FIGURE 1.—Trial profile. More patients in the combined-treatment group than in the methotrexate monotherapy group completed period 1, largely because of a larger number of withdrawals due to lack of efficacy in the monotherapy group. (Reprinted from Emery P, Breedveld FC, Hall S, et al. Comparison of methotrexate monotherapy with a combination of methotrexate and etanercept in active, early, moderate to severe rheumatoid arthritis (COMET): a randomised, double-blind, parallel treatment trial. *Lancet*. 2008;372:375-382, with permission from Elsevier Ltd.)

observation carried forward for missing data. This study is registered with ClinicalTrials.gov, number NCT00195494).

Findings.—274 participants were randomly assigned to receive combined treatment and 268 methotrexate alone. 132 of 265 (50%, 95% CI 44–56%) patients who took combined treatment and were available for assessment achieved clinical remission compared with 73 of 263 (28%, 23–33%) taking methotrexate alone (effect difference 22·05%, 95%CI 13·96–30·15%, p<0·0001). 487 evaluable patients had severe disease (DAS28 > 5·1). 196 of 246 (80%, 75–85%) and 135 of 230 (59%, 53–65%), respectively, achieved radiographic non-progression (20·98%, 12·97–29·09%, p < 0·0001). Serious adverse events were similar between groups.

Interpretation.—Both clinical remission and radiographic non-progression are achievable goals in patients with early severe rheumatoid arthritis within 1 year of combined treatment with etanercept plus methotrexate (Figs 1 and 2).

▶ This article details the results of the 1st year of the combination of methotrexate and etanercept in early rheumatoid arthritis (COMET) trial, a 24 month, double-blind randomized parallel group, multicenter, outpatient study.

During period 1 (the 1st 52 weeks), all patients received oral methotrexate starting at 7.5 mg once a week, titrating up to a maximum dose of 20 mg over 8 weeks, and were randomized to receive either weekly subcutaneous etanercept 50 mg or matching placebo injections. All patients received folate supplementation.

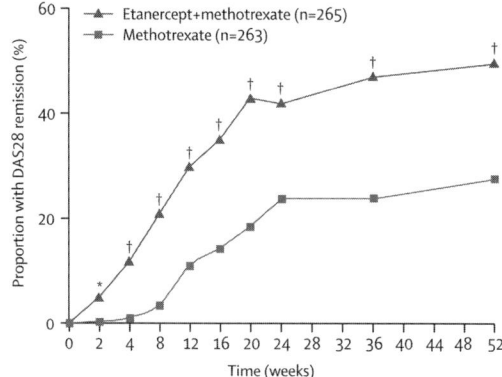

FIGURE 2.—DAS28 remission over 52 weeks of treatment. A significant difference in the proportion of patients in DAS28 remission was seen in week 2 and persisted for the study period. *p=0·002. †p<0·0001. (Reprinted from Emery P, Breedveld FC, Hall S, et al. Comparison of methotrexate monotherapy with a combination of methotrexate and etanercept in active, early, moderate to severe rheumatoid arthritis (COMET): a randomised, double-blind, parallel treatment trial. *Lancet*. 2008;372:375-382, with permission from Elsevier Ltd.)

Adult patients with active rheumatoid arthritis (RA) of between 3 months and 2 years duration who were methotrexate or TNF-inhibitor naive were eligible. Exclusion criteria included steroid injection or other DMARDs within 4 weeks of baseline visit, or other important medical diseases or comorbidities.

Prednisone ($\leq$ 10 mg/day) and nonsteroidal anti-inflammatory drugs (NSAIDs) were permitted if started at least 4 weeks prior to the baseline visit, but must remain at a constant dose throughout the first 24 weeks.

Coprimary endpoints were the proportion of patients who achieved remission (DAS28 < 2.6) at week 52, and the change in the van der Heijde modified total Sharp score (mTSS; joint erosion score plus joint space narrowing score) from baseline to week 52.

The patient demographics were similar between the 2 groups. Five hundred and fourty-two patients from 22 countries participated (87% from Europe and Australia and the remainder from Latin America and Asia).

Fig 1 illustrates the patient allocation and protocol completion details.

The mean disease duration was 9 months, and the mean DAS28 was 6.5 (indicating severe disease).

As illustrated in Fig 2, statistically, significantly more patients in the combined treatment group achieved a DAS28 remission than the monotherapy group as early as week 2. Furthermore, patients in the combined group had statistically significantly more patients who achieved radiographic nonprogression compared with the monotherapy group at week 52. Furthermore, fewer patients in the combination group missed work at least once compared with the monotherapy group (p = 0.004).

The 2 groups had similar safety profiles.

This trial substantiates the change in approach toward RA (and by extrapolation most noncrystalline inflammatory arthropathies), that early aggressive therapy outperforms the outdated pyramid approach. Furthermore, significant and compelling data exist indicating the superiority of TNF-inhibitor based combination regimens.

However, several questions remain:

1. Why did the investigators exclude American patients from this study?
2. I contend that RA is not a single immunologic disease. Therefore, if the data was reanalyzed according to country, continent, or ethnicity of patients, would the conclusions change?
3. If other DMARDs or DMARD combinations were substituted for MTX (ie, plaquenil, sulfasalazine, leflunomide), would the data and interpretations change?

S. M. Berney, MD

Effect of interleukin-6 receptor inhibition with tocilizumab in patients with rheumatoid arthritis (OPTION study): a double-blind, placebo-controlled, randomised trial
Smolen JS, for the OPTION Investigators (Med Univ of Vienna, Austria; et al)
Lancet 371:987-997, 2008

Background.—Interleukin 6 is involved in the pathogenesis of rheumatoid arthritis via its broad effects on immune and inflammatory responses. Our aim was to assess the therapeutic effects of blocking interleukin 6 by inhibition of the interleukin-6 receptor with tocilizumab in patients with rheumatoid arthritis.

Methods.—In this double-blind, randomised, placebo-controlled, parallel group phase III study, 623 patients with moderate to severe active rheumatoid arthritis were randomly assigned with an interactive voice response system, stratified by site with a randomisation list provided by the study sponsor, to receive tocilizumab 8 mg/kg (n=205), tocilizumab 4 mg/kg (214), or placebo (204) intravenously every 4 weeks, with methotrexate at stable pre-study doses (10–25 mg/week). Rescue therapy with tocilizumab 8 mg/kg was offered at week 16 to patients with less than 20% improvement in both swollen and tender joint counts. The primary endpoint was the proportion of patients with 20% improvement in signs and symptoms of rheumatoid arthritis according to American College of Rheumatology criteria (ACR20 response) at week 24. Analyses were by intention to treat. This trial is registered with ClinicalTrials.gov, number NCT00106548.

Findings.—The intention-to-treat analysis population consisted of 622 patients: one patient in the 4 mg/kg group did not receive study treatment and was thus excluded. At 24 weeks, ACR20 responses were seen in more patients receiving tocilizumab than in those receiving placebo (120 [59%] patients in the 8 mg/kg group, 102 [48%] in the 4 mg/kg group, 54 [26%] in the placebo group; odds ratio 4·0 [95% CI 2·6–6·1], p<0·0001 for 8 mg/kg *vs* placebo; and 2·6 [1·7–3·9],

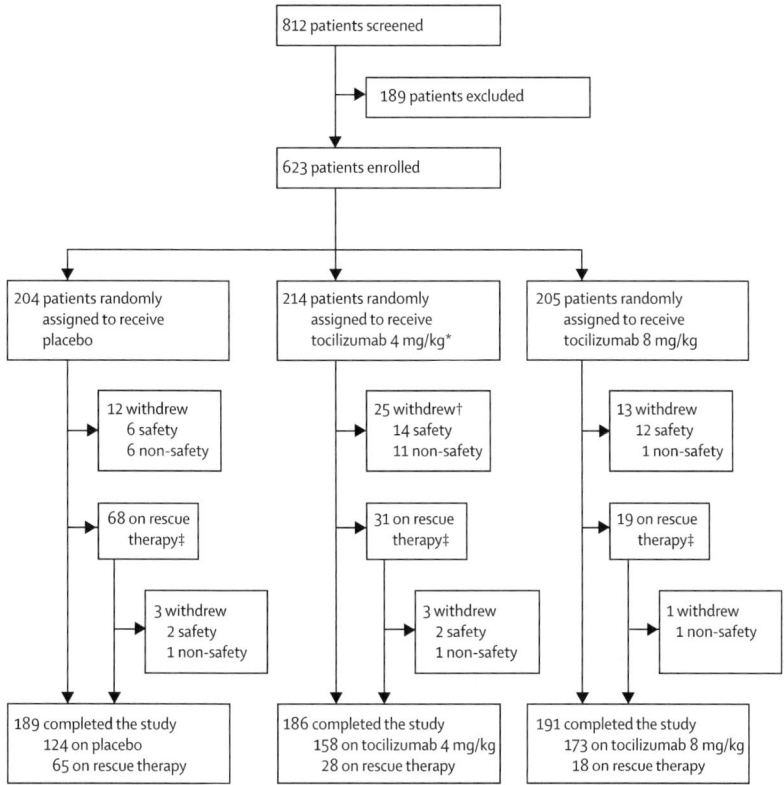

FIGURE 1.—Trial profile. *Includes one patient who was randomised to tocilizumab 4 mg/kg but received tocilizumab 8 mg/kg throughout the study. †Includes one patient who did not receive study treatment and was subsequently withdrawn. ‡Patient who did not achieve >20% improvement from baseline in both tender and swollen joint count at week 16 were offered rescue therapy. (Reprinted from Smolen JS, for the OPTION Investigators. Effect of interleukin-6 receptor inhibition with tocilizumab in patients with rheumatoid arthritis (OPTION study): a double-blind, placebo-controlled, randomised trial. *Lancet.* 2008;371:987-997.)

$p<0\cdot0001$ for 4 mg/kg *vs* placebo). More people receiving tocilizumab than those receiving placebo had at least one adverse event (143 [69%] in the 8 mg/kg group; 151 [71%] in the 4 mg/kg group; 129 [63%] in the placebo group). The most common serious adverse events were serious infections or infestations, reported by six patients in the 8 mg/kg group, three in the 4 mg/kg group, and two in the placebo group.

Interpretation.—Tocilizumab could be an effective therapeutic approach in patients with moderate to severe active rheumatoid arthritis (Fig 1, Tables 2 and 3).

▶ The authors undertook this study, the tOcilizumab Pivotal Trial in methotrexate Inadequate respONders (OPTION), to assess the efficacy of tocilizumab

TABLE 2.—Clinical Response to Treatment

	Tocilizumab 4 mg/kg (n = 213)	Tocilizumab 8 mg/kg (n = 205)	Placebo (n = 204)
ACR20			
Number of patients	102 (48%)	120 (59%)	54 (26%)
p value vs placebo*	p<0·0001	p<0·0001	NA
Odds ratio (vs placebo)†	2·6 (1·7–3·9)	4·0 (2·6–6·1)	NA
ACR50			
Number of patients	67 (31%)	90 (44%)	22 (11%)
p value vs placebo*	p<0·0001	p<0·0001	NA
Odds ratio (vs placebo)†	3·8 (2·3–6·5)	6·6 (3·9–11·2)	NA
ACR70			
Number of patients	26 (12%)	45 (22%)	4 (2%)
p value vs placebo*	p<0·0001	p<0·0001	NA
Odds ratio (vs placebo)†	7·0 (2·4–20·4)	14·2 (5·0–40·4)	NA
DAS28 <2·6			
Number of patients	21/156 (13%)	47/171 (27%)	1/121 (0·8%)
p value vs placebo*	p=0·0002	p<0·0001	NA
Odds ratio (vs placebo)†	18·8 (2·5–142·2)	45·0 (6·1–331·6)	NA
EULAR			
Good response	45 (21%)	78 (38%)	6 (3%)
Moderate response	87 (41%)	85 (41%)	65 (32%)
No response	81 (38%)	42 (20%)	133 (65%)
p value vs placebo*	p<0·0001	p<0·0001	NA
Odds ratio (vs placebo)†‡	3·1 (2·1–4·7)	7·6 (4·9–12·0)	NA

*Calculated with Cochran-Mantel-Haenszel χ^2 test with adjustment for site.
†Calculated with logistic regression, including region in the model (as algorithm fails to converge using site).
‡Good and moderate EULAR response compared with no response.
(Reprinted from Smolen JS, for the OPTION Investigators. Effect of interleukin-6 receptor inhibition with tocilizumab in patients with rheumatoid arthritis (OPTION study): a double-blind, placebo-controlled, randomised trial. *Lancet.* 2008;371:987-997.)

in patients with active rheumatoid arthritis (RA) also receiving methotrexate (MTX).

Adult patients with moderate to severe active RA of longer than 6 weeks duration who had an inadequate response to MTX were recruited. Active disease was defined as ≥ swollen joints, ≥ 8 tender joints, and a c-reactive protein (CRP) > 10 mg/l or an ESR ≥ 28 mm/h. Patients had received MTX for ≥ 12 weeks and were on a stable dose of 10 to 25 mg/week for ≥ 8 weeks. All other disease modifying antirheumatic drugs (DMARDs) were discontinued and washed out (however, the authors only mention leflunomide, anakinra, etanercept, infliximab, and adalimumab. What about sulfasalazine, hydroxychloroquine, and gold?) Oral prednisone (≤ 10 mg/day or equivalent dose) and NSAIDs were permitted if the doses were stable for the 6 weeks before inclusion. Patients were excluded if they had other autoimmune diseases, significant extra-articular manifestations of RA, function class IV RA, active or recurrent infections, hepatitis B or C, active liver disease (defined as AST or ALT ≥ 1.5 times upper limit of normal), or unsuccessful TNF inhibitor therapy. This phase III, 3 arm, randomized, double-blind placebo controlled parallel group, international study was conducted in 73 centers in 17 countries, during which time patients were enrolled and treated from 2/16/2005 and 11/13/2006.

TABLE 3.—Mean Changes in Core Variables from Baseline at Week 24 (Adjusted Means)

	Tocilizumab 4 mg/kg	Tocilizumab 8 mg/kg	Placebo
Swollen joint count	−8·5	−10·5	−4·3
Difference from placebo group	−4·2 (−6·1 to −2·3) p<0·0001	−6·2 (−8·1 to −4·2) p<0·0001	NA
Tender joint count	−14·5	−17·1	−7·4
Difference from placebo group	−7·0 (−10·0 to −4·1) p<0·0001	−9·6 (−12·6 to −6·7) p<0·0001	NA
Patient pain VAS (mm)	−25·0	−29·8	−14·0
Difference from placebo group	−11·0 (−17·0 to −5·0) p = 0·0004	−15·8 (−21·7 to −9·9) p<0·0001	NA
Patient global VAS (mm)	−28·8	−32·7	−17·8
Difference from placebo group	−10·9 (−17−1 to −4·8) p = 0·0005	−14·9 (−20·9 to −8·9) p<0·0001	NA
Physician global VAS (mm)	−38·3	−41·6	−32·7
Difference from placebo group	−5·6 (−10·5 to −0·8) p = 0·0229	−9·0 (−13·8 to −4·2) p=0·0002	NA
CRP (mg/L)	−16·6	−25·1	−3·5
Difference from placebo group	−13·0 (−20·1 to −5·9) p = 0·0004	−21·6 (−28·6 to −14·6) p<0·0001	NA
ESR (mm/h)	−25·5	−39·5	−7·1
Difference from placebo group	−18·3 (−24·3 to −12·4) p<0·0001	−32·3 (−38·2 to −26·5) p<0·0001	NA
HAQ	−0·52	−0·55	−0·34
Difference from placebo group	−0·18 (−0·34 to −0·02) p = 0·0296	−0·21 (−0·37 to −0·05) p = 0·0082	NA

Data are mean change from baseline, or mean difference from placebo (95% CI).

(Reprinted from Smolen JS, for the OPTION Investigators. Effect of interleukin-6 receptor inhibition with tocilizumab in patients with rheumatoid arthritis (OPTION study): a double-blind, placebo-controlled, randomised trial. *Lancet.* 2008;371:987-997.)

Patients on a stable dose of methotrexate (10-25 mg/week) were randomized to receive placebo, tocilizumab 4 mg/kg or 8 mg/kg intravenously at baseline and every 4 weeks for 24 weeks. They had regular efficacy and safety visits.

Fig 1 details and summarizes the trial profile regarding the number of patients randomized, withdrew, therapies received, and completed. As illustrated in Tables 2 and 3, 8 mg/kg was more effective than 4 mg/kg and both were statistically significantly better than placebo in multiple parameters when evaluated at week 24.

Although it appears that the tocilizumab groups had slightly more adverse events (such as infections and skin reactions), I am uncertain whether the authors performed a statistical analysis. Furthermore, the frequency of serious adverse events appears equal amongst the 3 treatment groups. However, the authors note that the tocilizumab patients had a higher frequency of transaminitis, hyperlipidemia, and neutropenia. The authors state that most of these abnormalities resolved spontaneously or after interruption of the treatment.

This article further supports the use of Tocilizumab for the treatment of RA. However, I am curious why the statistical analyses comparing the 4 mg/kg and 8 mg/kg doses were not included. It does not appear that significant infections or liver toxicity are a major issue yet. Only long term follow-up data specifically investigating or analyzing liver health will resolve the clinical significance of the transaminase abnormalities. Furthermore, while the data appears promising, until a study compares tocilizumab with the TNF inhibitors and proves either equality or superiority, I do not expect it to supplant this class of drugs as the gold standard of therapy for the inflammatory arthropathies, and may be relegated to "me too" status.

S. M. Berney, MD

Denosumab Treatment Effects on Structural Damage, Bone Mineral Density, and Bone Turnover in Rheumatoid Arthritis: A Twelve-Month, Multicenter, Randomized, Double-Blind, Placebo-Controlled, Phase II Clinical Trial
Cohen SB, Dore RK, Lane NE, et al (Metroplex Clinical Research Ctr, Dallas, TX; Anahcim, CA; Univ of California, Sacramento; et al)
Arthritis Rheum 58:1299-1309, 2008

Objective.—RANKL is essential for osteoclast development, activation, and survival. Denosumab is a fully human monoclonal IgG2 antibody that binds RANKL, inhibiting its activity. The aim of this multicenter, randomized, double-blind, placebo-controlled, phase II study was to evaluate the effects of denosumab on structural damage in patients with rheumatoid arthritis (RA) receiving methotrexate treatment.

Methods.—RA patients received subcutaneous placebo (n = 75), denosumab 60 mg (n = 71), or denosumab 180 mg (n = 72) injections every 6 months for 12 months. The primary end point was the change from baseline in the magnetic resonance imaging (MRI) erosion score at 6 months.

Results.—At 6 months, the increase in the MRI erosion score from baseline was lower in the 60-mg denosumab group (mean change 0.13; $P = 0.118$) and significantly lower in the 180-mg denosumab group (mean change 0.06; $P = 0.007$) than in the placebo group (mean change 1.75). A significant difference in the modified Sharp erosion score was observed as early as 6 months in the 180-mg denosumab group ($P = 0.019$) as compared with placebo, and at 12 months, both the 60-mg ($P = 0.012$) and the 180-mg ($P = 0.007$) denosumab groups were significantly different from the placebo group. Denosumab caused sustained suppression of markers of bone turnover. There was no evidence of an effect of denosumab on joint space narrowing or on measures of RA disease activity. Rates of adverse events were comparable between the denosumab and placebo groups.

Conclusion.—Addition of twice-yearly injections of denosumab to ongoing methotrexate treatment inhibited structural damage in patients with RA for up to 12 months, with no increase in the rates of adverse events as compared with placebo.

▶ Understanding that osteoclast activity mediated in part by RANK Ligand (RANKL) contributes to erosion formation in rheumatoid arthritis, the authors of this study set out to determine if the use of Denosumab, a fully human monoclonal antibody to RANKL, would slow the progression of structural damage in rheumatoid arthritis patients receiving methotrexate. This is a multicenter, randomized, double blind, placebo-controlled Phase II clinical trial. 218 patients with rheumatoid arthritis, diagnosed according to ACR 1987 criteria, for > 24 months, on a stable dose of methotrexate for > 8 weeks and the presence of > 6 swollen joints were randomized to receive either denosumab 60 mg, denosumab 180 mg or placebo subcutaneously every 6 months in 2 doses. The patients were evaluated with hand and wrist radiographs and MRIs, DEXA, blood and urine bone and cartilage biomarkers, and clinical assessments at several intervals within a 12-month period. The primary end point was the change in the MRI erosion score from baseline to 6 months. Of the 94% of patients who completed the study, those receiving denosumab 180 mg had statistically significant less change in their MRI erosion score. However, there was no effect of denosumab on the modified Sharp joint space narrowing score or the disease activity as measured by ACR response, HAQ, or DAS28. The denosumab groups also had decreases in the bone turnover markers and an increase in BMD over baseline. The authors concluded that denosumab augmented the methotrexate inhibited structural damage, improved the BMD, and suppressed bone turnover in patients with rheumatoid arthritis.

The prevention or slowing of structural damage in patients with rheumatoid arthritis is a goal for all rheumatologists treating this disease. With the introduction of biologic agents, we have had tremendous success in doing so. In this study, denosumab decreased bone destruction in patients taking methotrexate. A large percentage of rheumatoid arthritis patients are receiving TNF-alpha inhibitors, which appear to slow the progression of erosions. Denosumab may provide an alternative or complementary therapy, recognizing that it does not appear to decrease the synovitis, inflammation, or joint cartilage destruction. A next step in the investigation of denosumab could be to compare this drug to the TNF-alpha inhibitors or even to study its utility in combination with the TNF-alpha inhibitors.

N. Cotter, MD

Ocrelizumab, a Humanized Anti-CD20 Monoclonal Antibody, in the Treatment of Patients With Rheumatoid Arthritis: A Phase I/II Randomized, Blinded, Placebo-Controlled, Dose-Ranging Study

Genovese MC, Kaine JL, Lowenstein MB, et al (Stanford Univ, CA; Sarasota Arthritis Research Ctr, FL; Arthritis Ctr, Palm Harbor, FL; et al)
Arthritis Rheum 58:2652-2661, 2008

Objective.—Ocrelizumab, a humanized anti-CD20 monoclonal antibody, was studied in a first-in-human trial in rheumatoid arthritis (RA) patients receiving concomitant methotrexate (MTX).

Methods.—The ACTION trial was a combined phase I/II study of placebo plus MTX versus ocrelizumab plus MTX in 237 RA patients (intent-to-treat population). During phase I, 45 patients were treated with 1 of 5 escalating doses of study drug (infusions on days 1 and 15, 10–1,000 mg per each infusion). An additional 192 patients were randomized during phase II. Eligible patients had active disease, an inadequate response to treatment with at least MTX, rheumatoid factor positivity, and elevated levels of acute-phase reactants. The total study duration was 72 weeks. B cell pharmacodynamics over time was investigated.

Results.—Baseline demographics were similar among the treatment groups. Based on the entire 72-week data set, the incidence of serious adverse events in the ocrelizumab-treated patients was 17.9%, as compared with 14.6% in placebo-treated patients. The incidence of serious infections was 2.0% in all ocrelizumab-treated patients and 4.9% in placebo-treated patients. Infusion-associated adverse events were mostly grade 1 or grade 2 and were more frequent around the time of the first infusion. No serious infusion-associated adverse events were reported in the ocrelizumab group. Evidence of clinical activity was observed at all doses evaluated. Peripheral B cell depletion after infusion was rapid at all doses, with earlier repletion of B cells at doses of 10 mg and 50 mg. Human anti-human antibodies were detected in 19% and 10%, respectively, of those receiving 10 mg and 50 mg of ocrelizumab, compared with 0–5% of those receiving 200, 500, and 1,000 mg.

Conclusion.—Ocrelizumab therapy in combination with MTX was well tolerated. Doses of 200 mg (2 infusions) and higher showed better clinical responses, better reduction of C-reactive protein levels, and very low immunogenicity.

▶ The success of rituximab in the treatment of rheumatoid arthritis has illustrated the importance of B cells in the disease pathogenesis. This is a phase I/II randomized, blinded, placebo-controlled, dose-ranging study of ocrelizumab, a humanized anti-CD20 monoclonal antibody, in the treatment of patients with rheumatoid arthritis. In Phase I of the study, patients received ocrelizumab 10 mg in 2 infusions to determine its safety. In Phase II, 237 patients were randomized to receive placebo or ocrelizumab at doses of 10, 50, 200, 500, or 1000 mg in 2 infusions 2 weeks apart.

The results of this study show that B cell depletion was seen in all groups receiving ocrelizumab. Furthermore, more patients in the ocrelizumab groups achieved ACR20, ACR50, or ACR70 responses at week 24 compared with the placebo treated group. Maximum B cell depletion seemed to occur at the 200 mg dose, which correlated with the clinical response. Patients receiving ocrelizumab at doses of 200 mg and higher appeared to have a greater clinical benefit than the lower doses.

Rheumatoid arthritis is a complex disease that we do not fully understand, but through investigation of this disease many successful targeted therapies have emerged. B cell therapy has shown much promise thus far in the form of the rituximab, a chimeric monoclonal anti-CD20 antibody. Ocrelizumab is a humanized monoclonal antibody, but the advantages of the humanized antibody over chimeric, such as the development of antichimeric antibodies, are not addressed in this study. Further investigation comparing ocrelizumab with rituximab would be useful.

N. Cotter, MD

Golimumab in Patients With Active Rheumatoid Arthritis Despite Treatment With Methotrexate: A Randomized, Double-Blind, Placebo-Controlled, Dose-Ranging Study

Kay J, Matteson EL, Dasgupta B, et al (Massachusetts Gen Hosp, Boston, MA; Mayo Clinic College of Med, Rochester, MN; Southend Univ Hosp, West-clif, Essex, UK; et al)
Arthritis Rheum 58:964-975, 2008

Objective.—To assess the efficacy, safety, and pharmacology of subcutaneous administration of golimumab in patients with active rheumatoid arthritis (RA) despite treatment with methotrexate (MTX).

Methods.—Patients were randomly assigned in a double-blinded manner to receive injections of placebo plus MTX or 50 mg or 100 mg golimumab every 2 or 4 weeks plus MTX through week 48. Patients originally assigned to receive injections every 2 weeks had the interval increased to every 4 weeks starting at week 20. The primary end point was the proportion of patients meeting the American College of Rheumatology 20% improvement criteria (achieving an ACR20 response) at week 16. The study was powered to detect a difference in the primary end point when the combined golimumab groups and at least 1 of the individual dose groups were compared with placebo.

Results.—The primary end point was attained. Sixty-one percent of patients in the combined golimumab plus MTX dose groups achieved an ACR20 response at week 16 compared with 37% of patients in the placebo plus MTX group ($P = 0.010$). In addition, 79% of patients in the group receiving 100 mg golimumab every 2 weeks achieved an ACR20 response ($P < 0.001$ versus placebo). Through week 20 (after which patients receiving placebo were switched to active infliximab therapy), serious adverse events were reported in 9% of patients in the combined golimumab groups and in 6% of patients in the placebo group.

Conclusion.—Golimumab plus MTX effectively reduces the signs and symptoms of RA and is generally well tolerated in patients with an inadequate response to MTX.

▶ The essence of the age of biologics is the development of "smart weapons" targeted against individual molecules, which have been implicated in causing or contributing to a particular disease or inflammation. An IL-6 receptor antagonist, and small molecules targeting adenosine receptors and kinases, are on the horizon. An IL-1 receptor antagonist, anti-CD20, and CTLA4-Ig (which targets CD28) have each had some impact, but to date tumor necrosis factor (TNF) inhibitors have been the most successful target for suppression of rheumatoid arthritis (RA) and other inflammatory diseases. To extend that success, we now focus on refining the mechanism for inhibiting TNF action. The use of the 3 agents on the market has suggested that differences exist in the disease-specific efficacy and tolerability of the anti-TNF drugs. Trials of the fully human anti-TNF monoclonal antibody, Golimumab, will help delineate its role in RA treatment. This study was designed to establish the most effective dose of Golimumab and evaluate its safety.

This is a multi-center randomized, double blind, placebo-controlled, dose-ranging study including authors from Belgium, the United States, UK, and Australia. The patients had active RA (defined as at least 6 tender and 6 swollen joints) despite treatment with either oral or parenteral MTX.

The criteria required that patients receive at least 10 mg MTX/week for at least 3 months. Ten mg per week is a relatively low dose, though some patients are limited by side effects before achieving a more typical dose of 15 mg/week. The authors did not state the mean methotrexate dose.

All patients continued to receive at least 10 mg MTX/wk.

The 5 treatment groups received:

(1) placebo.

(2) Golimumab 50 mg every 4 weeks.

(3) Golimumab 50 mg every 2 weeks.

(4) Golimumab 100 mg every 4 weeks.

(5) Golimumab 100 mg every 2 weeks.

To maintain blinding, the q 4-week patients received placebo injections at the 2-week interim interval. At week 20, the placebo patients received 3 mg/kg of open-label infliximab every 8 weeks after the conventional loading procedure.

The primary end point was ACR 20% response at week 16. Secondary endpoints included DAS28, ACR-N (numeric index of the ACR response), and ACR20, ACR50, and ACR70 through week 52.

The groups were fairly well matched, though some notable outliers included the shorter disease duration for placebo (5.6%) and the 100 mg q 4 wk (6.3%) groups compared with the others (8.2%).

75% of patients completed the study. Strikingly, 40% of the MTX/placebo/Infliximab group discontinued their participation, most after the first 16 weeks (compared with only 21.2% in the Golim/MTX combined groups).

The Golimumab groups did not show a dose-dependent discontinuation.

The ACR 20% response is setting the bar low as an end point, given the kinds of responses we now expect from biologics, but the analysis also included ACR 50, -70, and -N, all of which showed significant responses.

Similar to numerous trials of other agents, approximately 50% of the Golim/MTX patients achieved an ACR50 response. Moreover, each dosing regimen had statistically greater proportions of ACR50 responders. Only 1 group had a statistically significant ACR20 improvement, perhaps because the ACR20 is such a low expectation and may represent the range of disease variation. The median ACR-N may be a better way to evaluate, and in this case the median ACR-N was 33.3% at week 16 with golimumab, but 0.0% in the placebo/MTX group.

With regard to serious infections, the frequency was similar between Remicade and golimumab.

Despite being a fully human antibody, 6.5% of the 107 golimumab-treated patients had antibodies to the drug, but there was no clear association with dosing or degree of response (ACR20, ACR50). Only one patient with antibodies had an injection site reaction, and none discontinued due to lack of efficacy.

The development of antinuclear antibodies was equivalent at week 52 (golimumab groups combined-21%, placebo/MTX/Remicade-18%), but no patients experienced a lupus-like syndrome. Three golimumab-treated patients had skin cancers, and a fourth was found to have a pre-existing chest X-ray abnormality later diagnosed as lung cancer.

Conclusions/Summary

The fully human anti-TNF Golimumab offers an alternative molecule for inhibition of TNF action in patients with RA. Antibodies to golimumab still occurred, but appear to be of little clinical significance. Larger placebo-controlled studies are being conducted to evaluate the safety and efficacy.

The benefits of TNF inhibitors are well proven, and will likely be a mainstay for treatment of inflammatory disorders for years to come. However, not all patients respond to the same TNFi, or to the first one they use, and some patients completely lose their response to TNF inhibitors, thus require a change to another type of biologic. With the broadening array of biologic therapies for RA, we hope to achieve ACR 70s and ACR-90s in an increasing number of patients.

In the future, identifying which patients will benefit from a particular therapeutic choice, would enable us to optimize our chances of maximizing the response while minimizing the risk.

D. L. Kimpel, MD, MA

Comparison of the Clinical Efficacy and Safety of Subcutaneous Versus Oral Administration of Methotrexate in Patients With Active Rheumatoid Arthritis: Results of a Six-Month, Multicenter, Randomized, Double-Blind, Controlled, Phase IV Trial

Braun J, Kästner P, Flaxenberg P, et al (Rheumazentrum Ruhrgebiet, Herne, Germany; Erfurt, Germany; Essen, Germany; et al)

Arthritis Rheum 58:73-81, 2008

Objective.—To compare the efficacy and safety of subcutaneous (SC) versus oral administration of methotrexate (MTX) in patients with active rheumatoid arthritis (RA).

Methods.—MTX-naive patients with active RA (Disease Activity Score in 28 joints ≥4) were eligible for the study if they had not previously taken biologic agents and had not taken disease-modifying antirheumatic drugs for 2 weeks prior to randomization. Patients were randomly assigned to receive 15 mg/week of MTX either orally (2 7.5-mg tablets plus a dummy prefilled syringe; n = 187 patients) or SC (prefilled syringe containing 10 mg/ml plus 2 dummy tablets; n = 188 patients) for 24 weeks. At week 16, patients who did not meet the American College of Rheumatology criteria for 20% improvement (ACR20) were switched from 15 mg of oral MTX to 15 mg of SC MTX and from 15 mg of SC

MTX to 20 mg of SC MTX for the remaining 8 weeks, still in a blinded manner. The primary outcome was an ACR20 response at 24 weeks.

Results.—At week 24, significantly more patients treated with SC MTX than with oral MTX showed ACR20 (78% versus 70%) and ACR70 (41% versus 33%) responses. Patients with a disease duration ≥12 months had even higher ACR20 response rates (89% for SC administration and 63% for oral). In 52 of the ACR20 nonresponders (14%), treatment was switched at week 16. Changing from oral to SC MTX and from 15 mg to 20 mg of SC MTX resulted in 30% and 23% ACR20 response rates, respectively, in these patients. MTX was well tolerated. The rate of adverse events was similar in all groups.

Conclusion.—This 6-month prospective, randomized, controlled trial is the first to examine oral versus SC administration of MTX. We found that SC administration was significantly more effective than oral administration of the same MTX dosage. There was no difference in tolerability.

▶ This study addresses one of the common clinical questions in rheumatology practice. "We do this, but do we really know if it is better?" Many rheumatologists, including this reviewer, have switched patients from oral to subcutaneous methotrexate (MTX) for reasons of tolerability or efficacy, with good results in many cases, but in the "N of 1" world of clinical practice, there has not been any intellectually satisfying "evidence basis" for doing this.

This is a prospective, placebo controlled, randomized clinical trial. Patients, doctors, and most staff were blinded to the treatment.

Appropriate groups were excluded (ie, individuals who were pregnant, individuals who had infectious hepatitis, etc), while some patients were added, such as patients with "extensive consumption of caffeine," based on previous reports that caffeine can interfere with the efficacy of MTX.

MTX is still the gold standard and comparator for the newer, more expensive biologics. Maximizing efficacy with our standard of care is a noble objective, given its well-established effectiveness and monitoring guidelines, low cost, and low toxicity. It is also the most commonly used agent in common with biologics for increased efficacy.

ACR70 response was significantly greater with SC MTX compared with oral MTX (41% vs 33%), as was the ACR20 response (78% vs 70%). ACR50 response was equivalent between the 2 groups (62% and 59%).

Similar adverse event rates were reported for both groups, 53% for SC, 48% for oral. Interestingly, gastrointestinal-related adverse events were equivalent between the 2 groups, with more diarrheas in the oral MTX group, and more anorexia in the SC MTX group.

When discussing therapy modifications with patients, clinicians now have evidence to support including injectable MTX in the discussion because of its enhanced efficacy and lower cost. Additionally, the increased efficacy does not bring with it any increase in adverse events.

D. L. Kimpel, MD, MA

An Explanation for the Apparent Dissociation Between Clinical Remission and Continued Structural Deterioration in Rheumatoid Arthritis

Brown AK, Conaghan PG, Karim Z, et al (Univ of Leeds, UK; et al)
Arthritis Rheum 58:2958-2967, 2008

Objective.—Achieving remission is the aim of treatment in rheumatoid arthritis (RA). This should represent minimal arthritis activity and ensure optimal disease outcome. However, we have previously demonstrated a high prevalence of imaging-detected synovial inflammation in RA patients who were in clinical remission. The purpose of this study was to evaluate the long-term significance of subclinical synovitis and its relationship to structural outcome.

Methods.—We studied 102 RA patients receiving conventional treatment who had been judged by their consultant rheumatologist to be in remission, as well as 17 normal control subjects. Subjects underwent clinical, laboratory, functional, and quality of life assessments over 12 months. In addition to standard radiography of the hands and feet, imaging of the hands and wrists was performed with musculoskeletal ultrasonography (US) and conventional 1.5T magnetic resonance imaging (MRI) at baseline and 12 months, using validated acquisition and scoring techniques.

Results.—Despite their being in clinical remission, 19% of the patients displayed deterioration in radiographic joint damage over the study period. Scores on musculoskeletal US synovial hypertrophy, power Doppler (PD), and MRI synovitis assessments in individual joints at baseline were significantly associated with progressive radiographic damage ($P = 0.032$, $P < 0.001$, and $P = 0.002$, respectively). Furthermore, there was a significant association between the musculoskeletal US PD score at baseline and structural progression over 12 months in totally asymptomatic metacarpophalangeal joints ($P = 0.004$) and 12 times higher odds of deterioration in joints with increased PD signal (odds ratio 12.21, $P < 0.001$).

Conclusion.—Subclinical joint inflammation detected by imaging techniques explains the structural deterioration in RA patients in clinical remission who are receiving conventional therapy. Our findings reinforce the utility of imaging for the accurate evaluation of disease status and the prediction of structural outcome.

▶ Data from recent clinical trials in rheumatoid arthritis (RA) indicate that disease remission is an obtainable goal of therapy. Remission has traditionally been defined by the Disease Activity Score 28-joint assessment (DAS28) and the American College of Rheumatology (ACR) remission criteria 1 to 3. These outcome measures are composite scores based on clinical and laboratory assessments, however, they do not always predict good outcome. Despite fulfilling these remission criteria, some patients continue to have radiographic progression. This finding may reflect the inadequate sensitivity of these techniques to identify persistent synovial inflammation. Previously, Brown et al showed that synovitis, as detected by musculoskeletal ultrasound (US) and magnetic resonance imaging (MRI), was present in patients who fulfilled the ACR and DAS28 remission criteria 4.

In this current study, the authors further explain the apparent dissociation between clinical remission and progressive joint damage. In this prospective longitudinal cohort study, RA patients in clinical remission and on conventional therapies were studied over 12 months. Subjects underwent clinical, laboratory, and radiographic assessments including US and MRI at baseline and 1 year. Despite satisfying the remission criteria, many patients had evidence of synovial inflammation on US and MRI at baseline. Furthermore, the authors showed that the baseline imaging findings were associated with a statistically significant likelihood of progressive joint damage. In particular, the presence of a power doppler (PD) signal and synovial hypertrophy by US, as well as synovitis on MRI, were associated with a higher likelihood of progression.

This study showed that structural progression occurs because subclinical synovitis is present in RA patients as detected by musculoskeletal ultrasound and MRI despite satisfying the criteria of clinical remission. The study also questions whether the current clinical, laboratory, and radiographic measures for assessing disease activity in RA are sensitive in detecting low levels of synovial inflammation, the apparent cause of progressive structural damage. This provocative study is sure to make rheumatologists question the adequacies of their current clinical practices when evaluating for disease activity in RA and should lead to redefining the criteria used in determining clinical remission.

For further reading on this subject I suggest article Pinals et al,[1] Van der Heijde et al,[2] Prevoo et al,[3] Brown et al.[4]

B. Hutton, MD

References

1. Pinals RS, Masi AT, Larsen RAand the Subcommittee for Criteria of Remission in Rheumatoid Arthritis of the American Rheumatism Association Diagnostic and Therapeutic Criteria Committee. Preliminary criteria for clinical remission in rheumatoid arthritis. *Arthritis Rheum.* 1981;24:1308-1315.
2. Van der Heijde DM, van't Hof MA, van Riel PL, Theunisse LM, Lubberts EW, van Leeuwen MA, et al. Judging disease activity in clinical practice in rheumatoid arthritis: first step in the development of a disease activity score. *Ann Rheum Dis.* 1990;49:916-920.
3. Prevoo ML, van 't Hof MA, Kuper HH, van Leeuwen MA, van de Putte LB, van Riel PL. Modified disease activity scores that include twenty-eight-joint counts: development and validation in a prospective longitudinal study of patients with rheumatoid arthritis. *Arthritis Rheum.* 1995;38:44-48.
4. Brown AK, Quinn MA, Karim Z, Conaghan PG, Peterfy CG, Hensor E, et al. Presence of significant synovitis in rheumatoid arthritis patients with disease-modifying antirheumatic drug–induced clinical remission: evidence from an imaging study may explain structural progression. *Arthritis Rheum.* 2006;54:3761-3773.

Biologic Treatment of Rheumatoid Arthritis and the Risk of Malignancy: Analyses From a Large US Observational Study
Wolfe F, Michaud K (Univ of Kansas School of Medicine, Wichita; Univ of Nebraska Med Ctr, Omaha)
Arthritis Rheum 56:2886-2895, 2007

Objective.—Induction of malignancy is a major concern when rheumatoid arthritis (RA) is treated with biologic therapy. A meta-analysis of RA biologic clinical trials found a general increased risk of malignancy, but this risk was not found in a large observational study. We undertook this study to assess the risk of malignancy among biologic-treated patients in a large US observational database.

Methods.—We studied incident cases of cancer among 13,001 patients during ~49,000 patient-years of observation in the years 1998–2005. Cancer rates were compared with population rates using the US National Cancer Institute SEER (Surveillance, Epidemiology, and End-Results) database. Assessment of the risk of biologic therapy utilized conditional logistic regression to calculate odds ratios (ORs) as estimates of the relative risk, further adjusted for 6 confounders: age, sex, education level, smoking history, RA severity, and prednisone use.

Results.—Biologic exposure was 49%. There were 623 incident cases of nonmelanotic skin cancer and 537 other cancers. The standardized incidence ratios and 95% confidence intervals (95% CIs) compared with SEER data were as follows: all cancers 1.0 (1.0–1.1), breast 0.8 (0.6–0.9), colon 0.5 (0.4–0.6), lung 1.2 (1.0–1.4), lymphoma 1.7 (1.3–2.2). Biologics were associated with an increased risk of nonmelanotic skin cancer (OR 1.5, 95% CI 1.2–1.8) and melanoma (OR 2.3, 95% CI 0.9–5.4). No other malignancy was associated with biologic use; the OR (overall risk) of any cancer was 1.0 (95% CI 0.8–1.2).

Conclusion.—Biologic therapy is associated with increased risk for skin cancers, but not for solid tumors or lymphoproliferative malignancies. These associations were consistent across different biologic therapies.

▶ There has been considerable interest over the past decade regarding the association between rheumatoid arthritis (RA) and malignancy. Numerous cohort studies have variably reported an increased risk of lymphoma, lung and skin cancers, and a reduced incidence of colorectal and breast cancer. Whether the disease processes itself or the immunomodulatory therapies used in its treatment are responsible for the increased risk of malignancy is still debated. In the past, DMARDs such as cyclophosphamide, methotrexate, and azathioprine used in the treatment of RA have been linked to an increased risk of cancer. Now, with the advent of biologics, there is rising concern as to the long-term safety of these immunomodulatory drugs and their risk of contributing to the development of cancer. These concerns have been underscored by recent observational studies and a meta-analysis demonstrating a potential association with antiTNF agents used in RA and malignancy.

The authors in this report attempted to address this issue. Using 2 national databases, Wolfe and Michaud conducted an observational study in which they compared cancer rates among rheumatoid arthritis patients with a history of biologic exposure with those of the general population. The main finding was the positive association between antiTNF therapy and skin cancer, both nonmelanotic and melanoma.

Despite these results, certain questions have to be raised. Inherent to all observational studies is the nonrandom assignment of treatment groups. If patients with more severe RA were selected to receive biologics, then disease severity may account for the increased risk of malignancy. This has been demonstrated with the risk of lymphoma in RA in the past. Another concern is that a history of cancer may affect a physician's decision to treat with an antiTNF, thus allowing again for confounding.

This study, however, may alleviate some fears regarding the association, or lack thereof, with both solid and hematologic malignancies. Biologics are still relatively new in the rheumatologist's armamentarium against RA and concerns of their long-term safety still exist. If the past is any determinant, undoubtedly, there will be many more studies attempting to answer this in the decade to come.

B. Hutton, MD

Patients With Pulmonary Tuberculosis Are Frequently Positive for Anti–Cyclic Citrullinated Peptide Antibodies, but Their Sera Also React With Unmodified Arginine-Containing Peptide
Kakumanu P, Yamagata H, Sobel ES, et al (Univ of Florida, Gainesville; National Hosp Organization, Musashi-Murayama, Tokyo)
Arthritis Rheum 58:1576-1581, 2008

Objective.—The anti-cyclic citrullinated peptide (anti–CCP) enzyme-linked immunosorbent assay (ELISA) has high sensitivity and specificity for rheumatoid arthritis (RA). However, detection of anti-CCP in patients with active pulmonary tuberculosis (TB) has recently been reported. To determine whether this activity was specific for the citrullinated residue, the specificity of anti-CCP–positive sera for CCP versus that for unmodified arginine-containing peptide (CAP) was examined in patients with TB and compared with that in patients with RA.

Methods.—Anti-CCP and anti-CAP in sera from patients with pulmonary TB (n = 49), RA patients (n = 36), and controls (n = 18) were tested by ELISA. Sera were available at diagnosis from most TB patients. All TB patients were treated with a combination of 2–4 antibiotics for at least 6 months, and sera were collected over time.

Results.—Anti-CCP was found in 37% of TB patients and in 43% of RA patients. CAP reactivity was more common in TB than in RA. High anti-CCP:anti-CAP ratios (>2.0) were seen far more commonly in anti-CCP-positive RA patients than in anti-CCP–positive TB patients (94% versus 22%). Anti-CCP was inhibited by CCP peptide in sera from RA patients, but not in sera from TB patients. A slight increase in anti-CCP was common after initiating treatment for TB, although the anti-CCP level decreased after 1–2 months.

Conclusion.—Anti-CCP is frequently present in patients with active TB. However, many anti-CCP–positive TB sera also reacted with CAP, and anti-CCP: anti-CAP ratios in TB sera were low. Anti-CCP:anti-CAP ratios should be useful clinically for distinguishing CCP-specific reactivity seen in RA from reactivity with both CCP and CAP frequently seen in pulmonary TB.

▶ Not only has the anti-cyclic citrullinated peptide antibody (anti-CCP) become a widely used serological marker for rheumatoid arthritis (RA), but it has also more recently been implicated in the pathogenesis of the disease itself. Citrullinated peptides are formed as part of a post-translation modification process during cellular events, such as apoptosis, and are associated with various inflammatory processes. Antibodies to these citrullinated peptides have been most frequently described in RA, however, anti-CCP have also been found in other autoimmune diseases, in smokers' lungs, and more recently in patients with active pulmonary tuberculosis (TB). Because patients with TB can exhibit arthropathy, some patients may actually mimic RA. Anti-CCP results in these patients may, therefore, be misleading. This poses a problem for rheumatologists similar to that seen in hepatitis C patients with arthropathy and rheumatoid factor.

The authors of this study attempted to determine the specificity of sera from patients with active pulmonary TB containing anti-CCP antibodies for CCP compared with similar unmodified arginine-containing peptide (CAP), because CAP does not react with anti-CCP in RA patients. Sera from patients with RA ($n = 36$), TB (49), and healthy controls ($n = 18$) were tested for anti-CCP and anti-CAP by enzyme-linked immunosorbent assay (ELISA). Anti-CCP was found in 37% of TB patients and 43% of RA patients. CAP reactivity was greater in anti-CCP positive TB patients. Consequently, anti-CCP positive RA patients demonstrated higher anti-CCP:anti-CAP ratios (> 2.0) than anti-CCP positive TB patients (94% vs 22%). A slight increase in anti-CCP titer was also seen when initiating TB therapy, although levels trended down within 1 to 2 months.

Consistent with previous results, this study demonstrates the high frequency of anti-CCP positivity in TB patients. Therefore, testing the sera of patients for CAP, where there is a suspicion for TB, may be useful. Unfortunately, this test is not commercially available, which limits the practicality of clinical testing currently. This study also provides some further understanding of the development of antibodies to citrullinated peptides in various inflammatory disorders. It also provides evidence that the anti-CCP antibody may not be as specific for RA as previously thought.

B. Hutton, MD

2 Systemic Lupus Erythematosus

Introduction

We chose 4 lupus articles that discuss: atherosclerotic morbidity and mortality in the LUMINA study; the association of erosive arthritis with anti-CCP antibodies in systemic lupus erythematosus; the use of mycophenolate mofetil in membranous nephritis; and the lack of predictive value of titers of antinuclear antibodies for the development of autoimmune diseases in the absence of the appropriate clinical history.

Seth Mark Berney, MD

Damage, Accelerated Atherosclerosis, and Mortality in Patients With Systemic Lupus Erythematosus: Lessons From LUMINA, a Multiethnic US Cohort
Durán S, González LA, Alarcón GS (The Univ of Alabama at Birmingham)
J Clin Rheumatol 13:350-353, 2007

Lupus in Minorities: Nature versus nurture (LUMINA) is a multiethnic cohort (Hispanics from Texas and the Island of Puerto Rico, African Americans, and Caucasians) of patients meeting at least 4 of the American

---

TABLE 1.—Predictors of the Occurrence of Vascular Arterial Events in LUMINA* Patients by Multivariable Logistic Regression Analysis

Variables	Odds Ratio	95% Confidence Interval	P
Age	1.075	1.037–1.114	<0.001
Smoking	3.731	1.391–10.000	0.009
Disease duration	1.452	1.223–1.725	<0.001
High-sensitive CRP†	3.356	1.264–8.929	0.015
aPL‡ antibodies	4.717	1.675–13.158	0.003

*Lupus in Minorities: Nature vs. nurture.
†C-reactive protein.
‡IgG and/or IgM and/or lupus anticoagulant. Modified from *Arthritis Rheum.* 2004;50:3947-3957.
(Reprinted from Durán S, González LA, Alarcón GS. Damage, accelerated atherosclerosis, and mortality in patients with systemic lupus erythematosus: lessons from LUMINA, a multiethnic US cohort. *J Clin Rheumatol.* 2007;13:350-353.)

TABLE 2.—Predictors of Damage in LUMINA* Patients by Cox Proportional Hazards Regression Analyses

Variables	Hazard Ratio	95% Confidence Interval	P
Hydroxychloroquine use†	0.73	0.52–1.00	0.0500
Propensity score	0.22	0.09–0.52	0.0006
Hydroxychloroquine use‡	0.55	0.34–0.87	0.0111
Propensity score	0.20	0.05–0.75	0.0172

*Lupus in Minorities: Nature vs. nurture.
†All patients included.
‡Only patients who had not developed any damage included. Modified from *Arthritis Rheum*. 2005;52:1473-1480.
(Reprinted from Durán S, González LA, Alarcón GS. Damage, accelerated atherosclerosis, and mortality in patients with systemic lupus erythematosus: lessons from LUMINA, a multiethnic US cohort. *J Clin Rheumatol*. 2007;13:350-353.)

College of Rheumatology (ACR) classification criteria for systemic lupus erythematosus (SLE). Patients had less than 5 years of disease duration at enrollment into the cohort and are living in the catchment areas of the participating institutions, The University of Alabama at Birmingham, The University of Texas Houston Health Sciences Center, and The University of Puerto Rico Medical Sciences Campus. The first patient was enrolled into LUMINA in the Spring of 1994; recruitment is ongoing. This review examines accelerated atherosclerosis, damage accrual, and mortality in this cohort (Tables 1 and 2).

▶ The Lupus in Minorities: Nature versus nurture (LUMINA) cohort is a multi-ethnic group of systemic lupus erythematosus (SLE) patients with less than 5 years disease duration from the catchment areas of University of Alabama at Birmingham, University of Texas Health Sciences Center at Houston, and University of Puerto Rico Medical Sciences Campus.

Previous articles from the LUMINA group have assessed factors associated with vascular events and mortality in SLE. The review article by Duran et al summarizes this previously published data.

Factors predicting vascular arterial events in 546 SLE patients are summarized in Table 1. The presence of antiphospholipid antibodies had the highest impact on their occurrence with an odds ratio of 4.717 ($P = .003$). This was followed by the highly sensitive C-reactive protein (CRP) with an odds ratio of 3.356 ($P = .015$). Disease duration had an odds ratio of 1.452 ($P < .001$).

The investigators have also assessed the LUMINA cohort for the impact of hydroxychloroquine on damage in SLE. They used the Systemic Lupus International Collaborating Clinics Damage Index (SDI) to document damage.[1] The SDI documents irreversible organ manifestations present for at least 6 months and is cumulative. Table 2 summarizes the data that suggests that patients with SLE who take hydroxychloroquine are at a decreased risk of damage compared with those who do not take hydroxychloroquine. Patients who had no damage at their initial evaluation had a lower hazard ratio than the entire cohort. Because the healthiest patients could have had a lower SDI and would never have accumulated damage irrespective of hydroxychloroquine, the authors calculated a "propensity" score to analyze this possibility.

The "propensity score" decreased their hazard ratio, but still showed a protective effect of hydroxychloroquine.

The final outcome that the authors reviewed was predictors of mortality in the LUMINA cohort. Poverty was a strong predictor with a hazard ratio of 2.109 ($P = .006$). Age, ethnicity, and sex were not statistically significant factors. To assess the impact of hydroxychloroquine on mortality, the authors performed a nested case-control analysis with a logistic regression, and concluded that their data indicates that hydroxychloroquine decreases mortality in SLE.

The LUMINA cohort is an important study group for SLE research because it is large and multiethnic. In this review, the most striking correlation is the impact of antiphospholipid antibodies on vascular arterial events.

The impact of hydroxychloroquine on damage accumulation is somewhat more complex. One limitation in their data collection is that there is no information regarding duration or dosage of hydroxychloroquine treatment. The data do suggest that hydroxychloroquine exhibits a protective effect on damage accumulation; however, this protective effect is significantly decreased with the "propensity" score to control for disease severity. Future studies should evaluate this protective effect within a moderate to severe SLE cohort, and attempt to define the mechanism of the benefits of hydroxychloroquine.

J. Sloane, MD

Reference

1. Gladman DD, Goldsmith CH, Urowitz MB, et al. The Systemic Lupus International Collaborating Clinics/American College of Rheumatology (SLICC/ACR) Damage Index for Systemic Lupus Erythematosus International Comparison. *J Rheumatol.* 2000;27:373-376.

Associations of Erosive Arthritis with Anti-Cyclic Citrullinated Peptide Antibodies and MHC Class II Alleles in Systemic Lupus Erythematosus

Chan MT, Owen P, Dunphy J, et al (Royal Natl Hosp for Rheumatic Diseases, Bath, UK; Bath Inst of Rheumatic Diseases, UK)

J Rheumatol 35:77-83, 2008

Objective.—To determine the associations of erosive arthritis (EA) with anti-cyclic citrullinated peptide (anti-CCP) antibodies and major histocompatibility class (MHC) II alleles in systemic lupus erythematosus (SLE).

Methods.—One hundred four patients with SLE were evaluated for arthritis and classified as EA, nonerosive arthritis, or no arthritis. EA was further classified as major or minor erosions. Sera from patients and 130 serum controls were tested for anti-CCP2 and rheumatoid factor (RF). Patients and 117 genetic controls were genotyped for HLA-DRB1 and HLA-DQB1. Statistical associations were tested using chi-square tests and odds ratios (OR) with 95% confidence intervals (CI).

Results.—Eight patients (8%) were anti-CCP+ and they accounted for 11% (8/71) of patients with synovitis. Twelve patients (11%) had EA.

Among patients with synovitis, EA was associated with anti-CCP (OR 28.5, 95% CI 4.7–173.8, p = 0.001), with a weaker association for RF (p = 0.3). Six patients with EA had major erosions and also met criteria for rheumatoid arthritis (RA). Four of these patients (67%) were anti-CCP+. HLA-DQB1*0302 was associated with EA (p = 0.01), with similar trends for HLA-DRB1*0401 and 2 copies of the shared epitope (SE). There were trends for associations of HLA-DQB1*0302 and 2 SE copies with anti-CCP production.

Conclusion.—The frequency of EA in SLE is likely to be higher than previously reported. Anti-CCP+ patients with SLE are more likely to have EA. Anti-CCP may be a useful serological marker for EA for patients presenting with synovitis. Anti-citrulline antibodies may have a pathogenic role in the development of major erosions, resulting in clinical features that overlap SLE with RA (rhupus).

▶ Chan et al intend to study the association of anti-CCP antibody and major histocompatibility class (MHC) 2 alleles with erosive arthritis in systemic lupus erythematosus (SLE). Erosive arthritis is considered uncommon in SLE (prevalence is approximately 5%).[1,2]

In this article's study population of 104 patients with lupus, 71 had synovitis, 12 of whom had bone erosions. Of the patients with erosions, 6 tested positive for the anti-CCP antibody. Two patients with nonerosive arthritis also had the anti-CCP antibody. The patients with erosive arthritis had fewer SLE criteria and all of the patients with major erosions met ACR criteria for rheumatoid arthritis (RA). The genetic markers associated with increased disease severity in RA, HLA DRB1*0401 and HLA DQB1*0302, were present in 67% and 100% of the SLE patients respectively with erosive arthritis. This genetic data raises the question of whether these patients actually had RA instead of SLE.

This publication is interesting because it raises the possibility of whether anti-CCP can serve as a serological marker for erosive arthritis in other rheumatologic diseases, and whether it could represent a way to identify patients who have the rare SLE/RA overlap syndrome know as Rhupus. Moreover, the presence of the anti-CCP antibody in these lupus patients may indicate that the specificity of this laboratory test for RA is not as high as has previously been reported.[3]

R. Dhawan, MD

References

1. Labowitz R, Schumacher HRJ. Articular manifestations of systemic lupus erythematosus. *Ann Intern Med.* 1971;74:911-921.
2. Alarcon-Segovia D, Abud-Mendoza C, Diaz-Jouanen E, Iglesias A, De los Reyes V, Hernandez-Ortiz J. Deforming arthropathy of the hands in systemic lupus erythematosus. *J Rheumatol.* 1988;15:65-69.
3. Bizzaro N, Mazzanti G, Tonutti E, Villalta D, Tozzoli R. Diagnostic accuracy of the anti-citrulline antibody assay for rheumatoid arthritis. *Clin Chem.* 2001; 47(6):1089-1093.

Mycophenolate mofetil as the primary treatment of membranous lupus nephritis with and without concurrent proliferative disease: a retrospective study of 29 cases
Kasitanon N, Petri M, Hass M, et al (Johns Hopkins Univ School of Medicine, Baltimore, MD; et al)
Lupus 17:40-45, 2008

Studies of immunosuppressive therapy, particularly mycophenolate mofetil (MMF), in membranous lupus nephritis (MLN) are limited. We report on our experience with primary (first-line) MMF therapy to induce and sustain renal remission in MLN with and without a concurrent proliferative lesion. Systemic lupus erythematosus (SLE) patients were studied, retrospectively, if treated with MMF for newly diagnosed MLN. Complete remission was defined as proteinuria less than 0.5 g/24 h, inactive urine sediment and normal estimated glomerular filtration rate. Response in pure MLN (Group I, $n = 10$) was compared with mixed MLN and proliferative lupus nephritis (Group II, $n = 19$). By 12 months, 4 (40%) patients in Group I and 7 (36.8%) in Group II achieved complete remission ($P = 0.87$). One (10%) patient in Group I and 2 (10.5%) in Group II had worsening renal disease ($P = 0.97$). Mean time to remission was more than seven months in both groups. The remaining patients had stable disease without improvement or worsening. Only 2 of 11 achieving initial remission had a relapse with an average of 28 months of follow-up after remission. Self-limited gastrointestinal symptoms occurred in 12 patients, none requiring withdrawal of the drug. Mycophenolate mofetil as a primary therapy in MLN was successful in inducing complete remission in about 40% of MLN, particularly in patients with mild proteinuria. However, 12 months of therapy was necessary for best outcomes. Response rate was not different in the presence or absence of a proliferative lesion.

▶ Membranous lupus nephritis is a common lupus renal lesion. However, despite its prevalence, there is no consensus approach to its treatment because most studies have focused on the therapy of the more severe and predictable proliferative nephritis. Mycophenolate mofetil (MMF) has recently demonstrated efficacy in treating proliferative glomerulonephritis. Evidence for its use in membranous nephritis, however, is limited. This small retrospective study of 29 patients in the Hopkins Lupus Cohort evaluates MMF as a first line therapy in membranous nephritis.

Patients in the study were divided into 2 groups, depending on their type of renal disease: pure membranous nephritis (International Society of Nephrology/Renal Pathology Society (ISN/RPS V)) ($n = 10$) (group 1), and mixed nephritis (III or IV + V) with new proteinuria (> 0.5 g/day) ($n = 19$) (group 2). Patients began MMF 2 g/day and increased the dose to 3 g/day after 1 month. All patients received similar doses of corticosteroids and could not have received other immunosuppressives within 6 months. The patient's prednisone dose was adjusted based on their extrarenal lupus manifestations.

Angiotensin-converting enzyme (ACE) inhibitors and angiotensin receptor blockers were allowed if the patients' blood pressures tolerated them. Complete remission was defined as proteinuria < 0.5 g/day, inactive urine sediment, and normal estimated glomerular filtration rate (eGFR).

At 12 months, 40% of patients in each group achieved complete remission, and only 1 patient in each group had worsening renal disease. The remaining patients' renal function remained stable. Gastrointestinal side effects most commonly reported, such as nausea, abdominal pain, and diarrhea, however, were self-limited, and none required drug cessation.

This small study presents data that supports the use of MMF as a first line therapy for membranous lupus nephritis. However, a long induction period of 12 months was required, suggesting a gradual response to therapy. This study will hopefully pave the way for larger randomized controlled trials to be performed to further evaluate the efficacy of MMF in the treatment of membranous lupus nephritis.

B. Hutton, MD

Increased titres of anti-nuclear antibodies do not predict the development of associated disease in the absence of initial suggestive signs and symptoms

Dinser R, Braun A, Jendro MC, et al (Justus-Liebig-Univ of Giessen; Univ Hosp of the Saarland, Homburg, Germany; et al)
Scand J Rheumatol 36:448-451, 2007

Objective.—To determine whether patients with elevated anti-nuclear antibodies (ANA), absent extractable nuclear antigen (ENA) reactivity, and no definite associated disease develop an ANA-associated disease (AAD).

Methods.—Patients with ANA titres of at least 1:320 and no ENA reactivity were identified by searching the database of our laboratory serving a tertiary care university hospital between 1998 and 2002. Medical records of this index time point were reviewed to exclude patients with active AAD at screening. Case patients were contacted by questionnaire between 2004 and 2005 and invited for a clinical visit to ascertain the individual disease status.

Results.—Seventy-six patients were evaluated after a median follow-up of 32 months. An AAD was diagnosed in eight patients: connective tissue disease (CTD) in three, autoimmune hepatitis in two, rheumatoid arthritis in one, encephalomyelitis disseminate in one, and lymphoma in one. The only predictive factor associated with the development of AAD was the suspicion of an autoimmune disease by the treating physician at the initial evaluation. In the absence of initial suspicion for an autoimmune disease, only two out of 54 patients developed AAD, whereas six out of 22 patients with initial disease suspicion developed a defined AAD.

Conclusion.—In the absence of a clinical suspicion, elevated ANA titres have a low positive predictive value of 4% for developing AAD for the upcoming 3 years.

▶ The authors sought to evaluate the value of high titer anti-nuclear antibodies (ANA) in the absence of antidsDNA, RNP, Sm, SS-A/Ro, SS-B/LaScl70, CENP-B, or Jo-1 antibodies in predicting the subsequent development of ANA associated disease.

Patients from the University hospital of Saarland with ANA titers of ≥1:320 without any of the above antibodies from 1/98 to 1/2002 were identified. These patients' clinical and laboratory data were analyzed to evaluate whether these patients had an ANA-associated diagnosis (AAD). If they did, they were excluded from further analysis. The remainder of the patients were contacted by mail and asked to fill out a questionnaire and add any other symptoms or new diagnoses. Furthermore, other physicians treating these patients were contacted for the clinical details. Patients with symptoms consistent with an undiagnosed AAD were invited for a follow-up clinical evaluation.

Seventy-six case subjects were identified, of whom 8 were diagnosed with definite AAD and 3 with persistently suspected AAD. However, when the investigators reanalyzed the data, regrouping the case subjects according to whether the individual had suspected AAD or unlikely AAD at the time the ANA was drawn, 9 of 22 of those suspected of having an AAD developed or were diagnosed with an AAD while only 2 of 54 from the unlikely group had an AAD.

The 9 suspected AAD patients with an AAD included: seronegative rheumatoid arthritis (RA), CREST, encephalomyelitis, systemic lupus erythematosus (SLE) (in 2), autoimmune hepatitis, and undifferentiated connective tissue disease (in 3).

The 2 unlikely AAD patients who had an AAD included: autoimmune hepatitis and cerebral lymphoma.

The only characteristic that was predictive of the development of an AAD was the initial clinical suspicion of an AAD (thus the ANA pretest probability). Therefore, the presence of only an ANA of at least 1:320 had a low predictive value for the development of an AAD within 3 years. In fact, if the practitioner had a clinical suspicion that a patient had an AAD, only 27% of ANA+ patients developed an AAD. However, if the practitioner had no clinical suspicion of the presence of an underlying AAD, only 4% of ANA+ patients developed a subsequent AAD.

This study is very important because it confirms what most rheumatologists know, and what nonrheumatologic colleagues have apparently forgotten – ANAs (as well as all of the autoantibody tests) are not worthwhile as screening tests. Furthermore, if we review the data again, 4 of the "AAD" are not even rheumatologic diagnoses, further reinforcing the lack of specificity of this test. The usage of all rheumatologic tests should be, and is, to confirm the practitioner's clinical suspicion.

S. M. Berney, MD

3   Vasculitis

Introduction

We chose 3 articles this year that analyze the responses to therapy with rituximab, infliximab, and azathioprine/methotrexate.

Seth Mark Berney, MD

Efficacy of Rituximab in Limited Wegener's Granulomatosis with Refractory Granulomatous Manifestations

Seo P, Specks U, Keogh KA, et al (Johns Hopkins Univ School of Medicine, Baltimore, MD)

J Rheumatol 35:2017-2023, 2008

Objective.—Patients with limited Wegener's granulomatosis (WG) may experience a relapsing and remitting course. How such patients should be treated, particularly when they are refractory to standard of care therapies, is not clear. Rituximab is a monoclonal anti-CD20 antibody that has been used successfully to treat multiple forms of autoimmune and rheumatic diseases, but its role in the treatment of limited WG remains uncertain.

Methods.—Eight patients with limited WG who were refractory to (or intolerant of) standard immunosuppressive therapies were evaluated at the Johns Hopkins Hospital or the Mayo Clinic Rochester, and were treated with rituximab using a standard lymphoma protocol.

Results.—Four men and 4 women with limited WG were treated with rituximab. Patients' mean age was 39 years. All patients had predominantly necrotizing granulomatous disease manifestations, including chronic sinusitis, pulmonary nodules, orbital pseudotumor, and subglottic stenosis. Patients had failed an average of 3 immunosuppressive agents, not including glucocorticoids. Six patients had failed (or were intolerant of) therapy with cyclophosphamide; all 8 had failed therapy with methotrexate. At the time of treatment, 3 of the 8 patients were antineutrophil cytoplasmic antibody-negative. Rituximab successfully induced disease remission in all 8 patients. Three patients were retreated preemptively with rituximab after return of peripheral blood B-cells. Five patients were successfully retreated with rituximab after disease flare.

Conclusion.—Rituximab is an effective therapy for patients with limited WG and may be sufficient to induce sustained remission, even among patients with refractory disease and predominantly necrotizing granulomatous disease manifestations.

▶ Wegener's granulomatosis (WGN) is a systemic autoimmune disease characterized by granulomatous inflammation and small to medium sized vessel vasculitis. In its generalized form, the disease typically presents with pulmonary capillaritis and glomerulonephritis, and is strongly associated with antineutrophil cytoplasmic antibodies (ANCA). However, WGN can present in a more limited form where granulomatous inflammation of the upper respiratory tract predominates. This form appears to be less life threatening because vasculitic involvement of the kidneys does not occur and ANCA positivity is variable. Researchers have recognized that patients with this subset of disease can be treated effectively with methotrexate.[1] However, in some cases, methotrexate may not maintain the patient's remission.

In this small study by Seo et al, 8 patients with refractory limited WGN were treated with rituximab. All patients had previously failed an average of 3 immunosuppressive agents such as azathioprine, cyclophosphamide, and chlorambucil, and at time of the treatment 3 of 8 were ANCA positive. Rituximab was administered using the standard lymphoma protocol (375 mg/m^2 IV weekly × 4 weeks), and was successful in inducing remission in all 8 patients. Three of the 8 patients were re-treated with rituximab preemptively after the return of peripheral B cells. Five patients were successfully re-treated with rituximab after recurrent disease flare.

In their discussion, the authors noted that previous studies involving rituximab and WGN had not been as successful. They also commented that only 3 patients in their study were ANCA positive, which suggests that the B cells' role in the disease is not limited to producing ANCAs. In fact, the observation that patients improve after anti-B cell therapy suggests that B cells may play a previously unrecognized role in the pathogenesis of the disease. Even though there is still much to be learned of this heterogeneous disease, the results of this study show promise for the use of rituximab.

B. Hutton, MD

Reference

1. Hoffman GS, Leavitt RY, Kerr GS, Fauci AS. The treatment of Wegener's granulomatosis with glucocorticoids and methotrexate. *Arthritis Rheum.* 1992;35:1322-1329.

Infliximab Treatment of Intravenous Immunoglobulin–Resistant Kawasaki Disease

Burns JC, Best BM, Mejias A, et al (Univ of California San Diego School of Medicine and Rady Children's Hosp San Diego; Univ of Texas Southwestern Med Ctr; et al)

J Pediatr 153:833-838, 2008

Objective.—To investigate the safety, tolerability, and pharmacokinetics of the anti–tumor necrosis factor-α monoclonal antibody infliximab in subjects with intravenous immunoglobulin (IVIG)-resistant Kawasaki disease (KD).

Study Design.—We conducted a multicenter, randomized, prospective trial of second IVIG infusion (2 g/kg) versus infliximab (5 mg/kg) in 24 children with acute KD and fever after initial treatment with IVIG. Primary outcome measures were the safety, tolerability, and pharmacokinetics of infliximab. Secondary outcome measures were duration of fever and changes in markers of inflammation.

Results.—Study drug infusions were associated with cessation of fever within 24 hours in 11 of 12 subjects treated with infliximab and in 8 of 12 subjects retreated with IVIG. No infusion reactions or serious adverse events were attributed to either study drug. No significant differences were observed between treatment groups in the change from baseline for laboratory variables, fever, or echocardiographic assessment of coronary arteries.

Conclusions.—Both infliximab and a second IVIG infusion were safe and well tolerated in the subjects with KD who were resistant to standard IVIG treatment. The optimal management of patients resistant to IVIG remains to be determined.

▶ Infliximab treatment of intravenous immunoglobulin (IVIG)-resistant Kawasaki disease (KD) primarily sought to determine the pharmacokinetics of infliximab in patients diagnosed with KD, in addition to its safety and tolerability. The secondary outcome measured efficacy based on fever duration, inflammatory markers, and coronary artery changes.

This prospective, randomized, nonblinded study was a pilot project between 6 institutions spanning 2 years. The subjects were required to meet the standard diagnostic criteria for KD, excluding atypical presentations. They all received the standard, initial dose of IVIG before their 15th day of fever, and all had incessant or recurrent fever within 48 hours to 7 days post-IVIG, indicating either a recurrence or inadequate suppression of the inflammatory process. Subjects were excluded for any risk factors increasing the likelihood of an adverse reaction to infliximab, including: known or suspected TB or fungal infection, evidence of recent pulmonary infection, immunization with BCG in the previous 6 months, or immunomodulatory therapy within the previous week. Twenty-four patients were enrolled. Twelve patients (group 1) received a second dose of IVIG at the standard dose of 2 g/kg, while the other 12 patients (group 2) received infliximab 5 mg/kg. Four patients in group 1 failed to defervesce, and subsequently received infliximab; 2 of whom further required additional medications due to their inadequate clinical response. One patient from the infliximab group had persistent fever and defervesced after a second IVIG administration.

Of the 3 primary objectives (pharmacokinetics, safety, and tolerability), the study was only adequately powered for the analysis of pharmacokinetics. Serious adverse events (SAEs) were reported in 5 patients, all of whom received infliximab. However, all of the SAEs were attributed to either KD or a previous drug exposure, thus they were considered unrelated to the infliximab. Forty-eight AEs occurred, none of which could be directly attributed to the therapies, due to a combination of patient crossover and limited exam information or patient co-operation with exams. Infliximab is considered relatively safe in children (although not formally established), and has been reviewed in studies involving juvenile rheumatoid arthritis and Crohn's disease patients.[1,2] Each of these studies showed a higher incidence of adverse reactions (infusion reactions, infections, hepatitis); however, each patient received several doses of infliximab with frequency and cumulative dose altering adverse event incidence. Unlike children with Crohn's disease and juvenile rheumatoid arthritis, the KD patient has an inherent risk of acute cardiac dysfunction. Because infliximab appears to increase mortality in severe congestive heart failure, I am curious why echocardiographic evaluation of cardiac function was not included in the safety evaluation, particularly because at least a basic function assessment is part of the standard ECHO evaluations performed on KD patients. Tolerability of infliximab was not exclusively defined. In the discussion, the authors surmise that the drug was safe and well tolerated without further commentary.

The secondary objective of efficacy of infliximab was not well established, due to small study size, confounding issue of multiple crossover patients, and uneven distribution of patients among institutions with varying laboratory techniques skewing the inflammatory marker outcomes. Even so, the similar fever durations in both groups and no statistical difference in the incidence of coronary involvement at least suggest infliximab is a viable alternate or adjunctive therapy.

I sense that this study was designed to lay a foundation for a more in-depth evaluation of efficacy, evaluating not only fever and inflammatory markers, but more importantly coronary artery changes. It will require a much larger multi-institutional study to collect an adequate number of patients, given the low incidence of treatment failure with IVIG. The true benefit of showing efficacy will be the ability to extend the results to the atypical and very high risk KD patients who are frequently the most challenging to treat and have the highest morbidity and mortality.

A. Wu, MD

References

1. Ruperto N, Lovell DJ, Cuttica R, et al. A randomized, placebo controlled trial of Infliximab plus methotrexate for the treatment of polyarticular-course juvenile rheumatoid arthritis. *Arthritis Rheum.* 2007;56:3096-3106.

2. Hyams J, Crandall W, Kugathasan S, et al. Induction and Maintenance Infliximab therapy for the treatment of moderate-to-severe Crohn's disease in Children. *Gastroenterology.* 2007;132:863-873.

Azathioprine or Methotrexate Maintenance for ANCA-Associated Vasculitis

Pagnoux C, Mahr A, Hamidou MA, et al (Université Paris Descartes, Hôpital Cochin; Centre Hospitalier Universitaire Hôtel-Dieu, Nantes; et al)
N Engl J Med 359:2790-2803, 2008

Background.—Current standard therapy for Wegener's granulomatosis and microscopic polyangiitis combines corticosteroids and cyclophosphamide to induce remission, followed by a less toxic immunosuppressant such as azathioprine or methotrexate for maintenance therapy. However, azathioprine and methotrexate have not been compared with regard to safety and efficacy.

Methods.—In this prospective, open-label, multicenter trial, we randomly assigned patients with Wegener's granulomatosis or microscopic polyangiitis who entered remission with intravenous cyclophosphamide and corticosteroids to receive oral azathioprine (at a dose of 2.0 mg per kilogram of body weight per day) or methotrexate (at a dose of 0.3 mg per kilogram per week, progressively increased to 25 mg per week) for 12 months. The primary end point was an adverse event requiring discontinuation of the study drug or causing death; the sample size was calculated on the basis of the primary hypothesis that methotrexate would be less toxic than azathioprine. The secondary end points were severe adverse events and relapse.

Results.—Among 159 eligible patients, 126 (79%) had a remission, were randomly assigned to receive a study drug in two groups of 63 patients each, and were followed for a mean ($\pm$SD) period of 29 ± 13 months. Adverse events occurred in 29 azathioprine recipients and 35 methotrexate recipients ($P = 0.29$); grade 3 or 4 events occurred in 5 patients in the azathioprine group and 11 patients in the methotrexate group ($P = 0.11$). The primary end point was reached in 7 patients who received azathioprine as compared with 12 patients who received methotrexate ($P = 0.21$), with a corresponding hazard ratio for methotrexate of 1.65 (95% confidence interval, 0.65 to 4.18; $P = 0.29$). There was one death in the methotrexate group. Twenty-three patients who received azathioprine and 21 patients who received methotrexate had a relapse ($P = 0.71$); 73% of these patients had a relapse after discontinuation of the study drug.

Conclusions.—These results do not support the primary hypothesis that methotrexate is safer than azathioprine. The two agents appear to be similar alternatives for maintenance therapy in patients with Wegener's granulomatosis and microscopic polyangiitis after initial remission.

▶ This article compares the safety and efficacy of methotrexate (MTX) and azathioprine (AZA) for the maintenance therapy of Wegener's granulomatosis and microscopic polyangiitis. One hundred and twenty-six patients who achieved remission induced by corticosteroids and monthly intravenous pulses of cyclophosphamide were randomized to receive either open label MTX or AZA to maintain their vasculitis remission. The primary endpoint was any adverse event leading to the discontinuation of the drug or death. Seven patients (11%) in the AZA group and 12 patients (19%) in the MTX group achieved the primary endpoint ($p = 0.21$). Although not statistically significant, this study identified a trend for more severe adverse events in the methotrexate group with a hazard ratio of 1.65. Contrary to studies performed in patients with Rheumatoid Arthritis and Sjogren's syndrome, the authors determined that methotrexate did not have a better toxicity profile than azathioprine.[1,2] Additionally, while relapse was not the primary endpoint, the data also suggests that both drugs were equally efficacious at maintaining remission.

I question whether the World Health Organization (WHO) toxicity criteria,[3] which the authors used, reflected drug toxicity or an actual disease flare? This is an oncology reference tool published by the WHO, which grades criteria for 28 toxic side effects, including hematological, GI, renal systems, etc. Drawbacks of this study include that many diagnoses were not biopsy proven for Wegener's granulomatosis or microscopic polyangiitis. Furthermore, the events that were considered relapses were not detailed. The Birmingham Vasculitis Activity score,[4] which is a clinical index of disease activity based on signs and symptoms in 9 different categories, reflects disease activity. However, these criteria are nonspecific and may actually reflect medication toxicity.

As stated by the study's authors, the choice of the drug is best decided by the patient's clinical situation, safety issues, and cost consideration.

R. Dhawan, MD

References

1. Singh G, Fries JF, Spitz P, Williams CA. Toxic effects of azathioprine in rheumatoid arthritis: a national post-marketing perspective. *Arthritis Rheum.* 1989;32: 837-843.
2. Price EJ, Rigby SP, Clancy U, Venables PJ. A double blind placebo controlled trial of azathioprine in the treatment of primary Sjögren's syndrome. *J Rheumatol.* 1998;25:896-899.
3. WHO Toxicity Criteria by Grade, http://www.fda.gov/cder/cancer/toxicityframe. htm Access date July 20, 2009.
4. Luqmani RA, Bacon PA, Moots RJ, et al. Birmingham Vasculitis Activity Score (BVAS) in systemic necrotizing vasculitis. *QJM.* 1994;87:671-678.

4 Fibromyalgia

Introduction

We chose 2 articles this year from the *Annals of Internal Medicine* and the *American Journal of Medicine* that may represent the best reviews to date on the pathophysiology and treatment of fibromyalgia.

Seth Mark Berney, MD

Narrative Review: The Pathophysiology of Fibromyalgia
Abeles AM, Pillinger MH, Solitar BM, et al (New York Univ Hosp for Joint Diseases; et al)
Ann Intern Med 146:726-734, 2007

Primary fibromyalgia is a common yet poorly understood syndrome characterized by diffuse chronic pain accompanied by other somatic symptoms, including poor sleep, fatigue, and stiffness, in the absence of disease. Fibromyalgia does not have a distinct cause or pathology. Nevertheless, in the past decade, the study of chronic pain has yielded new insights into the pathophysiology of fibromyalgia and related chronic pain disorders. Accruing evidence shows that patients with fibromyalgia experience pain differently from the general population because of dysfunctional pain processing in the central nervous system. Aberrant pain processing, which can result in chronic pain and associated symptoms, may be the result of several interplaying mechanisms, including central sensitization, blunting of inhibitory pain pathways, alterations in neurotransmitters, and psychiatric comorbid conditions. This review provides an overview of the mechanisms currently thought to be partly responsible for the chronic diffuse pain typical of fibromyalgia.

▶ Fibromyalgia is a chronic pain syndrome condition encountered frequently and diagnosed when the patient has widespread pain and tenderness to palpation of 11 of 18 specified points. Although the condition affects approximately 2% of the United States population, very little is known about the etiology, pathophysiology, or treatment. The authors reviewed the most recent and relevant articles published that have attempted to explain the pathophysiology of fibromyalgia.

The authors used the PubMed journal literature system to search for relevant English-language articles published from 1970 to 2006 using the following terms: fibromyalgia, fibrositis, chronic diffuse pain, chronic widespread pain, pathophysiology, etiology, mechanism(s), and central sensitization. Articles were selected based on quality, relevance to the disease, importance of the pathophysiologic mechanism, and the attention they had previously gained in the field.

The authors discuss the role of peripheral tissues versus the role of the CNS in the pathogenesis of fibromyalgia. The studies performed evaluate alterations in ADP/ATP in peripheral tissues and neuroimaging such as MRI and PET in fibromyalgia patients compared with controls. Several additional potential mechanisms of pathophysiology were discussed in the article, including the central sensitization (or the amplification of pain involving a phenomenon known as "wind-up" [repetitive painful stimuli become exaggerated]), improper down regulation of spinal cord responses to pain, glial cell involvement, dopamine involvement, and the hypothalamic- pituitary- adrenal axis involvement. Finally, the authors discuss the effect of depression, anxiety and posttraumatic stress disorder (PTSD) on the development of fibromyalgia.

Based on their review of the literature, the authors conclude that most of the evidence suggests that fibromyalgia is a disorder of central pain processing, involving several different mechanisms. However, no single mechanism can explain all aspects of the disease. This may in part be a result of the observation that many studies do not adequately separate fibromyalgia from other chronic pain syndromes. Fibromyalgia patients appear to experience pain differently than the general population in the absence of any other known disease. Just what exactly causes this is not yet known. Emotional and/or psychiatric disturbance may modify pain processing to produce fibromyalgia. Patients should be screened for PTSD or any history of verbal/physical/sexual abuse. Finally, more studies need to be done in order to develop targeted therapies.

This may represent the best review of the pathogenesis of fibromyalgia to date, and will hopefully lead to better research on the etiology and treatment of this condition.

M. Boyd, MD

Update on Fibromyalgia Therapy
Abeles M, Solitar BM, Pillinger MH, et al (The Univ of Connecticut School of Medicine, Farmington; New York Univ School of Medicine/NYU Hosp for Joint Diseases; et al)
Am J Med 121:555-561, 2008

Primary fibromyalgia, a poorly-understood chronic pain syndrome, is characterized by widespread musculoskeletal pain, nonrestorative sleep, fatigue, psychological distress, and specific regions of localized tenderness, all in the absence of otherwise apparent organic disease. While the etiology of fibromyalgia is unclear, accumulating data suggest that disordered central pain processing likely plays a role in the pathogenesis of symptoms.

Although various pharmacological treatments have been studied and espoused for treating fibromyalgia, no single drug or group of drugs has proved to be particularly useful in treating fibromyalgia patients as a whole, and only one drug to date has earned U.S. Food and Drug Administration approval for treating the syndrome in the United States. This review critically and systematically evaluates clinical investigations of medicinal and nonmedicinal treatments for fibromyalgia dating from 1970 to 2007.

▶ Fibromyalgia is a chronic pain syndrome of unclear etiology that is poorly understood by both the medical community and general public. Although it is a common condition, controlled trials are few and appropriate medical therapy is elusive. The authors of this article provide a review of 45 research articles of fibromyalgia treatments, divided into pharmacological, nonpharmacological, and complementary and alternative therapies, and concludes with recommendations for approaching the treatment of the fibromyalgia patient.

The authors discuss tricyclic agents, newer antidepressants, "other central nervous system-acting agents," anti-inflammatories, and pure analgesics in the treatment of fibromyalgia. The data for the efficacy of tricyclic antidepressants is mixed, although amitriptyline is the most extensively studied and has shown benefit in short-term studies.

Cyclobenzaprine showed no benefit over placebo. The newer antidepressants include selective serotonin reuptake inhibitors (SSRI) and serotonin-norepinephrine reuptake inhibitors (SNRI). SSRIs may have efficacy equal to that of amitriptyline; short-term studies of SNRIs were helpful, as reflected by the patient's Fibromyalgia Impact Questionnaire (FIQ). Milnacipran is a newer SNRI showing improvement in both the FIQ and global assessment. Other CNS-acting agents include pregabalin, the only FDA-approved drug for fibromyalgia at the time of this review, and gabapentin, both benefited fibromyalgia patients. Nonsteroidal anti-inflammatory drugs are commonly used, but not well studied and show no benefit over placebo. Corticosteroids are ineffective.

Tramadol in combination with acetaminophen appears to reduce pain. Nonpharmacological interventions, including exercise, physical therapy, cognitive behavioral therapy, and patient education, are an important part of the treatment of fibromyalgia. Unfortunately, well-controlled studies of these modalities are not available, but the authors believe they are important.

The data for complementary and alternative therapies are lacking. Meditation-based stress reduction and melatonin have both been evaluated in poor quality studies. Dehydroepiandrosterone showed no benefit, and the results for efficacy of acupuncture are mixed.

In this review, although there is a lack of evidence-based medicine to guide them, the authors recommend an approach to treating fibromyalgia. They realize that there is heterogeneity in fibromyalgia and that patient response to particular treatments will vary. A tricyclic agent remains first-line therapy. Tramadol can be used in patients whose primary complaint is generalized pain without other associated symptoms. SSRIs and SNRIs are good choices in patients with depression. Pregabalin or gabapentin can be considered in patients who have failed the above. Physical therapy is encouraged in the form of low-impact exercise, gradually increasing the amount over time. Support in the form of education, emotional support, and reassurance is also very important.

The treatment of fibromyalgia remains a challenge because of poor understanding of the etiology of the syndrome and lack of evidence-based medicine to guide therapy. The fibromyalgia patient should be reassured that their pain is real and encouraged to participate in a comprehensive treatment program that includes pharmacologic and nonpharmacologic therapies.

N. Cotter, MD

5 Scleroderma

Introduction

We review 3 scleroderma papers this year that reevaluate the utility of D-penicillamine in skin fibrosis; long-term follow-up of stem cell transplantation; and the effect of mycophenolate mofetil on scleroderma-related interstitial lung disease.

Seth Mark Berney, MD

A retrospective randomly selected cohort study of D-penicillamine treatment in rapidly progressive diffuse cutaneous systemic sclerosis of recent onset

Derk CT, Huaman G, Jimenez SA (Thomas Jefferson Univ, Philadelphia, PA)
Br J Dermatol 158:1063-1068, 2008

Background.—Several uncontrolled studies in systemic sclerosis have shown that D-penicillamine may cause improvement in skin sclerosis, decrease the rate of new visceral organ involvement, and improve overall survival.

Objectives.—To undertake a single-centre retrospective randomly selected cohort study to examine the effects of D-penicillamine treatment on skin and visceral organ involvement in patients with rapidly progressive systemic sclerosis of recent onset.

Methods.—Eighty-four patients with diffuse cutaneous systemic sclerosis who had received D-penicillamine within 24 months of clinically detectable onset of skin sclerosis were randomly selected from the systemic sclerosis cohort followed at the Scleroderma Center of Thomas Jefferson University. Employing a previously described severity scale, disease severity and skin involvement were compared from initiation of D-penicillamine to end of study and a correlated matched t-test was used to establish statistical significance.

Results.—At a mean ± SD duration of D-penicillamine therapy of 29.2 ± 5.5 months and at a median dose of 750 mg per day statistically significant improvement in skin ($P < 0.01$) and cardiac, pulmonary and renal involvement ($P < 0.05$) was observed. At last follow-up, 17 (20%) patients were still receiving D-penicillamine, 25 (30%) had discontinued it owing to disease improvement, and 18 (21%) had discontinued it owing to side-effects.

Conclusions.—In a population of patients with diffuse cutaneous systemic sclerosis, with progressive disease of recent onset, D-penicillamine treatment at a median dose of 750 mg per day caused a statistically significant reduction in skin involvement and improvement of renal, cardiac and pulmonary involvement.

▶ This is a retrospective analysis of a cohort of patients who had rapidly progressive systemic sclerosis. Eighty-four patients with diffuse cutaneous systemic sclerosis who had received D-Penicillamine within 24 months of clinically detectable onset of skin sclerosis were randomly selected from 1987 to 2002 at the Thomas Jefferson University Scleroderma Center. Patients were treated with D-Penicillamine with an escalating dose starting at 250 mg and increased to a max of 1250 mg for at least 3 consecutive months. Other concomitant medications were prednisone < 20 mg daily, calcium channel blockers, and low dose aspirin. This article contradicts another study[1] that compared low dose versus high dose D-Penicillamine, and failed to show a difference between the 2 treatment regimes. However, in the present investigation, Derk et al's patients were naive to the use of Penicillamine.

There was a statistically significant improvement in extent and severity of skin involvement as assessed by then modified Rodnan skin scores as well as improvement of renal, cardiac, and pulmonary involvement ($P < 0.05$) when D-Penicillamine was used at a median daily dose of 750 mg. The authors suggest further reevaluation of the potential benefits of D-Penicillamine. However, significant data exist regarding toxicity; therefore, newer drugs should be investigated.

S. Hayat, MD

Reference

1. Clements PJ, Furst DE, Wong WK, Mayes M, White B, Wigley F, et al. High-dose versus low-dose D-penicillamine in early diffuse systemic sclerosis: analysis of a two-year, double-blind, randomized, controlled clinical trial. *Arthritis Rheum.* 1999;42:1194-1203.

Long-term follow-up results after autologous haematopoietic stem cell transplantation for severe systemic sclerosis
Vonk MC, Marjanovic Z, van den Hoogen FHJ, et al (Radboud Univ Nijmegen Med Centre, The Netherlands; Hôpital Hôtel-Dieu, Paris, France; et al)
Ann Rheum Dis 67:98-104, 2008

Objective.—Systemic sclerosis (SSc) is a generalised autoimmune disease, causing morbidity and a reduced life expectancy, especially in patients with rapidly progressive diffuse cutaneous SSc. As no proven treatment exists, autologous haematopoietic stem cell transplantation (HSCT) is employed as a new therapeutic strategy in patients with a poor prognosis. This study reports the effects on survival, skin and major organ function of HSCT in patients with severe diffuse cutaneous SSc.

Patients and Methods.—A total of 26 patients were evaluated. Peripheral blood stem cells were collected using cyclophosphamide ($4 g/m^2$) and rHu G-CSF (5 to 10 µg/kg/day) and were reinfused after positive CD34+ selection. For conditioning, cyclophosphamide 200 mg/kg was used.

Results.—After a median follow-up of 5.3 (1–7.5) years, 81% (n = 21/26) of the patients demonstrated a clinically beneficial response. The Kaplan-Meier estimated survival at 5 years was 96.2% (95% CI 89–100%) and at 7 years 84.8% (95% CI 70.2–100%) and event-free survival, defined as survival without mortality, relapse or progression of SSc, resulting in major organ dysfunction was 64.3% (95% CI 47.9–86%) at 5 years and 57.1% (95% CI 39.3–83%) at 7 years.

Conclusion.—This study confirms that autologous HSCT in selected patients with severe diffuse cutaneous SSc results in sustained improvement of skin thickening and stabilisation of organ function up to 7 years after transplantation.

▶ This study shows autologous hematopoietic stem cell transplantation (HSCT) as a potential treatment in patients with severe scleroderma, and reports the long-term outcome and treatment effects for 5 years. A total of 26 patients were transplanted, 19 females and 7 males. After a median follow-up of 5.3 years, 81% (21/26) demonstrated a clinically beneficial response, and the estimated survival at 5 years was 96.2%; death from disease progression in 8% of the HSCT patients compared with the mortality of 40% in severe systemic sclerosis (SSC) patients without transplant. The study confirmed that autologous HSCT in patients with severe diffuse SSC with Modified Rodman Skin Scores > 20 and major organ involvement had sustained improvement of skin thickening and stabilization of organ function up to 7 years after transplantation. To date, this is the largest cohort of SSC patients studied after autologous HSCT, providing a rather good estimation of the long-term outcome and treatment effects at 5 years.

Infectious complications occurred in 19% of the patients, primarily caused by Herpes Zoster reactivation and atypical mycobacterium.

Altogether, event-free survival for patients with at least 6 months follow-up after HSCT was 64.3% at 5 years, and 57.1% at 7 years. Two patients died within 6 months of HSCT treatment related at 1 month for 1 patient and due to disease progression for another at 6 months after HSCT.

While these results are encouraging, this study has limitations. The study is small and will have to be confirmed in large numbers in the ongoing phase III randomized trials comparing autologous HSCT with monthly cyclophosphamide intravenously—in the European ASTIS trial and North American SCOT study.

S. Hayat, MD

Effect of Mycophenolate Mofetil on Pulmonary Function in Scleroderma-Associated Interstitial Lung Disease

Gerbino AJ, Goss CH, Molitor JA (Benaroya Res Inst, Seattle, WA; Univ of Washington, Seattle)
Chest 133:455-460, 2008

Objective.—We sought to determine the effectiveness of mycophenolate mofetil (MMF) in scleroderma-associated interstitial lung disease (SSc-ILD).

Methods.—We retrospectively identified patients who met criteria for systemic sclerosis, had evidence of SSc-ILD on chest CT, received > 1 g/d of MMF for ≥ 6 months, and had pulmonary function data available. Vital capacity (VC) and diffusion capacity of the lung for carbon monoxide (DLCO) at treatment onset were compared with VC and DLCO values 12 months before and 12 months after treatment onset. Twelve-month values were imputed from regression lines generated using all VC and DLCO measurements made in the 24-month period either prior to or following treatment onset.

Results.—Among 13 patients who met inclusion criteria, MMF was associated with a significant improvement in VC (mean, + 159 mL; confidence interval [CI], + 30 to + 289 mL; and + 4% of the predicted normal value; CI, + 2 to + 7%) after 12 months of treatment. In contrast, patients had a significant decrease in VC (mean, − 239 mL; CI, − 477 to − 0.5 mL; and − 5% of the predicted normal value; CI, − 11 to − 0.3%) in the 12 months prior to MMF treatment. DLCO did not change significantly during MMF treatment (mean, + 1% of the predicted normal value; CI, − 2 to + 5%) but decreased significantly in the 12 months prior to treatment (mean, − 5% of the predicted normal value; CI, − 10 to − 1%).

Conclusion.—These retrospective data suggest MMF improves VC in patients with SSc-ILD.

▶ Mycophenolate, an inosine monophosphate dehydrogenase inhibitor that blocks the proliferation of both B and T lymphocytes, has an established record of utility as a steroid-sparing agent for transplant recipients, and as an immuno-modulatory agent in autoimmune disease. Unfortunately, the utility of immuno-suppressives in the treatment of interstitial lung disease associated with scleroderma is not so clear. The roles of most agents in the treatment of scleroderma-associated interstitial lung disease are not well described,[1] and recent trials of cyclophosphamide[2,3] have not been overwhelmingly encouraging. Thus, the search for an effective agent continues.

Clinical trials testing therapeutics in scleroderma-associated interstitial lung disease present a difficult challenge for researchers, especially for those using retrospective data. The marked disease heterogeneity, especially of its progression,[4] is particularly relevant to understanding the implications of this manuscript. The authors[5] present data that seem to support the use of mycophenolate mofetil in the treatment of scleroderma-associated interstitial lung disease. In retrospect, they found 13 participants who had been treated for at least 6 months with mycophenolate mofetil who also had pulmonary function measures at treatment onset and during the therapy; a subgroup of 10 also had earlier pulmonary function. They observed that prior to treatment, lung function was declining (vital capacity on average 5.3 percentage points of predicted, or 228 mL, lower per year leading up to therapy), and that during therapy the vital capacity was higher (4.3 percentage points of predicted, or 129 mL, higher per year).

Under normal circumstances, there is significant variance in lung function measures when repeated at relatively short intervals; this short-term variance has led the American Thoracic Society[6] to state that "When there are only 2 tests available to evaluate change, the large variability necessitates relatively large changes to be confident that a significant change has in fact occurred." In fact, the within participant "noise" is such that a 12% week-to-week variance, and 15% year-to-year, is expected. The authors describe a "significant" change in lung function that lies well within the expected variability of the measure; in fact, only 2 subjects had an improvement in FVC of more than 10%. For the analysis of data from 13 subjects with a disease of highly variable course to result in "significant" between-group differences that fall within the expected, variation would suggest an overly sensitive analytic approach.

Given the variable course of interstitial lung disease in scleroderma,[7] retrospective case series that use highly variable outcomes are not sufficient to definitively define the role for any intervention. The authors are certainly correct that this report, combined with its predecessors, justifies a prospective trial of mycophenolate mofetil. The design of such a trial should choose its outcomes wisely and ensure that the study is appropriately powered.

R. Walter, MD, MPH

References

1. Henness S, Wigley FM, Henness S, et al. Current drug therapy for scleroderma and secondary Raynaud's phenomenon: evidence-based review. *Curr Opin Rheumatol.* 2007;19:611-618.
2. Tashkin DP, Elashoff R, Clements PJ, et al. Cyclophosphamide versus placebo in scleroderma lung disease. *N Engl J Med.* 2006;354:2655-2666.
3. Tashkin DP, Elashoff R, Clements PJ, et al. Effects of 1-year treatment with cyclophosphamide on outcomes at 2 years in scleroderma lung disease. *Am J Respir Crit Care Med.* 2007;176:1026-1034.
4. Vallance DK, Lynch JP III, McCune WJ. Immunosuppressive treatment of the pulmonary manifestations of progressive systemic sclerosis. *Curr Opin Rheumatol.* 1995;7:174-182.
5. Gerbino AJ, Goss CH, Molitor JA. Effect of mycophenolate mofetil on pulmonary function in scleroderma-associated interstitial lung disease. *Chest.* 2008;133: 455-460.
6. Pellegrino R, Viegi G, Brusasco V, et al. Interpretative strategies for lung function tests. *Eur Respir J.* 2005;26:948-968.
7. Renzoni EA. Interstitial lung disease in systemic sclerosis. *Monaldi Arch Chest Dis.* 2007;67:217-228.

6 Juvenile Idiopathic Arthritis

Introduction

We include 3 articles this year that evaluate the use of tocilizumab, adalimumab, and abatacept in juvenile idiopathic arthritis.

Seth Mark Berney, MD

Efficacy and safety of tocilizumab in patients with systemic-onset juvenile idiopathic arthritis: a randomised, double-blind, placebo-controlled, withdrawal phase III trial

Yokota S, Imagawa T, Mori M, et al (Yokohama City Univ School of Medicine, Japan; et al)

Lancet 371:998-1006, 2008

Background.—Systemic-onset juvenile idiopathic arthritis does not always respond to available treatments, including antitumour necrosis factor agents. We investigated the efficacy and safety of tocilizumab, an anti-interleukin-6-receptor monoclonal antibody, in children with this disorder.

Methods.—56 children (aged 2–19 years) with disease refractory to conventional treatment were given three doses of tocilizumab 8 mg/kg every 2 weeks during a 6-week open-label lead-in phase. Patients achieving an American College of Rheumatology Pediatric (ACR Pedi) 30 response and a C-reactive protein concentration (CRP) of less than 5 mg/L were randomly assigned to receive placebo or to continue tocilizumab treatment for 12 weeks or until withdrawal for rescue medication in a double-blind phase. The primary endpoint of the double-blind phase was an ACR Pedi 30 response and CRP concentration of less than 15 mg/L. Patients responding to tocilizumab and needing further treatment were enrolled in an open-label extension phase for at least 48 weeks. The analysis was done by intention to treat. This study is registered with ClinicalTrials.gov, numbers NCT00144599 (for the open-label lead-in and double-blind phases) and NCT00144612 (for the open-label extension phase).

Findings.—At the end of the open-label lead-in phase, ACR Pedi 30, 50, and 70 responses were achieved by 51 (91%), 48 (86%), and 38 (68%) patients, respectively. 43 patients continued to the double-blind phase and were included in the efficacy analysis. Four (17%) of 23 patients in the placebo group maintained an ACR Pedi 30 response and a CRP concentration of less than 15 mg/L compared with 16 (80%) of 20 in the tocilizumab group (p < 0·0001). By week 48 of the open-label extension phase, ACR Pedi 30, 50, and 70 responses were achieved by 47 (98%), 45 (94%), and 43 (90%) of 48 patients, respectively. Serious adverse events were anaphylactoid reaction, gastrointestinal haemorrhage, bronchitis, and gastroenteritis.

Interpretation.—Tocilizumab is effective in children with systemic-onset juvenile idiopathic arthritis. It might therefore be a suitable treatment in the control of this disorder, which has so far been difficult to manage.

▶ Systemic onset juvenile idiopathic arthritis (SOJIA) (very similar to adult-onset Still's disease) causes functional disability and growth abnormalities in up to 50% of the affected children. Furthermore, despite significant improvement with TNF inhibition, patients still have had disease progression and develop the potentially fatal macrophage activation syndrome. As a result, the authors performed a multicenter 3 phase randomized placebo controlled double blind trial to evaluate the efficacy and safety of the anti-interleukin-6 (IL-6) antibody, tocilizumab.

The authors present data that support the use of tocilizumab in the treatment of SOJIA. Although this is a relatively rare form of JIA, the patients become very sick and any addition to the therapeutic armamentarium can be very helpful, especially because tocilizumab appears relatively safe. This study may also serve as a justification for use in adult-onset Still's disease.

S. M. Berney, MD

Adalimumab with or without Methotrexate in Juvenile Rheumatoid Arthritis

Lovell DJ, for the Pediatric Rheumatology Collaborative Study Group and the Pediatric Rheumatology International Trials Organisation (Cincinnati Children's Hosp Med Ctr, OH; et al)

N Engl J Med 359:810-820, 2008

Background.—Tumor necrosis factor (TNF) has a pathogenic role in juvenile rheumatoid arthritis. We evaluated the efficacy and safety of adalimumab, a fully human monoclonal anti-TNF antibody, in children with polyarticular-course juvenile rheumatoid arthritis.

Methods.—Patients 4 to 17 years of age with active juvenile rheumatoid arthritis who had previously received treatment with nonsteroidal antiinflammatory drugs underwent stratification according to methotrexate use and received 24 mg of adalimumab per square meter of body-surface area (maximum dose, 40 mg) subcutaneously every other week for 16 weeks. We randomly assigned patients with an American College of Rheumatology Pediatric 30% (ACR Pedi 30) response at week 16 to receive adalimumab or placebo in a double-blind fashion every other week for up to 32 weeks.

Results.—Seventy-four percent of patients not receiving methotrexate (64 of 86) and 94% of those receiving methotrexate (80 of 85) had an ACR Pedi 30 response at week 16 and were eligible for double-blind treatment. Among patients not receiving methotrexate, disease flares (the primary outcome) occurred in 43% of those receiving adalimumab and 71% of those receiving placebo (P = 0.03). Among patients receiving methotrexate, flares occurred in 37% of those receiving adalimumab and 65% of those receiving placebo (P = 0.02). At 48 weeks, the

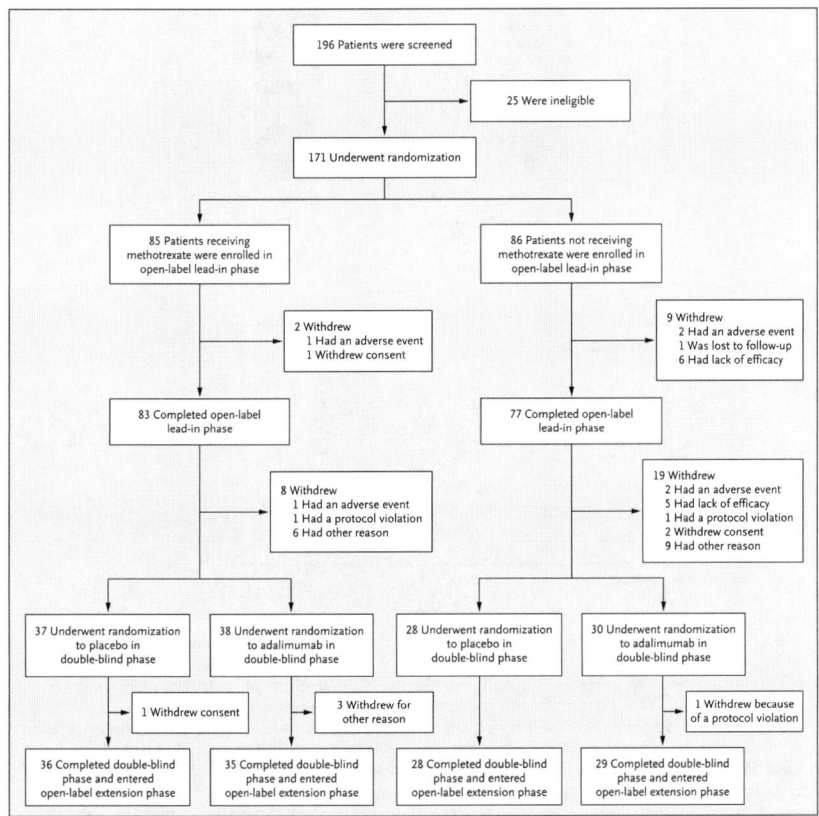

FIGURE 1.—Enrollment of Patients and Completion of the Study. (Reprinted from Lovell DJ, for the Pediatric Rheumatology Collaborative Study Group and the Pediatric Rheumatology International Trials Organisation. Adalimumab with or without methotrexate in juvenile rheumatoid arthritis. *N Engl J Med.* 2008;359:810-820, with permission from the Massachusetts Medical Society. All rights reserved.)

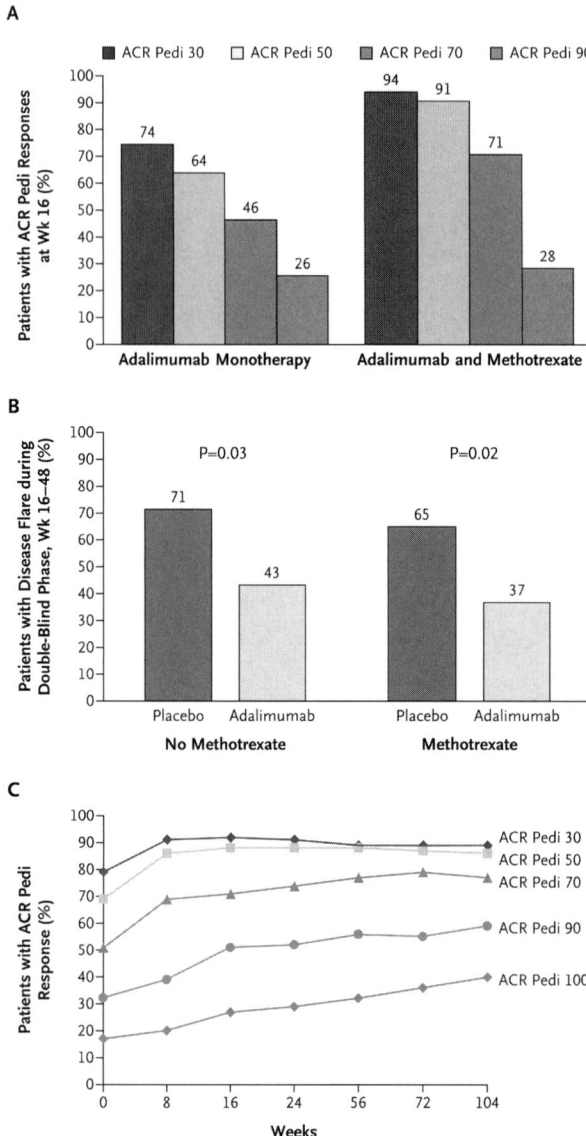

FIGURE 2.—Response to Treatment. Panel A shows American College of Rheumatology Pediatric (ACR Pedi) response levels among patients receiving open-label adalimumab at week 16 according to whether they were or were not receiving methotrexate. ACR Pedi 30, 50, 70, and 90 responses are defined as improvements of at least 30%, 50%, 70%, and 90%, respectively, in at least three of the six core criteria for juvenile rheumatoid arthritis, with worsening of 30% or more in no more than one criterion. Panel B shows the percentages of patients in the placebo and adalimumab groups with disease flare during the doubleblind phase of the study (weeks 16 through 48). Panel C shows ACR Pedi 30, 50, 70, 90, and 100 responses during the first 104 eeks of the open-label extension phase regardless of whether adalimumab was dosed according to body-surface area or body weight. The data are from the intention-to-treat population of 128 patients who entered the open-label extension phase of the study; for missing values, the last observation was carried forward. (Reprinted from Lovell DJ, for the Pediatric Rheumatology Collaborative Study Group and the Pediatric Rheumatology International Trials Organisation. Adalimumab with or without methotrexate in juvenile rheumatoid arthritis. *N Engl J Med.* 2008;359:810-820, with permission from the Massachusetts Medical Society. All rights reserved.)

TABLE 1.—Baseline Demographic and Clinical Characteristics of the Patients*

Characteristic	Open-Label Lead-in Phase		Double-Blind Phase			
	Methotrexate	No Methotrexate	Methotrexate		No Methotrexate	
	Adalimumab (N = 85)	Adalimumab (N = 86)	Placebo (N = 37)	Adalimumab (N = 38)	Placebo (N = 28)	Adalimumab (N = 30)
Age — yr	11.4 ± 3.3	11.1 ± 3.8	10.8 ± 3.4	11.7 ± 3.3	11.3 ± 3.8	11.1 ± 4.1
Age group — no. (%)						
4–8 yr	19 (22)	21 (24)	12 (32)	6 (16)	8 (29)	8 (27)
9–12 yr	30 (35)	32 (37)	10 (27)	17 (45)	7 (25)	10 (33)
13–17 yr	36 (42)	33 (38)	15 (41)	15 (40)	13 (46)	12 (40)
Female sex — no. (%)†	68 (80)	67 (78)	30 (81)	30 (79)	20 (71)	23 (77)
Race — no. (%)†						
White	81 (95)	76 (88)	36 (97)	36 (95)	27 (96)	26 (87)
Black	0	3 (3)	0	0	1 (4)	1 (3)
Other	4 (5)	7 (8)	1 (3)	2 (5)	0	3 (10)
Body weight — kg	43.8 ± 18.3	40.9 ± 19.3	44.3 ± 18.9	42.1 ± 17.9	45.4 ± 24.4	41.3 ± 17.3
Negative for rheumatoid factor — no./total no. (%)	64/83 (77)	67/85 (79)	30/36 (83)	27/37 (73)	21/27 (78)	24/30 (80)
Duration of juvenile rheumatoid arthritis — yr	4.0 ± 3.7	3.6 ± 4.0	4.0 ± 3.5	4.3 ± 4.1	2.9 ± 3.3	3.6 ± 4.0
Previous medication use — no. (%)						
Methotrexate	85 (100)	18 (21)	37 (100)	38 (100)	4 (14)	8 (27)
Other disease-modifying antirheumatic drugs	8 (9)	8 (9)	7 (19)	1 (3)	3 (11)	4 (13)
Methylprednisolone	4 (5)	2 (2)	2 (5)	2 (5)	1 (4)	0

*Plus-minus values are means ± SD.
†Race was determined by the patient or the parent.
(Reprinted from Lovell DJ, for the Pediatric Rheumatology Collaborative Study Group and the Pediatric Rheumatology International Trials Organisation. Adalimumab with or without methotrexate in juvenile rheumatoid arthritis. *N Engl J Med.* 2008;359:810-820, with permission from the Massachusetts Medical Society. All rights reserved.)

percentages of patients treated with methotrexate who had ACR Pedi 30, 50, 70, or 90 responses were significantly greater for those receiving adalimumab than for those receiving placebo; the differences between patients not treated with methotrexate who received adalimumab and those who received placebo were not significant. Response rates were sustained after 104 weeks of treatment. Serious adverse events possibly related to adalimumab occurred in 14 patients.

Conclusions.—Adalimumab therapy seems to be an efficacious option for the treatment of children with juvenile rheumatoid arthritis. (ClinicalTrials.gov number, NCT00048542.) (Figs 1, 2 and Table1).

▶ JRA, also referred to as Juvenile Idiopathic Arthritis (JIA), is the most common rheumatic disease of childhood, and is treated with methotrexate (MTX) at doses up to 15 mg/m^2 of surface area/week. However, as with the adult arthropathies, MTX has been inadequate. As a result, similar to RA, anti-TNF therapies have dramatically improved polyarticular JIA. This study details the efficacy and safety of adalimumab with or without MTX in patients with polyarticular JIA.

Methods: Patients aged 4 to 17 years with active polyarticular JIA disease (defined as $\geq$ 5 swollen joints and $\geq$ 3 joints with decreased range of motion) and an inadequate response to nonsteroidal anti-inflammatory drugs (NSAIDs) were eligible for inclusion in this randomized double-blind stratified placebo controlled multicenter medication withdrawal study. This trial is composed of a 16-week open-label lead-in phase, a 32 week double-blind withdrawal phase, and an open-label extension phase. Patients must also be either MTX naïve, inadequate responders, or have had an adverse reaction, which limited its use. At the beginning of the open-label lead-in phase, patients were separated based on their MTX exposure. Those who were MTX naïve or had discontinued MTX were assigned to the no-MTX group. Patients who received MTX at a stable dose of at least 10 mg/M^2/week for the 3-month period prior to screening, continued that dose throughout the open-label lead-in and double-blind phases.

During the open-label lead-in phase, all patients received 24 mg of the adalimumab/M^2 (to a max of 40 mg) sq q 2 week for 16 weeks. Stable doses of NSAIDs and corticosteroids $\leq$ 0.2 mg of prednisone or equivalent/kg/day (maximum dose of 10 mg/day) were permitted.

At week 16, patients who achieved an ACR Pediatric 30% entered the 32-week double-blind phase and underwent randomization at a 1:1 ratio within their MTX group, to receive q 2-week sq injections of either adalimumab or placebo.

Patients enrolled in this double-blind phase were eligible to receive open-label treatment with adalimumab in the extension phase of the study.

Results: Fig 1 illustrates the patient enrollment, withdrawal, and completion information. Table 1 contains the patient demographics of the patients during the first 2 phases of the study.

As we would have expected (based on the adult data), at the beginning and at the end of the initial open-label portion of the study, patients receiving MTX had less disease activity. Furthermore, the group receiving MTX appeared to have a larger response (no statistical analysis was performed—WHY?) than the group without MTX. However, Fig 2 indicates that all patients in the lead-in phase responded. Fig 2b also indicates that in the blinded part of the trial, patients receiving adalimumab had superior responses. Unfortunately, the authors do not report whether a statistically significant difference exists between the patients who received adalimumab and MTX compared with adalimumab without MTX.

The most commonly reported adverse events were infections and injection site reactions. Importantly, no patients died or developed opportunistic infections (including TB), malignancy, demyelinating disease or lupus-like reactions.

This is an important study because it further substantiates TNF blockade in JIA.

S. M. Berney, MD

Abatacept in children with juvenile idiopathic arthritis: a randomised, double-blind, placebo-controlled withdrawal trial
Ruperto N, for the Paediatric Rheumatology INternational Trials Organization (PRINTO) and the Pediatric Rheumatology Collaborative Study Group (PRCSG) (IRCCS G Gaslini, PRINTO, Genoa, Italy; et al)
Lancet 372:383-391, 2008

Background.—Some children with juvenile idiopathic arthritis either do not respond, or are intolerant to, treatment with disease-modifying anti-rheumatic drugs, including anti-tumour necrosis factor (TNF) drugs. We aimed to assess the safety and efficacy of abatacept, a selective T-cell costimulation modulator, in children with juvenile idiopathic arthritis who had failed previous treatments.

Methods.—We did a double-blind, randomised controlled withdrawal trial between February, 2004, and June, 2006. We enrolled 190 patients aged 6–17 years, from 45 centres, who had a history of active juvenile idiopathic arthritis; at least five active joints; and an inadequate response to, or intolerance to, at least one disease-modifying antirheumatic drug. All 190 patients were given 10 mg/kg of abatacept intravenously in the open-label period of 4 months. Of the 170 patients who completed this lead-in course, 47 did not respond to the treatment according to predefined American College of Rheumatology (ACR) paediatric criteria and were excluded. Of the patients who did respond to abatacept, 60 were randomly assigned to receive 10 mg/kg of abatacept at 28-day intervals for 6 months, or until a flare of the arthritis, and 62 were randomly assigned to receive placebo at the same dose and timing. The primary endpoint was time to flare of arthritis. Flare was defined as worsening of 30% or more in at least three of six core variables, with at least 30% improvement in no more than one variable. We analysed all patients who were treated as per protocol. This trial is registered, number NCT00095173.

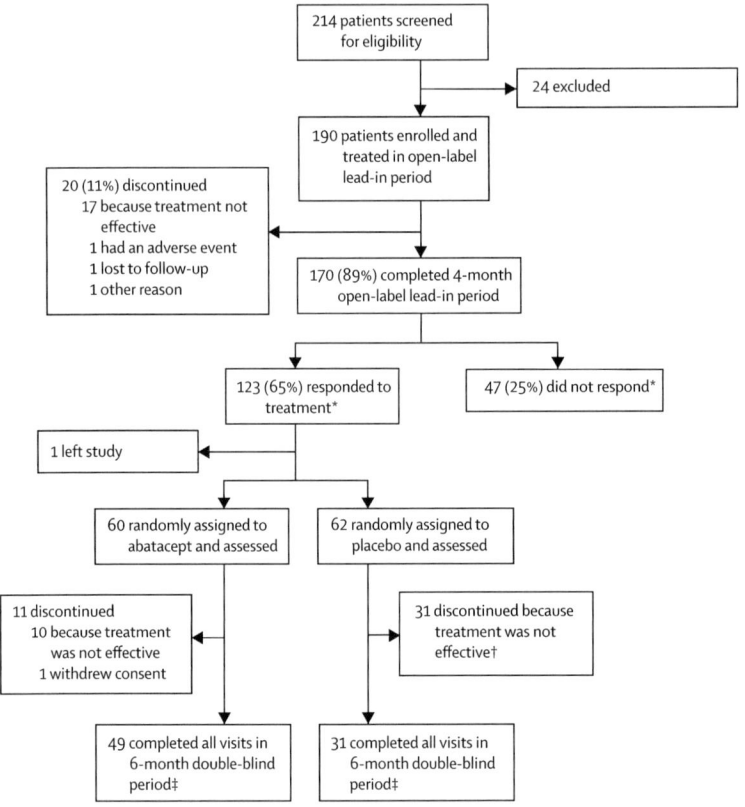

FIGURE 1.—Trial profile. *Response according to the American College of Rheumatology definition of improvement. †Two patients in the placebo group who discontinued because the treatment was not effective had no flare of arthritis. ‡One patient in the treatment group and two in the placebo group had a flare on the last visit during the double-blind period. (Reprinted from Ruperto N, for the Paediatric Rheumatology INternational Trials Organization (PRINTO) and the Pediatric Rheumatology Collaborative Study Group (PRCSG). Abatacept in children with juvenile idiopathic arthritis: a randomised, double-blind, placebo-controlled withdrawal trial. *Lancet.* 2008;372:383-391, with permission from Elsevier Ltd.)

Findings.—Flares of arthritis occurred in 33 of 62 (53%) patients who were given placebo and 12 of 60 (20%) abatacept patients during the double-blind treatment (p=0·0003). Median time to flare of arthritis was 6 months for patients given placebo (insufficient events to calculate IQR); insufficient events had occurred in the abatacept group for median time to flare to be assessed (p=0·0002). The risk of flare in patients who continued abatacept was less than a third of that for controls during that double-blind period (hazard ratio 0·31, 95% CI 0·16–0·95). During the double-blind period, the frequency of adverse events did not differ in the two treatment groups. Adverse events were recorded in 37 abatacept recipients (62%) and 34 (55%) placebo recipients (p=0·47); only two serious adverse events were reported, both in controls (p=0·50).

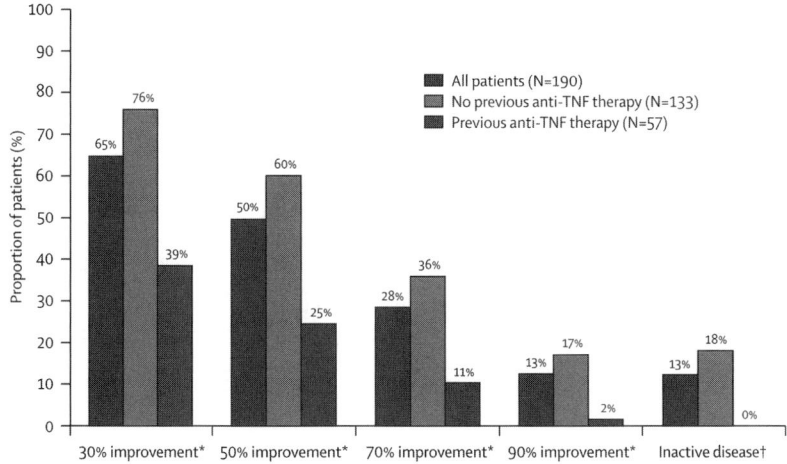

FIGURE 2.—Proportion of patients who had response rates of 30%, 50%, 70%, and 90%* after 4 months of open-label treatment in the lead-in period. *According to the American College of Rheumatology Paediatric responses. †Inactive disease defined as no joints with active arthritis, a physician's assessment of 10 or less on a 100 mm visual analogue scale, and a normal erythrocyte sedimentation rate. (Reprinted from Ruperto N for the Paediatric Rheumatology INternational Trials Organization (PRINTO) and the Pediatric Rheumatology Collaborative Study Group (PRCSG). Abatacept in children with juvenile idiopathic arthritis: a randomised, double-blind, placebo-controlled withdrawal trial. *Lancet.* 2008;372:383-391, with permission from Elsevier Ltd.)

Interpretation.—Selective modulation of T-cell costimulation with abatacept is a rational alternative treatment for children with juvenile idiopathic arthritis (Figs 1 and 2).

▶ Similar to adult inflammatory arthropathy, the childhood arthritides respond to methotrexate and the tumor necrosis inhibitors. However, not all patients respond completely. Therefore, this phase III, double-blind, randomized controlled withdrawal trial intends to evaluate the safety and efficacy of abatacept in children with juvenile idiopathic arthritis (JIA) who suboptimally improved.

Investigators enrolled patients aged 6 to 17 years with active JIA from 45 pediatric centers in Europe, Latin America, and the United States. For inclusion, patients must have had an inadequate response or intolerance to at least one disease modifying antirheumatic drugs (DMARD), including anti-TNF drugs. Furthermore, all DMARDs (except methotrexate) were withdrawn and prohibited during this trial. Patients were excluded if they had active uveitis, major concurrent illness, or were pregnant or lactating.

All patients received 10 mg/kg (max 1000 mg) abatacept via a 30 min intravenous infusion on days 1, 15, 29, 57, and 85. They also were permitted to continue their methotrexate and folic acid. Their oral corticosteroid dose was stabilized 4 weeks before enrollment at 10 mg/day or 0.2 mg/kg/day of prednisone equivalent (whichever was less). All other DMARDs and TNF inhibitors were washed out before enrollment.

At day 113, patients who improved by 30% (according to the ACR pediatric definition) were randomized to receive either abatacept or placebo (10 mg/kg), and at day 28 intervals for 6 months or a flare.

Patients were assessed before each infusion. The 1° endpoint was time to flare of the juvenile idiopathic arthritis.

During the 4-month open label period, 190 patients were enrolled. Fig 1 details the trial profile. Fig 2 illustrates the patient responses to the abatacept during the open label time.

During the double-blind period, the median time for the placebo group to flare was 6 months, during which 33 of 62 patients (53%) flared compared with 12 of 60 patients (20%) who received abatacept ($p = 0.0003$).

Additionally, 4 patients withdrew from the trial during the double-blind period (31 in the group) because of lack of an adequate response. Fig 5 in the original article shows the responses to the abatacept and placebo. The adverse events were similar between the placebo and abatacept groups.

This study indicates the T cell inhibitor, abatacept, is effective in children with JIA, and is also seemingly safe. It provides the rationale for using this drug in children and may be more effective in children who are TNF inhibitor naive.

The results of an abatacept versus TNF inhibitor trial would be very instructional. Unfortunately, I doubt any of the involved pharmaceuticals would sponsor or even voluntarily participate in such a trial because of the potential adverse effect a poor outcome would have on their share of the market.

S. M. Berney, MD

7   Osteoporosis

Introduction

This chapter contains 2 articles. The first addresses whether alendronate protects premenopausal women from glucocorticoid-induced bone loss and fracture. The other deals with the relative efficacy of osteoporosis medications on preventing nonvertebral fractures.

Seth Mark Berney, MD

Alendronate Protects Premenopausal Women from Bone Loss and Fracture Associated with High-dose Glucocorticoid Therapy

Okada Y, Nawata M, Nakayamada S, et al (Univ of Occupational and Environmental Health, Kitakyushu, Japan)
J Rheumatol 35:2249-2254, 2008

Objective.—We assessed the efficacy of bisphosphonate in premenopausal women (n = 47) commencing high-dose glucocorticoid (GC) therapy in protection against induced bone loss and bone fracture.

Methods.—Subjects had just developed systemic autoimmune diseases and were randomized to be treated with 1 mg/kg/day prednisolone and alfacalcidol 1 µg/day alone (alfacalcidol group; n = 22), or prednisolone and alfacalcidol 1 µg/day with alendronate 5 mg/day (alendronate group; n = 25), each for 18 months.

Results.—The percentage changes in lumbar spine bone mineral density (BMD) after 6 months of the therapy were −10.5% ± 0.8% in the alfacalcidol group, but only −2.1% ± 1.2% in the combined group. The rate of bone loss in the lumbar spine was significantly lower in the combined group than in the alfacalcidol group at 6 months. At 12 months of treatment, the percentage change in lumbar spine BMD was increased by 1.7% ± 1.4% in the combined group, but decreased by 9.9% ± 1.9% in the alfacalcidol group; the difference was significant. Bone fracture occurred at 12 months or later in 4 patients of the alfacalcidol groups, but not in the combined group, even at up to 18 months.

Conclusion.—Our results indicate that alendronate with alfacalcidol can maintain BMD and protects against high-dose GC-induced bone loss and bone fracture.

▶ This is a single-center, prospective, open-label controlled study to determine the efficacy of alendronate in the prevention of glucocorticoid-induced osteoporosis. 33 glucocorticoid-naïve patients with a newly diagnosed systemic autoimmune disease (systemic lupus erythematosus [SLE], mixed connective tissue disease [MCTD], dermatomyositis, and "other") requiring treatment with high-dose glucocorticoids (starting at ≥1 mg/kg/day, and no less than 7.5 mg/day after 6 months) were given alfacalcidol alone or in combination with alendronate, and followed for 18 months at the University of Occupational and Environmental Health in Japan. Dual-energy radiograph absorptiometry, radiographs, and metabolic bone markers were evaluated at baseline, 6, 12, and 18 months after starting treatment. The percentage change in bone mineral density (BMD) and metabolic bone markers were compared with baseline at each time interval.

Patients in the alfacalcidol group experienced a statistically significant decrease in BMD compared with the slight decrease in the alfacalcidol plus alendronate group at 6 months ($p < 0.001$). However, at 12 and 18 months, the mean lumbar BMD continued to decrease in the alfacalcidol group and actually increased in the combination group ($p < 0.001$). There were no statistical differences in the metabolic bone markers between the 2 groups at any time point. Four patients in the alfacalcidol group developed vertebral fractures. Based on these results, the investigators concluded that alendronate with alfacalcidol is worthwhile to prevent osteoporosis induced by high-dose glucocorticoid therapy.

Glucocorticoid-induced osteoporosis is an important morbidity in patients with diseases requiring systemic steroids. This study provides data supporting bisphosphonates as the primary prevention of glucocorticoid-induced osteoporosis. The study was small, with only 33 patients, and further investigation on a larger scale is needed to confirm the results. I note (though I am unsure of the significance) that the patients in this study were on very high doses of steroids, and the study specifically excluded patients treated with lower dose glucocorticoids. In addition to repeating this study, patients on lower doses of steroids should also undergo this evaluation.

N. Cotter, MD

Relative Effectiveness of Osteoporosis Drugs for Preventing Nonvertebral Fracture
Cadarette SM, Katz JN, Brookhart MA, et al (Brigham and Women's Hosp)
Ann Intern Med 148:637-646, 2008

Background.—Little information is available on the comparative effectiveness of osteoporosis pharmacotherapies.

Objective.—To compare the relative effectiveness of osteoporosis treatments to reduce nonvertebral fracture risk among older adults.

Design.—Cohort study.

Setting.—Enrollees in 2 statewide pharmaceutical benefit programs for persons age 65 years or older.

Patients.—43 135 new recipients of oral bisphosphonates, nasal calcitonin, and raloxifene who began treatment from 2000 to 2005. The mean age was 79 years (SD, 6.9), and 96% were women.

Measurements.—The primary outcome was nonvertebral fracture (hip, humerus, or radius or ulna) within 12 months of treatment initiation. Cox proportional hazard models stratified by state and adjusted for risk factors for fracture were used to compare fracture rates. Alendronate was the reference category in all analyses.

Results.—A total of 1051 nonvertebral fractures were observed within 12 months (2.62 fractures per 100 person-years). No large differences in fracture risk were found between risedronate (hazard ratio [HR], 1.01 [95% CI, 0.85 to 1.21]) or raloxifene (HR, 1.18 [CI, 0.96 to 1.46]) and alendronate. However, among those with a fracture history, raloxifene recipients experienced more nonvertebral fractures within 12 months (HR, 1.78 [CI, 1.20 to 2.63]) compared with alendronate recipients. Patients who received calcitonin experienced more nonvertebral fractures than those who received alendronate (HR, 1.40, [CI, 1.20 to 1.63]). Results were similar in sensitivity analyses that examined different lengths of follow-up (6 months and 24 months), were restricted to hip fracture as the outcome, and were completed in various subgroups.

Limitation.—Confounder adjustment was limited to health care utilization data, and the confidence bounds of some comparisons were too wide to rule out potential clinically important differences between agents.

Conclusion.—Differences in fracture risk between risedronate or raloxifene and alendronate were small. Nasal calcitonin recipients may have a higher risk for nonvertebral fractures compared with alendronate recipients. Future studies that can better adjust for possible confounding may further clarify these relationships.

▶ The goal of this study was to evaluate the impact of several osteoporosis medications on nonvertebral fractures.

This was a cohort study that used Medicare data to evaluate older patients who were new recipients of the antiresorptive medications: alendronate, risedronate, calcitonin, or raloxifene between April 1, 2000, and June 30, 2005. The study defined a new recipient of these medications as a patient who had not used any of these agents in the previous year and excluded patients who were nursing home residents and those who had a Medicare claim for Paget's disease. Patients were also excluded if they had received a bisphosphonate or teriparatide in the year before beginning the study.

The study's primary outcome was the incidence of nonvertebral fractures (defined as fractures of the hip, humerus, or radius or ulna) within 1 year of treatment initiation. The secondary outcomes included nonvertebral fractures within 6 and 24 months of treatment onset, as well as hip fracture within 6, 12, and 24 months of treatment onset. 43 135 patients were enrolled, 96% were women, the mean age was 78.7 years, and there was a similar distribution of patients with the diagnosis of osteoporosis among all study groups.

The study indicates that calcitonin recipients had more nonvertebral fractures at 12 months than those taking the other therapies. The calcitonin group also had more hip fractures than patients who received alendronate. The risk of a nonvertebral fracture was similar for patients taking either alendronate or risedronate in the first 12 months of treatment. Furthermore, patients who took raloxifene did not have a statistically different nonvertebral fracture risk than alendronate.

There were several drawbacks to this study. The patients taking calcitonin were older, and had more comorbid conditions and previous vertebral fractures than the patients taking the other therapies. Additionally, the raloxifene patients were younger and had fewer comorbid conditions and previous fractures. Moreover, we do not know whether the patients in each treatment group had statistically similar bone mineral densities before initiating therapy, nor did the investigators appear to standardize or control the calcium and vitamin D intake by patients, which complicates the data interpretation.

Despite the study's design limitations, it is important to note that there was a much higher risk for nonvertebral fractures for patients taking calcitonin versus bisphosphonate therapy. This reinforces the limited use of calcitonin as monotherapy for osteoporosis. Although this study involved a large patient population, additional studies should be performed to investigate this result further. Also, future studies will be needed to further determine the effect of raloxifene on nonvertebral fractures. These studies should include ibandronate, zoledronic acid, and teriparatide in the comparison of osteoporosis medications.

N. Cotter, MD

8 Spondyloarthropathies

Introduction

This chapter contains 4 articles. The first 2 describe the effect of using golimumab and etanercept in patients with ankylosing spondylitis. The remaining articles report on atherosclerosis in spondyloarthropathies.

Seth Mark Berney, MD

Efficacy and Safety of Golimumab in Patients With Ankylosing Spondylitis: Results of a Randomized, Double-Blind, Placebo-Controlled, Phase III Trial
Inman RD, Davis JC Jr, van der Heijde D, et al (Univ of Toronto, Japan; Univ of California, San Francisco; Leiden Univ Med Ctr, The Netherlands; et al)
Arthritis Rheum 58:3402-3412, 2008

Objective.—To evaluate the efficacy and safety of golimumab in patients with ankylosing spondylitis (AS) in the GO-RAISE study.

Methods.—Patients with active AS, a Bath AS Disease Activity Index (BASDAI) score ≥4, and a back pain score of ≥4 were randomly assigned in a 1.8:1.8:1 ratio to receive subcutaneous injections of golimumab (50 mg or 100 mg) or placebo every 4 weeks. The primary end point was the proportion of patients with at least 20% improvement in the ASsessment in AS (ASAS20) criteria at week 14.

Results.—At randomization, 138, 140, and 78 patients were assigned to the 50-mg, 100-mg, and placebo groups, respectively. After 14 weeks, 59.4%, 60.0%, and 21.8% of patients, respectively, were ASAS20 responders ($P < 0.001$). A 40% improvement in the ASAS criteria at week 24 occurred in 43.5%, 54.3%, and 15.4% of patients, respectively. Patients receiving golimumab also showed significant improvement in the physical and mental component summary scores of the Short Form 36 Health Survey, the Jenkins Sleep Evaluation Questionnaire score, the BASDAI score, and the Bath AS Functional Index score, but not the Bath AS Metrology Index score. Through week 24, 85.6% of golimumab-treated patients and 76.6% of patients in the placebo group had ≥1 adverse event, and 5.4% and 6.5% of patients, respectively, had ≥1 serious adverse event. Eight golimumab-treated patients and 1 placebo-treated patient had markedly abnormal liver enzyme values (≥100% increase from baseline and a value >150 IU/liter), which were transient.

Conclusion.—Golimumab was effective and well tolerated in a large cohort of patients with AS during a 24-week study period.

▶ Ankylosing spondylitis (AS) is a systemic autoimmune disease characterized by inflammation of the axial skeleton, sacroiliac joints, entheses, and peripheral joints, as well as various other extra-articular manifestations. To date, therapeutic options have been limited with only antitumor necrosis factor α (TNFα) agents demonstrating significant efficacy. Golimumab, a new anti-TNF agent, has been studied previously in the treatment of rheumatoid arthritis (RA) and psoriatic arthritis (PsA). In this phase III trial (the GO-RAISE study), the safety and efficacy of golimumab was evaluated in patients with AS.

This randomized, double blind, placebo-controlled trial evaluates patients with active AS, defined as a Bath AS Disease Activity Index (BASDAI) score ≥ 4 and a back pain score of ≥ 4 who were randomly assigned to receive subcutaneous golimumab (50 mg or 100 mg) or placebo every 4 weeks. Patients also had to have inadequately responded to either nonsteroidal anti-inflammatory drugs (NSAIDs) or disease-modifying antirheumatic drugs (DMARDs). Patients continued their concurrent treatment with methotrexate, sulfasalazine, hydroxychloroquine, corticosteroids, and NSAIDs at stable doses during the study. The primary end point was a 20% improvement in the assessment in AS (ASAS 20) criteria at week 14. Secondary end points included: ASAS 40% improvement (ASAS 40), ASAS partial remission, and 20% improvement in 5 of 6 ASAS domains (ASAS 5/6).[1]

The primary end point was achieved with 59.4% in the 50 mg group, and 60% in the 100 mg group achieving an ASAS 20 response at week 14 compared with 21.8% in the placebo group ($p < 0.001$). In addition, significantly more golimumab-treated patients achieved ≥50% improvement in the BASDAI score, compared with patients who received placebo. Golimumab was generally well tolerated. Nine patients developed transient liver enzyme abnormalities (≥100% increase from baseline and a value > 150 IU/liter), however, levels subsequently decreased in all patients, including those who continued the drug. Otherwise, the pattern of adverse events was consistent with the safety profile of the other antiTNF agents with golimumab-treated patients experiencing a slightly greater proportion of infections.

With safety and efficacy results of this study being similar to those of previous studies involving anti-TNF agents in AS and the convenience of once monthly dosing, golimumab is sure to become a popular choice amongst rheumatologists and their patients alike.

B. Hutton, MD

Reference

1. Van Der Heijde D, Bellamy N, Calin A, Dougados M, Khan MA, Van Der Linden Sand the Assessments in Ankylosing Spondylitis Working Group. Preliminary core sets for endpoints in ankylosing spondylitis. *J Rheumatol.* 1997;24:2225-2229.

Efficacy and safety of up to 192 weeks of etanercept therapy in patients with ankylosing spondylitis

Davis JC Jr, van der Heijde DM, Braun J, et al (Univ of California, San Francisco; Univ Hosp Maastricht, The Netherlands; et al)
Ann Rheum Dis 67:346-352, 2008

Objective.—Evaluate long-term safety and efficacy of etanercept treatment in patients with ankylosing spondylitis (AS).

Methods.—Patients with AS who previously participated in a randomised controlled trial (RCT) of etanercept were eligible to enrol in a 168-week open-label extension (OLE). Safety end points included rates of adverse events (AE), serious adverse events (SAE), infections, serious infections and death. Efficacy end points included Assessment in Ankylosing Spondylitis (ASAS20) response, ASAS 5/6 response and partial remission rates.

Results.—A total of 257 of 277 patients (92%) enrolled in the OLE. After up to 192 weeks of treatment with etanercept, the most common AEs were injection site reactions, headaches and diarrhoea. The exposure-adjusted rate of SAEs was 0.08 per patient-year. The rate of infections was 1.1 per patient-year, and the rate for serious infections was 0.02 per patient-year. No deaths were reported. Of patients who received etanercept in both the RCT and OLE and were still in the trial, 71% were ASAS20 responders at week 96, and 81% were responders at week 192. ASAS 5/6 response rates were 61% at week 96 and 60% at week 144, and partial remission response rates were 41% at week 96 and 44% at week 192. Placebo patients who switched to etanercept in the OLE showed similar patterns of efficacy maintenance.

Conclusions.—Etanercept was well tolerated for up to 192 weeks in patients with AS, with no unexpected AEs or SAEs observed. No deaths were reported. Improvements in the signs and symptoms of AS were maintained for up to 192 weeks.

▶ Tumor Necrosis Factor α (TNFα) is an integral cytokine involved in the inflammatory cascade with broad-ranging effects on both the innate and adaptive immune systems. The introduction of antiTNF agents has dramatically improved treatment options for a number of rheumatologic conditions. Etanercept, a soluble TNF receptor-Fc fusion protein, has been shown to be efficacious in the treatment of both rheumatoid arthritis and Ankylosing Spondylitis (AS). Controlled studies and their respective open label extensions (OLE) have demonstrated etanercept to be effective and well tolerated in patients with AS for up to 2 years. However, longer-term data have not been previously available.

In this current OLE, the safety and efficacy profiles of etanercept in patients with AS were evaluated. Eligible patients previously enrolled in a 24 week randomized controlled trial and OLE were enrolled in a second OLE, potentially extending etanercept exposure to 192 weeks. A total of 257 patients enrolled, of whom 126 patients (49%) completed the 168-week trial. Twenty-four

(13.7%) patients chose to not re-enroll. Only 7.8% of patients discontinued secondary due to a lack of efficacy. Adverse effects (AEs) (8.2%) made up the other most common reasons for withdrawal; these included injection site reactions (ISRs) and infections. ISRs were the most common AE and were generally mild, decreasing in frequency over time. Infections most commonly reported were upper respiratory (45%), sinusitis (16%), flu-like syndrome (15%), and bronchitis (11%).

No unexpected AEs, serious AEs (SAEs), serious infections, or deaths were reported. One case of TB was reported in a patient after 2.8 years of etanercept therapy – the patient previously had a negative PPD and chest radiograph. No SAEs related to the development of systemic lupus erythematosus, demyelinating disorders, or lymphoma were reported. Recurrent uveitis flares and new reported incidents of inflammatory bowel disease were lower in the etanercept groups than the placebo groups.

In this study, durable efficacy of etanercept was also indicated by sustained response rates over time for all clinical measures. Significant improvements were seen in disease index measures, inflammatory markers, back pain, AM stiffness and tender/swollen joint counts, which lasted for up to 192 weeks.

This OLE provides more evidence to support the durable long-term safety profile of etanercept. Etanercept, as well as the other anti-TNF therapies, have clearly revolutionized the treatment of inflammatory arthritides, such as AS, giving patients a safe and effective treatment option in addition to conventional disease-modifying antirheumatic drugs.

B. Hutton, MD

Spondyloarthritis: a strong predictor of early coronary artery bypass grafting
Hollan I, Saatvedt K, Almdahl SM, et al (The Feiring Heart Clinic AS, Norway; Rikshospitalet Univ Hosp, Oslo, Norway; et al)
Scand J Rheumatol 37:18-22, 2008

Objectives.—The main aim of the study was to examine whether patients with spondyloarthritides underwent their first coronary artery bypass grafting (CABG) at a younger age than those without spondyloarthritides.

Methods.—Patients who underwent their first CABG at the Feiring Heart Clinic during 2001–2005 were preoperatively screened for spondyloarthritides, and the cardiological assessment was registered. We compared the characteristics of patients with and without spondyloarthritides.

Results.—Of the 3852 patients undergoing their first CABG, 30 (0.78%) had spondyloarthritides. No statistically significant differences in traditional cardiovascular risk factors were found. The mean ages of patients with and without spondyloarthritides were 60.1 (SD = 8.7) and 66.9 (SD = 10.1) years, respectively. Spondyloarthritis was found by multivariate analysis to be a stronger independent predictor of early

CABG than traditional cardiovascular risk factors [adjusted beta −6.2, p < 0.001, 95% confidence interval (CI) −9.5 to −2.8]. Sixty per cent of spondyloarthritis patients and 52% of control patients had already suffered a myocardial infarction (p = 0.4).

Conclusion.—Spondyloarthritis was a stronger predictor of early CABG than most of the registered traditional cardiovascular risk factors. The prevalence of spondyloarthritis seemed to be higher in the CABG population than in the general population. These findings may indicate accelerated coronary artery disease (CAD) in spondyloarthritides (Tables 1 and 2).

▶ Recent studies have suggested that severe psoriasis increases the risk for myocardial infarction. While one may assume that patients with psoriatic arthritis also have an increased risk, few studies have assessed this specific correlation. Furthermore, little information exists about the association of ankylosing spondylitis and ischemic heart disease. Hollan et al performed a cross

TABLE 1.—Characteristics of the Study Population

	Control Group (n = 3822)	Spondyloarthritis Group (n = 30)	p
Age, years	66.9 ± 10.1	60.1 ± 8.7	<0.001
Male	2895 (75.7)	20 (66.7)	0.248
Body mass index, kg/m^2	26.9 ± 16.2	26.9 ± 4.3	0.995
Hypertension	1982 (51.9)	15 (50)	0.838
Positive family history of CAD	2564 (67.1)	20 (66.7)	0.958
Current smoking	858 (22.4)	11 (36.7)	0.063
Previous smoking	1601 (41.9)	13 (43.3)	0.874
DM	636 (16.7)	9 (30.0)	0.051
Hypercholesterolaemia	3132 (82)	26 (86.7)	0.505
Duration of CAD, months	63 ± 73	42 ± 43	0.659
History of MI	1994 (52.3)	18 (60)	0.402
Mean no. of MI	0.68 ± 0.80	0.73 ± 0.74	0.547
Mean NYHA class	2.9 ± 0.64	2.97 ± 0.77	0.580
No. of coronary arteries with significant stenosis	2.7 ± 0.5	2.5 ± 0.6	0.025
Left main coronary stenosis	907 (23.7)	9 (30)	0.422
Left ventricle ejection fraction (%)	64.3 ± 13.7	60.8 ± 13.8	0.165
Left ventricle hypertrophy	611 (16)	6 (20)	0.550
Lipid-lowering drugs	3089 (80.9)	26 (86.7)	0.427
Acetylsalicylic acid‡	3370 (88.3)	30 (100)	0.046
ACE inhibitors	1465 (38.4)	10 (33.3)	0.570
Beta-blockers	3180 (83.3)	27 (90)	0.328
Systemic glucocorticosteroids	113 (3.0)	4 (13.3)	0.012†
Aortic graft replacement at CABG	33 (0.9)	1 (3.3)	0.234†
Cardiac valve surgery at CABG	423 (11.1)	3 (10)	1.000†
Acute CABG	1162 (30.5)	13 (43.3)	0.128

CABG, coronary artery bypass graft surgery; DM, diabetes mellitus; MI, myocardial infarction; CAD, coronary artery disease; NYHA, New York Heart Association Functional Classification (class 1–4); ACE, angiotensin-converting enzyme. Numbers may not sum to total numbers because of missing data for some variables. Values are n (%) or mean ± SD.
†By Fisher's exact test.
‡Use of other platelet aggregation inhibiting drugs was similar in both groups.
(Reprinted from Hollan I, Saatvedt K, Almdahl SM, et al. Spondyloarthritis: a strong predictor of early coronary artery bypass grafting. *Scand J Rheumatol.* 2008;37:18-22.)

TABLE 2.—Predictors of a Younger Age at First CABG

| | Unadjusted | | | Adjusted | | | | | |
| | | | | Model I* | | | Model III‡ | | |
	beta	p	95% CI	beta	p	95% CI	beta	p	95% CI
Spondyloarthritis	-6.7	<0.001	-10.4 to -3.2	-6.2	<0.001	-9.5 to -2.8	-6.6	<0.001	-9.9 to -3.3
Female sex	5.2	<0.001	4.5–6.0	4.8	<0.001	4.1–5.5	4.7	<0.001	4.0–5.4
BMI	-0.04	<0.001	-0.06 to -0.02	-0.05	<0.001	-0.07 to -0.03	-0.05	<0.001	-0.07 to -0.03
Hypercholesterolaemia	-4.9	<0.001	-5.7 to -4.1	-4.2	<0.001	-5.0 to -3.4	-4.2	<0.001	-5.0 to -3.4
Hypertension	1.1	0.001	0.4–1.7	0.9	0.005	0.3–1.5	0.9	0.004	0.3–1.5
DM-insulin	-1.2	0.090	-2.6 to 0.2	-1.4	0.033	-2.7 to -0.1	-1.5	0.022	-2.7 to -0.2
DM-oral antidiabetics	0.8	0.198	-4.2 to 2.0	0.5	0.368	-0.6 to 1.6	0.5	0.391	-0.6 to 1.6
DM-diet	0.004	0.996	-1.7 to 1.7	-0.3	0.674	-2.0 to 1.2	-0.4	0.608	-2.0 to 1.2
Current smoking	-5.8	<0.001	-6.5 to -5.0	-5.7	<0.001	-6.5 to -5.0	-5.7	<0.001	-6.5 to -5.0
Previous smoking	0.8	0.011	0.2–1.5	-0.5	0.149	-1.2 to 0.2	-0.5	0.122	-1.2 to 0.1
Family history of CAD	-2.9	<0.001	-3.6 to -2.2	-2.6	<0.001	-3.3 to -2.0	-2.6	<0.001	-3.2 to -2.0
Systemic glucocorticosteroids	5.0	<0.001	3.2–6.9	—			4.8	<0.001	3.1–6.5

CABG, coronary artery bypass graft surgery; CI, confidence interval; BMI, body mass index; CAD, coronary artery disease; DM-insulin, diabetes mellitus treated with insulin; DM-oral antidiabetics, DM treated with oral antidiabetics; DM-diet, DM treated with diet. The results were similar for ankylosing spondylitis (AS) and psoriatic arthritis (PsA) subgroups.

*r^2 = 50.16.

†r^2 = 50.17.

(Reprinted from Hollan I, Saatvedt K, Almdahl SM, et al. Spondyloarthritis: a strong predictor of early coronary artery bypass grafting. *Scand J Rheumatol.* 2008;37:18-22.)

sectional analysis to examine the risk of seronegative spondyloarthropathy (SNSA) on a patient's age at their first coronary artery bypass graft (CABG).

There were 3852 patients undergoing their first CABG at a Norwegian medical clinic between May 2001 and January 2005 who were preoperatively screened for spondyloarthropathy by a rheumatologist. Fifteen patients were diagnosed with ankylosing spondylitis, 14 patients with psoriatic arthritis, and one patient with reactive arthritis. Table 1 compares the characteristics of the spondyloarthritis group to the control group.

Patients with SNSA were approximately 6 years younger than the control group ($P < .001$). Although not completely, but approaching statistical significance, patients with spondyloarthritis were more likely to smoke ($P = .063$), have diabetes mellitus ($P = .051$), and take aspirin ($P = .046$). Table 2 displays the multivariate analysis that assesses for risk factors that may impact on age at first CABG. Spondyloarthritis was a statistically significant predictor of early CABG ($P < .001$). Patients who were diagnosed with spondyloarthritis at a young age underwent CABG earlier than those diagnosed in later life ($P = .005$).

The data suggests that the diagnosis of spondyloarthropathy is an independent risk factor for earlier age of first CABG. However, the possibility of lead-time bias is a significant problem with this study. Perhaps patients with spondyloarthropathy were diagnosed with coronary artery disease at an earlier age secondary to closer medical attention and not the actual disease process. Another limitation is the small number of patients with spondyloarthropathy. Although not statistically significant, the increased percentage of diabetes and active smoking in the spondyloarthropathy group may have also impacted the data.

Future study should involve a larger index group so as to minimize confounding by traditional cardiovascular risk factors. It should also include an assessment of the degree of medical surveillance within the 2 groups. However, this appears to represent more support for the contention that systemic inflammatory disease contributes to the development of premature or accelerated atherosclerosis.

For further reading on this subject I suggest article by Gelfand et al,[1] and Peters et al.[2]

J. Sloane, MD

References

1. Gelfand JM, Neimann AL, Shin DB, Wang X, Margolis DJ, Troxel AB. Risk of myocardial infarction in patients with psoriasis. *JAMA*. 2006;296:1735-1741.
2. Peters MJ, Van Der Hortst-Bruinsma IE, Dijkmans BA, Nurmohamed MT. Cardiovacular risk profile of patients with spondyloarthropathies, particularly ankylosing spondylitis and psoriatic arthritis. *Semin Arth Rheum*. 2004;34:585-592.

Subclinical Atherosclerosis in Psoriatic Arthritis: A Case-Control Study

Eder L, Zisman D, Barzilai M, et al (Carmel Med Ctr, Haifa, Israel; Lin Med Ctr; Bnai Zion Med Ctr, Haifa, Israel)
J Rheumatol 35:877-882, 2008

Objective.—To investigate the prevalence of subclinical atherosclerosis among patients with psoriatic arthritis (PsA).

Methods.—Forty patients with PsA were enrolled. Controls were matched by age, sex, and atherosclerotic risk factors. AH patients and controls underwent duplex scan of the carotid arteries. Carotid intima-media thickness (IMT) was evaluated and the presence of atherosclerotic plaques was recorded. The plaques were graded and carotid plaque index was calculated.

Results.—Patients with PsA had a higher IMT (mean ± standard deviation, 1.04 ± 0.35 mm vs 0.88 ± 0.29 mm in controls; p = 0.03), and had a higher carotid plaque index than did matched controls (2.3 ± 2.6, compared to 1.12 ± 2.09; p = 0.03). Multivariate analysis demonstrated that PsA status as well as age and triglyceride levels were associated with the presence of carotid plaque. Other traditional risk factors were more prevalent among patients with PsA; however, they were not statistically significant.

Conclusion.—Our study demonstrates that patients with PsA may have an increased prevalence of subclinical atherosclerosis. These findings may

TABLE 1.—Characteristics of Patients with PsA and Healthy Controls

Characteristic	Patients with PsA, n = 40	Controls. n = 40	p
Age, mean (range), yrs	57.5 (43–76)	57.05 (34–79)	0.72
Females, n (%)	28 (70)	28 (70)	1
Diabetes mellitus, n (%)	5 (12.5)	5 (12.5)	1
Glucose level, mg/dl, mean ± SD	105 ± 40	97 ± 15	0.2
Hypertension, n (%)	19 (47.5)	19 (47.5)	1
Body mass index	28 ± 4	27 ± 3	0.3
Ever smoked cigarettes, n (%)	5 (12.5)	7 (17.5)	0.7
Hypercholesterolemia, n (%)	15 (37.5)	15 (37.5)	0.8
Total cholesterol level, mg/dl, mean ± SD	194 ± 47	211 ± 35	0.07
LDL cholesterol level, me/dl, mean ± SD	122 ± 34	131 ± 33	0.2
HDL cholesterol level, mg/dl, mean ± SD	46 ± 13	53 ± 12	0.02
Triglyceride level, mg/dl, mean ± SD	155 ± 97	149 ± 57	0.7
Use if statin, n (%)	13 ± (32.5)	6 (15)	0.11
Family history of cardiovascular disease, n (%)	9 (22.5)	7 (17.5)	0.7
ESR, mm/h, mean ± SD	38 ± 21	18 ± 9	0.04
CRP, mg/dl, mean ± SD	1.13 ± 1.28	0.25 ± 0.05	0.03

HDL: high density lipoprotein: CRP: C-reactive protein; LDL: low density lipoprotein; ESR: erythrocyte sedimentation rate; PsA: psoriatic arthritis.
(Reprinted from Eder L, Zisman D, Barzilai M, et al. Subclinical atherosclerosis in psoriatic arthritis: a case-control study. *J Rheumatol.* 2008;35:877-882.)

not be solely attributable to traditional risk factors alone. Special attention and strict control of atherosclerotic risk factors in patients with PsA is warranted (Table 1).

▶ In the past few years, researchers have begun to use the measurement of the carotid intima-media thickness (IMT) as a marker of systemic atherosclerosis. Multiple studies have correlated an increased IMT with vascular events.

Eder et al used high-resolution ultrasonography to assess the carotid IMT of a psoriatic arthritis population and compared it with the carotid IMT of normal controls.

Forty patients with psoriasis who met the Moll and Wright criteria for psoriatic arthritis were recruited consecutively from 3 outpatient clinics in Israel. Patients were excluded if they had experienced a previous atherosclerotic event. Forty control patients were recruited from a community-based clinic and matched to study patients. Table 1 displays the patient characteristics.

A single ultrasonographer measured and scored the IMT of the patients' bilateral carotid arteries. Plaques were scored as: Grade 1—single small plaque, Grade 2—single medium plaque or multiple small plaques, or Grade 3—large plaque or multiple medium plaques. The carotid plaque index was calculated and is the summation of the plaque scores.

Patients with psoriatic arthritis had statistically significant lower HDL cholesterol and higher ESR and CRP levels compared with normal controls. Although not statistically significant per the authors, study patients were twice as likely to be taking a statin (32.5% versus 15%).

Patients with psoriatic arthritis had a statistically significantly higher IMT ($P = .03$) and plaque index ($P = .011$) compared with normal controls. Logistic regression suggested a relationship between psoriatic arthritis and age with increased IMT thickness. Univariate analysis also suggested a correlation between age, triglyceride level, past prednisone use, and increased carotid plaque index. However, classic cardiovascular risk factors were not statistically associated with an increased IMT thickness or with the carotid plaque index.

This study is notable because it is one of the first to examine the IMT of patients with psoriatic arthritis. A large majority of patients with psoriasis and psoriatic arthritis have the "metabolic syndrome." This makes it difficult to separate the impact of psoriatic arthritis versus classic cardiovascular risk factors on atherosclerotic outcomes. Although the authors attempted to control for these variables by excluding patients with known atherosclerosis, the study population had a higher CRP, lower HDL, and higher use of statins in comparison with the control population. This profile suggests that the study population may have had a more atherogenic milieu, making the interpretation of the impact of psoriatic arthritis on the results more difficult. Furthermore, surprisingly, in this study, classic cardiovascular risk factors did not have a statistically significant relationship with increased IMT or plaque index. This makes their results difficult to interpret as one expects these risk factors should show a correlation.

Future studies should focus on a larger study population with tighter control over traditional risk factors.

J. Sloane, MD

9 Toxicities of Antirheumatic Agents

Introduction

The final chapter of this section contains 2 articles: one describes tumor necrosis factor inhibitor use in HIV patients; the other is about detecting latent tuberculosis utilizing a cytokine-based assay.

Seth Mark Berney, MD

The use of anti-tumour necrosis factor therapy in HIV-positive individuals with rheumatic disease
Cepeda EJ, Williams FM, Ishimori ML, et al (Univ of Texas-Houston Health Science Ctr; Cedars-Sinai Med Ctr, Los Angeles, CA)
Ann Rheum Dis 67:710-712, 2008

Objective.—The purpose of this study was to examine the safety and efficacy of anti-tumour necrosis factor (TNF) agents (etanercept, infliximab and adalimumab) in HIV-positive patients with rheumatic diseases refractory to standard therapy.

Methods.—Patients were treated with anti-TNF blocker with rheumatic diseases refractory to disease modifying antirheumatic drugs who had a CD4 count of >200 mm^3 and an HIV viral load of <60 000 copies/mm^3 and no active concurrent infections. Changes in CD4 counts, HIV viral loads, or other adverse effects while on anti-TNF agents and clinical response were monitored for 28.1 (SD 20.9) months (range 2.5–55).

Results.—Eight HIV-positive patients were treated with anti-TNF blockers (two patients with rheumatoid arthritis, three with psoriatic arthritis, one with undifferentiated spondyloarthritis, one with reactive arthritis and one with ankylosing spondylitis). No significant clinical adverse effect was attributed to this treatment in any patient. CD4 counts and HIV viral load levels remained stable in all patients. Three patients on etanercept therapy and two patients on infliximab had sustained clinical improvement in their rheumatic diseases.

Conclusions.—This retrospective series of eight patients suggests that treatment with anti-TNF-α therapy is a viable alternative in HIV patients without advanced disease with associated rheumatic diseases refractory to standard therapy.

▶ Rheumatologic disorders can be found in human immunodeficiency virus (HIV)-infected individuals, some of which may require antitumor necrosis factor (antiTNF) treatment. Tumor necrosis factor (TNF-α) is a proinflammatory cytokine whose primary role is regulation of immune cells and is synthesized primarily by macrophages and T-cells. Researchers have observed that exogenous TNF-α may enhance HIV replication in certain cell lines, thus contributing to HIV disease progression. Inhibition of TNF-α, may therefore be beneficial in HIV-infected patients. However, TNF-α plays a very important role in containing tuberculosis and fungal infections, which HIV-infected patients are particularly susceptible to. As a result, this study sought to analyze the safety and efficacy of anti-TNF treatment with etanercept, infliximab, and adalimumab in 8 HIV patients.

All patients had CD4 counts of at least 446 cells/mm^3, except one (268 cells/mm^3) and HIV viral loads under 425 copies/mm^3, except one (22 148 copies/mm^3). After 48 months of follow-up, no opportunistic infections or malignancies were observed (1 patient was on dapsone prophylaxis). In addition, the CD4 counts remained stable in all 8 patients. One out of 8 patients had a substantial increase in viral load, which decreased with temporary discontinuation of inflixmab and did not recur with reinfusion of the drug.

This study indicates the potential utility of antiTNF therapy in HIV patients who have inadequately responded to standard antirheumatic therapy. What remains unknown is the long-term effects of such therapy. Furthermore, the interactions of antiTNF therapy with highly active antiretroviral therapy (HAART) are not well described. Protease inhibitors, for example, enhance macrophage production of TNF-α, thus an inhibitor may have an adverse effect on HAART that includes a protease inhibitor. Finally, it is unclear what role antiTNF therapy will have in individuals with CD4 counts < 200 cells/mm3, as they are the riskiest population for opportunistic infections and AIDS-defining malignancies.

Nonetheless, this study, and several small previous studies, supports the findings of the short-term safety of antiTNF therapy in HIV-infected individuals with rheumatologic conditions. In addition, suppression of TNF-α may have other benefits in HIV-infected individuals where proinflammatory states have been associated with accelerated bone loss, HIV-myocarditis, AIDS-associated pulmonary interstitial and cystic disease, HIV pulmonary hypertension, HIV-neuropathy and tumorigenesis by inflammatory cytokines in Kaposi's sarcoma–mechanisms which remain poorly understood at this time.

For further reading on this subject I suggest article by Agostini etal,[1] Humbert et al,[2] Loiseau-Peres et al,[3] Walker et al,[4] yang et al,[5] and yoshioka et al.[6]

U. Wu, MD

References

1. Agostini C, Zambello R, Trentin L, et al. Alveolar macrophages from patients with AIDS and AIDS-related complex constitutively synthesize and release tumor necrosis factor alpha. *Am Rev Respir Dis.* 1991 Jul;144:195.
2. Humbert M, Monti G, Brenot F, et al. Increased interleukin-1 and interleukin-6 serum concentrations in severe primary pulmonary hypertension. *Am J Respir Crit Care Med.* 1995 May;151:1628.
3. Loiseau-Peres S, Delaunay C, Poupon S, et al. Osteopenia in patients infected by the human immunodeficiency virus. A case control study. *Joint, Bone, Spine.* 2002 Oct;69:482.
4. Walker UA, Tyndall A, Daikeler T. Rheumatic conditions in human immunodeficiency virus infection. *Rheumatology.* 2008;47:952.
5. Yang J, Hagan MK, Offermann MK. Induction of IL-6 gene expression in Kaposi's sarcoma cells. *J Immunol.* 1994 Jan 15;152:943.
6. Yoshioka M, Bradley WG, Shapshak P, et al. Role of immune activation and cytokine expression in HIV-1-associated neurologic diseases. *Adv Neuroimmunol.* 1995;5:335.

Detection of latent tuberculosis in immunosuppressed patients with autoimmune diseases: Performance of a *Mycobacterium tuberculosis* antigen-specific interferon γ assay

Matulis G, Jüni P, Villiger PM, et al (Univ of Bern, Switzerland)
Ann Rheum Dis 67:84-90, 2008

Objective.—To analyse the performance of a new *M tuberculosis*-specific interferon γ (IFNγ) assay in patients with chronic inflammatory diseases who receive immunosuppressive drugs, including tumour necrosis factor α (TNFα) inhibitors.

Methods.—Cellular immune responses to the *M tuberculosis*-specific antigens ESAT-6, CFP-10, TB7.7 were prospectively studied in 142 consecutive patients treated for inflammatory rheumatic conditions. Results were compared with tuberculin skin tests (TSTs). Association of both tests with risk factors for latent *M tuberculosis* infection (LTBI) and BCG vaccination were determined and the influence of TNFα inhibitors, corticosteroids, and disease modifying antirheumatic drugs (DMARDs) on antigen-specific and mitogen-induced IFNγ secretion was analysed.

Results.—126/142 (89%) patients received immunosuppressive therapy. The IFNγ assay was more closely associated with the presence of risk factors (odds ratio (OR) = 23.8 (95% CI 5.14 to 110) vs OR = 2.77 (1.22 to 6.27), respectively; p = 0.009), but less associated with BCG vaccination than the TST (OR = 0.47 (95% CI 0.15 to 1.47) vs OR = 2.44 (0.74 to (8.01), respectively; p = 0.025). Agreement between the IFNγ assay and TST results was low (κ = 0.17; 95% CI 0.02 to 0.32). The odds for a positive IFNγ assay strongly increased with increasing prognostic relevance of LTBI risk factors. Neither corticosteroids nor conventional DMARDs significantly affected IFNγ responses, but the odds for a positive IFNγ assay were decreased in patients treated with TNFα inhibitors (OR $= 0.21$ (95% CI 0.07 to 0.63), respectively; p $= 0.006$).

Conclusions.—These results demonstrate that the performance of the *M tuberculosis* antigen-specific IFNγ ELISA is better than the classic TST for detection of LTBI in patients receiving immunosuppressive therapy for treatment of systemic autoimmune disorders.

▶ Better tests for the detection of latent tuberculosis infection (LTBI) are needed, due to increased use of immunosuppressive therapies that may predispose patients to active tuberculosis. TNFα-inhibiting drugs, as well as systemic corticosteroids, increase a patients risk for reactivation of LTBI. Screening for LTBI is recommended before anti-TNF therapy is initiated, but it has been difficult due to the high rate of false-negatives in patients who are anergic as a result of previous or concurrent immunosuppressive therapy. In 2005, QuantiFERON TB-Gold received approval from the Food and Drug Administration to improve the diagnosis of latent tuberculosis infection as well as active tuberculosis. This in-vitro assay detects the release of IFNγ from sensitized lymphocytes re-exposed to the mycobacterial antigens named "early secretory antigenic target-6 (ESAT-6)" and "culture filtrate protein-10 (CFP-10)." The latest version of this test, the QFT-G In-Tube Assay (QFT-G) adds a peptide protein of another mycobacterium tuberculosis specific antigen "(TB 7.7)". The use of this assay should improve the specificity for latent infection compared with the tuberculin skin test (TST) using purified protein derivative (PPD) antigens because these antigens are not present in Bacille Calmette-Guerin (BCG) vaccines and many nontuberculous mycobacteria except *Mycobacterium kansasii*, *Mycobacterium szulgai*, and *Mycobacterium marinum*.

The authors intend to compare QFT-G with the TST for the detection of LTBI in patients with chronic inflammatory conditions on immunosuppressive drugs, including TNFα-inhibitors. This study indicated that this assay was more closely associated with the presence of LTBI risk factors and less associated with BCG vaccination status in contrast to the TST. However, in a multivariable linear regression analysis, the authors determined that TNFα-inhibitor treatment was associated with a decreased concentration of IFNγ for positive controls, which may influence the interpretation of true positive tests as indeterminate. Furthermore, even though there was 64% concordance between QFT-G and TST testing, there was a low kappa value for the measure of agreement, lower than what was found in previous studies. This may be in part due to the comparative tests not being performed simultaneously, up to 184 days apart. However, one cannot exclude concordance occurring by chance.

The centers for disease control has stated that the QFT-G test can be used in all circumstances the tuberculin skin test is used, and published recommendations of the interpretation and use of the assay exist. This assay can be used in patients on immunosuppressive agents, however, limited data on the use of QFT-G in immunosuppressed patients are available, and long-term studies in patients with impaired immune systems should be performed to further define the optimal use of these tests. Nonetheless, this study showed there appears to be a role for IFNγ release assays in the diagnosis of LTBI in patients with increased risk factors for LTBI, and should be considered instead of, or in conjunction with, TST, especially where false negatives are suspected.

For further reading on this subject I suggest an article by Mazurek et al.[1]

U. Wu, MD

Reference

1. Mazurek GH, et al. Guidelines for using the QunatiFERON-TB Gold test for detecting *Mycobacterium tuberculosis* infection, United States. *MMWR Recomm Rep.* 2005;54:49.

PART TWO

INFECTIOUS DISEASES

NANCY M. KHARDORI, MD

Introduction

Like last year, it was difficult to identify a relatively small number of scientific studies for inclusion in the Infectious Diseases section of the 2009 YEAR BOOK OF MEDICINE. It is not surprising given the global, evolving, and emerging nature of infectious diseases with impact on masses not just individual patients.

This year I have divided the selections into 9 chapters:

Pathogenesis of Infectious Diseases includes studies that demonstrate reasons why infections may not get diagnosed appropriately or respond to what currently would be considered appropriate management. In the first inclusion, the authors have demonstrated that *Streptococcus pneumoniae* forms surface attached communities (ie, biofilms) in the middle ear of experimentally infected chinchillas. The Centers for Disease Control and Prevention estimated that biofilm formation is responsible for 65% of the commonly treated infections including otitis media, nonhealing ulcers, and osteomyelitis. The role of carbohydrates (ie, exopolysaccharides) that allow *Staphylococcus epidermidis* to form biofilm on devices is well studied. The second inclusion demonstrates the correlation between carbohydrate availability, pneumococcal biofilm formation, nasopharyngeal colonization, and invasive disease in a mouse model. These studies, although done in animals, offer answers to a number of clinically relevant questions. The study on virulence of *Clostridium difficile* clearly shows that toxin B (not toxin A as shown in previous studies) is essential for virulence. The next selection discusses the early occurrence of infections in acute pancreatitis with significant impact on mortality.

Infectious Disease Management includes selections on changes in bacterial isolates and their antibiotic susceptibility from burn wounds, the clinical relevance of Candida colonization of central vascular catheters in noncandidemic, non-neutropenic patients, the effects of timing of administration and duration of antibiotics, interactions between antimicrobial agents and other drugs, antibiotics use for presumed nonbacterial respiratory tract infections, impact of early surgery on management of necrotizing soft tissue infections, mitral valve endocarditis, empyema and a clinical trial using polymixin B hemoperfusion in abdominal septic shock.

The Epidemiology and Management of Gram Positive Infections section includes new information on invasive Streptococcal infections, *Staphylococcus lugdunensis* (one of the lesser known coagulase negative Staphylococci) and *S. aureus* bacteremia.

The debate on when to start antiretroviral therapy, in my opinion, should be settled in favor of early initiation and is reiterated in 2 of the selections in the section on HIV Infection. The long-term control of HIV infection by CCR5 delta 32 stem-cell transplantation shown in one of the selections is exciting and full of potential, especially in light of another study that provides a model to understand how HIV-1 uses CCR5 to enter target cells.

With one third of the world population, 2 billion, infected with *Mycobacterium tuberculosis*, this disease remains unconquered. So any advances in its diagnosis and treatment would have tremendous public health impact. Unfortunately, the large number of interferon-based diagnostic tests that have made their way to the market has created a lot of confusion and limited usefulness as demonstrated by the few studies included in the section on Tuberculosis.

In the chapter on Health Care Associated Infections, the continued transmission of *C. difficile* and other infections in acute care hospitals attests to the lack of use of "common sense" in controlling the transmission. The presence of *C. difficile* on the hospital's computer keyboards demonstrated by one of the selections came as no surprise.

The selections on Parasitic Infections (ie, *Acanthamoeba keratitis* associated with contact lens solutions and cryptosporidiosis in the elderly population) are here to remind us about the presence of protozoa in the environment and their infection-causing potential everywhere, including the United States.

In the Vaccines chapter, the science of vaccines, the ultimate tool for control of infectious diseases, continues to advance steadily (although slowly), evidenced by expansion of age recommendations for HPV vaccine and experimental vaccines against tuberculosis and malaria—2 of the 10 biggest killers in the world. The use of group B streptococcal pilus components as vaccines opens the door to new direction in vaccine efforts. The disconcerting fact is the emergence of doubts about vaccines among parents. A selection in this section offers recommendations to overcome this hurdle in protecting our children against vaccine-preventable diseases—infections and infection-related cancers.

Influenza is the last but definitely not the least of selections in this section. This chapter provides clinically relevant information on the role of lymphocytes in viral clearance, resistance to antiviral drugs and the current ongoing pandemic of swine H1N1 influenza.

Most appropriately, I wish to close with the following quote:

"Modern adventurers like to up the ante, but even the most extreme sports wouldn't produce the adrenaline of a race against pandemic influenza or a cloud of anthrax at the Super Bowl. In the field of Infectious Diseases, reality is stranger than anything a writer could dream up. The most menacing bioterrorist is Mother Nature herself."

—Secret Agents: The Menace of Emerging Infections, *by Madeline Drexler, John Henry Press, 2002.*

Nancy Misri Khardori, MD

10 Pathogenesis of Infectious Diseases

Streptococcus pneumoniae Forms Surface-Attached Communities in the Middle Ear of Experimentally Infected Chinchillas

Reid SD, Hong W, Dew KE, et al (Wake Forest Univ School of Medicine, Winston-Salem, NC; et al)

J Infect Dis 199:786-794, 2009

Background.—*Streptococcus pneumoniae* (pneumococcus) causes respiratory and systemic infections that are a major public health problem worldwide. It has been postulated that pneumococci persist in vivo in biofilm communities.

Methods.—In this study, we analyzed whether pneumococci form biofilms in vivo, and if so, whether biofilms correlated with bacterial persistence. Chinchillas were infected with *S. pneumoniae* TIGR4 and euthanized at varying times after infection, after which the superior ear bullae were excised and examined by culture and microscopy.

Results.—Dense material, resembling the biofilms of other otitis media pathogens, was visible in the middle ear as late as 12 days after infection. Scanning electron microscopy revealed bacteria within an electron-dense matrix, similar to pneumococcal biofilms formed in vitro. Viability staining revealed groups of viable diplococci, as well as viable and nonviable host cells, attached to a fibrous matrix that was positive when stained with propidium iodide. Cryosections of biofilms were treated with polyclonal antibodies against the pneumococcal surface components pneumococcal surface protein A family 2, pneumococcal surface protein C, choline-binding protein, and neuraminidase, coupled with appropriate secondary antibody conjugates. Immunofluorescent staining showed the presence of pneumococcal communities within the material recovered from the middle ear chamber.

Conclusions.—On the basis of these data, we conclude that pneumococci form biofilms in vivo and that this process may be intertwined with the formation of neutrophil extracellular traps. These findings provide new insights into the potential causes of antibiotic treatment failure and bacterial persistence in chronic pneumococcal otitis media.

▶ Bacterial persistence in the form of adherent biofilms is now estimated to occur in 65% of infections, including persistent and recurrent otitis media.[1] The sessile mode of growth in the biofilms and the extracellular matrix contribute to the inefficacy of antimicrobial therapy, and to the inability of host immune responses to eradicate these bacteria. *Streptococcus pneumoniae* is one of the most frequently isolated bacteria from persistent and recurrent otitis media. The introduction of heptavalent conjugate pneumococcal vaccine has reduced the incidence of pneumococcal otitis media. However, an increase in the incidence of otitis media caused by pneumococcal serotypes not included in the vaccine is being reported. The role of bacterial components or variants in the formation of pneumococcal biofilms in vitro has been described recently.[2] This study extends these findings to an in vivo model. Healthy chinchillas were infected with *S pneumoniae* via transbullar infections. Middle ear chambers of animals euthanized 3 days, 7 days, and 12 days after injection showed visible microbial growth, bacteria within an electron-dense matrix by scanning electron microscopy, and staining of pneumococcal communities by antipneumococcal antibodies by immuno-fluorescence staining. The finding that pneumococci form biofilms in vivo provides new insight into the pathogenesis of persistent otitis media and antibiotic treatment failure.

N. M. Khardori, MD

References

1. Donlan RM. Biofilms: microbial life on surfaces. *Emerg Infect Dis.* 2002;8: 881-890.
2. Allegrucci M, Hu FZ, Shen K, et al. Phenotypic characterization of Streptococcus pneumoniae biofilm development. *J Bacteriol.* 2006;188:2325-2335.

Sialic Acid: A Preventable Signal for Pneumococcal Biofilm Formation, Colonization, and Invasion of the Host
Trappetti C, Kadioglu A, Carter M, et al (Università di Siena, Italy; Univ of Leicester, UK; et al)
J Infect Dis 199:1497-1505, 2009

The correlation between carbohydrate availability, pneumococcal biofilm formation, nasopharyngeal colonization, and invasion of the host has been investigated. Of a series of sugars, only sialic acid (i.e., N-acetylneuraminic acid) enhanced pneumococcal biofilm formation in vitro, at concentrations similar to those of free sialic acid in human saliva. In a murine model of pneumococcal carriage, intranasal inoculation of sialic acid significantly increased pneumococcal counts in the nasopharynx and instigated translocation of pneumococci to the lungs. Competition of both sialic acid–dependent phenotypes was found to be successful when evaluated using the neuraminidase inhibitors DANA (i.e., 2,3-didehydro-2-deoxy-N-acetylneuraminic acid), zanamivir, and oseltamivir. The association between levels of free sialic acid on mucosae, pneumococcal colonization, and development of invasive disease shows how a host-derived molecule can influence a colonizing microbe and also highlights a molecular mechanism that explains the epidemiologic correlation between respiratory infections due to neuraminidase-bearing viruses and bacterial pneumonia. The data provide a new paradigm for the role of a host compound in infectious diseases and point to new treatment strategies.

▶ Pneumococcal biofilm formation has been demonstrated in both in vitro and in vivo models.[1] The study by Trappetti et al is the first to demonstrate a causal association between carbohydrate availability (sialic acid at concentrations similar to those of free sialic acid in human saliva) and pneumococcal biofilm formation in vitro. In addition, intranasal inoculation of sialic acid in a murine model of pneumococcal carriage significantly increased pneumococcal counts in the nasopharynx and initiated translocation of pneumococci to the lungs. These data provide (1) the role of a host-derived molecule in pneumococcal colonization, biofilm formation, and development of invasive disease and (2) a possible mechanism for the epidemiologic correlation between respiratory infections due to neuraminidase-bearing viruses and bacterial pneumonia.

For further reading on this subject I suggest an article by Oggioni et al.[2]

N. M. Khardori, MD

References

1. Reid SD, Hong W, Dew KE, et al. Streptococcus pneumoniae forms surface-attached communities in the middle ear of experimentally infected chinchillas. *J Infect Dis.* 2009; 2009;785-794.
2. Oggioni MR, Trappett C, Kadioglu A, et al. Switch from planktonic to sessile life: a major event in pneumococcal pathogenesis. *Mol Microbiol.* 2006;61:1196-1210.

Toxin B is essential for virulence of *Clostridium difficile*
Lyras D, O'Connor JR, Howarth PM, et al (Monash Univ, Victoria, Australia)
Nature 458:1176-1179, 2009

Clostridium difficile is the leading cause of infectious diarrhoea in hospitals worldwide, because of its virulence, spore-forming ability and persistence. C. *difficile*-associated diseases are induced by antibiotic treatment or disruption of the normal gastrointestinal flora. Recently, morbidity and mortality resulting from C. *difficile*-associated diseases have increased significantly due to changes in the virulence of the causative strains and antibiotic usage patterns. Since 2002, epidemic toxinotype III NAP1/027 strains, which produce high levels of the major virulence factors, toxin A and toxin B, have emerged. These toxins have 63% amino acid sequence similarity and are members of the large clostridial glucosylating toxin family, which are monoglucosyltransferases that are pro-inflammatory, cytotoxic and enterotoxic in the human colon. Inside host cells, both toxins catalyse the transfer of glucose onto the Rho family of GTPases, leading to cell death. However, the role of these toxins in the context of a *C. difficile* infection is unknown. Here we describe the construction of isogenic *tcdA* and *tcdB* (encoding toxin A and B, respectively) mutants of a virulent *C. difficile* strain and their use in the hamster disease model to show that toxin B is a key virulence determinant. Previous studies showed that purified toxin A alone can induce most of the pathology observed after infection of hamsters with *C. difficile* and that toxin B is not toxic in animals unless it is co-administered with toxin A, suggesting that the toxins act synergistically. Our work provides evidence that toxin B, not toxin A, is essential for virulence. Furthermore, it is clear that the importance of these toxins in the context of infection cannot be predicted exclusively from studies using purified toxins, reinforcing the importance of using the natural infection process to dissect the role of toxins in disease.

▶ Recent increase in morbidity and mortality resulting from *Clostridiumdifficile*-associated disease has been attributed to antibiotic usage patterns and to the virulence of the causative strains.[1-3] Toxin production is the major virulence factor in *C difficile*. Epidemic toxinotype III NAP1/027 strains that produce high levels of the major virulence factors toxin A and toxin B emerged in 2002. Previous studies have shown purified toxin A to be responsible for most of the pathology in a hamster model of *C difficile* infection.

This study used isogenic *tcdA* and *tcdB* (encoding toxin A and B, respectively) mutants of a virulent *C difficile* strain in the hamster disease model. The results provide evidence that toxin B, not toxin A, is essential for virulence. This observation is reinforced by the fact that clinical isolates that lack toxin A are still capable of causing severe disease. Toxin B has been shown not to require the presence of toxin A for its in vivo activity. Naturally occurring toxin A and B isolates of *C difficile* have not been reported. The findings in this study represent a major shift in the understanding of pathogenesis of *C difficile* disease and underscore the importance of using the natural infection process (not isolated toxins or culture filtrates) in dissecting the role of toxins in disease pathogenesis. Most importantly, the diagnostic methods should focus on the detection of both toxins and on a cytotoxic assay that measures toxin B primarily.

N. M. Khardori, MD

References

1. Bartlett JG. Antibiotic-associated diarrhea. *N Engl J Med.* 2002;346:334-339.
2. Warny M, Pepin J, Fang A, et al. Toxin production by an emerging strain of Clostridium difficile associated with outbreaks of severe disease in North America and Europe. *Lancet.* 2005;366:1079-1084.
3. McDonald LC, Killgore GE, Thompson A, et al. An epidemic, toxin gene-variant strain of Clostridium difficile. *N Engl J Med.* 2005;353:2433-2441.

Timing and impact of infections in acute pancreatitis

Besselink MG, for the Dutch Acute Pancreatitis Study Group (Univ Med Ctr Utrecht, The Netherlands; et al)

Br J Surg 96:267-273, 2009

Background.—Although infected necrosis is an established cause of death in acute pancreatitis, the impact of bacteraemia and pneumonia is less certain.

Methods.—This was a cohort study of 731 patients with a primary episode of acute pancreatitis in 2004–2007, including 296 patients involved in a randomized controlled trial to investigate the value of probiotic treatment in severe pancreatitis. Time of onset of bacteraemia, pneumonia, infected pancreatic necrosis, persistent organ failure and death were recorded.

Results.—The initial infection in 173 patients was diagnosed a median of 8 (interquartile range 3–20) days after admission (infected necrosis, median day 26; bacteraemia/pneumonia, median day 7). Eighty per cent of 61 patients who died had an infection. In 154 patients with pancreatic parenchymal necrosis, bacteraemia was associated with increased risk of infected necrosis (65 *versus* 37.9 per cent; $P = 0.002$). In 98 patients with infected necrosis, bacteraemia was associated with higher mortality (40 *versus* 16 per cent; $P = 0.014$). In multivariable analysis, persistent organ failure (odds ratio (OR) 18.0), bacteraemia (OR 3.4) and age (OR 1.1) were associated with death.

Conclusion.—Infections occur early in acute pancreatitis, and have a significant impact on mortality, especially bacteraemia. Prophylactic strategies should focus on early intervention.

▶ The incidence of acute pancreatitis from many known and unknown causes continues to increase, and the overall mortality remains around 5%. Infectious complications, including infected pancreatic necrosis, bacteremia, and pneumonia, contribute significantly to mortality.[1] The use of prophylactic antibiotics or probiotics have not improved mortality. A post hoc analysis of the trial to investigate the use of probiotics in severe acute pancreatitis published in this study shows that infections occur early in acute pancreatitis, particularly bacteremia and pneumonia. The median time to bacteremia/pneumonia was 7 days compared with 26 days for infected necrosis. In patients with infected necrosis, bacteremia was associated with higher mortality. Persistent organ failure, advanced age, and bacteremia were associated with death.

N. M. Khardori, MD

Reference

1. Besselink MGH, Gooszen H. Trends in hospital volume and mortality for acute pancreatitis, 1997–2003. Dutch Acute Pancreatitis Study Group. *HPB (Oxford).* 2005;7:59.

Acute kidney injury in septic shock: clinical outcomes and impact of duration of hypotension prior to initiation of antimicrobial therapy
Bagshaw SM, The Cooperative Antimicrobial Therapy of Septic Shock (CATSS) Database Research Group (Univ of Alberta, Edmonton, Canada; et al)
Intensive Care Med 35:871-881, 2009

Objective.—To describe the incidence and outcomes associated with early acute kidney injury (AKI) in septic shock and explore the association between duration from hypotension onset to effective antimicrobial therapy and AKI.

Design.—Retrospective cohort study.

Subjects.—A total of 4,532 adult patients with septic shock from 1989 to 2005.

Setting.—Intensive care units of 22 academic and community hospitals in Canada, the United States and Saudi Arabia.

Measurements and Main Results.—In total, 64.4% of patients with septic shock developed early AKI (i.e., within 24 h after onset of hypotension). By RIFLE criteria, 16.3% had risk, 29.4% had injury and 18.7% had failure. AKI patients were older, more likely female, with more co-morbid disease and greater severity of illness. Of 3,373 patients (74.4%) with hypotension prior to receiving effective antimicrobial therapy, the median (IQR) time from hypotension onset to antimicrobial therapy was 5.5 h (2.0–13.3). Patients with AKI were more likely to have longer delays to receiving antimicrobial therapy compared to those with no AKI [6.0 (2.3–15.3) h for AKI vs. 4.3 (1.5–10.8) h for no AKI, $P < 0.0001$). A longer duration to antimicrobial therapy was also associated an increase in odds of AKI [odds ratio (OR) 1.14, 95% CI 1.10–1.20, $P < 0.001$, per hour (log-transformed) delay]. AKI was associated with significantly higher odds of death in both ICU (OR 1.73, 95% CI 1.60–1.9, $P < 0.0001$) and hospital (OR 1.62, 95% CI, 1.5–1.7, $P < 0.0001$). By Cox proportional hazards analysis, including propensity score-adjustment, each RIFLE category was independently associated with a greater hazard ratio for death (risk 1.31; injury 1.45; failure 1.56).

Conclusion.—Early AKI is common in septic shock. Delays to appropriate antimicrobial therapy may contribute to significant increases in the incidence of AKI. Survival was considerably lower for septic shock associated with early AKI, with increasing severity of AKI, and with increasing delays to appropriate antimicrobial therapy.

▶ Patients with septic shock continue to have a very high mortality despite significant advances in our diagnostic and therapeutic strategies. Early initiation of appropriate antibiotic therapy was shown to increase survival in septic shock, and is a key point in the current guidelines for the management of severe sepsis and septic shock.[1,2] Acute kidney injury (AKI) is a common occurrence in critically ill patients, including those with sepsis and septic shock. Patients with sepsis-associated AKI have higher in-hospital mortality and prolonged duration of stay compared with controls.[3]

In this multicenter retrospective analysis, Bagshaw et al[3] are investigating the association between the duration of hypotension before initiation of effective antimicrobial therapy and early AKI in patients admitted to the ICU with septic shock. The study is analyzing data from 4532 patients enrolled over a period of 16 years. Patients with baseline end-stage renal disease or no documentation of baseline creatinine values were excluded. The authors found a high incidence of early AKI (64.4%) in this population. Not surprisingly, patients with AKI had significantly longer duration from onset of hypotension to antibiotic therapy compared with those with no AKI. Longer duration between hypotension onset and the initiation of antimicrobial therapy was also associated with greater changes in serum creatinine and increased severity of AKI. The authors also studied the clinical outcomes associated with AKI and found an increase in both crude and covariate mortality in these patients.

There is no doubt that proper resuscitation and supportive therapy are extremely important in any type of shock, regardless of etiology. Generally, the alterations of the body homeostasis in shock are so great that therapies to reverse it are severely limited. For septic shock, antibiotics directed at the potential etiologic agent are an essential therapy, but they should be started within a very narrow window for maximal effectiveness. This study reiterates the relation between the delay in antimicrobial treatment and increased risk of organ failure (kidney failure in this case) and death in septic shock. This is an important parameter that deserves some emphasis in medical literature as "time to cath lab" for myocardial infarction, or "time to thrombolysis" for acute stroke.

C. A. Speil, MD

References

1. Kumar A, Roberts D, Wood KE, et al. Duration of hypotension before initiation of effective antimicrobial therapy is the critical determinant of survival in human septic shock. *Crit Care Med.* 2006;34:1589-1596.
2. Dellinger RP, Levy MM, Carlet JM, et al. Surviving Sepsis Campaign: international guidelines for management of severe sepsis and septic shock. *Crit Care Med.* 2008;36:296-327.
3. Bagshaw SM, George C, Bellomo R, ANZICS Database Management Committee. Early acute kidney injury and sepsis: a multicentre evaluation. *Crit Care.* 2008;12: R47. Epub 2008 Apr 10.

Fever and Leukocytosis in Critically Ill Trauma Patients: It is not the Blood
Claridge JA, Golob JF Jr, Fadlalla AMA, et al (Case Western Reserve Univ School of Medicine, Cleveland, OH; Cleveland State Univ Cleveland, OH)
Am Surg 75:405-410, 2009

The diagnosis of bacteremia in critically ill patients is classically based on fever and/or leukocytosis. The objectives of this study were to determine 1) if our intensive care unit obtains blood cultures based on fever and/or leukocytosis over the initial 14 days of hospitalization after trauma; and 2) the efficacy of this diagnostic workup. An 18-month retrospective cohort analysis was performed on consecutively admitted trauma patients.

Data collected included demographics, injuries, and the first 14 days maximal daily temperature, leukocyte count, and results of blood and catheter tip cultures. Fever was defined as a maximum daily temperature of 38.5°C or greater and leukocytosis as a leukocyte count 12,000/mm^3 or greater of blood. Five hundred ten patients were evaluated for a total of 3,839 patient-days. The mean age and injury severity score were 49 ± 1 years and 19 ± 1, respectively. Four hundred twenty-five blood culture episodes were obtained and 25 (6%) bacteremias were identified in 23 patients (5%). A significant association was found between obtaining blood cultures in patients with fever (relative risk [RR], 7.7), leukocytosis (RR, 1.3), and fever + leukocytosis (RR, 3.2). However, no significant association was found between these clinical signs and the diagnosis of bacteremia. In fact, fever alone was inversely associated with bacteremia. Our intensive care unit follows the common "fever workup" practice and obtains blood cultures based on the presence of fever and leukocytosis. However, fever and leukocytosis were not associated with bacteremia, suggesting inefficiency and that other factors are more important after trauma.

▶ Nosocomial infections are a common complication in surgical intensive care unit (ICU) patients, particularly among burn and trauma patients.[1] Blood cultures are considered a cornerstone for diagnosing systemic infections in these and other ICU patients. Typically, fever and/or leukocytosis in a hospitalized patient triggers an almost automated order for blood cultures from the health care provider. However, many critically ill trauma and burn patients have a systemic inflammatory response syndrome related to their initial injury, which often manifests with fever and leukocytosis.

In this retrospective study, Claridge et al evaluate fever and leukocytosis as predictors of bacteriemia in critically ill trauma patients during the first 2 weeks in the surgical and trauma ICU (STICU). Patients over 18 years old who spent at least 2 days in STICU, and were not admitted for more than 24 hours to another floor or hospital before the ICU admission, were included; 510 patients over 18 months met the inclusion criteria. There were 425 positive blood culture episodes in 202 patients, and 25 episodes of bacteriemia in 23 patients. Bacteriemia was defined as a positive blood culture with an organism not considered a contaminant. Organisms considered contaminants included diphtheroids, micrococci, coagulase negative staphylococci, and *Propionibacterium acnes* in a single bottle or in multiple bottles obtained from the same site in the absence of an obvious source like a positive catheter tip. The study found no association between fever, leukocytosis, or their combination and the presence of bacteriemia. Actually, fever without leukocytosis was inversely related to bacteriemia (relative risk [RR] 0.39). The mean temperature on the day of obtaining the blood culture in patients with bacteriemia was 38.7°C compared with 38.8°C in patients with a negative blood culture. The study also showed increased length of stay and mortality among the patients with bacteriemia, which is not surprising. The authors conclude that fever and leukocytosis do not seem to be associated with bacteriemia in this patient population, and recommend that no blood culture should be obtained in trauma patients within the first 48 hours of trauma. They also recommend that fever and/or leukocytosis should not be an automatic trigger for blood cultures in the first 14 days after trauma.

This study is important in outlining the difficulty in diagnosing infection in critically ill patients, in this case in a trauma unit. In managing these patients, the physician is caught between the threat of missing a potentially serious infection and the low specificity of classical signs such as fever and elevated WBC. In the end each patient is different and decisions should be made based on clinical judgment and common sense. Based on our day-to-day experience, this study's findings may be applied to other categories of critical care patients as well.

C. A. Speil, MD

Reference

1. National Nosocomial Infections Surveillance (NNIS) System Report, data summary from January 1992 through June 2004, issued October 2004. *Am J Infect Control*. 2004;32:470-485.

11 Infectious Disease Management

Changes in bacterial isolates from burn wounds and their antibiograms: A 20-year study (1986–2005)
Guggenheim M, Zbinden R, Handschin AE, et al (Univ Hosp Zurich, Switzerland; Univ of Zurich, Switzerland; et al)
Burns 35:553-560, 2009

Background.—Our aim is to elucidate shifts in the bacterial spectrum colonising burn wounds and corresponding antibiotic susceptibilities during a 20-year study period.

Methods.—Microbiological results from burn patients collected between 1986 and 2005 were analysed retrospectively.

Results.—*Staphylococcus aureus* was isolated most frequently (20.8%), followed by *Escherichia coli* (13.9%), *Pseudomonas aeruginosa* (11.8%), coagulase-negative staphylococci (CNS) (10.9%), *Enterococcus* sp. (9.7%), *Enterobacter cloacae* (5.6%), *Klebsiella pneumoniae* (5%), *Acinetobacter* sp. (3.2%), *Proteus mirabilis* (2%) and *Stenotrophomonas maltophilia* (1.4%). Susceptibility of *S. aureus* to broad-spectrum substances such as ciprofloxacin or penicillinase-stable penicillins has waned, others such as cotrimoxazole or netilmicin remained effective. Not a single resistance against vancomycin was recorded. Increases in methicillin-resistant *S. aureus* (MRSA) were pronounced (3% in 1986–1997 (the first of the three study periods) to 16% in 1998–2001 and 13% in 2002–2005). Results for methicillin-resistant CNS (MRCNS) show an even greater increase. *P. aeruginosa* has shown increasing susceptibility against netilmicin (1986–1989: 84%, 2002–2005: 95%). Susceptibility of *P. aeruginosa* to ceftazidime has decreased markedly. *S. maltophilia* has shown clinically relevant susceptibility mainly against ciprofloxacin. *Acinetobacter* sp. have shown little susceptibility to most antibiotics. Imipenem or meropenem have been very reliable reserve antibiotics throughout the study period for the fermenting *Enterobacteriaceae* (*E. coli*, *K. pneumoniae*, *E. cloacae* and *P. mirabilis*), with susceptibilities of or near 100%.

Conclusion.—In-depth knowledge of the bacteria causing infectious complications and of their antibiotic susceptibilities is a prerequisite for treating burn patients. Our study shows shifts in the microbial spectrum and their antibiogram, which mandate frequent reassessments.

▶ Improved initial care of patients with severe burns, including intensive care and early surgical intervention, has resulted in a decrease in early mortality. However, these patients have multiple risk factors for development of serious infections, including ventilator-associated pneumonia, blood stream infection, and wound infection. It is now estimated that 75% of the mortality in burn patients is related directly to infections.[1] The management of these infections is further complicated by the changing microbiology and evolving resistance to antimicrobial agents. Colonization of burn wounds by endogenous and exogenous microbial flora is the ongoing source of infections in these patients.

This study describes shifts in the bacterial spectrum colonizing burn wounds and corresponding antibiotic susceptibilities during a 20-year period. The 3 most commonly isolated gram-positive bacteria were *Staphylococcus aureus*, *Enterococcus* species, and coagulase-negative staphylococci (CNS). Resistance of *S aureus* to penicillinase-resistant penicillins (oxacillin or methicillin), *Enterococcus* to ampicillin, and CNS to multiple antibiotics increased steadily between 1980 and 2005. The 7 most commonly isolated gram-negative species were *Escherichia coli*, *Pseudomonas aeruginosa*, *Enterobacter cloacae*, *Klebsiella pneumoniae*, *Acinetobacter* species, *Proteus mirabilis*, and *Stenotrophomonas maltophilia*. With the exception of *P mirabilis*, all gram negatives have shown worsening antibiotic susceptibility patterns. I concur with the authors that burn units should assess the microbial spectrum and resistance patterns frequently to optimize antimicrobial therapy during any given period of time.

N. M. Khardori, MD

Reference

1. Anserminoi NM, Hemsley C. Intensive care management and control of infection. *Mol boil Rep.* 2004;329:220-223.

Is *Candida* colonization of central vascular catheters in non-candidemic, non-neutropenic patients an indication for antifungals?
Pérez-Parra A, Muñoz P, Guinea J, et al (Hosp General Universitario Gregorio Marañón, Madrid, Spain)
Intensive Care Med 35:707-712, 2009

Purpose.—To assess the influence of antifungal therapy on the outcome of non-candidemic adult patients with central vascular catheter (CVC) tips colonized by *Candida* species.

Methods.—A retrospective analysis of the outcome of patients with *Candida* colonization of their CVC tip and no concurrent candidemia was made over a 4-year period. Patients who either died or developed candidemia-invasive candidiasis (poor outcome) were compared with those who improved.

Results.—We finally included 58 patients for analysis. Almost all (91.4%) had to be admitted to the ICU during their hospital stay. Independent predictors for outcome were a McCabe and Jackson score corresponding to ultimately fatal underlying disease [odds ratio (OR) 11.98; 95% confidence interval (CI), 1.37–104.97; $P = 0.02$], and maximum severity corresponding to severe sepsis, septic shock or multiorgan failure (OR: 6.16, CI 95%: 1.00–37.93; $P = 0.05$). We were unable to demonstrate that antifungal therapy was an independent variable influencing outcome (OR 0.82; 95% CI, 0.27–2.47; $P = 0.73$).

Conclusions.—Our data suggest that, in non-neutropenic critically ill patients with no concomitant candidemia and with CVC tips colonized by *Candida*, antifungal therapy does not seem to have a significant influence on clinical outcome.

▶ Invasive candidiasis, a significant cause of morbidity and mortality in hospitalized patients, is difficult to diagnose, especially in noncandidemic patients.[1] Preemptive treatment for candidiasis is often based on clinical signs and colonization of mucosal or skin surfaces. Colonized intravenous catheters are responsible for a high proportion of candidemia or invasive candidiasis. The clinical significance of *Candida* colonization of a central venous catheter (CVC) tip in the absence of concomitant candidemia is not established, but often leads to initiation of antifungal therapy.

This is a retrospective study from a large tertiary care teaching hospital to review the outcome of noncandidemic patients with colonization of CVC tips over a 4-year period. A total of 58 patients were included in the analysis; 91.4% were in the intensive care unit during their hospital stay. Patients who died or developed invasive candidiasis (poor outcome) were compared with those who improved. Independent predictors for outcome were ultimately fatal underlying disease, severe sepsis, septic shock, or multiorgan failure. The data suggest that antifungal therapy for *Candida* species grown from CVC tips in the absence of candidemia in nonneutropenic critically ill patients does not have a significant influence on clinical outcome.

N. M. Khardori, MD

Reference

1. Dimopoulos G, Karabinis A, Samonis G, Falagas ME. Candidemia in immunocompromised and immunocompetent critically ill patients: a prospective comparative study. *Dur J Clin Microbiol Infect Dis.* 2007;26:377-384.

Delayed Administration of Antibiotics and Mortality in Patients With Community-Acquired Pneumonia

Cheng AC, Buising KL (Univ of Melbourne, Victoria, Australia; Centre for Clinical Res Excellence in Infectious Diseases, Melbourne, Victoria, Australia)
Ann Emerg Med 53:618-624, 2009

Study Objective.—Previous studies have demonstrated a crude association between the time to first antibiotic dose and mortality in patients with community-acquired pneumonia. We hypothesize that time to first antibiotic dose may affect mortality, particularly for patients at high risk of death, that is, patients hypoxic on presentation, patients in Pneumonia Severity Index class IV or V, and patients older than 65 years at our institution.

Methods.—We reviewed data from a prospectively collected database of patients with community-acquired pneumonia, excluding patients who had received antibiotics before presentation and palliative patients not receiving antibiotics. We examined time to first antibiotic dose in patients who died or had prolonged length of stay (all patients) and in specific subgroups regarded as high risk (age >65 years, Pneumonia Severity Index class IV or V, presence of hypoxia or hypotension).

Results.—In 501 patients, the median time to first antibiotic dose was 2.7 hours, with 91% of patients receiving antibiotics within 8 hours. Time to first antibiotic dose was not positively associated with mortality or prolonged length of stay in any of the subgroups examined. We found evidence that patients with severe pneumonia received antibiotics earlier than other patients.

Conclusion.—Most patients at this institution already receive timely antibiotic therapy. This finding may be due to either a true lack of association, in that minor delays in antibiotic administration, where antibiotics are generally administered within 8 hours, do not affect mortality. Additionally, there may be confounding by severity, such that patients at highest risk of death received antibiotics earlier.

▶ The importance of time to first dose of antibiotic in influencing outcomes in patients with community-acquired pneumonia (CAP) has been a subject of great debate for many years. Two large retrospective studies using Medicare databases showed improved survival with antibiotic administration within 8 and 4 hours of hospital arrival.[1,2] However, findings from other observational studies do not support this conclusion.[3]

Reflecting the ongoing controversy, the current guidelines for management of CAP from the Infectious Disease Society of America (IDSA) and the American Thoracic Society (ATS) advise administration of antibiotics as soon as possible after pneumonia is considered likely and (for emergency department [ED] patients) while the patient is still in the ED, but do not emphasize any timelines.[4] Meanwhile, the Joint Commission is using the median time to antibiotic and the number of patients receiving antibiotics within 6 hours of arrival as performance

measures (http://www.jointcommission.org/PerformanceMeasurement/
PerformanceMeasurement/Current + NHQM + Manual.htm).

The authors of this study are addressing this important issue in a prospectively collected data analysis of 501 patients presenting with CAP at a large teaching hospital in Melbourne, Australia. Patients who did not receive antibiotics, or who received antibiotics before presentation to the ED, were excluded from the study. Overall, 175 (35%), 346 (69%), and 454 (91%) patients received antibiotics within 2, 4, and 8 hours respectively of presentation. Overall, in-hospital mortality was 10.6%. The study did not find an association between the median time to antibiotic and mortality or length of stay. On the contrary, the time to antibiotic was shorter in the patients who died compared with survivors, probably because patients who had more severe illness tended to receive antibiotics earlier.

It is common sense to give antibiotics as soon as possible once an infectious disease is considered likely. Early administration of appropriate antibiotics saves many lives, and it is particularly important in severe infections or septic shock, as shown elsewhere in this book. However, based on the evolving data, it is not justified to recommend a specific timeline for antibiotic administration in CAP, but rather, as the IDSA/ATS guidelines advise, emphasize the general rule of antibiotic delivery as early as possible in the ED or even before hospital arrival (in the physician's office).

C. A. Speil, MD

References

1. Meehan TP, Fine MJ, Krumholz HM, et al. Quality of care, process, and outcomes in elderly patients with pneumonia. *JAMA.* 1997;278:2080-2084.
2. Houck PM, Bratzler DW, Nsa W, Ma A, Bartlett JG. Timing of antibiotic administration and outcomes for Medicare patients hospitalized with community-acquired pneumonia. *Arch Intern Med.* 2004;164:637-644.
3. Yu KT, Wyer PC. Evidence-based emergency medicine/critically appraised topic. Evidence behind the 4-hour rule for initiation of antibiotic therapy in community-acquired pneumonia. *Ann Emerg Med.* 2008;51:651-662.
4. Mandell LA, Wunderink RG, Anzueto A, et al. Infectious Diseases Society of America/American Thoracic Society consensus guidelines on the management of community-acquired pneumonia in adults. *Clin Infect Dis.* 2007;44:S27-S72.

Clinical Relevance of the Pharmacokinetic Interactions of Azole Antifungal Drugs with Other Coadministered Agents

Brüggemann RJM, Alffenaar J-WC, Blijlevens NMA, et al (Radboud Univ Nijmegen Med Centre, The Netherlands; Univ Med Centre Groningen, The Netherlands; et al)
Clin Infect Dis 48:1441-1458, 2009

There are currently a number of licensed azole antifungal drugs; however; only 4 (namely, fluconazole, itraconazole, posaconazole, and voriconazole) are used frequently in a clinical setting for prophylaxis or treatment of systemic fungal infections. In this article, we review the pharmacokinetic interactions of these azole antifungal drugs with other coadministered agents. We describe these (2-way) interactions and the extent to which metabolic pathways and/or other supposed mechanisms are involved in these interactions. This article provides an overview of all published drug-drug interactions in humans (either healthy volunteers or patients), and on the basis of these findings, we have developed recommendations for managing the specific interactions.

▶ The azole antifungals fluconazole, itraconazole, voriconazole, and posaconazole are important drugs used to treat systemic fungal infections; they are safe and well tolerated, but their use is somewhat limited by drug-drug interactions. This is particularly true in patients with multiple comorbidities, HIV infection, or malignancies, mostly because they are already receiving multiple other medications.[1]

These patients are typically the ones that benefit the most from the use of antifungal medications; sadly, they are also more prone to harm from side effects and drug interactions.

In this review article, Brüggemann et al are doing an excellent review of pharmacokinetics for the major triazole agents and clinically relevant drug interactions at multiple levels (absorption, metabolism, and excretion) with emphasis on their relations with the cytochrome P450 enzymes and the specific pathways involved. This article is supplemented with data from human studies, describing the clinically significant drug interactions by severity. Advice regarding how to manage each particular interaction is given.

This article is a useful tool for any physician prescribing azole antifungal drugs. First, it is a concise and practical review of the pharmacokinetics of the important members of the class, with emphasis on the differences between them. Second, the drug interaction tables provided could be used as a quick reference in clinical settings.

C. A. Speil, MD

Reference

1. Nivoix Y. Drug-drug interactions of triazole antifungal agents in multimorbid patients and implications for patient care. *Curr Drug Metab*. 2009;10:395-409.

The effect of limiting antimicrobial therapy duration on antimicrobial resistance in the critical care setting
Marra AR, de Almeida SM, Correa L, et al (Hosp Israelita Albert Einstein, São Paulo, Brazil; et al)
Am J Infect Control 37:204-209, 2009

Background.—Using antimicrobial agents for prolonged periods of time and/or in heavy densities is known to contribute to antimicrobial resistance.

Methods.—A quasiexperimental, before and after study to limit the duration of antimicrobial therapy to 14 days was conducted in a medical-surgical intensive care unit (ICU). An intervention to optimize antimicrobial therapy was performed when antimicrobial agents had been prescribed for more than 14 days. We then compared antimicrobial utilization using the defined daily dose (DDD) per 1000 patient-days, as well as resistance rates in selected organisms in the intervention phase to the previous 10-month period.

Results.—In the intervention phase, doctors approved to discontinue the antimicrobial therapy before 14 days in 89.8% (415/462) of the prescribed antibiotics in the ICU. Comparing the 2 time periods, we found a reduction in carbapenems (24.5% decrease), vancomycin (14.3% decrease), and cephalosporins (12.2% decrease) in the intervention phase. Imipenem resistance decreased in *Acinetobacter baumannii* from 88.5% to 20.0% ($P \leq .001$) and in *Klebsiella pneumoniae* from 54.5% to 10.7% ($P = .01$).

Conclusion.—These results suggest that an intervention to reduce the duration of antimicrobial therapy contributed to more rational use of antimicrobial agents and to the reduction of bacterial resistance in the critical care setting.

▶ Early appropriate empiric antimicrobial therapy for critically ill patients has been shown to decrease mortality.[1] Often, this is not followed by careful review of microbiological, radiographic, and clinical data resulting in continuation of initial broad-spectrum empiric antimicrobial therapy. This contributes to the misuse of antibiotics, leading to antibiotic resistance, which is strongly associated with adverse outcomes and increased resource use. The antibiotic choices now for some multidrug-resistance pathogens are nonexistent or limited to agents with significant toxicities.[2] The impact of duration of antimicrobial therapy on resistance in nosocomial pathogens has not been studied extensively.

In this quasi experimental pre- and post-study in a medical-surgical intensive care unit, the duration of antimicrobial therapy was limited to 14 days. This simple intervention led to the reduction of bacterial resistance and contributed to more rational use of antimicrobial agents. In my opinion, the concept of empiricism should be changed to one of presumptive antibiotic therapy based on patient and environmental factors as well as local antibiotic resistance patterns, and should be followed by streamlining and de-escalation as soon as microbiological data become available.

N. M. Khardori, MD

References

1. Kollef MH. Inadequate antimicrobial treatment: an important determinate of outcome for hospitalized patients. *Clin Infect Dis.* 2000;31:131-138.
2. Spelbergl B, Guidos R, Gilbert D, et al, for the Infectious diseases Society of America. The epidemic of antibiotic-resistant infections: a call to action for the medical community from the Infectious Diseases Society of America. *Clin Infect Dis.* 2008;46:155-164.

Emergence of Ciprofloxacin-Resistant *Neisseria meningitidis* in North America

Wu HM, Harcourt BH, Hatcher CP, et al (Natl Ctr for Immunization and Respiratory Diseases, Atlanta, GA; et al)
N Engl J Med 360:886-892, 2009

We report on three cases of meningococcal disease caused by ciprofflox-acin-resistant *Neisseria meningitidis*, one in North Dakota and two in Minnesota. The cases were caused by the same serogroup B strain. To assess local carriage of resistant *N. meningitidis*, we conducted a pharyngeal-carriage survey and isolated the resistant strain from one asymptomatic carrier. Sequencing of the gene encoding subunit A of DNA gyrase (*gyrA*) revealed a mutation associated with fluoroquinolone resistance and suggests that the resistance was acquired by means of horizontal gene transfer with the commensal *N. lactamica*. In susceptibility testing of invasive *N. meningitidis* isolates from the Active Bacterial Core surveillance system between January 2007 and January 2008, an additional ciprofloxacin-resistant isolate was found, in this case from California. Ciprofloxacin-resistant *N. meningitidis* has emerged in North America.

▶ *Neisseria meningitidis* is a redoubtable pathogen and invasive meningococcal infection is life-threatening even in immunocompetent individuals. Transient nasopharyngeal colonization is a well known prerequisite for infection. Although most carriers are asymptomatic, close contacts of infected patients are at higher risk for developing invasive disease and antimicrobial prophylaxis is indicated. Current guidelines recommend postexposure chemoprophylaxis with rifampin, ciprofloxacin, or ceftriaxone for persons at risk.[1] This article describes emergence of fluoroquinolone resistance in 4 clonally related isolates of *N meningitidis* in Minnesota and North Dakota. Three cases of invasive meningococcal disease caused by ciprofloxacin-resistant isolates were reported in the area between January 2007 and January 2008, which represented 9% of all confirmed cases. An epidemiological survey performed 2 to 3 weeks after the last case showed a carriage rate of 7.5%, including one close contact of patient 3. The isolates from the case patients and from the close contact of patient 3 showed identical pulsed field gel electrophoresis (PFGE) patterns. Based on the molecular analysis, the authors conclude the fluoroquinolone resistance was acquired through horizontal gene transfer from a local strain of *Neisseria lactamica*, which is a common commensal of the human respiratory tract.

Emerging fluoroquinolone resistance in *N meningitidis* raises questions about current recommendations for treatment and prophylaxis of meningococcal infections, which include fluoroquinolones as an alternative agent.[1,2] The potential similarity with the development of fluoroquinolone resistance in *Neisseria gonorrhoeae* is also concerning. Although Centers for Disease Control and Prevention (CDC) issued interim recommendations to avoid ciprofloxacin for chemoprophylaxis in certain counties in Minnesota and North Dakota, a high level of vigilance should be maintained for development of more widespread resistance. Alternative drugs, such as oral third generation cephalosporins, should be considered for study regarding chemoprophylaxis for meningococcal infection.

C. A. Speil, MD

References

1. Bilukha OO, Rosnstein N, National Center for Infectious Disease. Prevention and control of meningococcal disease: recommendations of the Advisory Committee on Immunization Practices (ACIP). *MMWR Recomm Rep.* 2005;54:1-21.
2. Tunkel AR, Hartman BJ, Kaplan SL, et al. Practice guidelines for the management of bacterial meningitis. *Clin Infect Dis.* 2004;39:1267-1284.

Influence of surgical treatment timing on mortality from necrotizing soft tissue infections requiring intensive care management
Boyer A, Vargas F, Coste F, et al (Hôpital Pellegrin-Tripode, Bordeaux cedex, France)
Intensive Care Med 35:847-853, 2009

Purpose.—Surgical treatment is crucial in the management of necrotizing soft tissue infections (NSTIs). The aim of this study was to determine the influence of surgical procedure timing on hospital mortality in severe NSTI.

Methods.—A retrospective study including 106 patients was conducted in a medical intensive care unit equipped with a hyperbaric chamber. Data regarding pre-existing conditions, intensive care and surgical management were included in a logistic regression model to determine independent factors associated with hospital mortality.

Results.—Overall hospital mortality was 40.6%. In multivariate analysis, underlying cardiovascular disease, SAPS II, abdominoperineal compared to limb localization, time from the first signs to diagnosis <72 h, and time from diagnosis to surgical treatment >14 h in patients with septic shock were independently associated with hospital mortality.

Conclusion.—In patients with NSTI and septic shock, hospital mortality is influenced by the timing of surgical treatment.

▶ Necrotizing soft-tissue infections are rapidly progressive and potentially fatal unless managed by a multidisciplinary approach of prompt surgical intervention, broad-spectrum antibiotics, and aggressive critical care.[1] Once diagnosed, surgical intervention is further delayed by the time required to stabilize the patient in the ICU. In patients with severe septic shock from necrotizing soft-tissue infection, the source must rapidly be removed by surgical intervention.[2]

This retrospective study used a logistic regression model to determine independent factors associated with hospital mortality in patients with necrotizing fasciitis. The overall hospital mortality in these patients with severe necrotizing soft-tissue infections was 40.6%. Among the independent variables associated with mortality was time of >14 hours from diagnosis to surgical treatment.

Early recognition of infection with surgery immediately following general ICU management along with broad-spectrum antimicrobial agents should be the gold standard therapy in patients with necrotizing soft-tissue infections.

N. M. Khardori, MD

References

1. Stevens DL, Bison AL, Chamber EF, et al. Practice guidelines for the diagnosis and management of skin and soft-tissue infections. *Clin Infect Dis.* 2005;41:1373-1406.
2. Russell JA. Management of sepsis. *N Engl J Med.* 2006;355:1699-1713.

Mitral Valve Infective Endocarditis: Benefit of Early Operation and Aggressive Use of Repair

Shang E, Forrest GN, Chizmar T, et al (Univ of Maryland Med Ctr, Baltimore, MD; The Oregon Health & Science Univ, Portland)

Ann Thorac Surg 87:1728-1734, 2009

Background.—In-hospital mortality rates for left-sided infective endocarditis (IE) exceed 20%. We investigated the outcomes of an aggressive approach to mitral valve IE that emphasizes early surgical intervention and preferential performance of mitral valve repair.

Methods.—We reviewed 89 consecutive operations in 87 patients for native mitral valve IE at a single institution from 2002 to 2007. Operations occurred promptly after completion of preoperative studies. Independent risk factors for death were investigated using multivariable logistic regression.

Results.—Mitral valve repair was accomplished in 56 of 89 patients (63%). Perioperative mortality was 4.4% (n = 4). Survival rates at 1 and 5 years were 89.9% (80 of 89) and 82.0% (73 of 90). There was a survival benefit for repair vs replacement at 1 ($p = 0.03$) and 5 years ($p = 0.0017$). Repair vs replacement (odds ratio [OR], 0.2; 95% confidence interval [CI], 0.06 to 0.72), diabetes (OR, 4.43; 95% CI, 1.18 to 16.66), and renal failure (OR, 3.65; 95% CI, 1.3 to 12.91) were independent risk factors for late mortality. Among 59 patients with active IE, preoperative head computed tomography (CT) showed 29 (49%) had abnormalities, including 12 (41%) with intracerebral hemorrhage. The median interval was 4 days from admission to operation. The rate of permanent postoperative stroke was 1.1% (1 of 89).

Conclusions.—These results support early surgical therapy for mitral valve IE. Head CT abnormalities do not warrant delay of operation. Mitral valve repair was associated with a long-term survival advantage compared with valve replacement.

▶ The mortality rates for infective endocarditis have not improved significantly since the 1960's, despite advances in antimicrobial and surgical therapy. However, early surgery for native valve endocarditis has been associated with improved long-term survival compared with medical therapy alone.[1] Indications for surgery include presence of large or anterior mitral leaflet vegetations, systemic embolization, lack of response to antimicrobial therapy, valvular dehiscence or large abscess, acute valvular insufficiency, and cardiac failure.[2] Regarding surgical therapy for mitral valve endocarditis, current surgical literature suggests a significant advantage of mitral valve repair over replacement, although no large randomized trials have been conducted.[3]

This study by Shang et al performs a retrospective analysis of 89 surgeries in 87 patients for native mitral valve endocarditis between July 2002 and June 2007. Most common etiologic agents were *Staphylococcus aureus* (41.6%) and *Streptococcus* subspecies. (30%). The reported outcomes were in-hospital or 30 days mortality (whichever was greater) and long-term (1 year and 5 years) mortality. The surgical team's approach favored repair of valve over replacement if technically feasible. Mitral valve repair was performed in 56 patients (63%). The type of surgery was not associated with a significant difference in short-term mortality, however at 1 year and 5 years, survival was significantly better for patients who underwent repair compared with replacement. This study's findings again show the long-term advantages of mitral valve repair over replacement in patients with infective endocarditis. Another important point is the low incidence of postoperative neurological complications, even in patients with abnormal head CT findings at the time of surgery (including 12 patients with intracerebral hemorrhage), suggesting that surgery should not be delayed in these patients. The main limitation is that patients who underwent mitral valve replacement were likely not candidates for repair, and therefore had more extensive valvular destruction. Nevertheless, this study again shows benefit for aggressive surgical therapy, particularly valve repair, in mitral valve infective endocarditis, and underscores the need for a team approach (ie, cardiologist, infectious disease specialist, and cardiac surgeon) in managing these challenging patients.

C. A. Speil, MD

References

1. Aksoy O, Sexton DJ, Wang A, et al. Early surgery in patients with infective endocarditis: a propensity score analysis. *Clin Infect Dis.* 2007;44:364-372.
2. Baddour LM, Wilson WR, Bayer AS, et al. Infective endocarditis: diagnosis, antimicrobial therapy, and management of complications: a statement for healthcare professionals from the Committee on Rheumatic Fever, Endocarditis, and Kawasaki Disease, Council on Cardiovascular Disease in the Young, and the Councils on Clinical Cardiology, Stroke, and Cardiovascular Surgery and Anesthesia, American Heart Association: endorsed by the Infectious Diseases Society of America. *Circulation.* 2005;111:e394-434.
3. Feringa HH, Shaw LJ, Poldermans D, et al. Mitral valve repair and replacement in endocarditis: a systematic review of literature. *Ann Thorac Surg.* 2007;83: 564-570.

Choice of First Intervention is Related to Outcomes in the Management of Empyema

Wozniak CJ, Paull DE, Moezzi JE, et al (Wright State Univ, Dayton, OH; Veterans Administration Med Ctr, Dayton, OH)

Ann Thorac Surg 87:1525-1531, 2009

Background.—The study determined whether the first procedure; simple drainage (tube thoracostomy, pigtail catheter) or operation (video-assisted thoracic surgery [VATS], thoracotomy) was related to outcomes in the management of empyema.

Methods.—Data were collected from 104 consecutive patients with empyema. Primary outcomes were additional procedures and death. Predictor variables included age, delay, Karnofsky performance status (KPS), Charlson comorbidity index (CCI), serum albumin, malignancy, Acute Physiology and Chronic Health Evaluation II score, loculations on computed tomography scan, empyema stage, and first procedure choice.

Results.—Advanced empyema (≥ stage IIA) was present in 84% of patients. Overall treatment success rates (no death, no additional drainage procedures) among evaluable patients for pigtail drainage, tube thoracostomy, VATS, and thoracotomy were 40% (4 of 10), 38% (14 of 37), 81% (13 of 16), and 89% (32 of 36), respectively. Five patients underwent miscellaneous procedures. Univariate variables associated with hospital death included KPS, CCI, and drainage as the first procedure. In multivariate analyses, KPS (coefficient, -0.06, $p = 0.002$) and failure of the first procedure (odds ratio [OR], 6.76; 95% confidence interval [CI], 1.45 to 31.4, $p = .01$) were independent predictors of death. Simple drainage as the first procedure was a strong, independent predictor of failure of the first procedure (OR, 11.1; 95% CI, 3.51 to 34.9; $p = .00004$).

Conclusions.—The choice of the first procedure is critical in the outcome for treatment of empyema, even with adjustment for confounding variables. VATS or thoracotomy as initial therapy for advanced empyema is associated with better outcomes.

▶ Managing a complicated parapneumonic effusion or empyema represents a very challenging task for the physician. Published guidelines by the American Association of Chest Physicians (AACP) help in making the initial decision between drainage and conservative treatment in parapneumonic effusions.[1] Once an effusion is considered an empyema there are several choices for evacuation of fluid, but the most important decision to be made lies between simple drainage by chest tube or via pigtail catheter with or without fibrinolytic therapy and surgical intervention that can be performed via thoracoscopy (video-assisted thoracic surgery [VATS]) or by open thoracotomy.

In this study, Wozniak et al sought to determine whether the choice of first procedure (drainage vs surgery) influenced the outcome in the management of empyema. Authors classified empyema in 3 stages using a modified American Thoracic Society classification system: stage I—early empyema with free flowing fluid and pH > 7.3, stage IIA—fibrinopurulent empyema with loculations, minimal, or no pleural peel and pH < 7.1, stage IIB—same as IIA with pleural peel and stage III with fibrothorax. Out of 106 patients with empyema, 2 patients with stage III disease where excluded. Most of remaining patients (84%) had advanced empyema (stage II). The most common organisms isolated from the pleural fluid where *Streptococcus* and *Staphylococcus* species in 31 patients. Treatment success was defined as no death and no need for subsequent drainage procedures. Simple drainage had an overall success rate of 38% to 40% compared with 81% for VATS and 89% for open thoracotomy. Drainage was much more effective with stage I disease versus stage II disease. The strongest predictor of in-hospital death was failure of the initial procedure. The authors conclude that choice of first intervention is essential in treatment success and survival in empyema, with surgery being a much better option than drainage, particularly in patients with advanced disease.

C. A. Speil, MD

Reference

1. Colice GL, Curtis A, Deslauriers J, et al. Medical and surgical treatment of parapneumonic effusions : an evidence-based guideline. *Chest.* 2000;118:1158-1171.

Early Use of Polymyxin B Hemoperfusion in Abdominal Septic Shock: The EUPHAS Randomized Controlled Trial
Cruz DN, Antonelli M, Fumagalli R, et al (St Bortolo Hosp and International Renal Res Inst Vicenza; Catholic Univ of Sacred Heart, Rome; Milano Bicocca Univ, St Gerardo dei Tintori Hosp, Monza; et al)
JAMA 301:2445-2452, 2009

Context.—Polymyxin B fiber column is a medical device designed to reduce blood endotoxin levels in sepsis. Gram-negative–induced abdominal sepsis is likely associated with high circulating endotoxin. Reducing circulating endotoxin levels with polymyxin B hemoperfusion could potentially improve patient clinical outcomes.

Objective.—To determine whether polymyxin B hemoperfusion added to conventional medical therapy improves clinical outcomes (mean arterial pressure [MAP], vasopressor requirement, oxygenation, organ dysfunction) and mortality compared with conventional therapy alone.

Design, Setting, and Patients.—A prospective, multicenter, randomized controlled trial (Early Use of Polymyxin B Hemoperfusion in Abdominal Sepsis [EUPHAS]) conducted at 10 Italian tertiary care intensive care units between December 2004 and December 2007. Sixty-four patients were enrolled with severe sepsis or septic shock who underwent emergency surgery for intra-abdominal infection.

Intervention.—Patients were randomized to either conventional therapy (n = 30) or conventional therapy plus 2 sessions of polymyxin B hemoperfusion (n = 34).

Main Outcome Measures.—Primary outcome was change in MAP and vasopressor requirement, and secondary outcomes were PaO_2/FIO_2 (fraction of inspired oxygen) ratio, change in organ dysfunction measured using Sequential Organ Failure Assessment (SOFA) scores, and 28-day mortality.

Results.—MAP increased (76 to 84 mm Hg; $P = .001$) and vasopressor requirement decreased (inotropic score, 29.9 to 6.8; $P < .001$) at 72 hours in the polymyxin B group but not in the conventional therapy group (MAP, 74 to 77 mm Hg; $P = .37$; inotropic score, 28.6 to 22.4; $P = .14$). The PaO_2/FIO_2 ratio increased slightly (235 to 264; $P = .049$) in the polymyxin B group but not in the conventional therapy group (217 to 228; $P = .79$). SOFA scores improved in the polymyxin B group but not in the conventional therapy group (change in SOFA, -3.4 vs -0.1; $P < .001$), and 28-day mortality was 32% (11/34 patients) in the polymyxin B group and 53% (16/30 patients) in the conventional therapy group (unadjusted hazard ratio [HR], 0.43; 95% confidence interval [CI], 0.20-0.94; adjusted HR, 0.36; 95% CI, 0.16-0.80).

Conclusion.—In this preliminary study, polymyxin B hemoperfusion added to conventional therapy significantly improved hemodynamics and organ dysfunction and reduced 28-day mortality in a targeted population with severe sepsis and/or septic shock from intra-abdominal gram-negative infections.

Trial Registration.—clinicaltrials.gov Identifier: NCT00629382.

▶ Endotoxin, a component of the outer cell membrane of gram-negative bacteria, has been considered for a long time an important factor in the pathogenesis of gram-negative sepsis and septic shock.[1] Consequently, different therapies that target endotoxin removal have been tried over the years. Polymixin B has a high affinity for endotoxin and has been used as an endotoxin adsorber in hemoperfusion devices. This type of therapy is widespread in Japan but not part of standard sepsis treatment in the United States or Western Europe.[2] A recent review of 28 studies showed benefit in using hemoperfusion with polymixin B for patients with sepsis or septic shock.[1] However, many of the studies reviewed were of lower quality and the authors concluded that larger randomized controlled trials (RCTs) are needed.

The Early Use of Polymyxin B Hemoperfusion in Abdominal Sepsis (EUPHAS) trial was a prospective randomized controlled multicenter study in patients with severe sepsis or septic shock due to intra-abdominal infections requiring emergency abdominal surgery. A total of 64 patients were randomized to standard therapy alone (30 patients) or standard therapy plus polymyxin B hemoperfusion (34 patients). Primary outcomes were changes in mean arterial pressure (MAP) and vasopressor requirements at 72 hours. Secondary end points were PaO_2/FiO_2 ratio, change in organ dysfunction, and 28-day mortality. At 72 hours, MAP significantly increased and the vasopressor requirements significantly decreased in the polymyxin B hemoperfusion group, but not in the conventional therapy group. The polymyxin B hemoperfusion group also had a significant reduction in the 28-day and in-hospital mortality rates compared with conventional therapy. The trial was stopped early due to the significant difference in mortality between the 2 arms observed at the interim analysis.

This study is the largest multicenter RCT to date on hemoperfusion with polymixin B in patients with septic shock caused by intra-abdominal infection. However, the trial refers to a specific population (patients with intra-abdominal infection who underwent surgery for source control) and findings may not be completely applicable to nonsurgical patients. Also, due to early termination, the number of patients analyzed was small, and therefore the statistical power of the study is significantly limited. As noted in the accompanying editorial in *JAMA*, a different outcome in only 1 patient would have eliminated the statistical significance of difference in mortality.[2] Nevertheless, based on this study and on the recent meta-analysis already mentioned, hemoperfusion using polymixin B appears promising. The authors conclude that a larger trial in a diverse population is indicated to confirm these findings. Considering that the therapy presented here is not used in the United States, another large randomized trial seems absolutely reasonable, despite the early termination of the European study.

C. A. Speil, MD

References

1. Cruz DN, Perazella MA, Bellomo R, et al. Effectiveness of polymyxin B-immobilized fiber column in sepsis: a systematic review. *Crit Care.* 2007;11:R47.
2. Kellum JA, Uchino S. International differences in the treatment of sepsis: are they justified? *JAMA.* 2009;301:2496-2497.

Antibiotic prescribing for presumed nonbacterial acute respiratory tract infections
Aspinall SL, Good CB, Metlay JP, et al (Ctr for Health Equity Res and Promotion, Pittsburgh, PA; et al)
Am J Emerg Med 27:544-551, 2009

Objective.—The objective of the study was to identify patient and provider factors associated with prescribing antibiotics for outpatients with acute respiratory tract infections of likely nonbacterial etiology.

Methods.—We identified outpatients who were diagnosed in the emergency department with nonspecific upper respiratory tract infections (URIs) and acute bronchitis at the VA Pittsburgh Healthcare System from June 15, 2003, to June 14, 2004, and the Philadelphia VA Medical Center from November 30, 2003, to March 31, 2004. Stepwise logistic regression was used to identify factors independently associated with antibiotic prescribing.

Results.—Overall, 26% of the 667 eligible patients with URIs and/or acute bronchitis received antibiotics. Antibiotics were prescribed significantly more frequently for acute bronchitis at one site (97% vs 65%, $P < .001$). Using multivariable analysis, the following factors were independently associated with antibiotic prescribing (odds ratio, 95%

confidence interval): presence of 1 or more comorbidities (2.1, 1.2-3.5), fever (2.5, 1.4-4.4), purulent sputum (2.5, 1.5-4.4), shortness of breath (2.8, 1.4-5.4), altered breath sounds (4.6, 2.4-8.6), diagnosis of acute bronchitis (15.9, 8.0-31.8), provider age ≥30 years (2.6, 1.1-6.3), and noninternal medicine specialty (2.7, 1.2-6.0).

Conclusions.—Antibiotic use was high and varied substantially for URIs and acute bronchitis. Specific signs and symptoms, a diagnosis of acute bronchitis, and provider age and specialty were associated with antibiotic prescribing. Interventions to decrease inappropriate prescribing should address the perceived utility of antibiotics in acute bronchitis and the accuracy of signs and symptoms in diagnosing a bacterial respiratory infection.

▶ Upper respiratory tract infections (URIs), including acute bronchitis account for a very large number of office and emergency department visits in the United States. Most of these infections have a viral etiology, and antibiotics are not an effective treatment.[1] Despite widely published guidelines, inappropriate antibiotic prescribing for URI, particularly acute bronchitis is common and leads to development of multidrug resistant bacteria and serious antibiotic-associated side effects.[2]

This analysis by Aspinall et al aimed to identify patient and provider-related factors associated with antibiotic prescription for URIs of probable nonbacterial etiology. Out of 2600 patients presenting with upper respiratory symptoms at 2 different VA facilities in Pennsylvania, 667 were enrolled in the study. Patients with possible bacterial infections, community-acquired pneumonia, and history of chronic obstructive pulmonary disease (COPD) were excluded. Overall, 26% with URIs received antibiotics, but the percentage went up significantly if acute bronchitis was diagnosed. Factors associated with increased antibiotic prescription included acute bronchitis (odds ratio 15.9), abnormal breath sounds (4.6), shortness of breath (2.8), self-reported fever (2.5), purulent sputum (2.5), presence of ≥1 comorbidities (2.1), provider age ≥30 (2.6), and provider specialty not internal medicine (2.7).

The authors conclude that although the antibiotics were generally overprescribed for URIs, this seemed to be a bigger issue with acute bronchitis. Overall, 78% of patients with acute bronchitis alone and 57% of patients who carried a diagnosis of both URI and acute bronchitis received antibiotics, compared with only 16% of patients diagnosed with URI alone. Based on this study and other published data, an intervention to decrease inappropriate antibiotic prescriptions for URIs should be particularly aimed at the proper diagnosis and management of acute bronchitis. The limited value of clinical signs and symptoms (ie, purulent sputum) in differentiating viral from bacterial infections should also be addressed, considering that many of these signs and symptoms are associated with an increase in the use of antibiotics.

C. A. Speil, MD

References

1. Stone S, et al. Antibiotic prescribing for patients with colds, upper respiratory tract infections, and bronchitis: a national study of hospital-based emergency departments. *Ann Emerg Med.* 2000;36:320-327.
2. Gonzales R, et al. Principles of appropriate antibiotic use for treatment of uncomplicated acute bronchitis: background. *Ann Intern Med.* 2001;134:521-529.

Statin Therapy Is Associated with Decreased Mortality in Patients with Infection

Donnino MW, Cocchi MN, Howell M, et al (Beth Israel Deaconess Med Ctr, Boston, MA; et al)
Acad Emerg Med 16:230-234, 2009

Objectives.—The objective was to investigate the association between statin therapy and mortality in emergency department (ED) patients with suspected infection.

Methods.—A secondary analysis of a prospective, observational cohort study was conducted at an urban, academic ED with approximately 50,000 annual visits. Data were collected between December 2003 and September 2004. Inclusion criteria consisted of age ≥ 18 years, clinical suspicion of infection, and hospital admission. Patients were divided by those receiving statin therapy and those not receiving statins while hospitalized. Medication data were collected from an inpatient pharmacy database. Comparisons were conducted with Fisher's exact test or Wilcoxon rank sum test. To adjust for baseline differences, multivariable logistic regression analysis controlling for gender, severity of illness (Mortality in Emergency Department Sepsis [MEDS] score), Charlson Comorbidity Index, and duration of statin therapy was performed.

Results.—Of 2,132 patients with suspected infection, 2,036 (95%) had interpretable pharmacy data and were analyzed. The cohort had a median age of 61 years (interquartile range [IQR] = 46–78 years) and a mortality of 3.9% (95% confidence interval [CI] = 3.1% to 4.8%). Patients who received statins ($n = 474$) had a lower unadjusted crude mortality (1.9%; 95% CI = 0.6% to 3.3%) compared to those who did not (4.5%; 95% CI = 3.4% to 5.4%; $p \leq 0.01$). When adjusting for gender, MEDS score, Charlson Comorbidity Index, and duration of statin therapy, the odds of death for statin patients was 0.27 (95% CI = 0.1 to 0.72; $p \leq 0.01$).

Conclusions.—Patients who were admitted to the hospital with infection and received statin therapy while hospitalized had a significantly lower in-hospital mortality compared to patients who did not receive a statin.

▶ Bacterial infections and the resulting sepsis syndrome are a leading cause of death worldwide. It is recognized that interventions trying to modify the course of sepsis syndrome should focus at least to some extent on modulating the inflammatory response.[1] Hydroxy-3-methylglutaryl (HMG) coenzyme A reductase inhibitors, known as statins, have been shown to have anti-inflammatory properties and protective effects on the endothelium, which may explain why they showed benefit in sepsis in a few observational studies.

The goal of this study by Donnino et al was to investigate the association between statin therapy and mortality in patients admitted to the hospital with presumed infection. The study analyzed data on 2036 patients with confirmed clinical infections. The overall in-hospital mortality for the group was 3.9%. Of these, 474 (23.3%) patients received a statin during their hospital stay. The patients' severity of disease and comorbidities were assessed by the Mortality in Emergency Department Sepsis (MEDS) score and by the Charlson Comorbidity Index (CCI) score, respectively. Patients who received a statin had a lower crude mortality rate than patients who did not (1.95% vs 4.5%, $P \leq .01$). After adjusting for gender, severity of disease, comorbidities, and duration of statin therapy, the odds of in-hospital death for patients who received statin therapy were 0.27.

Although this study cannot demonstrate cause and effect relationship due to its retrospective design, it showed a significantly decreased short-term mortality in the statin group despite the higher MEDS and CCI scores, which were probably a result of more severe preexisting illness in that group.

The possibly protective effects of statins in bacterial infections and sepsis are not well understood, but they may have clinical significance according to the current data. This study is an important part of the mounting evidence that may justify a larger, prospective randomized trial investigating the role of statin therapy in patients with bacterial infections and sepsis.

C. A. Speil, MD

Reference

1. Terblanche M, Almog Y, Rosenson RS, Smith TS, Hackam DG. Statins and sepsis: multiple modifications at multiple levels. *Lancet Infect Dis*. 2007;7:358-368.

12 Epidemiology and Management of Gram-Positive Infections

***Staphylococcus Aureus* Bacteremia Among Patients with Health Care-associated Fever**
Stryjewski ME, Kanafani ZA, Chu VH, et al (Duke Univ Med Ctr, Durham, NC; American Univ of Beirut Med Ctr, Lebanon; et al)
Am J Med 122:281-289, 2009

Background.—Although *Staphylococcus aureus* bacteremia is a common, serious infection, accurately identifying febrile patients with this diagnosis at the time of initial evaluation is difficult. The purpose of this investigation was to define clinical characteristics present at the time of the initial recognition of fever that were associated with the presence of any bloodstream infection and, in particular, with *S. aureus* bacteremia.

Methods.—All patients ≥18 years of age with a new episode of health care-associated fever (temperature ≥ 38°C) and at least one blood culture drawn were eligible for enrollment into this prospective multicenter cohort study. Multivariable analyses were conducted and internally validated scoring systems were developed to categorize the risk of bacteremia.

Results.—Of 1015 patients enrolled, 181 patients (17.8%) had clinically significant bacteremia, including 77 patients (7.6%) with *S. aureus* bacteremia. Clinical characteristics associated with *S. aureus* bacteremia were the presence of a hemodialysis graft or shunt (odds ratio [OR] 3.22; 95% confidence interval [CI], 1.85-5.61), chills (OR 2.38; 95% CI, 1.43-3.98), and a history of *S. aureus* infection (OR 2.68; 95% CI, 1.38-5.20). Peripheral vascular catheters were inversely associated with *S. aureus* bacteremia (OR 0.42; 95% CI, 0.26-0.69). Clinical characteristics associated with any bloodstream infection were central venous access, chills, history of S. *aureus* infection, and hemodialysis access.

Conclusions.—Among patients with health care-associated fever, the presence of easily recognizable clinical characteristics at the time of obtaining the initial blood cultures can help to identify patients at increased risk for any bloodstream infection, in particular for S. *aureus* bacteremia.

▶ *Staphylococcus aureus* remains among the most common causes of health care-associated bacteremia leading to substantial morbidity and mortality.[1] Initial decisions about antimicrobial therapy need to be made 24 to 48 hours before culture results are expected, and inappropriate empiric antibiotic treatment contributes to suboptimal outcomes. The decision making is particularly difficult in hospitalized patients who have multiple risk factors for gram-positive and gram-negative infection, and who have received or who are receiving antimicrobial therapy.

This prospective multicenter cohort study provides a number of easily recognizable clinical characteristics at the time of obtaining blood cultures for a new episode of fever (temperature > 38°C). Of the 181 patients with clinically significant positive blood cultures, 77 (8%) were *S aureus* followed by coagulase-negative staphylococci and *Enterococcus* species. The same factors have clinical characteristics associated with subsequent growth of *S aureus* from blood included hemodialysis graft or shunt, chills, and a history of *S aureus* infection. The same factors and or colonization with *S aureus* put the patients at the highest risk for recurrent *S aureus* bacteremia. These factors were common in both *S aureus* infection and any blood stream infection. However, they were more likely to be present in patients with *S aureus* bacteremia. This study validates the clinical observation that patients on hemodialysis and those with previous *S aureus* infection and or colonization with *S aureus* are at the highest risk for recurrent *S aureus* bacteremia.

N. M. Khardori, MD

Reference

1. Edmond MB, Wallace SE, McClish DK, Pfaller MA, Jones RN, Wenzel RP. Nosocomial bloodstream infections in United States hospitals: a three-year analysis. *Clin Infect Dis.* 1999;29:239-244.

Increasing Prevalence and Associated Risk Factors for Methicillin Resistant Staphylococcus Aureus Bacteriuria
Routh JC, Alt AL, Ashley RA, et al (Mayo Clinic, Rochester, MN)
J Urol 181:1694-1698, 2009

Purpose.—Infections due to methicillin resistant Staphylococcus aureus are becoming increasingly prevalent in hospitals and in the community. We reviewed our institutional experience to determine whether methicillin resistant S. aureus is becoming a more common cause of bacteriuria and to determine if there are specific risk factors that may predict the development of methicillin resistant S. aureus bacteriuria.

Materials and Methods.—We reviewed all urine cultures with a pure growth of a single organism obtained at our institution from 1997 and 2007. Patients with urine cultures positive for methicillin resistant S. aureus were compared to a cohort with cultures positive for methicillin sensitive S. aureus, and to a third cohort with cultures positive for Escherichia coli to determine patient characteristics and associated risk factors.

Results.—We identified 7,100 and 9,985 positive urine cultures performed in 1997 and 2007, respectively. The most common urinary organism was E. coli. The number of patients with methicillin resistant S. aureus bacteriuria increased from 18 (0.3%) to 74 (0.8%) (p < 0.001). On multivariate analysis older age (p = 0.004), catheter use (p = 0.004), hospital exposure (p < 0.001) and patient comorbidity (p < 0.001) were associated with methicillin resistant S. aureus bacteriuria compared with E. coli bacteriuria.

Conclusions.—Methicillin resistant S. aureus remains rare as a cause of bacteriuria but its incidence has increased during the last decade. Risk factors for methicillin resistant S. aureus bacteriuria include increased age, patient comorbidity, hospital exposure and catheter use. For patients with these risk factors and new onset urinary symptoms, methicillin resistant S. aureus should be considered a possible cause of urinary tract infection.

▶ Currently, more than 60% of staphylococcal infections in intensive care units in the United States are caused by methicillin-resistant *Staphylococcus aureus* (MRSA).[1] The distinction between health care associated and community-acquired MRSA strains has faded in recent years.[2] Invasive infections and skin and soft-tissue infections due to MRSA have been well documented in the recent literature. Bacteriuria due to MRSA in the absence of bacteremia has often been presumed to be secondary to contamination or colonization.

Routh et al in this study reviewed urine cultures with single organism growth at 2 time periods separated by 10 years (1997 and 2007). Symptomatic urinary tract infection (UTI) in patients with bacteriuria was defined by urinary symptoms, fever, or mental status changes and resolution of symptoms after appropriate antibiotic therapy. *Escherichia coli* remained the most common cause of UTI at both times, followed by *Enterococcus* species and *Klebsiella* species. Urine cultures growing methicillin-sensitive *S aureus* (MSSA) increased from 1% in 1997 to 1.4% in 2007. MRSA was grown from 0.3% urine cultures in 1997 compared with 0.8% in 2007. In patients with *Staphylococcus aureus* UTI, the likelihood of MRSA being the organism increased from 20% in 1997 to 35% in 2007 (*P* = .01). Patients with MRSA bacteriuria with risk factors like urinary catheter use, history of health care facility exposure, and new onset urinary symptoms should be treated for UTI.

N. M. Khardori, MD

References

1. Klevens RM, Edwards JR, Tenover FC, et al. Changes in the epidemiology of methicillin-resistant Staphylococcus aureus in intensive care units in US hospitals, 1992–2003. *Clin Infect Dis*. 2006;42:389.
2. Manian FA, Griesnauer S. Community-associated methicillin-resistant Staphylococcus aureus (MRSA) is replacing traditional health care-associated MRSA strains in surgical-site infections among inpatients. *Clin Infect Dis*. 2008;47:434.

Initial Low-Dose Gentamicin for *Staphylococcus aureus* Bacteremia and Endocarditis Is Nephrotoxic

Cosgrove SE, Vigliani GA, Fowler VG Jr, et al (Johns Hopkins Univ School of Medicine, Baltimore, MD; Beth Israel Deaconess Med Ctr, Boston, MA; et al)
Clin Infect Dis 48:713-721, 2009

Background.—The safety of adding initial low-dose gentamicin to anti-staphylococcal penicillins or vancomycin for treatment of suspected *Staphylococcus aureus* native valve endocarditis is unknown. This study evaluated the association between this practice and nephrotoxicity.

Methods.—We performed a prospective cohort study of safety data from a randomized, controlled trial of therapy for *S. aureus* bacteremia and native valve infective endocarditis involving 236 patients from 44 hospitals in 4 countries. Patients either received standard therapy (anti-staphylococcal penicillin or vancomycin) plus initial low-dose gentamicin ($n = 116$) or received daptomycin monotherapy ($n = 120$). We measured renal adverse events and clinically significant decreased creatinine clearance in patients (1) in the original randomized study arms and (2) who received any initial low-dose gentamicin either, as a study medication or ≤ 2 days before enrollment.

Results.—Renal adverse events occurred in 8 (7%) of 120 daptomycin recipients, 10 (19%) of 53 vancomycin recipients, and 11 (17%) of 63 antistaphylococcal penicillin recipients. Decreased creatinine clearance occurred in 9 (8%) of 113 of evaluable daptomycin recipients, 10 (22%) of 46 vancomycin recipients, and 16 (25%) of 63 antistaphylo-coccal penicillin recipients. An additional 21 patients received initial low-dose gentamicin ≤ 2 days before study enrollment. A total of 22% of patients who received initial low-dose gentamicin versus 8% of patients who did not receive initial low-dose gentamicin experienced decreased creatinine clearance ($P = .005$). Independent predictors of a clinically significant decrease in creatinine clearance were age ≥ 65 years and receipt of any initial low-dose gentamicin.

Conclusions.—Initial low-dose gentamicin as part of therapy for *S. aureus* bacteremia and native valve infective endocarditis is nephrotoxic and should not be used routinely, given the minimal existing data supporting its benefit.

▶ Based on the current American Heart Association guidelines, the addition of low-dose gentamicin to initial therapy of patients with *Staphylococcus aureus* endocarditis has become common. The concept that this approach achieves earlier clearance of blood cultures is based on in vitro data demonstrating synergy between antistaphylococcal penicillins or vancomycin and aminoglycosides. In vivo data from a rabbit model showed more rapid eradication of *S aureus* from cardiac vegetations when low-dose gentamicin is added to antistaphylococcal penicillins initially. Subsequently, it was shown that clearance time for methicillin-sensitive *S aureus* (MSSA) bacteremia decreased by 1 day in noninjection using patients with left-sided endocarditis, but it had no effect on morbidity or mortality.[1] Because patients receiving gentamicin for the first 2 weeks in addition to nafcillin in this study experienced significant renal impairment, the authors concluded that gentamicin should only be considered during the first 3 to 5 days of treatment. In spite of significant changes in host and pathogen factors, this practice has not been reevaluated in the past 25 years.

This prospective cohort study was undertaken to evaluate the safety of initial low-dose gentamicin for *S aureus* bacteremia and endocarditis. Gentamicin (1 mg/kg every 8 hours, with appropriate dose adjustment) for the first 4 days was added to nafcillin or vancomycin or daptomycin for high likelihood of left-sided endocarditis. Decreased creatinine clearance occurred in 22% of patients who received initial low-dose gentamicin compared with 8% of patients who did not. The demonstrated nephrotoxicity of this approach is significant considering the minimal data supporting a small nonsignificant benefit.

N. M. Khardori, MD

Reference

1. Korzeniiowshi O, Sande MA. Combination antimicrobial therapy for Staphylococcal aureus endocarditis in patients addicted to parenteral drugs and in nonaddicts: a prospective study. *Ann Intern Med.* 1982;97:496-503.

Staphylococcus lugdunensis, a Common Cause of Skin and Soft Tissue Infections in the Community
Böcher S, Tønning B, Skov RL, et al (Viborg Hosp, Denmark; Statens Serum Institut, Copenhagen, Denmark)
J Clin Microbiol 47:946-950, 2009

Staphylococcus lugdunensis, a rare cause of severe infections such as native valve endocarditis, often causes superficial skin infections similar to *Staphylococcus aureus* infections. We initiated a study to optimize the identification methods in the routine laboratory, followed by a population-based epidemiologic analysis of patients infected with *S. lugdunensis* in Viborg County, Denmark. Recognition of a characteristic *Eikenella corrodens*-like odor on Columbia sheep blood agar combined with colony pleomorphism and prominent β-hemolysis after 2 days of incubation, confirmed by API-ID-32 Staph, led to an 11-fold increase in the detection of *S. lugdunensis*. By these methods we found 491 *S. lugdunensis* infections in 4 years, corresponding to an incidence of 53 per 100,000 per year, an increase from 5 infections per 100,000 inhabitants in the preceding years. Seventy-five percent of the cases were found in general practice; these were dominated by skin abscesses (36%), wound infections (25%), and paronychias (13%). Fifty-six percent of the infections occurred below the waist, and toes were the most frequently infected site (21%). Only 3% of the patients suffered from severe invasive infections. The median age was 52 years, and the male/female ratio was 0.69. Our study shows that *S. lugdunensis* is a common cause of skin and soft-tissue infections (SSTI) and is probably underrated by many laboratories. *S. lugdunensis* should be accepted as a significant pathogen in SSTI and should be looked for in all routine bacteriological examinations, and clinicians should be acquainted with the name and the pathology of the bacterium.

▶ Coagulase-negative staphylococci (CoNS) as a group are often considered contaminants, colonizers, or low virulence opportunistic pathogens, and are seldom identified to species level. *Staphylococcus lugdunensis*, one of the CoNS, behaves more like *Staphylococcus aureus* than other members of CoNS. It causes native and prosthetic valve endocarditis, osteomyelitis, peritonitis, intravascular catheter infections, prosthetic joint infections, urinary tract infections, and intertriginous skin and soft-tissue infections (SSTI).[1]

This bench to bedside study reports improved microbiological methods to speciate CoNS, which led to an 11-fold increase in the detection of *S lugdunensis* corresponding to 491 *S lugdunensis* infections in 4 years. Severe invasive infection occurred in 3%. Skin abscesses (36%), wound infections (25%), and paronychias (13%) comprised 75% of the infections caused by *S lugdunensis*. This clinical correlation with cultures implicates *S lugdunensis* as a significant pathogen in SSTI, which should be looked for in all routine bacteriological specimens. The significance of *S lugdunensis* growing from clinical specimens should be conveyed to the clinicians.

N. M. Khardori, MD

Reference

1. Bellamy R, Barkham T. Staphylococcus lugdunensis infection sites; predominance of abscesses in the pelvic girdle region. *Clin. Infect. Dis.* 2002;35:E32-E34.

Outbreak of Invasive Group A Streptococcal Disease Among Children Attending a Day-Care Center

Agüero J, Ortega-Mendi M, Eliecer Cano M, et al (Univ Hosp Marqués de Valdecilla, Spain; General Directorate of Public Health, Govern of Cantabria; et al)
Pediatr Infect Dis J 27:602-604, 2008

Background.—Most cases of invasive group A streptococcal (GAS) disease arise sporadically in the community, but outbreaks of severe invasive GAS infections have been reported in closed environments, such as military populations, family communities and hospitals. An outbreak of invasive GAS disease involving 3 cases of streptococcal toxic shock syndrome (TSS), one with a fatal course, occurred among children attending a day-care center located in Cantabria, Northern Spain.

Objective.—To determine the characteristics of GAS isolates obtained from the outbreak environment.

Methods.—GAS isolates obtained from children attending the same day-care facility, staff members, and family contacts were assayed for *emm* typing, pulse-field gel electrophoresis (PFGE), and toxin-gene content. One isolate obtained from the fatal case was also characterized by multilocus sequence typing. Antimicrobial susceptibility testing was done. Strains from patients unrelated to the outbreak were included for comparison.

Results.—All GAS isolates from children attending the day-care center, including those from streptococcal TSS cases, shared the same *emm* type 4, genomic pattern by PFGE (A) and toxin-gene profile. Neither the *emm* type nor the PFGE pattern or toxin gene profile of the outbreak-associated strains were encountered among GAS isolated from household or staff contacts.

Conclusions.—A clone of GAS belonging to *emm* type 4 and characterized by a specific PFGE pattern and toxin-gene profile was responsible for a community outbreak of streptococcal TSS disease in a child day-care center in Spain. This is the first day-care outbreak reported in our country.

▶ Group A *Streptococcus* (GAS) or *Streptococcus pyogenes*, a common cause of pharyngitis, can also cause potentially fatal invasive infections like necrotizing fasciitis and toxic shock syndrome.[1] Although most cases are spread out, sporadic cases, outbreaks of invasive GAS disease have been described in closed environments, including families, nursing homes, and hospitals.[2]

This study reports an outbreak of invasive GAS disease in a child day-care center. At the epicenter of the outbreak were 3 children 15 to 39 months old who presented with multiorgan failure – one of whom died. Pharyngeal samples of all 40 children attending the day care, 189 household contacts, and 4 staff members were cultured. GAS isolates from necropsy specimens from the fatal case, blood samples from case 3, and throat samples from 10 out of 37 asymptomatic children all belonged to *emm* type 4 and all had the same specific pulse-field gel electrophoresis (PFGE) pattern and toxin-gene profile.

The outbreak clone was different from 13 GAS isolates from 166 family contacts to the asymptomatic children. Varicella, a known risk factor for invasive GAS disease, had been diagnosed in the fatal case 18 days before. This report extends outbreak invasive GAS disease to day care centers, and justifies notification and surveillance of this potentially fatal disease.

N. M. Khardori, MD

References

1. Stevens DL. Streptococcal toxic shock syndrome associated with necrotizing fasciitis. *Annu Rev Med.* 2000;51:271-288.
2. Ichiyama S, Nakashima K, Shimokata K, et al. Transmission of Streptococcus pyogenes causing toxic shock like syndrome among family members and confirmation by DNA macrorestriction analysis. *J Infect Dis.* 1997;175:723-726.

Population-Based Study of Invasive Disease Due to β-Hemolytic Streptococci of Groups Other than A and B
Broyles LN, Van Beneden C, Beall B, et al (Emory Univ School of Medicine, Atlanta, GA; Ctrs for Disease Control and Prevention; et al)
Clin Infect Dis 48:706-712, 2009

Background.—β-Hemolytic streptococci of groups other than A and B(NABS) are increasingly recognized as causes of clinically significant disease, but precise information about this heterogeneous group is lacking. We report the incidence of NABS infection and describe the epidemiologic and clinical characteristics.

Methods.—Active, population-based surveillance for invasive NABS was performed over a 2-year period in the 8-county metropolitan Atlanta, Georgia, area and the 3-county San Francisco Bay, California, area. Clinical records were reviewed, and available isolates were sent to the Centers for Disease Control and Prevention (Atlanta) for additional microbiologic characterization. Incidences were calculated using year-appropriate US Census Bureau data.

Results.—A total of 489 cases of invasive NABS infection were identified (3.2 cases per 100,000 population). The median age of patients was 55 years; 64% of patients were males, and 87% had underlying diseases. The incidence was higher among black persons than white persons (4.0 vs. 2.5 cases per 100,000 population; $P < .01$) and increased with age among all races. Infections were community acquired in 416 cases (85%). Among the 450 patients (94%) with NABS infection who were hospitalized, 55 (12%) died. Of 266 isolates (54%) speciated at the Centers for Disease Control and Prevention, 212 (80%) were *Streptococcus dysgalactiae* subspecies *equisimilis*; 46 (17%) were members of the *Streptococcus anginosus* group. *S. dysgalactiae* subspecies *equisimilis* primarily presented as skin and soft-tissue infection in older patients, whereas individuals with invasive *S. anginosus* group infections were more likely to be younger patients with intra-abdominal infections.

Conclusions.—NABS comprise multiple distinct species that cause a significant number of community-acquired invasive infections. Clinical manifestations differ by species. Thus, speciation of invasive NABS may be warranted in clinical settings.

▶ Non-A and non-B β-hemolytic streptococci (NABS), including groups C, G, F, and L are capable of causing significant disease. Groups G and C are the most common.[1] Group G β-hemolytic streptococci have surpassed group A streptococci as a leading cause of invasive streptococcal infection in some areas.[2] The true burden of NABS infection in the United States is not known because not all laboratories identify NABS isolates to species level and infections they cause are not reportable.

In this active, population-based surveillance for invasive NABS infections over a 2-year period in Atlanta, Georgia and San Francisco, California Bay area, a total of 489 cases were identified (3.2 cases per 100 000 population). Skin and soft-tissue infections in older patients and intra-abdominal infections in younger patients were common presentations. Mortality rate in the hospitalized patients was 12%. The NABS isolates from this surveillance were uniformly susceptible to penicillins and cephalosporins, but had significant resistance to erythromycin and tetracycline. Speciation of this heterogeneous group of bacteria and in vitro antimicrobial susceptibility testing are needed for clinical decision making and optimal management, in addition to improving understanding of NABS epidemiology.

N. M. Khardori, MD

References

1. Skogberg K, Simonen H, Renkonen O, Valtonen V. Beta-haemolytic group A, B, C, and G streptococcal septicaemia: a clinical study. *Scand J Infect Dis*. 1988;20: 119-125.
2. Sylvetsky N, Raveh D, Schlesinger Y, Rudensky B, Yinnon AM. Bacteremia due to β-hemolytic Streptococcus group G: increasing incidence and clinical characteristics of patients. *Am J Med*. 2002;112:622-626.

13 Human Immunodeficiency Virus

Effect of Early versus Deferred Antiretroviral Therapy for HIV on Survival
Kitahata MM, for the NA-ACCORD Investigators (Univ of Washington, Seattle; et al)
N Engl J Med 360:1815-1826, 2009

Background.—The optimal time for the initiation of antiretroviral therapy for asymptomatic patients with human immunodeficiency virus (HIV) infection is uncertain.

Methods.—We conducted two parallel analyses involving a total of 17,517 asymptomatic patients with HIV infection in the United States and Canada who received medical care during the period from 1996 through 2005. None of the patients had undergone previous antiretroviral therapy. In each group, we stratified the patients according to the CD4+ count (351 to 500 cells per cubic millimeter or >500 cells per cubic millimeter) at the initiation of antiretroviral therapy. In each group, we compared the relative risk of death for patients who initiated therapy when the CD4+ count was above each of the two thresholds of interest (early-therapy group) with that of patients who deferred therapy until the CD4+ count fell below these thresholds (deferred-therapy group).

Results.—In the first analysis, which involved 8362 patients, 2084 (25%) initiated therapy at a CD4+ count of 351 to 500 cells per cubic millimeter, and 6278 (75%) deferred therapy. After adjustment for calendar year, cohort of patients, and demographic and clinical characteristics, among patients in the deferred-therapy group there was an increase in the risk of death of 69%, as compared with that in the early-therapy group (relative risk in the deferred-therapy group, 1.69; 95% confidence interval [CI], 1.26 to 2.26; P < 0.001). In the second analysis involving 9155 patients, 2220 (24%) initiated therapy at a CD4+ count of more than 500 cells per cubic millimeter and 6935 (76%)

deferred therapy. Among patients in the deferred-therapy group, there was an increase in the risk of death of 94% (relative risk, 1.94; 95% CI, 1.37 to 2.79; P < 0.001).

Conclusions.—The early initiation of antiretroviral therapy before the CD4+ count fell below two prespecified thresholds significantly improved survival, as compared with deferred therapy.

▶ The current guidelines from the Department of Health and Human Services recommend starting antiretroviral therapy in adults with HIV infection with a CD4+ count of 350 or less, but the optimal timing of initiating therapy is unknown.[1]

This is an observational study involving a very large number of asymptomatic HIV patients from the United States and Canada who were treated between 1996 and 2005. The patients were stratified in 2 groups based on baseline CD4+ count (351-500 and above 500). Within each group, the patients who started antiretroviral therapy within 6 months from the measurement (early therapy) were compared with the patients who deferred therapy, the primary outcome being death from any cause. The authors found a significantly increased risk of death in both deferred therapy groups, even after adjustment for known risk factors such as hepatitis C virus (HCV) coinfection or IV drug use. Interestingly, the most deaths in all groups were from nonAIDS related illnesses, including nonAIDS defining cancers.

There is currently a trend in favor of starting antiretroviral therapy earlier, based on numerous observations, including the fact that even nonAIDS related illnesses such as cardiovascular disease are associated with lower CD4+ counts. The benefits of early therapy include increased control of viral replication, more complete immune restoration, and possibly even less side effects from antiretroviral medications. However, there is the potential of developing viral resistance, and the long-term side effects of antiretroviral therapy are not well defined. The authors show significantly increased risk of death of any cause even in patients with a CD4+ count above 500 who deferred antiretroviral therapy. This study makes a major contribution to the increasing amount of evidence showing benefit of early antiretroviral therapy, even in patients with very high CD4+ counts, and it is likely that the new HIV treatment guidelines will reflect the changes in our understanding of HIV infection.

C. A. Speil, MD

Reference

1. Department of Health and Human Services Panel on Antiretroviral Guidelines for Adults and Adolescents. Guidelines for the use of antiretroviral agents in HIV-1-infected adults and adolescents, http://www.aidsinfo.nih.gov/ContentFiles/AdultandAdolescentGL.pdf. Accessed November 3, 2008.

Incomplete Peripheral CD4+ Cell Count Restoration in HIV-Infected Patients Receiving Long-Term Antiretroviral Treatment

Kelley CF, Kitchen CMR, Hunt PW, et al (Emory Univ, Atlanta, GA; Univ of California at Los Angeles; Univ of California, San Francisco; et al)

Clin Infect Dis 48:787-794, 2009

Background.—Although antiretroviral therapy has the ability to fully restore a normal CD4+ cell count (>500 cells/mm^3) in most patients, it is not yet clear whether all patients can achieve normalization of their CD4+ cell count, in part because no study has followed up patients for > 7 years.

Methods.—Three hundred sixty-six patients from 5 clinical cohorts who maintained a plasma human immunodeficiency virus (HIV) RNA level ≤ 1000 copies/mL for at least 4 years after initiation of antiretroviral therapy were included. Changes in CD4+ cell count were evaluated using mixed-effects modeling, spline-smoothing regression, and Kaplan-Meier techniques.

Results.—The majority (83%) of the patients were men. The median CD4+ cell count at the time of therapy initiation was 201 cells/mm^3 (interquartile range, 72–344 cells/mm^3), and the median age was 47 years. The median follow-up period was 7.5 years (interquartile range, 5.5–9.7 years). CD4+ cell counts continued to increase throughout the follow-up period, albeit slowly after year 4. Although almost all patients (95%) who started therapy with a CD4+ cell count ≥ 300 cells/mm^3 were able to attain a CD4+ cell count ≥ 500 cells/mm^3, 44% of patients who started therapy with a CD4+ cell count <100 cells/mm^3 and 25% of patients who started therapy with a CD4+ cell count of 100–200 cells/mm^3 were unable to achieve a CD4+ cell count >500 cells/mm^3 over a mean duration of follow-up of 7.5 years; many did not reach this threshold by year 10. Twenty-four percent of individuals with a CD4+ cell count <500 cells/mm^3 at year 4 had evidence of a CD4+ cell count plateau after year 4. The frequency of detectable viremia ("blips") after year 4 was not associated with the magnitude of the CD4+ cell count change.

Conclusions.—A substantial proportion of patients who delay therapy until their CD+ cell count decreases to <200 cells/mm^3 do not achieve a normal CD4+ cell count, even after a decade of otherwise effective antiretroviral therapy. Although the majority of patients have evidence of slow increases in their CD4+ cell count over time, many do not. These individuals may have an elevated risk of non–AIDS-related morbidity and mortality.

▶ CD4+ count is the most important marker of immunological response to treatment in HIV-infected patients. Lower CD4+ counts on therapy have been associated with increased morbidity and mortality, both AIDS and non-AIDS related in this population.[1] Moreover, it was shown that patients who achieve cell counts of > 500/mm^3 have mortality rates similar to the general population.[2] It is because of this that increasing CD4$^+$ count has become the principal goal of antiretroviral treatment.

This study is focusing on analyzing the immune restoration in HIV-infected patients who achieved long-term viral suppression on therapy. The authors followed 366 HIV-infected patients from 5 different clinical cohorts who were able to maintain HIV RNA levels <1000 copies/mL for at least 4 years following initiation of antiretroviral treatment. Baseline CD4$^+$ cell count and age were found to be important predictors of immune restoration (as measured by increase in CD4$^+$ cells) in this cohort. While 95% of patients with a baseline CD4$^+$ > 300/mm^3 were able to eventually achieve a CD4$^+$ count > 500/mm^3, only 75% of patients with CD4$^+$ of 100 to 200/mm^3, and 56% of patients with CD4$^+$ < 100/mm^3 did so. The authors conclude that delay of antiretroviral therapy until CD4$^+$ cell count falls below 200/mm^3 is clearly associated with decreased immune reconstitution and all the dire consequences that result from it. The study adds important evidence in favor of early initiation of antiretroviral therapy as emphasized in the current guidelines. These findings were also discussed in the accompanying editorial.[3]

C. A. Speil, MD

References

1. Baker JV, et al. CD4+ count and risk of non-AIDS diseases following initial treatment for HIV infection. *AIDS.* 2008;22:841-848.
2. Lewden C, et al. Agence Nationale de Recherches sur le Sida et les Hepatites Virales (ANRS) CO8 APROCO-COPILOTE Study Group; Agence Nationale de Recherches sur le Sida et les Hepatites Virales (ANRS) CO3 AQUITAINE Study Group. HIV-infected adults with a CD4 cell count greater than 500 cells/mm^3 on long-term combination antiretroviral therapy reach same mortality rates as the general population. *J Acquir Immune Defic Syndr.* 2007;46:72-77.
3. Julg B, Walker BD. The paradox of incomplete CD4 cell count restoration despite successful antiretroviral treatment and the need to start highly active antiretroviral therapy early. *Clin Inf Dis.* 2009;48:795-797.

Long-Term Control of HIV by *CCR5* Delta32/Delta32 Stem-Cell Transplantation

Hütter G, Nowak D, Mossner M, et al (Campus Benjamin Franklin, Berlin, Germany; et al)
N Engl J Med 360:692-698, 2009

Infection with the human immunodeficiency virus type 1 (HIV-1) requires the presence of a CD4 receptor and a chemokine receptor, principally chemokine receptor 5 (CCR5). Homozygosity for a 32-bp deletion in the *CCR5* allele provides resistance against HIV-1 acquisition. We transplanted stem cells from a donor who was homozygous for *CCR5* delta32 in a patient with acute myeloid leukemia and HIV-1 infection. The patient remained without viral rebound 20 months after transplantation and discontinuation of antiretroviral therapy. This outcome demonstrates the critical role *CCR5* plays in maintaining HIV-1 infection.

▶ Despite significant advances in our understanding and treatment of HIV infection it remains incurable and continues to cause significant morbidity and mortality worldwide. HIV disease represents a major public health problem everywhere, but it takes catastrophic proportions in countries with limited resources. Infection with HIV requires the presence of the CD4 receptor and another chemokine receptor on the surface of target cells, either chemokine receptor 5 (CCR5) on macrophages or CXC chemokine receptor (CXCR4) on T lymphocytes. Most often, the wild type virus is macrophage tropic or *CCR5* variant, therefore, individuals who lack this receptor are unusually resistant to infection with HIV and, if infected, may have a slower progression of disease.[1] This is supported by observations in long-term nonprogressors and in people that remained seronegative after being repeatedly exposed to the virus. About 1% to 3% of the Western population is homozygous for the *CCR5* deletion.[2]

In this study by Hütter et al, the investigators have performed an allogeneic stem-cell transplant (SCT) in a patient with HIV-1 infection and acute myeloid leukemia (AML). The cells were obtained from a human leukocyte antigen (HLA)-compatible, unrelated donor who was homozygous for the *CCR5* delta32 deletion. Sequence analysis of the patient's HIV showed *CCR5* coreceptor use; however, ultradeep sequencing analysis showed a small proportion of virus (2.9%) to be X4 and dual tropic. The patient had a relapse of the AML at 332 days after the SCT, and a second transplant was performed from the same donor. The second procedure resulted in remission of the AML, and the patient remained disease free at 20 months follow-up. The patient's highly active antiretroviral therapy (HAART) was discontinued 1 day before the first SCT, and the levels of HIV-1 RNA remained undetectable for all of the follow-up period. The patient's CD4+ count was above 400 at the 20 months follow-up in the absence of any antiretroviral therapy.

This study again shows the major importance of the chemokine receptors, particularly *CCR5*, in the pathogenesis and progression of HIV infection, and it should encourage further research into *CCR5*-directed therapy such as blocking or modifying the *CCR5* receptors at the gene level. The only *CCR5*-directed therapy so far, the antiviral drug maraviroc, has shown good results, but has to be given with other antiretroviral medications, and of course it is only applicable for *CCR5* tropic viruses.

C. A. Speil, MD

References

1. Liu R, Paxton WA, Choe S, et al. Homozygous defect in HIV-1 coreceptor accounts for resistance of some multiply-exposed individuals to HIV-1 infection. *Cell.* 1996;86:367-377.
2. Levy AJ. Not an HIV Cure, but encouraging new directions [editorial]. *N Engl J Med.* 2009;360:724.

14 Tuberculosis

Mycobacterium tuberculosis and polymorphonuclear pleural effusion: Incidence and clinical pointers

Lin M-T, The TAMI Group (Natl Taiwan Univ Hosp, Taipei; et al)
Respir Med 103:820-826, 2009

Background.—Delayed diagnosis and treatment of a polymorphonuclear cell (PMN)-predominant pleural effusion due to *Mycobacterium tuberculosis* (MTB) are associated with poor outcome and the risk of tuberculosis transmission. We investigated the clinical differences of PMN-predominant pleural effusion due to MTB or other microorganisms.

Methods.—From January 2000 to April 2007, a total of 354 patients with tuberculous pleurisy were identified. Among them, 39 (11.0%) adults had PMN-predominant pleural effusion (MTB group). Their clinical characteristics were compared with the 117 age-/gender-matched controls (1:3) selected from 715 patients with PMN-predominant pleural effusion due to other microorganisms.

Results.—Among patients with PMN-predominant septic pleural effusion, 5.2% were due to MTB. The in-hospital mortality rate in the MTB group was 36%, similar to that of the control group. Sputum samples were culture-positive for MTB in 41%. Weight loss ($p = 0.006$), initial leukocyte count $\leq 11,000/\mu L$ ($p = 0.007$), and poor clinical response to empirical antibiotics in the first 3 days ($p = 0.002$) were independent factors suggestive of tuberculous pleurisy. A shift toward mononuclear cell predominance of pleural effusions within 1 week was significantly associated with tuberculous pleurisy. In the MTB group, if anti-tuberculous treatment was started more than 14 days after the initial visit, there was a worse prognosis ($p = 0.034$). Among those with delayed treatment, 96.2% had finding(s) suggestive of tuberculous pleurisy.

Conclusions.—A high index of clinical suspicion can identify MTB in about 5.2% of patients presenting with PMN-predominant septic pleural effusions. Awareness of the clinical pointers can lead to early diagnosis and improved clinical outcome.

▶ Early diagnosis and treatment of pleural effusion caused by *Mycobacterium tuberculosis* are important for both patient outcome and preventing further transmission. It is generally accepted that pleural effusion with mononuclear cell predominance favors a chronic disease process, including tubercular pleurisy.[1] It is, therefore, easy not to consider a diagnosis of early tuberculosis pleurisy in patients with predominantly polymorphonuclear cells (PMN) in the pleural fluid. *M tuberculosis* is cultured from sputum samples of 52% of patients with tuberculosis pleurisy, even in the absence of chest X-ray abnormalities. These patients are infectious and able to transmit tuberculosis.[2]

This retrospective study conducted in a tuberculosis high prevalence area investigated clinical features with the potential of differentiating PMN-predominant pleural effusion due to *M tuberculosis* from that due to other organisms. In 5.2% of PMN-predominant pleural effusion, it was due to tuberculosis with a mortality rate of 36%. Sputum samples were positive for *M tuberculosis* in 41%. The clinical features that were independently suggestive of tubercular pleurisy included initial peripheral leukocyte count < 11 000 µL, weight loss, poor response to empiric antibiotics in the first 3 days, and a shift toward mononuclear cell predominance at repeat analysis of pleural fluid within 1 week. Based on these data, in patients with risk factors for tuberculosis a follow-up study of pleural fluid within 1 week might lead to earlier treatment of tubercular pleurisy.

N. M. Khardori, MD

References

1. Light RW. Management of pleural effusions. *J Formos Med Assoc.* 2000;99: 523-531.
2. Conde MB, Loivos AC, Rezende VM, et al. Yield of Sputum induction in the diagnosis of plural tuberculosis. *Am J Respir Crit Care Med.* 2003;167:723-725.

Comparative Performance of Tuberculin Skin Test, QuantiFERON-TB-Gold In Tube Assay, and T-Spot.*TB* Test in Contact Investigations for Tuberculosis

Diel R, Loddenkemper R, Meywald-Walter K, et al (Univ of Düsseldorf, Germany; German Central Committee Against Tuberculosis; Public Health Dep Hamburg-Central, Germany; et al)
Chest 135:1010-1018, 2009

Rationale.—*Mycobacterium tuberculosis* (MTB)-specific interferon-γ release assays (IGRAs) are an alternative or adjunct to the tuberculin skin test (TST) in identifying recent contacts with latent tuberculosis infection (LTBI), but there are scarce data directly comparing performance of the tests.

Objective.—To evaluate the agreement between both IGRAs and to determine which contacts were most likely to represent LTBI, the Quanti-FERON-TB-Gold In Tube assay (QFT) and the T-Spot.*TB* test (T-Spot) were compared in TST-positive persons recently exposed to pulmonary tuberculosis cases.

Methods.—Prospectively enrolled close contacts (n = 812) of 123 culture-confirmed tuberculosis source cases underwent IGRA testing using standardized collected data. Factors independently influencing the risk of MTB infection and their interactions with each other were evaluated by multivariate analysis.

Results.—Five variables were found to significantly predict a positive IGRA test result (age, source case acid-fast bacilli positive and/or coughing, cumulative exposure time, foreign origin). There was excellent agreement between the two IGRAs (93.9%, κ = 0.85), with QFT finding 30.2% of contacts positive and T-Spot finding 28.7%. Assuming positivity to both IGRAs as true infection, sensitivity of the TST at > 10 mm was 72% and at > 15 mm was 39.7%. The use of either IGRA as a replacement for the TST would decrease the number of LTBI suspects to be investigated by approximately 70%.

Conclusions.—IGRAs are a more accurate indicator of the presence of LTBI than the TST. Both QFT and T-Spot appear to be valuable public health tools, showing excellent agreement with each other.

▶ With the goal of improving the diagnosis of latent tuberculosis infection (LTBI), a number of in vitro assays measuring (Mycobacterium tuberculosis [MTB])-specific interferon-γ release assays (IGRAs) have recently become available. Treatment of recently infected patients (eg, those detected during contact investigations) is central to tuberculosis control in low-incidence countries like the United States. The in vivo correlate of delayed type hypersensitivity as detected by tuberculin skin test (TST) has a high negative predictive value in nonimmunocompromised patients. But cross-reactive immune response to BCG vaccination or infection with mycobacteria other than *M tuberculosis* limits its usefulness as a diagnostic test. IGRAs have been shown to be at least as sensitive as TST (without the cross reactivity with other mycobacteria) for active tuberculosis.[2]

This study compared QuantiFERON TB Gold in tube assay and T-spot TB tests in a large cohort of TST-positive (> 5 mm) close contacts of active tuberculosis cases. Both tests in previous studies have been shown to be positive in association with measures of exposure and infection risk. The overall agreement between the 2 tests was excellent (93.9%) in this study. Using these tests as the comparator, the specificity of TST was 64.5%, 72%, and 39.7% respectively, using a cutoff of > 15 mm, > 10 mm, and > 5 mm. The positive rate for both IGRAs increased with higher TST cutoffs the contacts who reported coughing in their source case, cumulative exposure time of contacts, and in contacts of acid-fast bacilli (AFB)-positive source cases.

Although data from this study are encouraging, a number of questions remain unanswered. IGRAs may not detect latent or active TB in patients with lymphocytopenia, they have a low positive predictive value in active TB, and the results may be indeterminate in some patients. This study and other current literature indicate that IGRAs have improved diagnostic yield of noninvasive TB testing but are not yet optimal.

For further reading on this subject I suggest an article by the American Thoracic Society.[1]

N. M. Khardori, MD

References

1. American Thoracic Society. Targeted tuberculin testing and treatment of latent tuberculosis infection. *Am J Respir Crit Care Med.* 2000;161:S221-S247.
2. Mori T, Sakatani M, Yamagishih F, et al. Specific detection of tuberculosis infection: an interferon-γ-based assay using new antigens. *Am J Respir Crit Care Med.* 2004;170:59-64.

Within-Subject Variability and Boosting of T-Cell Interferon-γ Responses after Tuberculin Skin Testing

van Zyl-Smit RN, Pai M, Peprah K, et al (Univ of Cape Town, South Africa; McGill Univ, Montreal, Canada; et al)

Am J Respir Crit Care Med 180:49-58, 2009

Rationale.—The optimal strategy for the diagnosis of latent tuberculosis infection is controversial. Adoption of a two-step strategy (tuberculin skin test [TST] followed by an IFN-γ release assay [IGRA], compared with an IGRA alone), may be limited by TST-mediated boosting of subsequent IGRA responses. Assessment of within subject IGRA variability will aid in establishing thresholds for conversions and reversions, and interpretation of serial testing results.

Objectives.—To determine short-term IGRA variability and the impact of TST on subsequent IGRA results.

Methods.—Within-subject variability and TST-mediated boosting of IGRA responses were evaluated in 26 South African participants with varying exposure risk. IGRAs (T-SPOT.*TB*, QuantiFERON-TB Gold In-Tube [QuantiFERON-TB-GIT], PPD, and heparin-binding hemagglutinin) were repeated four times over 21 days pre-TST, and on Days 3, 7, 28, and 84 post-TST administration.

Measurements and Main Results.—All participants showed within-subject IGRA variability. Changes of ± 3 spots (T-SPOT.*TB*) or ± 80% from the mean IFN-γ response (QuantiFERON-TB-GIT) over 3 weeks explained 95% of the variability. Spontaneous conversions/ reversions occurred in 7 of 26 subjects (27%) (6 for T-SPOT.*TB* and 1 for Quanti-FERON-TB-GIT [$P = 0.049$]) during the within-patient variability studies (pre-TST). After the TST eight subjects (33%) boosted above the defined baseline variability. By Day 7 post-TST, but not Day 3, 2 (12.5%) initially IGRA-negative test subjects converted. By contrast, boosting of PPD and heparin-binding hemagglutinin occurred by Day 3 post-TST.

Conclusions.—When using a two-step screening strategy it appears safe to perform a QuantiFERON-TB-GIT or T-SPOT.*TB* IGRA within 3 days of performing the TST. A 3-spot or 80% IFN-γ response variation, on either side of baseline values, explains 95% of the short-term variability and may be useful for interpreting conversions and reversions, and values close to the cut-point.

▶ This article looks at Interferon-γ release assays (IGRAs) that use peripheral blood-derived T-cell responses to *Mycobacterium tuberculosis* specific proteins, early secreted antigenic target 6 (ESAT-6), culture filtrate protein-10 (CFP-10), and TB7.7 (p4).[1] These proteins are absent in BCG vaccines and most other nontubercular bacteria (except *Mycobacterium kansasii, Mycobacterium marinum*, and *Mycobacterium szulgai*). IGRAs have been shown to be sensitive and specific laboratory markers of presumed latent tuberculosis infection (LTBI).[2] The views on how the tuberculin skin test (TST) and IGRAs can be used for LTBI screening are divergent. The United States Centers for Disease Control and Prevention (CDC) guidelines recommend that a single IGRA can replace the TST. The United Kingdom based National Institute for Health and Clinical Excellence (NICE) and revised Canadian guidelines recommend that a positive TST be followed by an IGRA (up to 6 weeks after TST in the United Kingdom guidelines). The NICE recommendation takes into account cost-benefit analysis and the rationale that the equally sensitive and more widely available test (TST) should precede the use of a more specific but complex assay (IGRA). The PPD RT-23, a culture filtrate of *M tuberculosis,* contains many antigens, including ESAT-6 and CFP-10 (used in commercially available IGRA tests), as well as other TB-specific antigens such as heparin-binding hemagglutinin (HBHA). Because of the antigen sharing between TST and IGRA reagents, it is a reasonable hypothesis that previous TST could result in a "false positive" boosted IGRA result. Based on the results published in this study in South Africa, provision for the boosting effect and within-subject variability should be made when using a 2-step screening strategy. The authors conclude that it is safe to perform IGRAs within 3 days of performing TST, and short-term within-subject variability may be useful in interpreting conversions and reversions.

N. M. Khardori, MD

References

1. Schoepfer AM, Flogerzi B, Fallegger S, et al. Comparison of interferon-gamma release assay versus tuberculin skin test for tuberculosis screening in inflammatory bowel disease. *Am J Gastroenterol.* 2008;103:2799-2806.
2. Pai M, Zwerling A, Menzies D. Systematic review: T-cell-based assays for the diagnosis of latent tuberculosis infection: an update. *Ann Intern Med.* 2008;149:177-194.

Latent Tuberculosis Diagnosis in Children by Using the QuantiFERON-TB Gold In-Tube Test

Lighter J, Rigaud M, Eduardo R, et al (New York Univ School of Medicine)
Pediatrics 123:30-37, 2009

Background.—The QuantiFERON-TB Gold test was the first blood test to be approved for the diagnosis of latent tuberculosis infection. Although it has been shown to be sensitive and specific in adults, limited data on its performance in children are available.

Methods.—This was a prospective study of children receiving health care in New York, New York. Each child was assessed for risk factors for *Mycobacterium tuberculosis* infection, underwent tuberculin skin testing, and had a QuantiFERON-TB Gold In-Tube test performed. The concordance between tuberculin skin test and QuantiFERON-TB Gold In-Tube test results was calculated, and the results were analyzed according to the likelihood of exposure to *M tuberculosis*.

Results.—Data for 207 children with valid tuberculin skin test and QuantiFERON-TB Gold In-Tube test results were analyzed. There was excellent correlation between negative tuberculin skin test results and negative QuantiFERON-TB Gold In-Tube test results; however, only 23% of children with positive tuberculin skin test results had positive QuantiFERON-TB Gold In-Tube test results. Positive QuantiFERON-TB Gold In-Tube test results were associated with increased likelihood of M tuberculosis exposure, and interferon γ levels were higher in children with known recent exposure to *M tuberculosis*, compared with children with older exposure histories. Younger children produced lower interferon γ levels in response to the mitogen (phytohemagglutinin) control used in the QuantiFERON-TB Gold In-Tube test, but indeterminant results were low for children of all ages. Performance characteristics were similar across all age groups.

Conclusion.—The QuantiFERON-TB Gold In-Tube test is a specific test for M tuberculosis exposure in children, with performance characteristics similar to those for adults residing in regions with low levels of endemic disease. Concerns about test sensitivity, especially for children < 2 years of age, will require additional prospective long-term evaluation.

▶ An improved screening method for latent tuberculosis infection (LTBI) in children would be extremely useful because tuberculosis causes > 450 000 cases per year in children. Also, children are more likely to develop disseminated and serious disease. The QuantiFERON-TB Gold test was the first blood test to be approved for the diagnosis of LTBI; the test has been shown to be sensitive and specific in adults.[1,2]

Lighter et al are reporting a study done in children less than 18 years who were receiving care at a public hospital in New York City. The children were assessed for risk factors for *Mycobacterium tuberculosis* infection and underwent tuberculin skin test (TST) and QuantiFERON-TB Gold In-Tube Testing. This is an area with low levels of endemic tuberculosis with an incidence of

4.6 cases per 100 000 population reported in 2006. The authors report performance characteristics in this cohort of children comparable with those for adults residing in regions with low levels of endemic disease. Although indeterminate results were low for all ages, children less than 2 years of age produced lower interferon-γ levels in response to the control mitogen (phytohemagglutinin). This could mean more false negative interferon γ-releasing assays (IGRAs) in this age group, leading to risk for developing active tuberculosis. However, using a more specific test than TST, such as IGRA, fewer children will receive isoniazid prophylaxis.

N. M. Khardori, MD

References

1. Mazurek GH, Zajdowicz MJ, Hankinson AL, et al. Detection of Mycobacterium tuberculosis infection in United States Navy recruits using the tuberculin skin test or whole-blood Interferon-γ release assays. *Clin Infect Dis.* 2007;45:826-836.
2. Arend SM, Thijsen SF, Leyten EM, et al. Comparison of two Interferon-γ assays and tuberculin skin test for tracing tuberculosis contacts. *Am J Respir Crit Care Med.* 2007;175:618-627.

Screening of tuberculosis by interferon-γ assay before biologic therapy for rheumatoid arthritis
Murakami S, Takeno M, Kirino Y, et al (Yokohama City Univ Graduate School of Medicine, Japan; et al)
Tuberculosis 89:136-141, 2009

Infection with *Mycobacterium tuberculosis* (*M. tuberculosis*) is a critical complication in anti-TNF therapies. In 141 BCG vaccinated healthy individuals and 71 rheumatoid arthritis (RA) patients as screening before anti-TNF therapies, *M. tuberculosis* specific immune responses were evaluated by tuberculin skin test (TST) and enzyme-linked immunospot assay (ELISPOT), which detected antigen specific IFN-γ secreting cells in peripheral blood mononuclear cells simulated with either purified protein derivative (PPD), early secretory antigen target 6 (ESAT-6) or culture filtrate protein 10 (CFP-10). Induration over 5 mm in TST was found in 87.9% of controls and 21.4% of RA patients. Erythema size in TST was significantly suppressed in RA patients, especially those receiving prednisolone (PSL), whereas the PPD specific IFN-γ secretion was less attenuated. Significant responses to either ESAT-6 or CFP-10 in ELISPOT were detected in 14.1% of RA patients including those having positive TST, while the ELISPOT assay was negative in all healthy individuals and 73.3% of RA patients having positive TST. Of ELISPOT positive RA patients, mean dosage of PSL was 4.58 mg and 1.25 mg in TST negative and positive patients, respectively. Thus, ELISPOT is useful for screening of tuberculosis in RA patients, even in those receiving corticosteroids.

▶ The use of antitumor necrosis factor (TNF) therapy has added to the groups at risk for reactivation of latent tuberculosis (TB), which is observed within 6 months of initiation.[1] The estimated incidence of TB in patients receiving inflix-imab was 24.4 cases per 100 000 patient-year compared with 6.2 cases in the United States general population. Similar data were reported from Spain, Portugal, Greece, and Japan. Tuberculin skin test (TST) and chest X-ray are recommended to screen for latent TB before antiTNF therapy. TST is known to cause a false-negative reaction in immunosuppressed patients. Interferon-γ release assays (IGRAs) distinguish between patients with TB and BCG-vaccinated individuals.[2] The sensitivity of these assays is high enough to detect responses in immunocompromised HIV infected patients and malnourished infants.[2]

The study by Murakami et al from Japan provides data on the usefulness of an interferon-based enzyme-linked immunospot assay (ELISPOT) in screening for TB before biologic therapy for rheumatoid arthritis. The test was found useful in this patient group, including those receiving corticosteroids for rheumatoid arthritis.

N. M. Khardori, MD

References

1. Keane J, Gershon S, Wise RP, et al. Tuberculosis associated with infliximab, a tumor necrosis factor alpha-neutralizing agent. *N Engl J Med.* 2001;345:1098-1104.
2. Ferrara G, Losi M, D'Amico R, et al. Use in routine clinical practice of two commercial blood tests for diagnosis of infection with Mycobacterium tuberculosis: a prospective study. *Lancet.* 2007;367:1328-1334.

Risk of sensitization in healthy adults following repeated administration of rdESAT-6 skin test reagent by the Mantoux injection technique
Lillebaek T, Bergstedt W, Tingskov PN, et al (Univ of Copenhagen, Denmark; Statens Serum Institut (SSI), Copenhagen, Denmark)
Tuberculosis 89:158-162, 2009

Limited specificity of the tuberculin skin test incited the development of the intradermal *Mycobacterium tuberculosis*-specific rdESAT-6 skin test. Animal studies have shown, however, that there is a possible risk of sensitization when repeated injections of rdESAT-6 are given. The aim of this phase 1 open clinical trial was to assess the sensitization risk and safety of repeated administration of rdESAT-6 reagent in 31 healthy adult volunteers. Three groups of volunteers received two fixed doses of 0.1 μg rdESAT-6 28, 56 or 112 days apart, respectively. After the second injection, the diameter of induration and/or redness at the injection site was measured and taken as a possible sensitization reaction if >5 mm. In vitro interferon γ (IFN-γ) responses were measured as supportive evidence. Local adverse reactions at the injection site and adverse events were recorded. One out of 31 (3%) volunteers showed a positive skin reaction (sensitization) upon a second injection of rdESAT-6 after 28 days and an increased IFN-γ response to ESAT-6. For 7 (23%) of the volunteers, local adverse reactions related to the product were registered, but all reactions were mild and predictable. In conclusion, repeated injections of the rdESAT-6 skin test reagent are safe, and sensitization occurs at a low rate, especially if the time span between succeeding doses is wide.

▶ A large number of published studies have demonstrated the usefulness of interferon-γ release assays (IGRAs) using *Mycobacterium tuberculosis* specific antigens for screening of latent TB infection (LTBI) and diagnosis of active TB.[1] They have also been shown to discriminate between TB infection and BCG vaccination-induced cell mediated immune responses.[2] Although not optimal yet, they have the potential of improving detection of TB infection in adults and children, including those who have received previous BCG vaccination. However, these assays are dependent on the availability of advanced laboratory facilities and trained personnel. This limits their use in many areas of the world that most need them, ie, TB high-burden and resource-limited countries. A new and improved skin test (based on the current tuberculin skin test [TST]) would be more feasible and therefore more useful in these countries.

The early secretory antigen target-6 (ESAT-6) is a protein expressed by *M tuberculosis*, *M bovis*, and *M africanum*.[3] A new skin test using a recombinant dimer of ESAT-6 (rdESAT-6) has been shown to elicit large delayed type hypersensitivity (DTH) skin reactions in guinea pigs infected with *M tuberculosis*, but not those sensitized with bacille Calmette-Guérin (BCG) or *M avium*. This study presents the findings of a phase 1 open clinical trial looking at the immunogenicity and safety of rdESAT-6 in healthy adult volunteers. The immune response was measured by in vivo skin reaction (sensitization) and by in vitro interferon-γ (IFN-γ) production after 2 injections of rdESAT-6 separated by 28, 56, or 112 days. Only 3% (1 out of 31) of volunteers showed a positive skin reaction and an increased IFN-γ; response to ESAT-6 following a second injection of rdESAT-6 after 28 days. Local reactions in 23% of volunteers were mild and predictable. Based on this well done study, repeated injections of rdESAT-6 skin reagents are safe with low sensitization rates especially if the doses are widely spaced.

N. M. Khardori, MD

References

1. Madhukar P, Riley LW, Colford JM Jr. Interferon-γ; assays in the immune-diagnosis of tuberculosis: a systematic review. *Lancet Infect Dis.* 2004;4:761-776.
2. Arend SM, Franken WPJ, Aggerbeck H, et al. Double-blind randomized phase 1 study comparing rdESAT-6 to tuberculin as skin test reagent in the diagnosis of tuberculosis infection. *Tuberculosis.* 2007;88:249-261.
3. Andersen P, Munck ME, Pollock JI, Doherty TM. Specific immune-based diagnosis of tuberculosis. *Lancet.* 2000;356:1099-1104.

15 Health Care Associated Infections

Health Care–Associated *Clostridium difficile* Infection in Adults Admitted to Acute Care Hospitals in Canada: A Canadian Nosocomial Infection Surveillance Program Study
Gravel D, Canadian Nosocomial Infection Surveillance Program (Public Health Agency of Canada, Ottawa, Ontario)
Clin Infect Dis 48:568-576, 2009

Background.—*Clostridium difficile* infection (CDI) is the most frequent cause of health care–associated infectious diarrhea in industrialized countries. The only previous report describing the incidence of health care–associated CDI (HA CDI) in Canada was conducted in 1997 by the Canadian Nosocomial Infection Surveillance Program. We re-examined the incidence of HA CDI with an emphasis on patient outcomes.

Methods.—A prospective surveillance was conducted from 1 November 2004 through 30 April 2005. Basic demographic data were collected, including age, sex, type of patient ward where the patient was hospitalized on the day HA CDI was identified, and patient comorbidities. Data regarding severe outcome were collected 30 days after the diagnosis of HA CDI; severe outcome was defined as an admission to the intensive care unit because of complications of CDI, colectomy due to CDI, and/or death attributable to CDI.

Results.—A total of 1430 adults with HA CDI were identified in 29 hospitals during the 6-month surveillance period. The overall incidence rate of HA CDI for adult patients admitted to these hospitals was 4.6 cases per 1000 patient admissions and 65 per 100,000 patient-days. At 30 days after onset of HA CDI, 233 patients (16.3%) had died from all causes; 31 deaths (2.2%) were a direct result of CDI, and 51 deaths (3.6%) were indirectly related to CDI, for a total attributable mortality rate of 5.7%.

Conclusions.—The rates are remarkably similar to those found in our previous study; although we found wide variations in HA CDI among the participating hospitals. However, the attributable mortality increased almost 4-fold (5.7% vs. 1.5%; $P < .001$).

▶ Infection caused by *Clostridium difficile* remains the most frequent cause of health care associated infectious diarrhea in industrialized countries.[1] Recently several countries have reported an increase in the incidence and severity of *C difficile* infection (CDI).[2,3] In addition, CDI is an independent predictor of increased length of hospital stay and cost to both patients and hospitals. Since the 2002 epidemic caused by strain NAP1/027 in Quebec, Canada, several hospitals in that region have experienced a dramatic increase in the incidence, severity, and recurrences of hospital-associated CDI.

This report is a prospective surveillance conducted from November 2004 to April 2005 in 29 teaching hospitals in Canada. The results from this surveillance were compared with those from the previous comprehensive report from 1997. The overall rates of CDI were remarkably similar to that of the previous surveillance, perhaps indicating that after the epidemic, rates have leveled off again. However, the attributable mortality in this study was 5.7% compared with 1.5% in 1997. This robust national database has a number of future advantages, including the longitudinal assessment of factors associated with CDI in the hospital setting.

N. M. Khardori, MD

References

1. McFarland LV. Epidemiology of infectious and iatrogenic nosocomial diarrhea in a cohort of general medicine patients. *Am J Infect Control.* 1995;23:295-305.
2. Zilberberg MD, Shorr AF, Kollef MH. Increase in adult Clostridium difficile-related hospitalizations and case-fatality rate, United States, 2000–2005. *Emerg Infect Dis.* 2008;14:1487-1489.
3. Money H. Annual incidence of MRSA falls in England, but *C. difficile* continues to rise. *BMJ.* 2007;335:958.

What is on that keyboard? Detecting hidden environmental reservoirs of *Clostridium difficile* during an outbreak associated with North American pulsed-field gel electrophoresis type I strains
Dumford DM III, Nerandzic MM, Eckstein BC, et al (Univ Hosps of Cleveland, OH; Res Service, Cleveland, OH; et al)
Am J Infect Control 37:15-19, 2009

Background.—Numerous studies have demonstrated that environmental surfaces in the rooms of patients with *Clostridium difficile* infection (CDI) are often contaminated with spores. However, less information is available regarding the frequency of contamination of environmental surfaces outside of CDI isolation rooms.

Methods.—We performed a point-prevalence culture survey for *C difficile* in rooms of patients not in isolation for CDI, in physician and nurse work areas, and on portable equipment, including pulse oximetry devices, electrocardiogram machines, mobile computers, and medication distribution carts. Isolates were characterized by assessment of toxin production, polymerase chain reaction (PCR) ribotyping, and PCR for binary toxin genes.

Results.—Of 105 nonisolation rooms, 17 (16%) were contaminated with toxin-producing *C difficile*, with the highest rate of contamination on the spinal cord injury unit (32%). Of 87 surfaces cultured outside of patient rooms, 20 (23%) were contaminated, including 9 of 29 (31%) in physician work areas, 1 of 10 (10%) in nurse work areas, and 9 of 43 (21%) portable pieces of equipment, including a pulse oximetry finger probe, medication carts, and bar code scanners on medication carts. Of 26 isolates subjected to typing, 19 (73%) matched ribotype patterns detected in stool samples from CDI patients and 13 (50%) were epidemic, binary toxin-positive strains.

Conclusion.—In the context of a CDI outbreak, we found that environmental contamination was common in nonisolation rooms, in physician and nurse work areas, and on portable equipment. Further research is needed to determine whether contamination in these areas plays a significant role in transmission.

▶ Considering the human and financial burden of *Clostridium difficile* infection (CDI) in hospitalized patients, methods to interrupt transmission are of paramount importance. To pursue this goal, the areas in the hospital environment that harbor this hardy organism become a focus of attention.

Using a point prevalence culture survey during an outbreak, this study demonstrated contamination by *C difficile* spores in nonisolation patient rooms, physician work areas, nurse work areas, portable pieces of equipment, medication carts, and bar code scanners on medication carts. Of the isolates typed, 73% matched with ribotypes in the stool samples of patients with CDI and 50% were epidemic, binary toxin-positive strains. Although this study does not address the transmissibility of *C difficile* from these environmental sources, common sense dictates that this is highly likely.

N. M. Khardori, MD

Use of surgical face masks to reduce the incidence of the common cold among health care workers in Japan: A randomized controlled trial
Jacobs JL, Ohde S, Takahashi O, et al (Univ of Hawaii John A. Burns School of Medicine, Honolulu; St. Luke's Life Science Inst Ctr for Clinical Epidemiology, Tokyo, Japan; et al)
Am J Infect Control 37:417-419, 2009

Background.—Health care workers outside surgical suites in Asia use surgical-type face masks commonly. Prevention of upper respiratory infection is one reason given, although evidence of effectiveness is lacking.

Methods.—Health care workers in a tertiary care hospital in Japan were randomized into 2 groups: 1 that wore face masks and 1 that did not. They provided information about demographics, health habits, and quality of life. Participants recorded symptoms daily for 77 consecutive days, starting in January 2008. Presence of a cold was determined based on a previously validated measure of self-reported symptoms. The number of colds between groups was compared, as were risk factors for experiencing cold symptoms.

Results.—Thirty-two health care workers completed the study, resulting in 2464 subject days. There were 2 colds during this time period, 1 in each group. Of the 8 symptoms recorded daily, subjects in the mask group were significantly more likely to experience headache during the study period ($P < .05$). Subjects living with children were more likely to have high cold severity scores over the course of the study.

Conclusion.—Face mask use in health care workers has not been demonstrated to provide benefit in terms of cold symptoms or getting colds. A larger study is needed to definitively establish noninferiority of no mask use.

▶ Health care workers outside surgical suites, and more recently the general public in Japan, use surgical-type face masks commonly. The assumed rationale is prevention of respiratory infections, including the common cold. A meta-analysis of published literature did not provide conclusive evidence.[1]

To validate a common practice in Japanese health care workers with a face value rationale, Jacobs et al conducted a randomized study. The group wearing face masks was compared with the group not wearing one over 77 consecutive days. Risk factors for cold and the number of colds based on a previously validated measure of self-reported symptoms were compared. No benefit was demonstrated for the group wearing face masks. Judging from the scene at United States airports, it seems that based on the face mask use by people in Japan and other countries in Asia, an industry for "custom face masks" is being created.

N. M. Khardori, MD

Reference

1. Jefferson T, Foxlee R, Del Mar C, et al. Physical interventions to interrupt or reduce the spread of respiratory viruses: a systematic review. *BMJ.* 2008;336: 77-80.

16 Parasitic Infections

Acanthamoeba Keratitis Associated with Contact Lens Wear in Singapore
Por YM, Mehta JS, Chua JLL, et al (Singapore Natl Eye Centre; et al)
Am J Ophthalmol 148:7-12, 2009

Purpose.—To describe an outbreak of Acanthamoeba keratitis (AK) cases among contact lens wearers.

Design.—Retrospective cohort study.

Methods.—Patients with AK were included. Relevant demographic and clinical data were obtained from case records, and patients were interviewed using a standardized questionnaire. Contact lens practices, including type of contact lens and solution used, were noted. In addition, clinical features at presentation, management, and clinical outcomes were recorded.

Results.—Forty-two patients (affecting 43 eyes) treated between 2000 and 2007 were included. Diagnosis was made by microbiologic culture in 35 cases and by microbiologic and histologic analysis in 2 cases, whereas the remainder were diagnosed based on clinical features and response to treatment. There was a gradual increase in cases since 2005, with a sharp increase in 2007, when 8 local patients were treated. Of 30 patients where contact lens solution data were available, 18 reported using a Complete brand Multipurpose solution (Advanced Medical Optics, Santa Ana, California, USA) before the infection. Among resident cases treated since February 2006, 7 (63%) of 11 patients used a Complete brand solution. Suboptimal hygiene practices were found in all patients interviewed. Fifteen patients required corneal grafting, with 11 undergoing therapeutic deep lamellar keratoplasty (DLK), 2 undergoing optical penetrating keratoplasty (PK), 1 undergoing optical DLK, and 1 undergoing therapeutic PK. The remainder were treated successfully medically with combination antiamebic therapy. The average duration of therapy was 116.2 days (range, 15 to 283 days). Of patients with radial keratoneuritis with or without epithelial disease, 83.3% achieved final vision of 20/40 or better, whereas this was achieved in 41.7% of those with ring infiltrate. Twenty-five percent of patients with ring infiltrate had final visual acuity of counting fingers or worse, whereas no patient with keratoneuritis and epithelial disease had final vision worse than counting fingers.

Conclusions.—There was an increase in the number of contact lens users with AK seen in the major eye departments of Singapore. Most of our patients also reported using a Complete brand Multipurpose solution before infection, and this parallels a similar outbreak in the United States. Increasing severity of infection was associated with worse visual outcome.

▶ *Acanthamoeba* subspecies is a ubiquitous, free-living protozoan parasite with worldwide distribution and causes a potentially blinding ocular infection. Most cases of amoebic keratitis (AK) occur in immunocompetent contact lens wearers. Outbreaks of AK have been linked to contact lens solutions contaminated with the protozoan or to those that fail to effectively decontaminate lenses. A multistate outbreak of AK affecting 138 people occurred in the United States between 2005 and 2007.[1] In that outbreak investigation, preliminary analysis indicated that the odds of having ever used Advanced Medical Optics Complete MoisturePlus (AMOCMP) multipurpose contact lens solution were 20 times greater in AK patients than for healthy controls. The company voluntarily recalled AMOCMP from domestic and international markets. Further investigation into this outbreak suggested that the solution was not intrinsically contaminated, but its antiacanthamoeba activity (tested before marketing) became insufficient over time.

This study reports a similar outbreak of AK seen in patients in the major eye departments in Singapore between 2000 and 2007. Similar to the United States outbreak, many patients (60%-63%) were using AMOCMP. Other prominent risk factors were swimming, showering, and sleeping with contact lenses on.

N. M. Khardori, MD

Reference

1. Verani JR, Lorick SA, Yoder JS, et al. National outbreak of acanthamoeba keratitis associated with use of a contact lens solution, United States. *Emerg Infect Dis.* 2009;15:1236-1242.

Laboratory Diagnosis of Amoebic Keratitis: Comparison of Four Diagnostic Methods for Different Types of Clinical Specimens
Boggild AK, Martin DS, Lee TY, et al (Toronto General Hosp, Ontario, Canada; Ontario Agency for Health Protection and Promotion, Etobicoke, Canada; et al)
J Clin Microbiol 47:1314-1318, 2009

Amoebic keratitis causes significant ocular morbidity in contact lens wearers. Current diagnostic methods for amoebic keratitis are insensitive and labor-intensive and have poor turnaround time. We evaluated four laboratory methods for detection of acanthamoebae in clinical specimens. Deidentified, delinked consecutive specimens from patients with suspected amoebic keratitis were assayed for acanthamoebae by direct smear analysis, culture, and PCR using two different primer sets specific for *Acanthamoeba* ribosomal DNA. The consensus reference standard was considered fulfilled when the results for any two of the four tests were positive, and the outcome measures were sensitivity and specificity. Of 107 specimens assayed over an 18-month period, 20 were positive for acanthamoebae. The sensitivity and specificity of each assay were as follows, respectively: for smear analysis, 55% (95% confidence interval [CI], 33.2 to 76.8%) and 100%; for culture, 73.7% (95% CI, 54.4 to 93.0%) and 100%; for PCR using Nelson primers, 90% (95% CI, 76.9 to 100%) and 90.8% (95% CI, 84.7 to 96.9%); and for PCR using JDP primers, 65% (95% CI, 44.1 to 85.9%) and 100%. Nelson primer PCR demonstrated a single-organism level of analytic sensitivity. The performance characteristics of the assays varied by specimen type, with contact lenses and casings showing the highest rates of detectable acanthamoebae and the highest diagnostic sensitivities for direct smear analysis, culture, and JDP primer PCR, though these results are based on small numbers and should be interpreted cautiously. These findings have important implications for clinicians collecting diagnostic specimens and for diagnostic laboratories, especially in outbreak situations.

▶ Amoebic or Acanthamoeba keratitis (AK) occurs sporadically in patients who have corneal trauma or use tap water or other homemade preparations to clean contact lenses. As described in the previous commentary, most outbreaks have been linked to contact lens solutions contaminated with *Acanthamoeba* or by those that fail to retain effective decontaminating activity post-marketing. A recent study compared the efficacy of 11 different contact lens solutions against cysts of 3 different species of *Acanthamoeba*.[2] The 2 contact lens solutions that contained hydrogen peroxide were the only solutions that showed any disinfection ability against 2 of the 3 common species that cause AK. Delayed diagnosis, mainly because of the clinical resemblance of AK to viral, bacterial, and fungal keratitis, has been associated with more severe clinical progression and poor visual outcome.[1] Patients who develop polymicrobial keratitis, ie, infectious crystalline keratopathy (ICK) superimposed on AK, are at an even higher risk of developing disabling pain and corneal scarring.[3] Even when considered as a diagnostic possibility, current laboratory methods for AK are insensitive or have long turnaround time.

This study compares conventional methods of smear analysis and cultures with PCR using 2 different primer sets specific for *Acanthamoeba* ribosomal DNA. The sensitivity and specificity of 55% and 100% for smear, 73.7% and 100% for culture, and 65% to 95% and 97% to 100% for the 2 PCR based tests was observed. With much shorter turnaround time the PCR test, especially in combination with the smear analysis, would provide early laboratory diagnosis. From a clinical point of view, AK should be included in the differential especially in contact lens wearers.

N. M. Khardori, MD

References

1. Marciano-Cabral G, Cabral G. Acanthamoeba spp. As agents of disease in humans. *Clin Microbiol Rev.* 2003;16:273-307.
2. Johnston SP, Sriram R, Qvarnstrom Y, et al. Resistance of Acanthamoeba cysts to disinfection in multiple contact lens solutions. *J Clin Microbiol.* 2009;47: 2040-2045.
3. Tu EY, Joslin CE, Nijm LM, Feder RS, Jain S, Shoff ME. Polymicrobial keratitis: Acanthamoeba and Infectious crystalline keratopathy. *Am J Ophthalmol.* 2009; 148:13-19.

Cryptosporidiosis in the Elderly Population of the United States
Mor SM, DeMaria A Jr, Griffiths JK, et al (Tufts Cummings School of Veterinary Medicine, North Grafton, MA; Tufts Med School; Massachusetts Dept of Public Health; et al)
Clin Infect Dis 48:698-705, 2009

Background.—Although cryptosporidiosis has been a nationally notifiable disease since 1995, surveillance estimates are undermined by limited diagnostic testing and incomplete reporting of cases to health authorities. Further, existing surveillance systems do not capture the specific risks of cryptosporidiosis to sensitive populations, such as the elderly population. The Centers for Medicare and Medicaid Services databases present a novel means to investigate the cryptosporidiosis burden in the US elderly population.

Methods.—We abstracted records for all Medicare-covered persons aged ≥ 65 years who received a diagnosis of a cryptosporidiosis-related illness between 1991 and 2004 ($n = 1304$) in the United States. Annual rates of cryptosporidiosis-related hospitalization were calculated and compared with surveillance data published by the Centers for Disease Control and Prevention. The total burden of disease and outcomes of hospitalization were also assessed.

Results.—Cryptosporidiosis- related hospitalizations increased during the study period at a rate of 0.15–0.39 cases per 100,000 elderly persons each year; this increase was probably attributable to increased awareness and testing. Comparison between cryptosporidiosis-related hospitalization and Centers for Disease Control and Prevention surveillance data revealed considerable state-to-state variation. The rate of hospitalization among persons aged ≥ 85 years was more than double that among persons aged 65–74 years. Volume depletion and noninfectious diseases of the digestive system were common concurrent diagnoses. The highest case-fatality rates were among persons aged ≥ 85 years (7.8%) and among persons infected with HIV (10.3%).

Conclusions.—Although awareness of cryptosporidiosis has increased, underdiagnosis and underreporting of cases remains a major barrier to accurate surveillance in many states. Infection among elderly persons is associated with volume depletion and negative hospital outcomes, including death.

▶ Cryptosporidiosis is an important cause of diarrhea worldwide. It is transmitted via fecal-oral route, and also through fomites and contaminated water. It usually causes a self-limited disease in immunocompetent individuals, but may cause life-threatening infection in immunocompromised patients, and it has been occasionally associated with large outbreaks in the United States.[1] People with the acquired immunodeficiency syndrome (AIDS) are at particular risk for chronic infection and more severe disease. The elderly and debilitated may also be at increased risk for infection-related complications and mortality. In the United States, cryptosporidiosis has been a notifiable disease since 1995, but reporting requirements vary by state. Routine testing of stool for ova and parasites does not identify *Cryptosporidium*, which may be a cause for underdiagnosis.[1]

In this study, Siobhan et al investigate the prevalence and outcomes of cryptosporidiosis in persons aged ≥65 years using records from the Centers for Medicare and Medicaid Services (CMS) databases for a 14-year period (between January 1, 1991 through December 31, 2004). A total of 1304 records with a diagnosis of cryptosporidiosis-related illness were found. Cryptosporidiosis-related hospitalization increased with age for both men and women, being more than double in persons aged ≥85 years compared with persons aged 65 to 74 years. Hospital duration of stay was also higher for age≥85 years compared with the other groups. Overall, in-hospital death was 5.4%, but the death rate was significantly higher in persons aged ≥85 years (7.8%) and in patients with HIV infection/AIDS (10.3%). The authors also observed a general upward trend in cryptosporidiosis related hospitalizations, but they attributed it to increased awareness and testing for the disease rather than truly increased incidence or severity.

This study is important because it increases our awareness of a commonly neglected disease. While it is more often than not a self-limited infection, it may have devastating consequences in AIDS patients and in the elderly. Physicians also need to know that ordering stool for ova and parasites may not include identification of *Cryptosporidium*, but immunofluorescent assays also using stool are available and have good sensitivity and specificity.

C. A. Speil, MD

Reference

1. Chen XM, Keithly JS, Paya CV, LaRusso NF. Cryptosporidiosis. *N Engl J Med*. 2002;346:1723-1731.

17 Vaccines

Safety, immunogenicity, and efficacy of quadrivalent human papillomavirus (types 6, 11, 16, 18) recombinant vaccine in women aged 24–45 years: a randomised, double-blind trial
Muñoz N, Manalastas R Jr, Pitisuttithum P, et al (Natl Inst of Cancer, Bogotá, Colombia; Philippine General Hosp, Manila; Mahidol Univ, Bangkok, Thailand; et al)
Lancet 373:1949-1957, 2009

Background.—Although the peak incidence of human papillomavirus (HPV) infection occurs in most populations within 5–10 years of first sexual experience, all women remain at risk for acquisition of HPV infections. We tested the safety, immunogenicity, and efficacy of the quadrivalent HPV (types 6, 11, 16, 18) L1 virus-like-particle vaccine in women aged 24–45 years.

Methods.—Women aged 24–45 years with no history of genital warts or cervical disease were enrolled from community health centres, academic health centres, and primary health-care providers into an ongoing multicentre, parallel, randomised, placebo-controlled, double-blind study. Participants were allocated by computer-generated schedule to receive quadrivalent HPV vaccine (n = 1911) or placebo (n = 1908) at day 1, and months 2 and 6. All study site investigators and personnel, study participants, monitors, and central laboratory personnel were blinded to treatment allocation. Coprimary efficacy endpoints were 6 months' or more duration of infection and cervical and external genital disease due to HPV 6, 11, 16, 18; and due to HPV 16 and 18 alone. Primary efficacy analyses were done in a per-protocol population, but intention-to-treat analyses were also undertaken. This study is registered with Clinical-Trials.gov, number NCT00090220.

Findings.—1910 women received at least one dose of vaccine and 1907 at least one dose of placebo. In the per-protocol population, efficacy against the first coprimary endpoint (disease or infection related to HPV 6, 11, 16, and 18) was 90·5% (95% CI 73·7–97·5, four of 1615 cases in the vaccine group *vs* 41/1607 in the placebo group) and 83·1% (50·6–95·8, four of 1601 cases *vs* 23/1579 cases) against the second coprimary endpoint (disease or infection related to HPV 16 and 18 alone).

In the intention-to-treat population, efficacy against the first coprimary endpoint was 30·9% (95% CI 11·1–46·5, 108/1886 cases *vs* 154/1883 cases) and against the second coprimary endpoint was 22·6% (−2·9 to 41·9, 90/1886 cases *vs* 115/1883 cases), since infection and disease were present at baseline. We recorded no vaccine-related serious adverse events.

Interpretation.—The quadrivalent HPV vaccine is efficacious in women aged 24–45 years not infected with the relevant HPV types at enrolment.

▶ A number of infectious agents, including human papillomavirus (HPV) and hepatitis B virus, are associated with cancers. After the hepatitis B vaccine, HPV is the second vaccine for cancer prevention studied and introduced for clinical use. Based on phase II trials conducted in North America, Latin America, Asia, and Europe on 15 000 women aged 16 to 26 years, the quadrivalent HPV (type 6, 11, 16, and 18) vaccine was shown to be highly effective in prevention of cervical, vulvar, or vaginal intraepithelial neoplasia related to HPV 6, 11, 16, or 18, and adenocarcinoma in situ in women who were naive to the respective HPV types at enrollment.[1,2] Using immunogenicity bridging studies in younger females (9-15 years), the vaccine was approved for ages 9 to 26 years. The earlier vaccination was recommended based on the peak incidence of HPV infection within 5 to 10 years of first sexual experience (age 15-25 years). Changes in sexual behaviors, increasing divorce rates and acquisition of new sexual partners during middle age, and a second peak of HPV infection after menopause, all favor the use of this vaccine in older women.

This multicenter, randomized, placebo-controlled, double-blind study reports on the safety, immunogenicity, and efficacy of quadrivalent HPV recombinant vaccine in women aged 24 to 45 years. The vaccine was shown to be safe and efficacious in women 24 to 45 years not infected with the relevant HPV type at enrollment.

N. M. Khardori, MD

References

1. Garland SM, Hernandez-Avila M, Wheeler CM, et al. Quadrivalent vaccine against human papillomavirus to prevent anogenital diseases. *N Engl J Med.* 2007;356:1928-1943.
2. The FUTURE II Study Group. Quadrivalent vaccine against human papillomavirus to prevent high-grade cervical lesions. *N Engl J Med.* 2007;356:1915-1927.

Safety and Immunogenicity of a New Tuberculosis Vaccine, MVA85A, in *Mycobacterium tuberculosis*–infected Individuals
Sander CR, Pathan AA, Beveridge NER, et al (Univ of Oxford, UK; et al)
Am J Respir Crit Care Med 179:724-733, 2009

Rationale.—An effective new tuberculosis (TB) vaccine regimen must be safe in individuals with latent TB infection (LTBI) and is a priority for global health care.

Objectives.—To evaluate the safety and immunogenicity of a leading new TB vaccine, recombinant Modified Vaccinia Ankara expressing Antigen 85A (MVA85A) in individuals with LTBI.

Methods.—An open-label, phase I trial of MVA85A was performed in 12 subjects with LTBI recruited from TB contact clinics in Oxford and London or by poster advertisements in Oxford hospitals. Patients were assessed clinically and had blood samples drawn for immunological analysis over a 52-week period after vaccination with MVA85A. Thoracic computed tomography scans were performed at baseline and at 10 weeks after vaccination. Safety of MVA85A was assessed by clinical, radiological, and inflammatory markers. The immunogenicity of MVA85A was assessed by IFNγ and IL-2 ELISpot assays and FACS.

Measurements and Main Results.—MVA85A was safe in subjects with LTBI, with comparable adverse events to previous trials of MVA85A. There were no clinically significant changes in inflammatory markers or thoracic computed tomography scans after vaccination. MVA85A induced a strong antigen-specific IFN-γ and IL-2 response that was durable for 52 weeks. The magnitude of IFN-γ response was comparable to previous trials of MVA85A in bacillus Calmette-Guérin–vaccinated individuals. Antigen 85A–specific polyfunctional CD4+ T cells were detectable prior to vaccination with statistically significant increases in cell numbers after vaccination.

Conclusions.—MVA85A is safe and highly immunogenic in individuals with LTBI. These results will facilitate further trials in TB-endemic areas. Clinical trial registered with www.clinicaltrials.gov (NCT00456183).

▶ With one-third (2 billion) of the world's population estimated to be latently infected with *Mycobacterium tuberculosis* latent TB infection (LTBI), based on tuberculin skin testing (TST), 9 million people developing tuberculosis disease per year, and 2 million tuberculosis related deaths per year, tuberculosis remains an unconquered disease.

Patients with LTBI have a lifetime risk of 5% to 10% for reactivation and development of postprimary disease. If reactivation occurs, these patients change from reservoirs to source patients capable of transmitting TB. Therefore, a vaccine more effective than the currently available BCG vaccine, which also works well in patients with known or unknown LTBI, would have a significant impact on the global burden of tuberculosis. Vaccination with newer and more effective tuberculosis vaccines may be unavoidable and possibly desirable in clinical practice outside of clinical trials that have so far been designed primarily as preexposure vaccines. Recombinant modified vaccinia virus Ankara expressing antigen 85A (MVA85A) was shown to boost BCG-primed and naturally acquired antimycobacterial immunity in humans.[1]

This open label phase 1 trial of MVA85A was performed in 12 subjects with LTBI and showed that this vaccine is safe and highly immunogenic in this patient population.

N. M. Khardori, MD

Reference

1. McShane H, Pathan AA, Sander CR, et al. Recombinant modified vaccine virus Ankara expressing antigen 85A boosts BCG-primed and naturally acquired antimycobacterial immunity in human. *Nat Med.* 2004;10:1240-1244.

Post-exposure vaccination against *Mycobacterium tuberculosis*
Henao-Tamayo M, Palaniswamy GS, Smith EE, et al (Colorado State Univ, Fort Collins; et al)
Tuberculosis 89:142-148, 2009

Enhancing immunity to tuberculosis in animal models after exposure to the infection has proved difficult. In this study we used a newly described flow cytometric technique to monitor changes in cell populations accumulating in the lungs of guinea pigs challenged by low-dose aerosol infection with *Mycobacterium tuberculosis* and vaccinated 10 days later. On day 40 after infection the fusion protein F36 and a pool of Ag85A and ESAT6 vaccines had significant effects on the bacterial load, showed increased expression of the activation marker CD45+ on CD4+ T cells, and reduced numbers of heterophils. Lung pathology and pathology scores were marginally improved in animals given these vaccines, but lymph node pathology was not influenced. Despite early effects no changes in long-term survival were seen. These results suggest that a single post-exposure vaccination can initially slow the disease process. However, this effect is transient, but this could be of use in an multidrug resistant/extremely drug resistant outbreak situation because it could potentially slow the infection long enough to complete drug susceptibility testing and initiate effective chemotherapy.

▶ Postexposure immunotherapy for *Mycobacterium tuberculosis* in the context of an outbreak situation would be a logical approach to improve the burden of tuberculosis in the world. Animal studies with immunotherapeutic vaccines so far have shown either an absence of changes in bacterial load and pathology or, in the case of repeated heat shock protein DNA vaccination, a worsened disease state.[1,2] The explanations given for these results are: (i) vaccines do not boost existing immunity once the animal is well into the chronic phase of the infection; and (ii) if antigen specific T-cells could potentially be expanded by post-exposure vaccination, the degeneration and necrosis in the lung may prevent adequate penetration of these cells into the infected area. The Ag85A, ESAT6 mixture, and F36 fusion vaccines given postexposure to guinea pigs showed protective effects, but whether they were transient and improved long-term survival was not evident. This initial transient effect might still be useful as a component of first approach to outbreak situations.

In this study, BCG vaccine was compared with a number of experimental vaccines in a postexposure guinea pig model. The vaccines were given 10 days after a low-dose aerosol infection with *M tuberculosis*. Two of the candidate vaccines showed marginal improvement in lung pathology, no effect on lymph node pathology, or long-term survival. The cost of development of such vaccines would not justify the potential limited use except perhaps in drug-resistant tuberculosis while awaiting susceptibility results.

N. M. Khardori, MD

References

1. Turner J, Rhoades ER, Keen M, Belisle JT, Frank AA, Orme IM. Effective pre-exposure tuberculosis vaccines fail to protect when they are given in an immuno-therapeutic mode. *Infect Immun.* 2000;68:1706-1709.
2. Taylor JL, turner OC, Basaraba RJ, Belisle JT, Huygen K, Orme IM. Pulmonary necrosis resulting from DNA vaccination against tuberculosis. *Infect Immun.* 2003;71:2192-2198.

Safety and Immunogenicity of RTS,S/ASO2D Malaria Vaccine in Infants

Abdulla S, Oberholzer R, Juma O, et al (Bagamoyo Res and Training Centre of Ifakara Health Inst, Tanzania; et al)
N Engl J Med 359:2533-2544, 2008

Background.—The RTS,S/AS malaria vaccine is being developed for delivery through the World Health Organization's Expanded Program on Immunization (EPI). We assessed the feasibility of integrating RTS,S/AS02D into a standard EPI schedule for infants.

Methods.—In this phase 2B, single-center, double-blind, controlled trial involving 340 infants in Bagamoyo, Tanzania, we randomly assigned 340 infants to receive three doses of either the RTS,S/AS02D vaccine or the hepatitis B vaccine at 8, 12, and 16 weeks of age. All infants also received a vaccine containing diphtheria and tetanus toxoids, whole-cell pertussis vaccine, and conjugated *Haemophilus influenzae* type b vaccine (DTPw/Hib). The primary objectives were the occurrence of serious adverse events during a 9-month surveillance period and a demonstration of noninferiority of the responses to the EPI vaccines (DTPw/Hib and hepatitis B surface antigen) with coadministration of the RTS,S/AS02D vaccine, as compared with the hepatitis B vaccine. The detection of antibodies against *Plasmodium falciparum* circumsporozoite and efficacy against malaria infection were secondary objectives.

Results.—At least one serious adverse event was reported in 31 of 170 infants who received the RTS,S/AS02D vaccine (18.2%; 95% confidence interval [CI], 12.7 to 24.9) and in 42 of 170 infants who received the hepatitis B vaccine (24.7%; 95% CI, 18.4 to 31.9). The results showed the noninferiority of the RTS,S/AS02D vaccine in terms of antibody responses to EPI antigens. One month after vaccination, 98.6% of infants receiving the RTS,S/AS02D vaccine had seropositive titers for anticircumsporozoite antibodies on enzyme-linked immunosorbent assay (ELISA). During the 6-month period after the third dose of vaccine, the efficacy of the

RTS,S/AS02D vaccine against first infection with *P. falciparum* malaria was 65.2% (95% CI, 20.7 to 84.7; P = 0.01).

Conclusions.—The use of the RTS,S/AS02D vaccine in infants had a promising safety profile, did not interfere with the immunologic responses to coadministered EPI antigens, and reduced the incidence of malaria infection. (ClinicalTrials.gov number, NCT00289185.)

▶ Like tuberculosis, malaria persists as a major global infectious disease, and the best hope for its eradication seems to be through vaccination, particularly in children. The RTS,S vaccine with the adjuvant system AS02D has been studied in infants and children aged 3 to 4 years living in a highly endemic area.[1,2] A protection rate of 65% against new infection and efficacy against breakthrough infections was associated with reductions in both mild and severe malaria episodes. Because this vaccine contains hepatitis B surface antigen, a response to hepatitis B surface antigen was induced which in fact was higher than that of the licensed hepatitis B vaccine. This vaccine is being developed for delivery through the World Health Organization's Expanded Program on Immunization (EPI).

This phase 2B double-blind controlled trial, studies the interplay of RTS,S/AS vaccine with other vaccines given routinely through EPI, including diphtheria and tetanus toxoids, whole-cell pertussis vaccine, and conjugated *Haemophilus influenzae* type b vaccine. RTS,S/AS vaccine or hepatitis B vaccine was given at 8, 12, and 16 weeks of age along with DTPw/Hib. The malaria vaccine did not interfere with the response to coadministered routine vaccines, and showed an efficacy of 65.2% against first infection with *Plasmodium falciparum*. As in the previous trials of this vaccine, the integrated vaccination approach did not pose any obvious safety concerns.

N. M. Khardori, MD

References

1. Aponte JJ, Aide P, Renom M, et al. Safety of the RTS,S/AS02D candidate malaria vaccine in infants living in a highly endemic area of Mozambique: a double blind randomized controlled phase 1/11b trial. *Lancet.* 2007;37:1543-1551.
2. Macete EV, Sacarlal J, Aponte JJ, et al. Evaluation of two formulations of adjuvanted RTS, S malaria vaccine in children aged 3 to 5 year living in a malaria-endemic region of Mozambique: a phase 1/11b randomized double-blind bridging trial. *Trials.* 2007;8:11.

Preventing Bacterial Infections with Pilus-Based Vaccines: the Group B Streptococcus Paradigm
Margarit I, Rinaudo CD, Galeotti CL, et al (Novartis Vaccines, Siena; et al)
J Infect Dis 199:108-115, 2009

We recently described the presence of 3 pilus variants in the human pathogen group B streptococcus (GBS; also known as *Streptococcus agalactiae*), each encoded by a distinct pathogenicity island, as well as the ability of pilus components to elicit protection in mice against homologous challenge. To determine whether a vaccine containing a combination of proteins from the 3 pilus types could provide broad protection, we analyzed pili distribution and conservation in 289 clinical isolates. We found that pilus sequences in each island are conserved, all strains carried at least 1 of the 3 islands, and a combination of the 3 pilus components conferred protection against all tested GBS challenge strains. These data are the first to indicate that a vaccine exclusively constituted by pilus components can be effective in preventing infections caused by GBS, and they pave the way for the use of a similar approach against other pathogenic streptococci.

▶ The acquisition of maternal opsonizing antibodies and the presence of maternal antibody against capsular polysaccharide (CPS) of *Streptococcus agalactiae* (group B streptococcus [GBS]) in infants are inversely correlated with their risk of developing early as well as late onset disease. Raising the amount of such antibodies in the mother by vaccination against GBS would be expected to improve morbidity and mortality from GBS in infants. CPS from GBS conjugated to tetanus toxoid has been shown to be safe and immunogenic. Such vaccines, however, would not be protective against the increasing number of nontypeable strains that do not possess CPS. Vaccines made of protein antigens common to all strains offer the possibility of protection against typeable and nontypeable strains.[1] These protective antigens have been shown to constitute pilus-like structures.[2]

Using a novel approach to vaccine development, this study used a combination of proteins from 3 pilus types of GBS (all strains contain at least one of them). The vaccine conferred protection to mice against infection with all tested GBS strains. Because pili are known to be present in other pathogenic streptococci, this approach has wide potential usefulness.

For further reading on this subject I suggest an article by Paoletti et al.[3]

N. M. Khardori, MD

References

1. Maione D, Margarit I, Rinaudo CD, et al. Identification of a universal Group B Streptococcus vaccine by multiple genome screens. *Science.* 2005;309:148-150.
2. Lauer P, Rinaudo CD, Soriani M, et al. Genome analysis reveals pili in Group B. *Science.* 2005;309:105.
3. Paoletti LC, Kasper D. Conjugate vaccines against group B Streptococcus types IV and VII. *J Infect Dis.* 2002;186:123-126.

18 Influenza

Prolonged Influenza Virus Infection during Lymphocytopenia and Frequent Detection of Drug-Resistant Viruses

Gooskens J, Jonges M, Claas ECJ, et al (Leiden Univ Med Ctr, The Netherlands; Natl Inst of Public Health and the Environment, Bilthoven, The Netherlands)

J Infect Dis 199:1435-1441, 2009

The factors that cause prolonged human influenza virus respiratory tract infection and determine its clinical impact and the development of drug-resistant viruses are unclear. During a 3-year period, symptomatic influenza virus excretion for ≥ 2 weeks was observed among 8 immuno-compromised patients and found to be associated with lymphocytopenia at onset (8 of 8 patients) more often than with granulocytopenia (2 of 8 patients) or monocytopenia (2 of 8 patients). Six (75%) of 8 patients developed influenza lower respiratory tract infection (10 episodes), and receipt of oseltamivir treatment was significantly associated with clinical improvement (8 of 8 episodes vs. 0 of 2 untreated episodes; $P = .02$). Complete viral clearance was strongly correlated with lymphocyte recon-stitution ($P = .04$) but was never observed during the first 2 weeks after oseltamivir treatment. Neuraminidase inhibitor–resistant influenza viruses emerged in 2 (67%) of 3 patients eligible for resistance analysis. In conclusion, prolonged influenza virus infection was associated with lymphocyto-penia, influenza lower respiratory tract infection, and frequent development of drug resistance during antiviral therapy. Clinical improve-ment in influenza lower respiratory tract infection is observed during oseltamivir treatment, but complete viral clearance is dependent on lymphocyte reconstitution, irrespective of receipt of antiviral medication.

▶ Newer antiviral drugs have been shown to be effective for treatment and prevention of influenza.[1] As would be expected, with more use, resistance to various antivirals is becoming evident and clinically relevant. Development of resistance during antiviral therapy would be expected to delay viral clearance even if patients experience clinical improvement. Few published reports have documented the occurrence of prolonged influenza virus infection among immunocompromised patients.[2] However, the factors associated with prolonged influenza virus infection (viral excretion for > 2 weeks) and consequent drug resistance are not well understood.

This study of 8 immunocompromised patients shows that lymphocytopenia (8/8) is a major risk factor for prolonged symptomatic viral excretion for > 2 weeks. Of the 8 patients, 6 developed influenza viral infection of lower respiratory tract. Oseltamivir was used to treat 5 out of 8 patients. Authors were able to do antiviral resistance testing for 3 of the 5 paired viruses. Neuraminidase inhibitor resistance (both oseltamivir and zanamavir) was demonstrated in 2 out of the 3 viruses. One reverted back to wild-type virus 3 weeks after discontinuation of oseltamivir and the other reverted to zanamavir sensitive and oseltamivir reduced susceptibility. Complete viral clearance correlated strongly with reconstitution of lymphocyte count. These data point to the significance of host factors in the natural history of influenza illness and the risk of development of antiviral resistance during therapy.

N. M. Khardori, MD

References

1. Moscona A. Neuraminidase inhibitors for influenza. *N Encl J med*. 2005;353: 1363-1373.
2. Ison MG, Gubareva LV, Atmar RL, Treanor J, Hayden FG. Recovery of drug-resistance influenza virus from immunocompromised patients: a case series. *J Infect Dis*. 2007;193:760-764.

Infections With Oseltamivir-Resistant Influenza A(H1N1) Virus in the United States

Dharan NJ, for the Oseltamivir-Resistance Working Group (Ctrs for Disease Control and Prevention, Atlanta, GA; et al)
JAMA 301:1034-1041, 2009

Context.—During the 2007-2008 influenza season, oseltamivir resistance among influenza A(H1N1) viruses increased significantly for the first time worldwide. Early surveillance data suggest that the prevalence of oseltamivir resistance among A(H1N1) viruses will most likely be higher during the 2008-2009 season.

Objectives.—To describe patients infected with oseltamivir-resistant influenza A(H1N1) virus and to determine whether there were any differences between these patients and patients infected with oseltamivir-susceptible A(H1N1) virus in demographic or epidemiological characteristics, clinical symptoms, severity of illness, or clinical outcomes.

Design, Setting, and Patients.—Influenza A(H1N1) viruses that were identified and submitted to the Centers for Disease Control and Prevention by US public health laboratories between September 30, 2007, and May 17, 2008, and between September 28, 2008, and February 19, 2009, were tested as part of ongoing surveillance. Oseltamivir resistance was determined by neuraminidase inhibition assay and pyrosequencing analysis. Information was collected using a standardized case form from patients with oseltamivir-resistant A(H1N1) infections and a comparison group of patients with oseltamivir-susceptible A(H1N1) infections during 2007-2008.

Main Outcome Measures.—Demographic and epidemiological information as well as clinical information, including symptoms, severity of illness, and clinical outcomes.

Results.—During the 2007-2008 season, influenza A(H1N1) accounted for an estimated 19% of circulating influenza viruses in the United States. Among 1155 influenza A(H1N1) viruses tested from 45 states, 142 (12.3%) from 24 states were resistant to oseltamivir. Data were available for 99 oseltamivir-resistant cases and 182 oseltamivir-susceptible cases from this period. Among resistant cases, median age was 19 years (range, 1 month to 62 years), 5 patients (5%) were hospitalized, and 4 patients (4%) died. None reported oseltamivir exposure before influenza diagnostic sample collection. No significant differences were found between cases of oseltamivir-resistant and oseltamivir-susceptible influenza in demographic characteristics, underlying medical illness, or clinical symptoms. Preliminary data from the 2008-2009 influenza season identified resistance to oseltamivir among 264 of 268 influenza A(H1N1) viruses (98.5%) tested.

Conclusions.—Oseltamivir-resistant A(H1N1) viruses circulated widely in the United States during the 2007-2008 influenza season, appeared to be unrelated to oseltamivir use, and appeared to cause illness similar to oseltamivir-susceptible A(H1N1) viruses. Circulation of oseltamivir-resistant A(H1N1) viruses will continue, with a higher prevalence of resistance, during the 2008-2009 season.

▶ Subsequent to the significant increase in resistance to adamantanes (amantidine and rimantidine) among influenza A (H3N2) during the 2005-2006 influenza season, neuraminidase inhibitors (NAIs) (oseltamivir and zanamavir) became the only class of antiviral agents recommended for the treatment and prophylaxis of influenza in the United States.[1] Before this, the resistance rates of influenza viruses to (NAIs) worldwide was less than 1%, and was reported typically among persons who had received oseltamivir. Human-to-human transmission of NAI-resistant virus had not been documented. During the 2007-2008 influenza season, increased resistance to oseltamivir was reported worldwide, including in the United States, and was identified in influenza A (H1N1).

This study describes patients infected with oseltamivir-resistant influenza A (H1N1) identified during the 2007-2008 influenza surveillance in the United States. The resistance to oseltamivir appeared to be unrelated to oseltamivir use, and the illness caused by the resistant and susceptible viruses was similar. Nosocomial transmission of the resistant virus was shown to be associated with significant morbidity and mortality in high-risk patients.[2] The national adjusted overall proportion of oseltamivir resistance was 2%, based on which national recommendations for use of antiviral agents were not changed during 2007-2008. Surveillance studies from Europe and other countries revealed oseltamivir resistance in up to 67% of H1N1 viruses. In a study from Japan, phylogenetic analysis showed that 1 resistant virus belonged to the lineage of oseltamivir-resistant viruses isolated in Europe and North America, and the other 2 emerged independently in Japan. Oseltamivir is used widely in Japan.[3] Early surveillance data from the 2008-2009 influenza season estimated oseltamivir resistance among influenza A (H1N1) to be > 90%, and led to the change in recommendations for antiviral use against influenza.[4] Resistance to zanamavir did not change. Initial testing of the 2009 pandemic (novel) influenza A (H1N1) found it susceptible to neuraminidases and resistant to adamantanes. On August 6, 2009, the United States Centers for Disease Control and Prevention (CDC) detected oseltamivir resistance in pandemic influenza A (H1N1) from Seattle, Washington,[5] and as of September 4, 2009, 9 cases of oseltamivir-resistant pandemic H1N1 have been reported from the United States, and sporadic cases have been reported worldwide.

N. M. Khardori, MD

References

1. Centers for Disease Control and Prevention (CDC). High levels of adamantine resistance among influenza A (H3N2) viruses and interim guidelines for use of antiviral agents – United States, 2005–06 influenza season. *MMWR Morb Moral Wkly Rep.* 2006;55:44-46.
2. Gooskens J, Jonges M, Claas E, Meijer A, van den Brock PJ, Kroes A. Morbidity and Mortality associated with nosocomial transmission of oseltamivir-resistant influenza A (H1N1) virus. *JAMA.* 2009;301:1042-1046.
3. Tamura D, Mitamura K, Yamazaki M, et al. Oseltamivir-resistant influenza A viruses circulating in Japan. *J of Clinic Microb.* 2009;47:1425-1427.
4. Centers for Disease Control and Prevention (CDC). Issues Interim recommendations for the use of influenza antiviral medications in the setting of oseltamivir resistance among circulating influenza A (H1N1) viruses, 2008–09 Influenza season, http://www2acdc.gov/HAN/ArchiveSys/viewMsgV.asp?AlertNum=00279. Accessed January 2, 2009.
5. Centers for Disease Control and Prevention (CDC). Oseltamivir-resistant novel influenza A (H1N1) virus infection in two immunosuppressed patients – Seattle, Washington, 2009. *MMWR Morb Moral Wkly Rep.* 2009;58:893-897.

Triple-Reassortant Swine Influenza A (H1) in Humans in the United States, 2005–2009
Shinde V, Bridges CB, Uyeki TM, et al (Ctrs for Disease Control and Prevention, Atlanta, GA; et al)
N Engl J Med 360:2616-2625, 2009

Background.—Triple-reassortant swine influenza A (H1) viruses — containing genes from avian, human, and swine influenza viruses — emerged and became enzootic among pig herds in North America during the late 1990s.

Methods.—We report the clinical features of the first 11 sporadic cases of infection of humans with triple-reassortant swine influenza A (H1) viruses reported to the Centers for Disease Control and Prevention, occurring from December 2005 through February 2009, until just before the current epidemic of swine-origin influenza A (H1N1) among humans. These data were obtained from routine national influenza surveillance reports and from joint case investigations by public and animal health agencies.

Results.—The median age of the 11 patients was 10 years (range, 16 months to 48 years), and 4 had underlying health conditions. Nine of the patients had had exposure to pigs, five through direct contact and four through visits to a location where pigs were present but without contact. In another patient, human-to-human transmission was suspected. The range of the incubation period, from the last known exposure to the onset of symptoms, was 3 to 9 days. Among the 10 patients with known clinical symptoms, symptoms included fever (in 90%), cough (in 100%), headache (in 60%), and diarrhea (in 30%). Complete blood counts were available for four patients, revealing leukopenia in two, lymphopenia in one, and thrombocytopenia in another. Four patients were hospitalized, two of whom underwent invasive mechanical ventilation. Four patients received oseltamivir, and all 11 recovered from their illness.

Conclusions.—From December 2005 until just before the current human epidemic of swine-origin influenza viruses, there was sporadic infection with triple-reassortant swine influenza A (H1) viruses in persons with exposure to pigs in the United States. Although all the patients recovered, severe illness of the lower respiratory tract and unusual influenza signs such as diarrhea were observed in some patients, including those who had been previously healthy.

▶ Febrile respiratory illness caused by influenza virus in pigs was identified in 1931, 3 years before influenza viruses were identified as a cause of illness in humans. Pigs seem to act as a mixing vessel for reassortant of avian, swine, and human influenza viruses, and thus play an important role in the emergence of novel influenza viruses capable of causing human pandemics.[1] The most commonly circulating swine influenza virus among pigs—classic swine influenza A (H1N1)–underwent little change between the 1930s and 1990s. By the late 1990s multiple strains and subtypes (H1N1, H3N2, and H1N2) of triple assortant swine influenza A emerged and became predominant among North American pig herds. The genomes of these viruses included combinations of avian, human, and swine influenza virus gene segments. In the past 35 years only about 50 cases of swine influenza virus infection in humans (most due to classic swine influenza virus A H1N1) have been reported worldwide. Serological studies suggest that people with occupational swine exposure are at highest risk for infection. Until April 2009, human-to-human transmission of swine influenza virus was limited and nonsustained. The first human infection with triple reassortant swine influenza A (H1) in the United States occurred in December 2005.[2] Human infection in the United States with a novel influenza A virus (including those of animal origin) was classified as a nationally notifiable infectious disease in June 2007. By February 2009, 11 notifications of confirmed human infection with triple reassortant swine influenza (H1),

8 of which occurred after June 2007, were received by the Centers for Disease Control and Prevention (CDC). Nine of the 11 patients had exposure to pigs, and all 11 recovered from their illness as reported in this study.

N. M. Khardori, MD

References

1. Ma W, Kahn RE, Richt JA. The pig as a mixing vessel for influenza viruses: human and veterinary implications. *J Mol Genet Med.* 2009;3:158-166.
2. Newman AP, Reisdort E, Beinemann J, et al. Human case of swine influenza A (H1N1) triple reassortant virus infection, Wisconsin. *Emerg Infect Dis.* 2008; 14:1470-1472.

Emergence of a Novel Swine-Origin Influenza A (H1N1) Virus in Humans
Novel Swine-Origin Influenza A (H1N1) Virus Investigation Team (Ctrs for Disease Control and Prevention, Atlanta, GA)
N Engl J Med 360:2605-2615, 2009

Background.—On April 15 and April 17, 2009, novel swine-origin influenza A (H1N1) virus (S-OIV) was identified in specimens obtained from two epidemiologically unlinked patients in the United States. The same strain of the virus was identified in Mexico, Canada, and elsewhere. We describe 642 confirmed cases of human S-OIV infection identified from the rapidly evolving U.S. outbreak.

Methods.—Enhanced surveillance was implemented in the United States for human infection with influenza A viruses that could not be subtyped. Specimens were sent to the Centers for Disease Control and Prevention for real-time reverse-transcriptase–polymerase-chain-reaction confirmatory testing for S-OIV.

Results.—From April 15 through May 5, a total of 642 confirmed cases of S-OIV infection were identified in 41 states. The ages of patients ranged from 3 months to 81 years; 60% of patients were 18 years of age or younger. Of patients with available data, 18% had recently traveled to Mexico, and 16% were identified from school outbreaks of S-OIV infection. The most common presenting symptoms were fever (94% of patients), cough (92%), and sore throat (66%); 25% of patients had diarrhea, and 25% had vomiting. Of the 399 patients for whom hospitalization status was known, 36 (9%) required hospitalization. Of 22 hospitalized patients with available data, 12 had characteristics that conferred an increased risk of severe seasonal influenza, 11 had pneumonia, 8 required admission to an intensive care unit, 4 had respiratory failure, and 2 died. The S-OIV was determined to have a unique genome composition that had not been identified previously.

Conclusions.—A novel swine-origin influenza A virus was identified as the cause of outbreaks of febrile respiratory infection ranging from self-limited to severe illness. It is likely that the number of confirmed cases underestimates the number of cases that have occurred.

▶ The background on human infections caused by triple-reassortant swine influenza virus consisted of 11 cases (one more case pending confirmation) in the United States between 2005 and 2009.[1] The Centers for Disease Control identified 2 cases of human infection with a swine-origin influenza A (H1N1) virus (S-OIV) on April 15, 2009 and April 17, 2009. The virus is characterized by a unique combination of gene segments that had not been identified previously among human or swine influenza A cases. Subsequently, cases of human infection with the same novel virus have also been identified in Mexico, Canada, and elsewhere. The World Health Organization (WHO) on April 2, 2009, labeled the event as WHO-designated pandemic phase at level 3 (no sustained human-to-human transmission), changed it to phase 4 on April 27, 2009 (human-to-human transmission verified), and upgraded it to phase 5 (same identified virus causing sustained community-level outbreaks in multiple countries) on April 29, 2009. If sustained human-to-human transmission is verified in all countries and/or the substantial increase in case count continues, the WHO pandemic level may be changed to the highest—phase 6.[2]

This study describes the first 642 confirmed cases of human S-OIV infection from the rapidly evolving United States outbreak. Similar to previous pandemics, rates of infection are higher in younger age groups (40% between 10 and 18 years of age and only 5% in 51 years of age and older). Clusters of confirmed S-OIV infection were identified early in the investigation in schools and universities in the United States, school staff, and contacts of students. The illness ranged from self-limited to severe.

Further published reports have (1) identified pregnancy as a high risk for complications from pandemic H1N1 virus infections and recommended prompt treatment of pregnant patients with anti-influenza drugs,[3] and (2) shown an increase in the rate of severe pneumonia with a shift in the age distribution (71% of severe pneumonia cases between 5 and 59 years of age).[4] These data suggest a rationale for focusing prevention efforts (including vaccination) on the younger population. The concept of "original antigenic sin," in which the immune response is greatest to antigens to which first exposure occurred in childhood, was described by Francis in 1960.[5] In this instance, that would mean that persons born before 1957 who were exposed to influenza A (H1N1) viruses in childhood might be better protected against this subtype than those who were first exposed to other influenza A subtypes (H2N2 and H3N2).

I am tempted to end this discussion by saying that in the world of infectious disease truth is always stranger than fiction, and science fiction writers do not need to create the materials they subject the rest of us to.

N. M. Khardori, MD

References

1. Shinde V, Bridges CB, Uyeki TM, et al. Triple-reassortant swine influenza A (H1) in humans in the United States, 2005-2009. *N Engl J Med.* 2009;360:2616-2625.
2. Katz R. Use of revised international health regulations during influenza A (H1N1) Epidemic, 2009. *Emerg Inf Dis.* 2009;15:1165-1170.
3. Jamieson DJ, Honein MA, Rasmussen SA, et al. H1N1 2009 influenza virus infection during pregnancy in the USA. *Lancet.* 2009;374:451-458.
4. Chowell G, Bertozzi SM, Colchero MA, et al. Severe respiratory disease concurrent with the circulation of H1N1 influenza. *N Engl J Med.* 2009;361:674-679.
5. Francis JT. On the doctrine of original antigenic sin. *Proc Am Philo Soc.* 1960;104: 572-578.

PART THREE

HEMATOLOGY AND ONCOLOGY

JAMES TATE THIGPEN, MD

19 Cancer Prevention

A Randomized, Controlled Trial of Financial Incentives for Smoking Cessation

Volpp KG, Troxel AB, Pauly MV, et al (Philadelphia Veterans Affairs Med Ctr, PA; Leonard Davis Inst of Health Economics, Philadelphia, PA; et al)
N Eng J Med 360:699-709, 2009

Background.—Smoking is the leading preventable cause of premature death in the United States. Previous studies of financial incentives for smoking cessation in work settings have not shown that such incentives have significant effects on cessation rates, but these studies have had limited power, and the incentives used may have been insufficient.

Methods.—We randomly assigned 878 employees of a multinational company based in the United States to receive information about smoking-cessation programs (442 employees) or to receive information about programs plus financial incentives (436 employees). The financial incentives were $100 for completion of a smoking-cessation program, $250 for cessation of smoking within 6 months after study enrollment, as confirmed by a biochemical test, and $400 for abstinence for an additional 6 months after the initial cessation, as confirmed by a biochemical test. Individual participants were stratified according to work site, heavy or nonheavy smoking, and income. The primary end point was smoking cessation 9 or 12 months after enrollment, depending on whether initial cessation was reported at 3 or 6 months. Secondary end points were smoking cessation within the first 6 months after enrollment and rates of participation in and completion of smoking-cessation programs.

Results.—The incentive group had significantly higher rates of smoking cessation than did the information-only group 9 or 12 months after enrollment (14.7% vs. 5.0%, P<0.001) and 15 or 18 months after enrollment (9.4% vs. 3.6%, P<0.001). Incentive-group participants also had significantly higher rates of enrollment in a smoking-cessation program (15.4% vs. 5.4%, P<0.001), completion of a smoking-cessation program (10.8% vs. 2.5%, P<0.001), and smoking cessation within the first 6 months after enrollment (20.9% vs. 11.8%, P<0.001).

Conclusions.—In this study of employees of one large company, financial incentives for smoking cessation significantly increased the rates of smoking cessation. (ClinicalTrials.gov number, NCT00128375.)

▶ The authors have demonstrated the difficulty in obtaining satisfactory smoking cessation rates. They randomized patients in a multinational company based in the United States to smoking cessation versus smoking cessation with a financial incentive. Smokers were randomized into the 2 groups, and could have earned up to $750 if they participated in smoking cessation counseling ($100), 6 months of abstinence ($250), and 12 months of abstinence ($400).

The study demonstrated that money did motivate individuals to quit over those individuals that were not offered a financial incentive at 6 and 12 months (20.9% vs 11.8%, $P < .001$ and 14.7% vs 5%, $P < .001$, respectively).

There are several concerns about applying this study to the general population. The study population was of a primarily higher socioeconomic group (64% of participants earning more than 5 times the national poverty level annually) and 90% were white. The study demonstrates that a $750 incentive achieved a surprisingly low 15-month abstinence rate of 9.4%. The authors quote studies demonstrating a cost of $3400 annually to employers for smoking employees in the form of extra smoking related costs. This does demonstrate that paying employees to stop may make some financial sense, but pay to quit does not replace more aggressive counseling programs.

T. L. Bauer II, MD

Effect of Selenium and Vitamin E on Risk of Prostate Cancer and Other Cancers: The Selenium and Vitamin E Cancer Prevention Trial (SELECT)
Lippman SM, Klein EA, Goodman PJ, et al (Univ of Texas M. D. Anderson Cancer Ctr, Houston; Cleveland Clinic, OH; Southwest Oncology Group Statistical Center, Seattle, WA; et al)
JAMA 301:39-51, 2009

Context.—Secondary analyses of 2 randomized controlled trials and supportive epidemiologic and preclinical data indicated the potential of selenium and vitamin E for preventing prostate cancer.

Objective.—To determine whether selenium, vitamin E, or both could prevent prostate cancer and other diseases with little or no toxicity in relatively healthy men.

Design, Setting, and Participants.—A randomized, placebo-controlled trial (Selenium and Vitamin E Cancer Prevention Trial [SELECT]) of 35 533 men from 427 participating sites in the United States, Canada, and Puerto Rico randomly assigned to 4 groups (selenium, vitamin E, selenium + vitamin E, and placebo) in a double-blind fashion between August 22, 2001, and June 24, 2004. Baseline eligibility included age 50 years or older (African American men) or 55 years or older (all other men), a serum prostate-specific antigen level of 4 ng/mL or less, and a digital rectal examination not suspicious for prostate cancer.

Interventions.—Oral selenium (200 μg/d from *L*-selenomethionine) and matched vitamin E placebo, vitamin E (400 IU/d of *all rac-α*-tocopheryl acetate) and matched selenium placebo, selenium + vitamin E, or placebo + placebo for a planned follow-up of minimum of 7 years and a maximum of 12 years.

Main Outcome Measures.—Prostate cancer and prespecified secondary outcomes, including lung, colorectal, and overall primary cancer.

Results.—As of October 23, 2008, median overall follow-up was 5.46 years (range, 4.17-7.33 years). Hazard ratios (99% confidence intervals [CIs]) for prostate cancer were 1.13 (99% CI, 0.95-1.35; n = 473) for vitamin E, 1.04 (99% CI, 0.87-1.24; n = 432) for selenium, and 1.05 (99% CI, 0.88-1.25; n = 437) for selenium + vitamin E vs 1.00 (n = 416) for placebo. There were no significant differences (all *P* > .15) in any other prespecified cancer end points. There were statistically nonsignificant increased risks of prostate cancer in the vitamin E group (*P* = .06) and type 2 diabetes mellitus in the selenium group (relative risk, 1.07; 99% CI, 0.94-1.22; *P* = .16) but not in the selenium + vitamin E group.

Conclusion.—Selenium or vitamin E, alone or in combination at the doses and formulations used, did not prevent prostate cancer in this population of relatively healthy men.

Trial Registration.—clinicaltrials.gov identifier: NCT00006392.

▶ This long-awaited article failed to demonstrate that selenium or vitamin E prevents prostate cancer or any cancer for that matter. For years, when asked by patients what they could do to prevent disease, I told them to give these a shot based on strong, epidemiologic evidence that they worked as well as phase III trials in other diseases that demonstrated a hint that they were protective. This study proved that I was wrong.

So which is correct, the earlier epidemiologic data, or the current randomized trial? Maybe (but not certainly) both. Treatment with a mineral or vitamin for a relative short time in an older population probably stacks the deck against the treatment. If nutrients are going to work, they probably will have to be ingested early in life, for a prolonged period of time and as foods not as isolated minerals/vitamins. In other words, there is no substitute for taking care of yourself when you are young by eating healthy. While this message may not always resonate with the American public, it is probably close to the truth.

A. S. Kibel, MD

20 Cancer Screening

Sensitivity and specificity of multimodal and ultrasound screening for ovarian cancer, and stage distribution of detected cancers: results of the prevalence screen of the UK Collaborative Trial of Ovarian Cancer Screening (UKCTOCS)

Menon U, Gentry-Maharaj A, Hallett R, et al (Univ College London Elizabeth Garrett Anderson Inst for Women's Health, UK; et al)

Lancet Oncol 10:327-340, 2009

Background.—Ovarian cancer has a high case–fatality ratio, with most women not diagnosed until the disease is in its advanced stages. The United Kingdom Collaborative Trial of Ovarian Cancer Screening (UKCTOCS) is a randomised controlled trial designed to assess the effect of screening on mortality. This report summarises the outcome of the prevalence (initial) screen in UKCTOCS.

Methods.—Between 2001 and 2005, a total of 202 638 postmenopausal women aged 50–74 years were randomly assigned to no treatment (control; n=101 359); annual CA125 screening (interpreted using a risk of ovarian cancer algorithm) with transvaginal ultrasound scan as a second-line test (multimodal screening [MMS]; n=50 640); or annual screening with transvaginal ultrasound (USS; n=50 639) alone in a 2:1:1 ratio using a computer-generated random number algorithm. All women provided a blood sample at recruitment. Women randomised to the MMS group had their blood tested for CA125 and those randomised to the USS group were sent an appointment to attend for a transvaginal scan. Women with abnormal screens had repeat tests. Women with persistent abnormality on repeat screens underwent clinical evaluation and, where appropriate, surgery. This trial is registered as ISRCTN22488978 and with ClinicalTrials.gov, number NCT00058032.

Findings.—In the prevalence screen, 50 078 (98·9%) women underwent MMS, and 48 230 (95·2%) underwent USS. The main reasons for withdrawal were death (two MMS, 28 USS), non-ovarian cancer or other disease (none MMS, 66 USS), removal of ovaries (five MMS, 29 USS), relocation (none MMS, 39 USS), failure to attend three appointments for the screen (72 MMS, 757 USS), and participant changing their mind (483 MMS, 1490 USS). Overall, 4355 of 50 078 (8.7%) women in the

MMS group and 5779 of 48 230 (12·0%) women in the USS group required a repeat test, and 167 (0·3%) women in the MMS group and 1894 (3·9%) women in the USS group required clinical evaluation. 97 of 50 078 (0·2%) women from the MMS group and 845 of 48 230 (1·8%) from the USS group underwent surgery. 42 (MMS) and 45 (USS) primary ovarian and tubal cancers were detected, including 28 borderline tumours (eight MMS, 20 USS). 28 (16 MMS, 12 USS) of 58 (48·3%; 95% CI 35·0–61·8) of the invasive cancers were stage I/II, with no difference (p=0·396) in stage distribution between the groups. A further 13 (five MMS, eight USS) women developed primary ovarian cancer during the year after the screen. The sensitivity, specificity, and positive-predictive values for all primary ovarian and tubal cancers were 89·4%, 99·8%, and 43·3% for MMS, and 84·9%, 98·2%, and 5·3% for USS, respectively. For primary invasive epithelial ovarian and tubal cancers, the sensitivity, specificity, and positive-predictive values were 89·5%, 99·8%, and 35·1% for MMS, and 75·0%, 98·2%, and 2·8% for USS, respectively. There was a significant difference in specificity (p<0·0001) but not sensitivity between the two screening groups for both primary ovarian and tubal cancers as well as primary epithelial invasive ovarian and tubal cancers.

Interpretation.—The sensitivity of the MMS and USS screening strategies is encouraging. Specificity was higher in the MMS than in the USS group, resulting in lower rates of repeat testing and surgery. This in part reflects the high prevalence of benign adnexal abnormalities and the more frequent detection of borderline tumours in the USS group. The prevalence screen has established that the screening strategies are feasible. The results of ongoing screening are awaited so that the effect of screening on mortality can be determined.

▶ Among gynecologic cancers, ovarian carcinoma accounts for 54% of all deaths because it is the only one of the major 3 without a means for early detection. This study by Menon et al randomized 202 638 women to 1 of 3 arms: a no-screening control arm, an arm screening patients annually with transvaginal ultrasound, or a multimodality approach to screening for ovarian carcinoma that used annual CA-125 screening interpreted with a risk of ovarian cancer algorithm, which triggered the subsequent use of transvaginal ultrasound. The bottom line of the study was that screening with ultrasound only yielded a positive predictive value of 2.8%, whereas the multimodality screening produced a positive predictive value of 35.1%, which, if confirmable, would suggest that this approach would eventually be expected to reduce mortality from ovarian carcinoma.

An accompanying editorial in *The Lancet Oncology* detailed a number of problems with the trial. The most important of these was the fact that the impact on mortality is not yet clear. Without this, one cannot conclude that this approach to screening should be used outside of clinical trial. In short, these data are interesting and provocative, but we still have no valid screening approach that can be routinely recommended.

J. T. Thigpen, MD

Results From Four Rounds of Ovarian Cancer Screening in a Randomized Trial
Partridge E, for the PLCO Project Team (Univ of Alabama, Birmingham; et al)
Obstet Gynecol 113:775-782, 2009

Objective.—To test whether annual screening with transvaginal ultrasonography and CA 125 reduces ovarian cancer mortality.

Methods.—Data from the first four annual screens, denoted T0–T3, are reported. A CA 125 value at or above 35 units/mL or an abnormality on transvaginal ultrasonography was considered a positive screen. Diagnostic follow-up of positive screens was performed at the discretion of participants' physicians. Diagnostic procedures and cancers were tracked and verified through medical records.

Results.—Among 34,261 screening arm women without prior oophorectomy, compliance with screening ranged from 83.1% (T0) to 77.6% (T3). Screen positivity rates declined slightly with transvaginal ultrasonography, from 4.6 at T0 to 2.9–3.4 at T1–T3; CA 125 positivity rates (range 1.4–1.8%) showed no time trend. Eighty-nine invasive ovarian or peritoneal cancers were diagnosed; 60 were screen detected. The positive predictive value (PPV) and cancer yield per 10,000 women screened on the combination of tests were similar across screening rounds (range 1.0–1.3% for PPV and 4.7–6.2 for yield); however, the biopsy (surgery) rate among screen positives decreased from 34% at T0 to 15–20% at T1–T3. The overall ratio of surgeries to screen-detected cancers was 19.5:1. Seventy-two percent of screen-detected cases were late stage (III/IV).

Conclusion.—Through four screening rounds, the ratio of surgeries to screen-detected cancers was high, and most cases were late stage. However, the effect of screening on mortality is as yet unknown.

Clinical Trial Registration.—ClinicalTrials.gov, www.clinicaltrials.gov, NCT00002540.

▶ This article reports the initial results of a major randomized trial evaluating screening for ovarian cancer. The study reported here is part of the Prostate, Lung, Colorectal and Ovarian (PLCO) study from the National Cancer Institute of the United States. Partridge et al report the results of the first 4 annual screens with CA-125, plus transvaginal ultrasound; 34 261 patients were randomized to screening or no screening. The bottom line was a positive predictive value of 1.3, and a very high ratio of surgeries as a result of screening to number of invasive cancers diagnosed (19.5-1). These results lend little credence to the value of this approach for the early detection of ovarian cancer. In addition, the data are premature for the determination of impact on overall mortality, the real bottom line for any screening test. One cannot, on the basis of these results, recommend screening with annual CA-125 plus transvaginal ultrasound.

J. T. Thigpen, MD

RNAi screen for rapid therapeutic target identification in leukemia patients
Tyner JW, Deininger MW, Loriaux MM, et al (Oregon Health and Science Univ Knight Cancer Inst, Portland; et al)
Proc Natl Acad Sci U S A 106:8695-8700, 2009

Targeted therapy has vastly improved outcomes in certain types of cancer. Extension of this paradigm across a broad spectrum of malignancies will require an efficient method to determine the molecular vulnerabilities of cancerous cells. Improvements in sequencing technology will soon enable high-throughput sequencing of entire genomes of cancer patients; however, determining the relevance of identified sequence variants will require complementary functional analyses. Here, we report an RNAi-assisted protein target identification (RAPID) technology that individually assesses targeting of each member of the tyrosine kinase gene family. We demonstrate that RAPID screening of primary leukemia cells from 30 patients identifies targets that are critical to survival of the malignant cells from 10 of these individuals. We identify known, activating mutations in JAK2 and K-RAS, as well as patientspecific sensitivity to downregulation of FLT1, CSF1R, PDGFR, ROR1, EPHA4/5, JAK1/3, LMTK3, LYN, FYN, PTK2B, and N-RAS. We also describe a previously undescribed, somatic, activating mutationin the thrombopoietin receptor that is sensitive to downstream pharmacologic inhibition. Hence, the RAPID technique can quickly identify molecular vulnerabilities in malignant cells. Combination of this technique with whole-genome sequencing will represent an ideal tool for oncogenic target identification such that specific therapies can be matched with individual patients.

▶ Past approaches to the identification of potential therapeutic targets has been mostly a "best candidate" or "best guess" event. In reality, this has actually worked quite well in identification and pharmacologic or immunologic targeting following through into clinical trials, and, in some instances, approved drugs and new standards of care. However, with the advent of new generation sequencing and high throughput screenings approaches, whether with aptamers, siRNAS, peptide libraries, or other methods, the potential to significantly increase the pace of discovery is palpable. Using an RNAi-based, high-throughput screen directed against tyrosine kinases, Tynner et al identified in myeloid leukemia several key targets, some of which were already known to be important and others considered to be novel. A critical next step is to determine to what extent these pathways are relevant to a larger number of acute myeloid leukemia (AML) samples, and to develop robust models for further testing. These studies also raise the incredible importance of early and close linkage to pharmaceutical and biotechnology companies or drug development teams, for it is the small-molecule drugs that are likely to be most important in exploiting such lovely preclinical work into changing clinical outcomes.

R. J. Arceci, MD, PhD

Screening and Prostate-Cancer Mortality in a Randomized European Study
Schröder FH, for the ERSPC Investigators (Erasmus Med Ctr, Rotterdam, The Netherlands)
N Engl J Med 360:1320-1328, 2009

Background.—The European Randomized Study of Screening for Prostate Cancer was initiated in the early 1990s to evaluate the effect of screening with prostate-specific–antigen (PSA) testing on death rates from prostate cancer.

Methods.—We identified 182,000 men between the ages of 50 and 74 years through registries in seven European countries for inclusion in our study. The men were randomly assigned to a group that was offered PSA screening at an average of once every 4 years or to a control group that did not receive such screening. The predefined core age group for this study included 162,243 men between the ages of 55 and 69 years. The primary outcome was the rate of death from prostate cancer. Mortality follow-up was identical for the two study groups and ended on December 31, 2006.

Results.—In the screening group, 82% of men accepted at least one offer of screening. During a median follow-up of 9 years, the cumulative incidence of prostate cancer was 8.2% in the screening group and 4.8% in the control group. The rate ratio for death from prostate cancer in the screening group, as compared with the control group, was 0.80 (95% confidence interval [CI], 0.65 to 0.98; adjusted P=0.04). The absolute risk difference was 0.71 death per 1000 men. This means that 1410 men would need to be screened and 48 additional cases of prostate cancer would need to be treated to prevent one death from prostate cancer. The analysis of men who were actually screened during the first round (excluding subjects with noncompliance) provided a rate ratio for death from prostate cancer of 0.73 (95% CI, 0.56 to 0.90).

Conclusions.—PSA-based screening reduced the rate of death from prostate cancer by 20% but was associated with a high risk of overdiagnosis. (Current Controlled Trials number, ISRCTN49127736.)

▶ This study and the study by Andriole et al[1] attempt to put the question of prostate-specific–antigen (PSA) testing to rest. Unfortunately, things are just more confusing than ever. Schröder et al examined 182000 men between the ages of 50 and 74 from 7 different European studies who were randomized to either screen or not be screened for prostate cancer. The endpoint of this study was overall mortality, and to cut to the chase, this study demonstrated an improvement in overall survival, which was statistically significant with a rate ratio for death from prostate cancer 0.73 (95% CI, 0.56 to 0.90). Andriole et al randomized roughly 76000 patients in the United States to either annual PSA screening or standard of care. At a median follow up of 7 years, they did not demonstrate an improvement in overall survival with a risk ratio of death of 1.13 (95% CI, 0.75 to 1.70).

Why the different results? Both studies have large sample size, although impressively this abstracted study from Europe had more than twice the number of patients. Perhaps there was possibly contamination in the control arm. In Andriole et al,[1] a significant percentage of the patients in the control arm were actually undergoing PSA screening (roughly 50%). This may have been enough to alter the results. In contrast, in this European study there was relatively little crossover between the patients who received screening and those who did not.

The main problem with this European study (and possibly PSA screening) is that at the relatively short follow up of approximately 9 years, there were not a lot of deaths from prostate cancer. Their estimates were that to prevent 1 prostate cancer death, 1410 men would have to be screened and 48 men would have to be treated. Clearly, this is a lot of men requiring screening and treatment to save 1 life. While I am sure that the man saved benefited, there continues to be concern that we are over treating a significant number of patients.

What does this all mean? Well, the PSA screening debate will continue. I think there are those in the camp that believe that PSA screening benefits all patients, and there are those who are convinced that PSA screening benefits none. I believe there is a middle ground where there are some patients who benefit and some patients who do not. My hope is that in the coming years we identify this cohort of patients. It may simply be on the basis of age or family history or genetic testing. Only the future will tell us.

A. S. Kibel, MD

Reference

1. Andriole GL, Grubb RL 3rd, Buys SS, et al. Mortality results from a randomized prostate-cancer screening trial. *N Engl J Med.* 2009;360:1310-1319.

Mortality Results from a Randomized Prostate-Cancer Screening Trial
Andriole GL, for the PLCO Project Team (Washington Univ School of Medicine, St. Louis; et al)
N Engl J Med 360:1310-1319, 2009

Background.—The effect of screening with prostate-specific–antigen (PSA) testing and digital rectal examination on the rate of death from prostate cancer is unknown. This is the first report from the Prostate, Lung, Colorectal, and Ovarian (PLCO) Cancer Screening Trial on prostate-cancer mortality.

Methods.—From 1993 through 2001, we randomly assigned 76,693 men at 10 U.S. study centers to receive either annual screening (38,343 subjects) or usual care as the control (38,350 subjects). Men in the screening group were offered annual PSA testing for 6 years and digital rectal examination for 4 years. The subjects and health care providers received the results and decided on the type of follow-up evaluation. Usual care sometimes included screening, as some organizations have recommended. The numbers of all cancers and deaths and causes of death were ascertained.

Results.—In the screening group, rates of compliance were 85% for PSA testing and 86% for digital rectal examination. Rates of screening in the control group increased from 40% in the first year to 52% in the sixth year for PSA testing and ranged from 41 to 46% for digital rectal examination. After 7 years of follow-up, the incidence of prostate cancer per 10,000 person-years was 116 (2820 cancers) in the screening group and 95 (2322 cancers) in the control group (rate ratio, 1.22; 95% confidence interval [CI], 1.16 to 1.29). The incidence of death per 10,000 person-years was 2.0 (50 deaths) in the screening group and 1.7 (44 deaths) in the control group (rate ratio, 1.13; 95% CI, 0.75 to 1.70). The data at 10 years were 67% complete and consistent with these overall findings.

Conclusions.—After 7 to 10 years of follow-up, the rate of death from prostate cancer was very low and did not differ significantly between the two study groups. (ClinicalTrials.gov number, NCT00002540.)

▶ This study and the study by Schröder et al[1] attempt to put the question of prostate-specific–antigen (PSA) testing to rest. Unfortunately, things are just more confusing than ever. Schröder et al[1] examined 182 000 men between the ages of 50 and 74 from 7 different European studies who were randomized to either screen or not be screened for prostate cancer. The endpoint of this study was overall mortality, and to cut to the chase, this study demonstrated an improvement in overall survival, which was statistically significant with a rate ratio for death from prostate cancer 0.73 (95% CI, 0.56 to 0.90). This study by Andriole et al randomized roughly 76 000 patients in the United States to either annual PSA screening or standard of care. At a median follow up of 7 years, they did not demonstrate an improvement in overall survival with a risk ratio of death of 1.13 (95% CI, 0.75 to 1.70).

Why the different results? Both studies have large sample size, although impressively the study from Europe[1] had more than twice the number of patients. Perhaps there was possibly contamination in the control arm. In this study by Andriole et al, a significant percentage of the patients in the control arm were actually undergoing PSA screening (roughly 50%). This may have been enough to alter the results. In contrast, in the European study[1] there was relatively little crossover between the patients who received screening and those who did not.

The main problem with the European study[1] (and possibly PSA screening) is that at the relatively short follow up of approximately 9 years, there were not a lot of deaths from prostate cancer. Their estimates were that to prevent 1 prostate cancer death, 1410 men would have to be screened and 48 men would have to be treated. Clearly, this is a lot of men requiring screening and treatment to save 1 life. While I am sure that the man saved benefited, there continues to be concern that we are over treating a significant number of patients.

What does this all mean? Well, the PSA screening debate will continue. I think there are those in the camp that believe that PSA screening benefits all patients, and there are those who are convinced that PSA screening benefits none. I believe there is a middle ground where there are some patients who benefit and some patients who do not. My hope is that in the coming years we identify this cohort of patients. It may simply be on the basis of age or family history or genetic testing. Only the future will tell us.

A. S. Kibel, MD

Reference

1. Schröder FH, Hugosson J, Roobol MJ, et al. Screening and prostate-cancer mortality in a randomized European study. *N Engl J Med.* 2009;360:1320-1328.

21 Gynecologic Cancer

Oregovomab Maintenance Monoimmunotherapy Does Not Improve Outcomes in Advanced Ovarian Cancer

Berek J, Taylor P, McGuire W, et al (Stanford Univ School of Medicine, CA; Univ of Virginia, Charlottesville; Franklin Square Hosp, Baltimore, MD; et al)

J Clin Oncol 27:418-425, 2009

Purpose.—This phase III study tested the hypothesis that the CA-125–specific murine monoclonal antibody, oregovomab, administered as a monoimmunotherapy after front-line therapy in a selected ovarian cancer population would prolong time to relapse (TTR) and, ultimately, survival.

Patients and Methods.—Patients with stage III to IV ovarian cancer with preoperatively elevated CA-125 and objectively defined characteristics were randomly assigned 4 to 12 weeks after front-line carboplatin and paclitaxel chemotherapy to maintenance monoimmunotherapy in a fully blinded protocol. Two mg of oregovomab or placebo was infused over 20 minutes at weeks 0, 4, and 8 and then 12 weeks until recurrence or up to year 5. Patients were evaluated with serial imaging and clinical evaluation for evidence of recurrence at quarterly visits. TTR was the primary end point.

Results.—Three hundred seventy-three patients were accrued at more than 60 centers; 251 patients were assigned to oregovomab and 120 patients were assigned to placebo. The treatment arms were well balanced. There were no differences in the clinical outcomes between treatment groups. Median TTR measured from randomization after completion of chemotherapy for the integrated study was 10.3 months (95% CI, 9.7 to 13.0 months) for oregovomab and 12.9 months (95% CI, 10.1 to 17.4 months) for placebo ($P = .29$, log-rank test). The treatment was well tolerated. Grade 3 to 4 toxicity was reported in 24.6% of patients in the placebo group and 20.1% of patients in the oregovomab group, respectively.

Conclusion.—Although oregovomab has demonstrated bioactivity, the strategy of monoimmunotherapy is not effective as maintenance therapy after front-line treatment of a favorable subset of patients with advanced ovarian cancer. Future studies of this or other tumor-antigen specific immunization strategies should seek ways to further augment induced immunity.

▶ The estimated overall clinical complete response rate for stages III to IV ovarian carcinoma approaches 75%; yet 75% of the clinical complete responders will relapse if no further therapy is given. To date, only one randomized trial has demonstrated an advantage for maintenance therapy in ovarian carcinoma.[1] That study demonstrated a highly significant progression-free survival advantage for 12 additional cycles of paclitaxel in those with a clinical complete response after 6 cycles of front-line paclitaxel plus carboplatin. A number of ongoing randomized phase III trials are evaluating maintenance bevacizumab or, in one case, maintenance cediranib. This trial evaluates the value of maintenance therapy with a monoclonal antibody against CA-125. No improvement in progression-free survival was observed; in fact, the trend observed was in the opposite direction. One can safely conclude that this antibody, at least at this dose and schedule, has no role as maintenance therapy in ovarian carcinoma.

J. T. Thigpen, MD

Reference

1. Markman M, Liu PY, Wilczynski S, et al. Phase III randomized trial of 12 versus 3 months of single agent paclitaxel in patients with advanced ovarian cancer who attained a clinically-defined complete response to platinum/paclitaxel-based chemotherapy: a Southwest Oncology Group and Gynecologic Oncology Group trial. *J Clin Oncol.* 2003;21:2460-2465.

Serous Tubal Intraepithelial Carcinoma: Its Potential Role in Primary Peritoneal Serous Carcinoma and Serous Cancer Prevention
Carlson JW, Miron A, Jarboe EA, et al (Brigham and Women's Hosp and Harvard Med School; Dana-Farber Cancer Inst, Boston, MA)
J Clin Oncol 26:4160-4165, 2008

Purpose.—A diagnosis of primary peritoneal serous carcinoma (PPSC) requires exclusion of a source in other reproductive organs. Serous tubal intraepithelial carcinoma (STIC; stage 0) has been described in asymptomatic women with *BRCA* mutations and linked to a serous cancer precursor in the fimbria. This study examined the frequency of STIC in PPSC and its clinical outcome in *BRCA*-positive women.

Patients and Methods.—Presence or absence of STIC was recorded in consecutive cases meeting the 2001 WHO criteria for PPSC, including 26 patients with nonuniform sampling of the fallopian tubes (group 1) and 19 patients with complete tubal examination (group 2; sectioning and extensively examining the fimbriated end, or SEE-FIM protocol). In selected cases, STIC or its putative precursor and the peritoneal tumor were analyzed for *p53* mutations (exons 1 to 11). Outcome of STIC was ascertained by literature review.

Result.—Thirteen (50%) of 26 PPSCs in group 1 involved the endosalpinx, with nine STICs (35%). Fifteen (79%) of 19 cases in group 2 contained endosalpingeal involvement, with nine STICs (47%). STIC was typically fimbrial and unifocal, with variable invasion of the tubal wall. In five of five cases, the peritoneal and tubal lesion shared an identical *p53* mutation. Of 10 reported STICs in *BRCA*-positive women, all patients were without disease on follow-up.

Conclusion.—The fimbria is the source of nearly one half of PPSCs, suggesting serous malignancy originates in the tubal mucosa but grows preferentially at a remote peritoneal site. The generally low risk of recurrence in stage 0 (STIC) disease further underscores STIC as a possible target for early serous cancer detection and prevention.

▶ This article is one of several that have suggested that the source of origin for a substantial proportion of primary peritoneal serous carcinomas is in fact the fallopian tube. Previous studies of primary peritoneal carcinomas have suggested that these lesions respond to systemic therapy exactly as do serous carcinomas of ovarian origin; in fact, most studies of celomic epithelial carcinoma of the ovary include primary peritoneal carcinomas and fallopian tube carcinomas. These observations support the concept that what we now refer to as "garden variety ovarian carcinoma" is simply one form of celomic epithelial carcinoma, and that management of these lesions is essentially the same regardless of focus of origin within the peritoneal cavity. Where focus of origin becomes important is when the focus is on early detection prior to the advent of spread. The data from this article suggest that it may be feasible to detect tubal lesions early and thus to intervene with surgical resection alone. What remains is to demonstrate that any approach actually results in early detection. Such an approach has not yet been identified, so management of most celomic epithelial carcinomas will continue to focus for the immediate future on bulk reduction and systemic therapy for advanced disease.

J. T. Thigpen, MD

Randomized phase 3 trial of interferon gamma-1b plus standard carboplatin/paclitaxel versus carboplatin/paclitaxel alone for first-line treatment of advanced ovarian and primary peritoneal carcinomas: Results from a prospectively designed analysis of progression-free survival
Alberts DS, Marth C, Alvarez RD, et al (Univ of Arizona, Tucson; Innsbruck Med Univ, Austria; The Univ of Alabama at Birmingham; et al)
Gynecol Oncol 109:174-181, 2008

Objectives.—Interferon gamma (IFN-γ) is a pleiotropic cytokine with antiproliferative, immunostimulatory, and chemosensitization properties. This trial was designed to evaluate IFN-γ 1b plus carboplatin and paclitaxel in treatment-naive ovarian cancer (OC) and primary peritoneal carcinoma (PPC) patients.

Methods.—Eligible patients were randomized to 6 cycles of carboplatin/paclitaxel every 3 weeks or the same in combination with IFN-γ 1b (100 µg 3 × /wk subcutaneously). The primary endpoint was overall survival (OS) time (target hazard ratio (HR) = 0.77). Secondary endpoints included progression-free survival (target HR = 0.7), based on blinded review of serial imaging scans, physical exams, and CA-125 levels.

Results.—847 patients were enrolled (OC 774, PPC 73) in Europe ($n = 539$) and North/South America ($n = 308$) from January 29, 2002 to March 31, 2004 and stratified according to: optimal debulking ($n = 271$) versus suboptimal debulking with plans for interval debulking (PID) ($n = 238$) or no PID ($n = 338$). The study stopped early following a protocol-defined second interim analysis which revealed significantly shorter OS time in patients receiving IFN-γ 1b plus chemotherapy compared to chemotherapy alone (1138 days vs. not estimable, HR = 1.45, 95% CI = 1.15–1.83). At the time of the analysis, 169 of 426 (39.7%) patients in the IFN-γ 1b plus chemotherapy group had died compared to 128 of 421 (30.4%) in the chemotherapy alone group. Serious adverse events were more common in the IFN-γ 1b plus chemotherapy group (48.5% vs. 35.4%), primarily due to a higher incidence of serious hematological toxicities (34.5% vs. 22.7%).

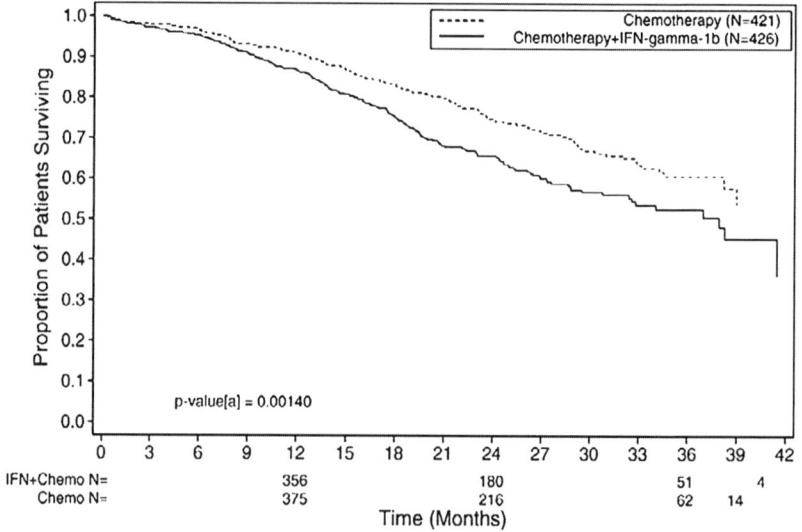

FIGURE 1.—Kaplan–Meier estimates for overall survival time by treatment group: ITT population. [a] Log-rank test with randomization stratification factor in the model. Analysis based on 9Nov2005 phone contact database. (Reprinted from Alberts DS, Marth C, Alvarez RD, et al. Randomized phase 3 trial of interferon gamma-1b plus standard carboplatin/paclitaxel versus carboplatin/paclitaxel alone for first-line treatment of advanced ovarian and primary peritoneal carcinomas: results from a prospectively designed analysis of progression-free survival. *Gynecol Oncol.* 2008;109:174-181.)

Conclusions.—Treatment with IFN-γ 1b in combination with carboplatin/paclitaxel does not have a role in the first-line treatment of advanced ovarian cancer (Fig 1).

▶ The basis for the evaluation of the addition of low-dose gamma interferon to paclitaxel/carboplatin as front-line therapy for advanced ovarian carcinoma was substantial activity of single-agent gamma interferon in several phase II trials from the early 1990s, combined with a small Austrian phase III trial in advanced ovarian carcinoma comparing cisplatin/cyclophosphamide ± gamma interferon. The small phase III trial showed a significant improvement in progression-free survival; events for survival were insufficient to reach meaningful conclusions. A phase II trial showed that it was feasible to combine paclitaxel/carboplatin with the same dose of gamma interferon. Surprisingly, gamma interferon combined with paclitaxel/carboplatin produced a significantly inferior survival in the large phase III trial (Fig 1). Further studies of gamma interferon have been abandoned as a result of this outcome. The results of this trial provide reason for oncologists to be cautious about adopting promising new approaches outside of clinical trials without data from adequately powered phase III trials confirming the value of the new approach.

J. T. Thigpen, MD

Ovarian cancer and oral contraceptives: collaborative reanalysis of data from 45 epidemiological studies including 23 257 women with ovarian cancer and 87 303 controls
Collaborative Group on Epidemiological Studies of Ovarian Cancer (Cancer Res UK Epidemiology Unit, Oxford)
Lancet 371:303-314, 2008

Background.—Oral contraceptives were introduced almost 50 years ago, and over 100 million women currently use them. Oral contraceptives can reduce the risk of ovarian cancer, but the eventual public-health effects of this reduction will depend on how long the protection lasts after use ceases. We aimed to assess these effects.

Methods.—Individual data for 23 257 women with ovarian cancer (cases) and 87 303 without ovarian cancer (controls) from 45 epidemiological studies in 21 countries were checked and analysed centrally. The relative risk of ovarian cancer in relation to oral contraceptive use was estimated, stratifying by study, age, parity, and hysterectomy.

Findings.—Overall 7308 (31%) cases and 32 717 (37%) controls had ever used oral contraceptives, for average durations among users of 4·4 and 5·0 years, respectively. The median year of cancer diagnosis was 1993, when cases were aged an average of 56 years. The longer that women had used oral contraceptives, the greater the reduction in ovarian cancer risk (p<0·0001). This reduction in risk persisted for more than 30 years after oral contraceptive use had ceased but became somewhat attenuated over time—the proportional risk reductions per 5 years of use were 29% (95% CI 23–34%) for use that had ceased less than 10 years previously, 19% (14–24%) for use that had ceased 10–19 years previously, and 15% (9–21%) for use that had ceased 20–29 years previously. Use during the 1960s, 1970s, and 1980s was associated with similar proportional risk reductions, although typical oestrogen doses in the 1960s were more than double those in the 1980s. The incidence of mucinous tumours (12% of the total) seemed little affected by oral contraceptives, but otherwise the proportional risk reduction did not vary much between different histological types. In high-income countries, 10 years use of oral contraceptives was estimated to reduce ovarian cancer incidence before age 75 from 1·2 to 0·8 per 100 users and mortality from 0·7 to 0·5 per 100; for every 5000 woman-years of use, about two ovarian cancers and one death from the disease before age 75 are prevented.

Interpretation.—Use of oral contraceptives confers long-term protection against ovarian cancer. These findings suggest that oral contraceptives have already prevented some 200 000 ovarian cancers and 100 000 deaths from the disease, and that over the next few decades the number of cancers prevented will rise to at least 30 000 per year (Fig 2).

▶ This meta-analysis of epidemiologic data on risk reduction for ovarian cancer with the use of oral contraceptives confirms what has been reported in

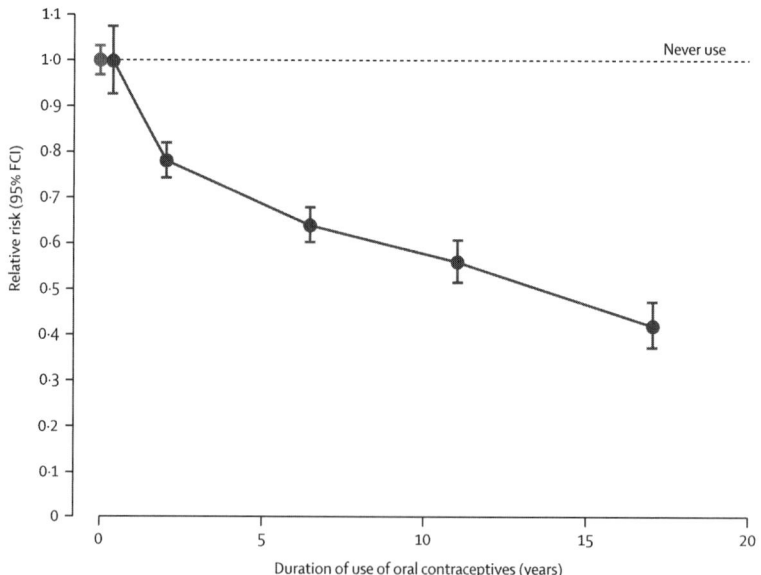

FIGURE 2.—Relative risk* of ovarian cancer by duration of use of oral contraceptives. *Stratified by study, age, parity, and hysterectomy. (Reprinted from Collaborative Group on Epidemiological Studies of Ovarian Cancer. Ovarian cancer and oral contraceptives: collaborative reanalysis of data from 45 epidemiological studies including 23 257 women with ovarian cancer and 87 303 controls. *Lancet.* 2008;371:303-314, with permission from Elsevier Ltd.)

individual articles: prolonged use of oral contraceptives lowers the risk for ovarian cancer by a substantial margin (Fig 2). The degree of risk reduction is about 29% per 5 years of use, but this risk reduction is attenuated over time when oral contraceptives have been stopped. The estrogen dose contained in the particular preparation does not seem to matter because there was no difference in risk reduction with earlier preparations, which contained up to twice as much estrogen as later preparations. The only histologic type of ovarian carcinoma not affected by oral contraceptive use was the category of mucinous coelomic epithelial carcinomas, which, in the United States, constitute less than 10% of all coelomic epithelial carcinomas. While all of these sounds very good, not discussed in the article is the downside – an increased risk for breast carcinoma, which may vary from 1.2- to 1.4-fold. As a result, the use of oral contraceptives solely to decrease the risk of developing ovarian cancer is generally not recommended; oral contraceptives could possibly be recommended in women who face a high risk of ovarian cancer because of a familial disorder associated with ovarian cancer (BRCA1, BRCA2, etc).

J. T. Thigpen, MD

Evaluation of New Platinum-Based Treatment Regimens in Advanced-Stage Ovarian Cancer: A Phase III Trial of the Gynecologic Cancer InterGroup

Bookman MA, Brady MF, McGuire WP, et al (The Fox Chase Cancer Ctr, Philadelphia, PA; Gynecologic Oncology Group Statistical and Data Ctr, Buffalo, NY; Franklin Square Hosp, Baltimore, MD; et al)
J Clin Oncol 27:1419-1425, 2009

Purpose.—To determine if incorporation of an additional cytotoxic agent improves overall survival (OS) and progression-free survival (PFS) for women with advanced-stage epithelial ovarian carcinoma (EOC) and primary peritoneal carcinoma who receive carboplatin and paclitaxel.

Patients and Methods.—Women with stages III to IV disease were stratified by coordinating center, maximal diameter of residual tumor, and intent for interval cytoreduction and were then randomly assigned among five arms that incorporated gemcitabine, methoxypolyethylene glycosylated liposomal doxorubicin, or topotecan compared with carboplatin and paclitaxel. The primary end point was OS and was determined by pairwise comparison to the reference arm, with a 90% chance of detecting a true hazard ratio of 1.33 that limited type I error to 5% (two-tail) for the four comparisons.

Results.—Accrual exceeded 1,200 patients per year. An event-triggered interim analysis occurred after 272 events on the reference arm, and the study closed with 4,312 women enrolled. Arms were well balanced for demographic and prognostic factors, and 79% of patients completed eight cycles of therapy. There were no improvements in either PFS or OS associated with any experimental regimen. Survival analyses of groups

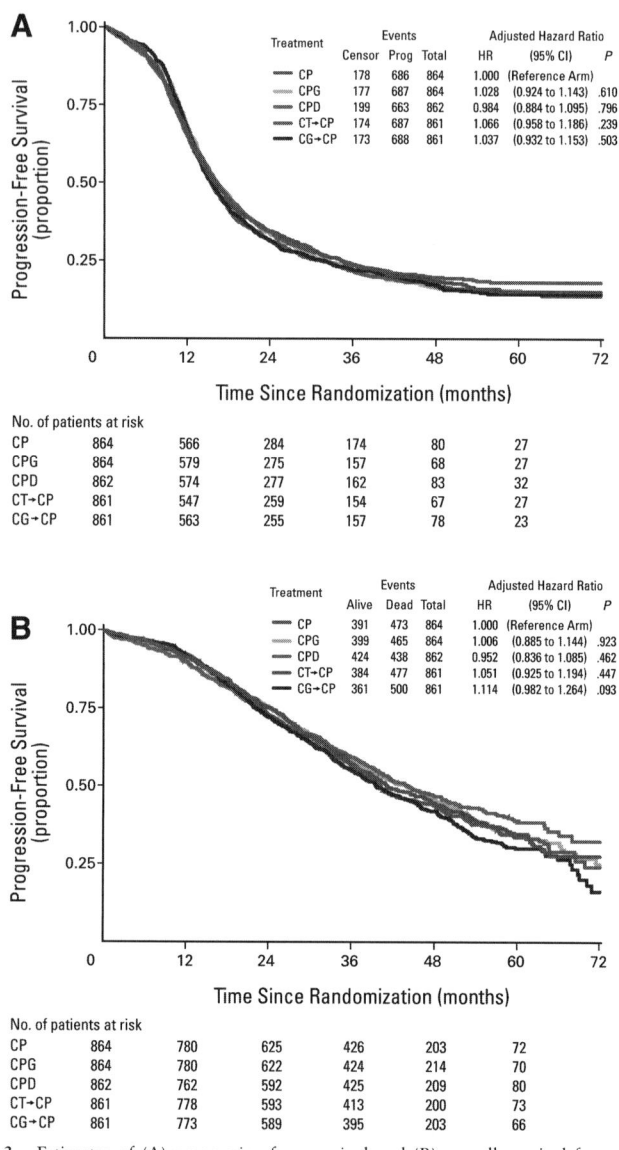

FIGURE 3.—Estimates of (A) progression-free survival and (B) overall survival for each treatment arm, including the cumulative number of events, the number of patients at risk, and a summary of hazard ratios; *P* values were adjusted for extent of residual disease and participating cooperative group. Median progression-free survival rates varied from 15.4 to 16.4 months, and median overall survival rates varied from 39.6 to 44.2 months. CP, carboplatin and paclitaxel; CPG, carboplatin, paclitaxel, and gemcitabine; CPD, carboplatin, paclitaxel, and doxorubicin; CT-CP, carboplatin plus topotecan, then carboplatin plus paclitaxel; CG-CP, carboplatin plus gemcitabine, then carboplatin plus paclitaxel. (Reprinted from Bookman MA, Brady MF, McGuire WP, et al. Evaluation of new platinum-based treatment regimens in advanced-stage ovarian cancer: a phase III trial of the Gynecologic Cancer Intergroup. *J Clin Oncol.* 2009;27:1419-1425, with permission from the American Society of Clinical Oncology.)

defined by size of residual disease also failed to show experimental benefit in any subgroup.

Conclusion.—Compared with standard paclitaxel and carboplatin, addition of a third cytotoxic agent provided no benefit in PFS or OS after optimal or suboptimal cytoreduction. Dual-stage, multiarm, phase III trials can efficiently evaluate multiple experimental regimens against a single reference arm. The development of new interventions beyond surgery and conventional platinum-based chemotherapy is required to additionally improve outcomes for women with advanced EOC (Fig 3).

▶ This is the largest study of ovarian carcinoma ever reported. The study evaluates whether adding a third cytotoxic agent to the international standard therapy of paclitaxel plus carboplatin enhances the outcome of patients with advanced ovarian carcinoma. The standard doublet of paclitaxel/carboplatin (PC) was compared with 2 triplets (PC plus gemcitabine and PC plus pegylated liposomal doxorubicin [PLD]) and 2 sequential doublet regimens (topotecan plus carboplatin or gemcitabine plus carboplatin for 4 cycles followed by paclitaxel plus carboplatin for 4 cycles). Toxicity was increased with both triplets, and there was no evidence of improvement in either progression-free or overall survival. The design of the study permits an adequate evaluation of the 2 gemcitabine-containing regimens, but the PLD was given at a dose of 30 mg/m^2 every 6 weeks, and the topotecan was given as a 3-day regimen of 0.75 mg/m^2/d. Although one could argue that neither PLD nor topotecan was given a fair test, the overall study results are not encouraging for the potential value of adding a third cytotoxic agent to frontline therapy.

This study demonstrates one other important fact. When study designs are simple and straightforward, patient accrual to ovarian cancer studies can permit large trials to be completed successfully. This trial accrued at greater than 1200 patients per year, by far the most rapid accrual of patients with ovarian cancer ever reported.

As a side note, the regimens in this trial used 8 cycles of therapy solely for the purpose of keeping all regimens symmetrical in treatment duration. There is no evidence that 8 cycles of therapy yield a result superior to the more commonly used 6 cycles of therapy, hence, one should not recommend 8 cycles of therapy because this was what was done in this particular trial.

J. T. Thigpen, MD

22 Breast Cancer

American College of Radiology Appropriateness Criteria® on Conservative Surgery and Radiation: Stages I and II Breast Carcinoma
White JR, Halberg FE, Rabinovitch R, et al (Med College of Wisconsin, Milwaukee; Marin Cancer Inst, Greenbrae, CA; Univ of Colorado Cancer Ctr, Denver, CO; et al)
J Am Coll Radiol 5:701-713, 2008

Background.—During the past 2 decades, breast conservation therapy (BCT) has become firmly established as a standard therapeutic approach for eligible women with early-stage breast cancer. Breast radiation after conservative surgery is an integral component of BCT, resulting in comparable local control and equivalent survival to mastectomy. Successful breast conservation relies on understanding key elements for patient selection, evaluation, treatment contraindications, radiation therapy methods, and integration with systemic therapy.

Methods.—The Appropriateness Criteria Committee of the American College of Radiology convened an expert panel to examine BCT for early-stage breast cancer. By using a modified Delphi technique to generate consensus, the expert panel responded to questionnaires on 9 clinical cases that address various key elements of breast conservation. A literature review on BCT led to the generation of an evidence table to support the consensus and overview.

Results.—Consensus for appropriateness criteria for BCT was produced for various clinical scenarios commonly encountered in practice. These topics include radiation oncology management issues related to young patient age, sentinel node biopsy, elderly patients, other histology, positive margins, extensive intraductal component, node-positive breast cancer, genetic breast cancer, partial breast irradiation, and systemic therapy. Radiation methods for BCT are reviewed.

Conclusion.—The Breast Cancer Panel has generated a consensus of up-to-date guidelines for the appropriate use of radiation for BCT by using a modified Delphi process for the American College of Radiology Appropriateness Criteria.

▶ Standards of care for surgery, radiation, and/or chemotherapy are difficult to develop because all too often there is not enough science and too many opinions to achieve a consensus. The American College of Radiology (ACR) has developed multiple documents outlining standards of care for a wide variety of diseases. The most recent is this article on appropriateness criteria for breast conservation in Stage I and II breast cancer.

The authors of this and the other pre-existing ACR standards are to be commended for the vast amount of work that goes into evaluating realms of literature on every aspect of the topic and further commended on their tenacity to work through the tedious, but very important process of modified Delphi technique to generate consensus.

Appropriateness criteria such as these need to be digested by all radiation oncologists who treat Stage I and II breast carcinoma. This allows the oncologist to be as certain as possible that they are treating patients at the current standards of care (quality) level.

C. A. Lawton, MD

Ten-Year Follow-Up of 3 Years of Oral Adjuvant Clodronate Therapy Shows Significant Prevention of Osteoporosis in Early-Stage Breast Cancer
Saarto T, Vehmanen L, Blomqvist C, et al (Helsinki Univ Central Hosp, Finland)
J Clin Oncol 26:4289-4295, 2008

Purpose.—We have previously reported that 3-year adjuvant clodronate treatment prevents bone loss in breast cancer patients. Here we report the 10-year follow-up data of clodronate in the prevention of treatment-related osteoporosis in women with early-stage breast cancer.

Patients and Methods.—Two hundred sixty-eight pre- and postmenopausal, node-positive breast cancer patients were randomly assigned to clodronate, 1.6 g orally administered daily, or to control groups for 3 years. Premenopausal women were treated with adjuvant CMF chemotherapy; and postmenopausal women were treated with antiestrogens, either 20 mg tamoxifen or 60 mg toremifene, for 3 years. The bone mineral density (BMD) of the lumbar spine and hip was measured before treatment and at 1, 2, 3, 5, and 10 years after therapy.

Results.—Eighty-nine disease-free patients were included in the analyses of osteoporosis-free survival. During the 10-year period, 24 of 89 patients were diagnosed with osteoporosis. Fourteen patients developed spinal osteoporosis (three of 41 in the clodronate group, and 11 of 48 in the control group), and 14 of 89 patients were diagnosed with hip osteoporosis (seven of 41 in the clodronate group, and seven of 48 in the control group). The 10-year spinal, osteoporosis-free survival rate was 92.7% in the clodronate group, and 77.0% in the control group ($P = .035$). No difference was seen in the frequency of hip osteoporosis (85.4% v 82.9%; $P = .92$). Baseline BMD measurement had a predictive value of 18 of 24 patients (75%) who developed osteoporosis had osteopenia of the lumbar spine at baseline.

Conclusion.—Three years of clodronate therapy significantly reduces the incidence of lumbar spine osteoporosis. Patients at risk of developing osteoporosis are among those who have pretreatment osteopenia, that is, baseline BMD measurement has predictive value.

▶ Osteoporosis is a possible toxicity for breast cancer patients who receive antiestrogens and/or chemotherapy. Fractures as a result of osteoporosis are a significant clinical problem in that they decrease quality of life secondary to the pain that they can cause and hip fractures, if they occur, are associated with an increase in mortality.

Methods to decrease the potential for osteoporosis and associated fractures in breast cancer patients have been studied. Bisphosphonates, in particular, are a class of drugs that have been shown to help maintain bone density in women receiving systemic therapy for breast cancer. The challenge for most of the studies showing the benefit of these drugs in breast cancer patients is that the follow-up is short. These authors present 10-year follow-up of a study of 268 women randomly assigned to 3 years of an oral bisphosphonate versus no treatment. There was a benefit to the therapy with regard to 10-year spinal osteoporosis-free survival, but no benefit to treatment with regard to 10-year hip osteoporosis-free survival.

Unfortunately, fracture rate was not evaluated. It is really the fracture itself that is the problem for the patient with osteoporosis. Yet, knowing that osteoporosis is associated with increased fracture risk and that lower bone mineral density at the time of randomization showed a benefit to the oral bisphosphonate in terms of osteoporosis risk, patients with osteopenia prebreast cancer therapy should be counseled as to the potential benefit of bisphosphonate therapy.

C. A. Lawton, MD

Endocrine Therapy plus Zoledronic Acid in Premenopausal Breast Cancer
Gnant M, Mlineritsch B, Schippinger W, et al (Med Univ of Vienna, Austria; Paracelsus Med Univ Salzburg; Med Univ of Graz; et al)
N Engl J Med 360:679-691, 2009

Background.—Ovarian suppression plus tamoxifen is a standard adjuvant treatment in premenopausal women with endocrine-responsive breast cancer. Aromatase inhibitors are superior to tamoxifen in postmenopausal patients, and preclinical data suggest that zoledronic acid has antitumor properties.

Methods.—We examined the effect of adding zoledronic acid to a combination of either goserelin and tamoxifen or goserelin and anastrozole in premenopausal women with endocrine-responsive early breast cancer. We randomly assigned 1803 patients to receive goserelin (3.6 mg given subcutaneously every 28 days) plus tamoxifen (20 mg per day given orally) or anastrozole (1 mg per day given orally) with or without zoledronic acid (4 mg given intravenously every 6 months) for 3 years. The primary end point was disease-free survival; recurrence-free survival and overall survival were secondary end points.

Results.—After a median follow-up of 47.8 months, 137 events had occurred, with disease-free survival rates of 92.8% in the tamoxifen group, 92.0% in the anastrozole group, 90.8% in the group that received endocrine therapy alone, and 94.0% in the group that received endocrine therapy with zoledronic acid. There was no significant difference in disease-free survival between the anastrozole and tamoxifen groups (hazard ratio for disease progression in the anastrozole group, 1.10; 95% confidence interval [CI], 0.78 to 1.53; P = 0.59). The addition of zoledronic acid to endocrine therapy, as compared with endocrine therapy without zoledronic acid, resulted in an absolute reduction of 3.2 percentage points and a relative reduction of 36% in the risk of disease progression (hazard ratio, 0.64; 95% CI, 0.46 to 0.91; P = 0.01); the addition of zoledronic acid did not significantly reduce the risk of death (hazard ratio, 0.60; 95% CI, 0.32 to 1.11; P = 0.11). Adverse events were consistent with known drug-safety profiles.

Conclusions.—The addition of zoledronic acid to adjuvant endocrine therapy improves disease-free survival in premenopausal patients with estrogen-responsive early breast cancer. (ClinicalTrials.gov number, NCT00295646.)

▶ This trial looks at the comparative efficacy of tamoxifen versus anastrozole and the role of bisphosphonates in premenopausal women on adjuvant endocrine therapy for limited breast cancer. None of the patients had known bone involvement at the time of initiation of therapy on study. A statistically significant 36% reduction in the likelihood of disease progression was observed in the group assigned to receive zoledronic acid 4 mg every 6 months (the first 254 patients received 4 mg every 4 weeks). There was no observed difference between tamoxifen and anastrozole. No improvement in overall survival was noted, but there were only 42 events for survival at the time of this report. No osteonecrosis was observed on the study. These data show that the observed advantage of aromatase inhibitors over antiestrogens in postmenopausal women could not be confirmed in premenopausal women; hence, the use of tamoxifen in premenopausal remains reasonable first hormonal therapy. The data also suggest that a bisphosphonate should be included in the management of these patients who do not have observable bone involvement.

J. T. Thigpen, MD

Estimated Risk of Radiation-Induced Breast Cancer From Mammographic Screening for Young *BRCA* Mutation Carriers

Berrington de Gonzalez A, Berg CD, Visvanathan K, et al (Johns Hopkins Bloomberg School of Public Health, Baltimore, MD; Natl Cancer Inst, Rockville, MD)
J Natl Cancer Inst 101:205-209, 2009

BRCA mutation carriers are recommended to start mammographic screening for breast cancer as early as age 25–30 years. We used an excess relative risk model (based on a pooled analysis of three cohorts with 7600 subjects who received radiation exposure) to estimate the lifetime risk of radiation-induced breast cancer from five annual mammographic screenings in young (<40 years) *BRCA* mutation carriers. We then estimated the reduction in breast cancer mortality required to outweigh the radiation risk. Breast cancer rates for mutation carriers were based on a pooled analysis of 22 pedigree studies with 8139 subjects. For *BRCA1* mutation carriers, the estimated lifetime risk of radiation-induced breast cancer mortality per 10 000 women resulting from annual mammography was 26 (95% confidence interval [CI] = 14 to 49) for screening at age 25–29 years, 20 (95% CI = 11 to 39) for screening at age 30–34 years, and 13 (95% CI = 7 to 23) for screening at age 35–39 years. To outweigh these risks, screening would have to reduce breast cancer mortality by 51% (95% CI = 27% to 96%) at age 25–29 years, by 12% (95% CI = 6% to 23%) at age 30-34 years, and by 4% (95% CI = 2% to 7%) at age 35–39 years; estimates were similar for *BRCA2* mutation carriers. If we assume that the mortality reduction from mammography is 15%–25% or less for young women, these results suggest that there would be no net benefit from annual mammographic screening of *BRCA* mutation carriers at age 25–29 years; the net benefit would be zero or small at age 30–34 years, but there should be some net benefit at age 35 or older. These results depend on a number of assumptions due to the absence of empiric data. The impact of varying these assumptions was therefore examined.

▶ The study seeks to determine whether the recommendation for an early start to regular mammography in patients with *BRCA* mutations results in a high enough estimated risk of radiation-induced breast cancer to offset any advantage gained. The authors conclude that there is little evidence of a benefit from the starting regular mammography before age 35, despite the high risk of breast cancer in such patients. These conclusions, however, are based on some rather significant assumptions. The most important of these is the assumption that the risk of radiation-induced cancer is best represented by a linear no-threshold model. This essentially means that patients have an increased risk at even very low levels of radiation exposure. Simply put, the data do not support such a view.

No study has ever actually demonstrated an increased risk below a cumulative exposure above background radiation of 10 Roentgen Equivalent Man. Instead, all estimates of increased risk below this level are the result of extrapolation from higher exposures based on a no-threshold model. Such a model fails to take into account the fact that cells have a tremendous capacity for repair of radiation-induced damage that must be overcome before risk actually increases. The authors' conclusions must therefore be regarded as suspect and based on unwarranted assumptions, at least on the basis of current actual data.

J. T. Thigpen, MD

23 Prostate Cancer

Long-term results of the M. D. Anderson randomized dose-escalation trial for prostate cancer

Kuban DA, Tucker SL, Dong L, et al (Univ of Texas M. D. Anderson Cancer Ctr, Houston, et al)

Int J Radiat Oncol Biol Phys 70:67-74, 2008

Purpose.—To report the long-term results of a randomized radiotherapy dose escalation trial for prostate cancer.

Methods and Materials.—From 1993 to 1998, a total of 301 patients with stage T1b to T3 prostate cancer were accrued to a randomized external beam dose escalation trial using 70 Gy versus 78 Gy. The median follow-up is now 8.7 years. Kaplan-Meier analysis was used to compute rates of prostate-specific antigen (PSA) failure (nadir + 2), clinical failure, distant metastasis, disease-specific, and overall survival as well as complication rates at 8 years post-treatment.

Results.—For all patients, freedom from biochemical or clinical failure (FFF) was superior for the 78-Gy arm, 78%, as compared with 59% for the 70-Gy arm ($p = 0.004$, and an even greater benefit was seen in patients with initial PSA >10 ng/ml (78% vs. 39%, $p = 0.001$). The clinical failure rate was significantly reduced in the 78-Gy arm as well (7% vs. 15%, $p = 0.014$). Twice as many patients either died of prostate cancer or are currently alive with cancer in the 70-Gy arm. Gastrointestinal toxicity of grade 2 or greater occurred twice as often in the high dose patients (26% vs. 13%), although genitourinary toxicity of grade 2 or greater was less (13% vs. 8%) and not statistically significantly different. Dose-volume histogram analysis showed that the complication rate could be significantly decreased by reducing the amount of treated rectum.

Conclusions.—Modest escalation in radiotherapy dose improved freedom from biochemical and clinical progression with the largest benefit in prostate cancer patients with PSA >10 ng/ml.

▶ Appropriate doses to treat localized prostate cancer have been studied extensively over the last decade. The group at MD Anderson published 1 of the first randomized trials of dose escalation for localized disease. Subsequent groups have shown similar findings in that the biochemical non-evidence of disease (bNED) control is improved; yet survival has not been impacted to date with dose escalation for certain patients. In the case of this trial, 70 versus 78 Gy delivered to isocenter, the patients who benefit the most are the patients whose initial prostate-specific antigen (PSA) was >10.0 ng/mL. This places these patients into the intermediate-risk group. As with all dose escalation, there are potential increased risks and increased gastrointestinal toxicity as was seen in the dose-escalated group. Based on these and other studies of dose escalation, it is appropriate for intermediate-risk patients, but has to be carefully designed to avoid excessive toxicity. Low-risk patients who are very unlikely to succumb to their disease may need to use more caution when considering dose escalation, as not all of the randomized trials have shown a benefit to it.

C. A. Lawton, MD

Measuring the Quality of Care in Radiation Oncology
Hayman JA (Univ of Michigan, Ann Arbor, MI)
Semin Radiat Oncol 18:201-206, 2008

Quality care is one of the dominant issues in health care today. In this article, we will review the key concepts underlying quality measures and discuss how measures are developed and defined. We will next examine how these measures are currently being used and will conclude with some thoughts regarding the steps necessary to use quality measures to improve the quality of care in radiation oncology.

▶ Quality of care in radiation oncology is the degree to which radiation oncology services for patients result in the desired and expected cancer control rate and is consistent with state-of-the-art of radiation oncology for the given cancer. This topic is of ever-increasing interest because the cost of all health care including radiation oncology services continues to increase in the United States despite no clear evidence of increase in cure rates relative to other countries who spend far less per patient. Quality of care has become a forefront issue for patients, employers, and payers alike. All of us want good value for the dollars we spend, especially in health care where the costs are so high. The big challenge for increase in quality of care in the United States is to develop appropriate measures to evaluate quality. The American College of Radiology has developed practice guidelines to help identify quality measurements in radiation oncology for multiple disease sites such as breast and prostate. The current "pay for performance" is an effort on behalf of the government to measure and subsequently reward quality, yet the process is slow and bureaucratic. As this author points out, we as oncologists need to use the practice standards that exists and measure quality, or lack thereof, on a large scale such as is done by the Quality Research in Radiation Oncology (QRRO) initiative (previously patterns of care). In the end, quality must be present or payment should be lessened or even withheld until quality improves.

C. A. Lawton, MD

Multiple newly identified loci associated with prostate cancer susceptibility
Eeles RA, Kote-Jarai Z, Giles GG, et al (The Inst of Cancer Res, Surrey, UK)
Nat Genet 40:316-321, 2008

Prostate cancer is the most common cancer affecting males in developed countries. It shows consistent evidence of familial aggregation, but the causes of this aggregation are mostly unknown. To identify common alleles associated with prostate cancer risk, we conducted a genome-wide association study (GWAS) using blood DNA samples from 1,854 individuals with clinically detected prostate cancer diagnosed at ≤ 60 years or with a family history of disease, and 1,894 population-screened controls with a low prostate-specific antigen (PSA) concentration (<0.5 ng/ml). We analyzed these samples for 541,129 SNPs using the Illumina Infinium platform. Initial putative associations were confirmed using a further 3,268 cases and 3,366 controls. We identified seven loci associated with prostate cancer on chromosomes 3, 6, 7, 10, 11, 19 and X ($P = 2.7 \times 10(-8)$ to $P = 8.7 \times 10(-29)$). We confirmed previous reports of common loci associated with prostate cancer at 8q24 and 17q. Moreover, we found that three of the newly identified loci contain candidate susceptibility genes: MSMB, LMTK2 and KLK3.

▶ Genetic variants in the gene for PSA (*KLK3*) have been linked to an increased risk of prostate cancer. While PSA is an important marker for prostate cancer, it is important to recognize that it is not a tumor suppressor gene or an oncogene, ie, it does not cause cancer. This raises the intriguing possibility that these variants in the PSA gene are not associated with an increased risk of developing prostate cancer but simply associated with an increased risk of being diagnosed with prostate cancer. By this, I mean that an increase in PSA because of the genetic background possibly could increase the likelihood that an individual undergoes a biopsy, which in turn increases the likelihood the patient is diagnosed with prostate cancer. Ahn et al[1] examined a large cohort of patients to determine if these variants were associated with an increased risk of prostate cancer or an increased risk of having an elevated PSA. They confirmed previous studies by demonstrating that there was a strong association between the variants and being diagnosed with prostate cancer. However, when they controlled for PSA, they found this association completely disappeared. Importantly, when they examined the control population in the PLCO Study (ie, those not diagnosed with prostate cancer), they found that the variants implicated previously were associated with high PSA levels.

This does not mean that PSA variants don't have potential clinical utility. Patients predisposed to a higher PSA (irrespective of whether they have prostate cancer or not), might under biopsies only for a higher PSA. I suspect that there are other variants in genes, which may not alter a patient's risk of cancer, but might alter our screening parameters.

A. S. Kibel, MD

Reference

1. Ahn J, Berndt SI, Wacholder S, et al. Variation in KLK genes, prostate-specific antigen and risk of prostate cancer. *Nat Genet.* 2008;40:1032-1034.

Endocrine treatment, with or without radiotherapy, in locally advanced prostate cancer (SPCG-7/SFUO-3): an open randomised phase III trial
Widmark A, for the Scandinavian Prostate Cancer Group Study 7 and the Swedish Association for Urological Oncology 3 (Umeå Univ, Sweden; et al)
Lancet 373:301-308, 2009

Background.—Several studies have shown the efficacy of endocrine therapy in combination with radiotherapy in high-risk prostate cancer. To assess the effect of radiotherapy, we did an open phase III study comparing endocrine therapy with and without local radiotherapy, followed by castration on progression.

Methods.—This randomised trial included men from 47 centres in Norway, Sweden, and Denmark. Between February, 1996, and December, 2002, 875 patients with locally advanced prostate cancer (T3; 78%; PSA<70; N0; M0) were centrally randomly assigned by computer to endocrine treatment alone (3 months of total androgen blockade followed by continuous endocrine treatment using flutamide; 439 patients), or to the same endocrine treatment combined with radiotherapy (436 patients). The primary endpoint was prostate-cancer-specific survival, and analysis was by intention to treat. This study is registered as an international standard randomised controlled trial, number ISRCTN01534787.

Findings.—After a median follow-up of 7·6 years, 79 men in the endocrine alone group and 37 men in the endocrine plus radiotherapy group had died of prostate cancer. The cumulative incidence at 10 years for prostate-cancer-specific mortality was 23·9% in the endocrine alone group and 11·9% in the endocrine plus radiotherapy group (difference 12·0%, 95% CI 4·9–19·1%), for a relative risk of 0·44 (0·30–0·66). At 10 years, the cumulative incidence for overall mortality was 39·4% in the endocrine alone group and 29·6% in the endocrine plus radiotherapy group (difference 9·8%, 0·8–18·8%), for a relative risk of 0·68 (0·52–0·89). Cumulative incidence at 10 years for PSA recurrence was substantially higher in men in the endocrine-alone group (74·7% *vs* 25·9%, p<0·0001; HR 0·16; 0·12–0·20). After 5 years, urinary, rectal, and sexual problems were slightly more frequent in the endocrine plus radiotherapy group.

Interpretation.—In patients with locally advanced or high-risk local prostate cancer, addition of local radiotherapy to endocrine treatment halved the 10-year prostate-cancer-specific mortality, and substantially decreased overall mortality with fully acceptable risk of side-effects compared with endocrine treatment alone. In the light of these data, endocrine treatment plus radiotherapy should be the new standard.

▶ Does local control improve survival of patients with high-risk localized prostate cancer, or should we just be looking to systemic treatment? In other words should we use radiation therapy or surgery on these patients or just go straight to hormone therapy? Once again, the Swedes have succeeded in answering this question. This multicenter study examines 875 patients with locally advanced prostate cancer. Half of the men received androgen deprivation plus radiation therapy and the other half just androgen deprivation. The authors found that prostate specific antigen (PSA) recurrence, prostate cancer specific mortality, and overall mortality were all improved in the group of patients who received the radiation therapy in addition to the androgen depravation therapy. This provided strong level I evidence that local control improves the outcomes of patients with locally advanced disease.

This study has the potential to profoundly alter our management of patients with high-risk localized disease. It provides a strong rationale for not simply treating patients with hormone therapy alone but taking patients with advance T3 and T4 disease and giving them radiation therapy and possibly taking patients with less advanced T3 disease and high PSAs and treating them with radical prostatectomy. While the decision to proceed with radical prostatectomy is an extrapolation from the article, I personally believe that radical prostatectomy does a better job of providing local control and, therefore, has the potential to actually do a better job than radiation therapy in this high-risk patient population.

A. S. Kibel, MD

24 Lung Cancer

Extent of Lymphadenectomy and Outcome for Patients With Stage I Nonsmall Cell Lung Cancer
Varlotto JM, Recht A, Nikolov M, et al (Beth Israel Deaconess Med Ctr, Boston, MA; et al)
Cancer 115:851-858, 2009

Background.—It is uncertain whether lymphadenectomy (LA) affects overall survival (OS) or disease-free survival (DFS) rates for patients with stage I nonsmall cell lung cancer (NSCLC), as is the optimal number of lymph nodes that should be recovered.

Methods.—There were 24,273 patients with stage I NSCLC diagnosed from 1992 to 2002 who were included in the Surveillance, Epidemiology, and End Results database and who underwent a definitive surgical procedure. Median follow-up was 35 months.

Results.—For the entire population, having LA was associated with an increase in the 5-year OS rate from 41.6% to 58.4% ($P < .0001$) and in DFS from 58.0% to 73.09%, compared with not having LA. Outcome improved with increasing number of recovered lymph nodes, with a plateau at 11 or more lymph nodes. For patients diagnosed from 1998 to 2002 undergoing only N1 or only N2 dissections, LA was also associated with statistically significant improvements in OS in both groups and a significant difference and trend for improved DFS in the 2 groups, respectively. The maximum differences in both OS and DFS between those with no LA and those with LA occurred when 11 to 16 lymph nodes were removed for the former group or 7 to 10 lymph nodes for the latter group, respectively.

Conclusions.—LA was associated with increased rates of OS and DFS, compared with no LA. Our results also suggest the minimum number of recovered lymph nodes needed to see the maximum staging accuracy conferred by LA.

▶ Several organizations and publications have mentioned the desired levels of lymph nodes to be at least sampled surgically when resecting nonsmall cell lung cancer (NSCLS). The authors have demonstrated the survival benefit to resecting lymph nodes. Using the surveillance, epidemiology, and end results (SEER) database, they identified 24 273 patients with stage I NSCLC from 1992 to

2002. Their median followup on these patients was 35 months. Lymph adenectomy (LA) was associated with improved overall survival (OS) at 5 years, from 41.6% to 58.4% (p < 0.0001). LA was also associated with improved disease-free survival (DFS) from 58.0% to 73.09%.

The greatest improvement in OS and DFS in patients undergoing only N1 node removal occurred when greater than 11 lymph nodes were removed compared with no lymph nodes (4 year OS 40% vs 68.2%; DFS 40% vs 78.6%). Patients with 11 or more N2 nodes had a worse OS than those with 7 to 10 lymph nodes removed (p = 0.023). The 90-day crude mortality was 5.6% and 1.8%, respectively.

T. L. Bauer II, MD

Menstrual and Reproductive Factors in Association With Lung Cancer in Female Lifetime Nonsmokers
Weiss JM, Lacey JV Jr, Shu X-O, et al (International Epidemiology Inst, Rockville, MD)
Am J Epidemiol 168:1319-1325, 2008

Cigarette smoking is irrefutably the strongest risk factor for lung cancer; however, approximately 25% of cases worldwide occur among nonsmokers. The age-adjusted annual incidence rate of lung cancer in Shanghai, a region where relatively few women smoke cigarettes, is one of the highest in the world. To help further elucidate the etiology of lung cancer among nonsmokers, the authors examined hormonal factors among women who were lifetime nonsmokers. They analyzed data from the prospective Shanghai Women's Health Study, which recruited Chinese women aged 40–70 years between 1996 and 2000 from selected urban communities. The current analysis included 71,314 women ($n = 220$ cases) who were lifetime nonsmokers and had no history of cancer at baseline. Later age at menopause (≥ 51 vs. <46 years; hazard ratio (HR) = 0.63, 95% confidence interval (CI): 0.40, 1.00), longer reproductive period (≥ 36 vs. <31 years; HR = 0.60, 95% CI: 0.39, 0.93), higher parity (≥ 4 vs. 0 children; HR = 0.42, 95% CI: 0.19, 0.90), and intrauterine device use (HR = 0.59, 95% CI: 0.41, 0.86) were associated with decreased risks of lung cancer. This large prospective study suggests a potential role for hormonal factors in the etiology of lung cancer among nonsmoking women.

▶ Ten to 15% of all lung cancer in females occurs among nonsmokers. Weiss et al confirm a statistically significant decreased risk of lung cancer in women with later age of menopause, longer length of reproductive years, higher parity, and intrauterine device use. Their findings suggest a protective role of hormones in the development of lung cancer among nonsmoking females.

The strength of this study is in its size (> 70 000 participants) and focus on only nonsmokers. Previous studies have been modest in size with inclusion of smokers. Passive smoke exposure and age of life events may be subject to recall bias, but the authors expected this to be random.

I agree with the authors' conclusion of a potential protective role, and encourage further investigation of hormonal factors (ie, estrogen) in the etiology of lung cancer among nonsmoking females.

A. S. Galler, MD
T. L. Bauer II, MD

25 Geriatric Oncology

Active Surveillance of Renal Masses in Elderly Patients
Abouassaly R, Lane BR, Novick AC (Glickman Urological and Kidney Inst, Cleveland, OH)
J Urol 180:505-509, 2008

Purpose.—We identify and report on a large number of patients treated with active surveillance for incidentally diagnosed renal masses at our institution.

Materials and Methods.—We identified all patients 75 years or older evaluated in our department for a renal mass between January 2000 and December 2006. A total of 110 patients with enhancing renal masses were initially treated with active surveillance and this group made up the cohort for our study. Medical records were reviewed for clinical and radiological followup, and vital status was obtained from the Social Security Death Index. Clinical and radiographic followup was available for review on 104 and 89 patients, respectively.

Results.—Patients had a median age of 81 years (range 76 to 95) with a median Charlson comorbidity index of 2 (range 0 to 7) at diagnosis. Patients had as many as 9 tumors being followed (median of 1) with a median tumor size of 2.5 cm (range 0.9 to 11.2). During a median followup of 24 months (range 1 to 90) mean tumor growth rate was 0.26 cm per year. Of the 89 patients with radiological followup 38 (43%) exhibited no tumor growth on active surveillance. Comparison of the clinical and radiographic features of patients with tumor growth and those with stable disease revealed no statistical differences. Four patients (3.6%) were treated as a result of disease progression 12 to 54 months after diagnosis. At the conclusion of the study 34 patients (31%) were deceased. To our knowledge the renal mass did not contribute to the cause of death in any patient.

Conclusions.—Active surveillance of incidental renal masses appears to be a viable option for older patients with multiple medical comorbidities and a limited life expectancy.

▶ The management of incidentally found renal masses is a somewhat controversial issue because surgical extirpation via nephrectomy or other means

203

(such as radiofrequency ablation) has the potential to cure many patients with this cancer. Unfortunately, not all patients are candidates for surgical or aggressive nonsurgical management, given their comorbidities. The authors in this study reviewed records for elderly patients with incidentally found renal masses and determined that the rate of progression was exceedingly slow in most patients, and few required intervention. In all cases where death occurred, the renal mass was not suspected as a cause or associated event. This study is important because physicians often distress over the management of otherwise curable disease. In the setting of prostate cancer we have acquiesced to the fact that the slow rate of progression in elderly individuals often allows a watchful waiting approach to cancer care because the prostate cancer often does not contribute to the patient's mortality. If a similar scenario exists for incidental renal cell carcinoma (RCC), then this would provide the rationale for observation as opposed to intervention. Clearly, this study was specific for the patients with incidentally found renal lesions and diagnostic biopsies were not typically performed (though enhancing lesions, in the kidneys are rarely anything but RCC). It is not clear that the same approach can be taken for patients with symptomatic renal masses, and hence the risk-benefit ratio needs to be considered for all cases.

M. S. Gordon, MD

Adjuvant Chemotherapy in Older Women with Early-Stage Breast Cancer
Muss HB, for the CALGB Investigators (Univ of Vermont, Burlington; et al)
N Engl J Med 360:2055-2065, 2009

Background.—Older women with breast cancer are underrepresented in clinical trials, and data on the effects of adjuvant chemotherapy in such patients are scant. We tested for the noninferiority of capecitabine as compared with standard chemotherapy in women with breast cancer who were 65 years of age or older.

Methods.—We randomly assigned patients with stage I, II, IIIA, or IIIB breast cancer to standard chemotherapy (either cyclophosphamide, methotrexate, and fluorouracil or cyclophosphamide plus doxorubicin) or capecitabine. Endocrine therapy was recommended after chemotherapy in patients with hormone-receptor-positive tumors. A Bayesian statistical design was used with a range in sample size from 600 to 1800 patients. The primary end point was relapse-free survival.

Results.—When the 600th patient was enrolled, the probability that, with longer follow-up, capecitabine therapy was highly likely to be inferior to standard chemotherapy met a prescribed level, and enrollment was discontinued. After an additional year of follow-up, the hazard ratio for disease recurrence or death in the capecitabine group was 2.09 (95% confidence interval, 1.38 to 3.17; $P<0.001$). Patients who were randomly assigned to capecitabine were twice as likely to have a relapse and almost twice as likely to die as patients who were randomly assigned to standard chemotherapy ($P = 0.02$). At 3 years, the rate of relapse-free survival was 68% in the capecitabine group versus 85% in the standard-chemotherapy group, and the overall survival rate was 86% versus 91%. Two patients in the capecitabine group died of treatment-related complications; as compared with patients receiving capecitabine, twice as many patients receiving standard chemotherapy had moderate-to-severe toxic effects (64% vs. 33%).

Conclusions.—Standard adjuvant chemotherapy is superior to capecitabine in patients with early-stage breast cancer who are 65 years of age or older. (ClinicalTrials.gov number, NCT00024102.)

▶ There has long been a tendency among oncologists to regard chronological age as an indicator of tolerance to chemotherapy and other more aggressive treatment approaches to cancer. Many have advocated that less aggressive, perhaps better tolerated regimens, ought to be considered in patients over the age of 65. This phase III trial of breast cancer treatment in older women evaluates such an approach. Capecitabine alone is compared with standard adjuvant chemotherapy consisting of either cyclophosphamide, methotrexate, and fluorouracil (CMF) or FAC. The study shows clearly that such attempts to give less aggressive chemotherapy results in inferior outcomes in regard to relapse-free survival. This should not be surprising because previous studies have shown that dose reductions in standard chemotherapy yield inferior results. The investigators make the very valid point in their discussion that treatment of patients, regardless of age, should be based on published results and not an ad hoc approach that arbitrarily modifies treatment regimens without regard to whether these modifications have been appropriately evaluated in phase III trials. In addition to this point, the other major message of this trial is that patients should be treated based on their physiological status rather than their chronological age. While age certainly should be considered, it should not lead to untested alterations in regimens to make the regimen more tolerable for the older patient.

J. T. Thigpen, MD

Adjuvant Treatments do not Alter the Quality of Life in Elderly Patients With Colorectal Cancer: A Population-based Study

Bouvier A-M, Jooste V, Bonnetain F, et al (Univ of Bourgogne, Dijon, France; French-Speaking Federation of Digestive Oncology, Dijon, France; et al)
Cancer 113:879-886, 2008

Background.—The current study was performed to longitudinally assess the impact of adjuvant treatments on the quality of life (QoL) of elderly colorectal cancer survivors.

Methods.—The Burgundy Digestive Cancer Registry was used to select all patients aged ≥75 years who were diagnosed with colorectal cancer between 2003 and 2005. A total of 209 patients were asked to complete questionnaires during the first year after diagnosis: at the time of inclusion in the study (Q0), at 3 months after the initial diagnosis (Q3), at 6 months after the initial diagnosis (Q6), and at 12 months after the initial diagnosis (Q12) using the European Organization for Research and Treatment of Cancer (EORTC) QLQ-C30. A total of 125 patients (60%) responded. Mixed model analyses of variance for repeated measurement were used to compare QoL scores according to therapeutic schemes. Interactions between time of follow-up and treatment were tested.

Results.—Patient sex, age, location of the tumor, and TNM stage of disease did not appear to differ significantly between respondents and nonrespondents. Global Health and Emotional Functioning improved for colon cancer survivors between Q0 and Q12, and were noted to improve between Q3 and Q12 for rectal cancer patients. According to French recommendations, patients who received chemotherapy for stage III colon cancer ($P = .176$) or radiotherapy for rectal cancer ($P = .959$) reported no significant changes in Global Health compared with those patients not receiving adjuvant therapies. Patients treated with chemotherapy reported better Physical Functioning than patients who did not received chemotherapy ($P = .0113$).

Conclusions.—To the authors' knowledge, the current study is the first to examine trends over time with regard to the influence of adjuvant treatments for colon and rectal cancers on QoL in a general aged population. Providing evidence that adjuvant chemotherapy for colon cancer has no negative impact on the QoL of elderly patients is of great significance in encouraging clinicians to treat this population.

▶ The subjective exclusion of elderly patients from what may be viewed as aggressive treatment, is a phenomenon that has recently garnered more attention in the literature. This mechanism may also result in the under-representation of the elderly in clinical trials, despite the absence of age restrictive language in the study protocol. Over the past several years, there has been more information emerging, which essentially demonstrates that fit elderly patients may tolerate radiation and/or chemotherapy as well as fit younger patients. In fact, fit elderly patients may tolerate these treatments better than nonfit (eg, poor performance status, multiple comorbidities) nonelderly patients.

This study, using patients in the Burgundy Digestive Cancers Registry, assessed with a European Organization for Research and Treatment of Cancer (EORTC) QoL tool, confirms that the elderly do tolerate and can benefit from adjuvant therapy for colorectal cancer. The assessment included patients receiving either adjuvant radiation therapy or chemotherapy. The so-called elderly received this treatment with no decrement in quality of life. The underlying message is that one has to be alive to have a quality of life, thus, underscoring the importance of not excluding these patients from adjuvant therapy just because they have surpassed an arbitrary chronologic landmark. Perception of what is elderly is somewhat dependent on the age of the beholder. What's important is to first assess performance status and comorbidities and then look at age. Also, as pointed out in the Firat[1] performance status is not a surrogate for comorbidities; both are independent predictors of treatment tolerance and outcome.

R. W. Byhardt, MD

Reference

1. Firat S, Pleister A, Byhardt RW, Fore E. Age is independent of comorbidity influencing patient selsction for combined modality therapy for treatment of stage III nonsmall cell lung cancer (NSCLC). *Am J Clin Oncol.* 2006;29:252-257.

26 Supportive Care

A 12-week randomised study comparing intravenous iron sucrose versus oral ferrous sulphate for treatment of postpartum anemia
Westad S, Backe B, Salvesen KÅ, et al (Innlandet Hosp Trust, Lillehammer, Norway; St Olav Hosp, Trondheim, Norway; et al)
Acta Obstet Gynecol Scand 87:916-923, 2008

Objective.—To analyze the effect of intravenous ferrous sucrose compared with oral ferrous sulphate on hematological parameters and quality of life in women with postpartum anemia.

Design.—Open randomised controlled trial.

Setting.—Multicentre study comprising five obstetrical departments in Norway.

Population.—Hundred and twenty-eight postpartum women with hemorrhagic anemia (Hb between 6.5 g/100 ml and 8.5 g/100 ml). The intervention group (59 women) received 600 mg iron sucrose intravenously followed by 200 mg iron sulphate daily from week 5. The control group (70 women) were given 200 mg iron sulphate daily.

Methods.—Randomisation and start of treatment occurred within 48 hours of the delivery. Participants were followed up at 4, 8 and 12 weeks.

Main Outcome Measures.—Hemoglobin, ferritin and quality of life assessed with the Medical Outcomes Study Short Form 36 (SF-36) and the Fatigue Scale.

Results.—After 4 weeks the mean hemoglobin values in both groups were similar (11.9 g/100 ml vs. 12.3 g/100 ml, $p = 0.89$). The mean serum ferritin value after 4 weeks was significantly higher in the intervention group with 13.7 µg/L vs. 4.2 µg/L in the control group ($p < 0.001$). At 8 and 12 weeks the hematological parameters were similar. The total fatigue score was significantly improved in the intervention group at week 4, 8 and 12, whereas SF-36 scores did not differ.

Conclusion.—Women who received 600 mg intravenous iron sucrose followed by standard oral iron after four weeks, replenished their iron stores more rapidly and had a more favorable development of the fatigue score indicating improved quality of life.

▶ This trial addresses an important consideration for patients with iron deficiency anemia. That is, whether induction with intravenous (IV) iron sucrose therapy accelerates the recovery from anemia in patients with an uncomplicated anemia due to blood loss. Unlike patients with chronic illnesses such as auto-immune disorders or inflammatory conditions where mobilization of iron stores may be a problem, postpartum anemia is related to iron deficiency in a normal host. In this study, subjects received 3 doses of iron sucrose followed by oral maintenance therapy compared with oral replacement from day 1 in the standard-of-care group. Compliance was monitored by pill count, and both groups were equally compliant. Not surprisingly, the IV experimental arm was found to have a faster recovery of iron stores compared with oral replacement. In addition, this group had less fatigue, although no differences in the Short Form (SF)-36 quality of life scores were noted. Subjectively, the IV group did not recover their hemoglobin any faster than the oral group, and there was no difference at longer time points. Hence, initial IV iron induction was not associated with any subjective benefit in terms of the major endpoint, which was hemoglobin recovery. Explanation for the improvement in fatigue may well lie with the fact that the 2 arms were not double blinded, and, hence, patients receiving IV iron may have experienced an improvement in their fatigue due to the impression that the experimental arm would be superior. This trial is an excellent example for the need for double blinding. One cannot conclude that IV iron, clearly more expensive, provides any objective evidence of benefit in this patient population with normal bone marrow function.

M. S. Gordon, MD

Estimation of the Warfarin Dose with Clinical and Pharmacogenetic Data
The International Warfarin Pharmacogenetics Consortium (Stanford, CA)
N Engl J Med 360:753-764, 2009

Background.—Genetic variability among patients plays an important role in determining the dose of warfarin that should be used when oral anticoagulation is initiated, but practical methods of using genetic information have not been evaluated in a diverse and large population. We developed and used an algorithm for estimating the appropriate warfarin dose that is based on both clinical and genetic data from a broad population base.

Methods.—Clinical and genetic data from 4043 patients were used to create a dose algorithm that was based on clinical variables only and an algorithm in which genetic information was added to the clinical variables. In a validation cohort of 1009 subjects, we evaluated the potential clinical value of each algorithm by calculating the percentage of patients whose predicted dose of warfarin was within 20% of the actual stable therapeutic dose; we also evaluated other clinically relevant indicators.

Results.—In the validation cohort, the pharmacogenetic algorithm accurately identified larger proportions of patients who required 21 mg of warfarin or less per week and of those who required 49 mg or more per week to achieve the target international normalized ratio than did the clinical algorithm (49.4% vs. 33.3%, P<0.001, among patients requiring ≤21 mg per week; and 24.8% vs. 7.2%, P<0.001, among those requiring ≥49 mg per week).

Conclusions.—The use of a pharmacogenetic algorithm for estimating the appropriate initial dose of warfarin produces recommendations that are significantly closer to the required stable therapeutic dose than those derived from a clinical algorithm or a fixed-dose approach. The greatest benefits were observed in the 46.2% of the population that required 21 mg or less of warfarin per week or 49 mg or more per week for therapeutic anticoagulation.

▶ The use of warfarin for chronic anticoagulation is associated with risk of both under- and over-anticoagulation such that patients may be at risk for either recurrent thrombotic events or excessive bleeding. The development of algorithms, designed to characterize patients based on either clinical or clinical and pharmacogenetic data hold the potential to improve anticoagulation strategies compared with empiric dosing. In this article, the authors assessed the development of a warfarin dosing algorithm based on either clinical data alone or clinical data in conjunction with pharmacogenetic data. Data from over 4000 patients were used to create the data set, and they were then tested in a validation cohort of over 1000 patients. Ultimately, and not surprisingly, the pharmacogenetic algorithm accurately identified those patients who required far less or far more warfarin for anticoagulation than would have been predicted based on the clinical alone dosing algorithm.

This trial is one of a number that have been working toward the development of a uniform standard for a warfarin dosing algorithm. Given the frequency of the use of warfarin, the ability to rapidly test patients for specific PG determinants is critical to being able to enact such an algorithm.

M. S. Gordon, MD

27 Miscellaneous Topics

Adjuvant therapy with pegylated interferon alfa-2b versus observation alone in resected stage III melanoma: final results of EORTC 18991, a randomised phase III trial

Eggermont AMM, for the EORTC Melanoma Group (Erasmus Univ Med Ctr, Rotterdam, Netherlands; et al)

Lancet 372:117-126, 2008

Background.—Any benefit of adjuvant interferon alfa-2b for melanoma could depend on dose and duration of treatment. Our aim was to determine whether pegylated interferon alfa-2b can facilitate prolonged exposure while maintaining tolerability.

Methods.—1256 patients with resected stage III melanoma were randomly assigned to observation (n=629) or pegylated interferon alfa-2b (n=627) 6 µg/kg per week for 8 weeks (induction) then 3 µg/kg per week (maintenance) for an intended duration of 5 years. Randomisation was stratified for microscopic (N1) versus macroscopic (N2) nodal involvement, number of positive nodes, ulceration and tumour thickness, sex, and centre. Randomisation was done with a minimisation technique. The primary endpoint was recurrence-free survival. Analyses were done by intention to treat. This study is registered with ClinicalTrials.gov, number NCT00006249.

Findings.—All randomised patients were included in the primary efficacy analysis. 608 patients in the interferon group and 613 patients in the observation group were included in safety analyses. The median length of treatment with pegylated interferon alfa-2b was 12 (IQR $3 \cdot 8$–$33 \cdot 4$) months. At $3 \cdot 8$ ($3 \cdot 2$–$4 \cdot 2$) years median follow-up, 328 recurrence events had occurred in the interferon group compared with 368 in the observation group (hazard ratio $0 \cdot 82$, 95% CI $0 \cdot 71$–$0 \cdot 96$; p=$0 \cdot 01$); the 4-year rate of recurrence-free survival was $45 \cdot 6$% (SE $2 \cdot 2$) in the interferon group and $38 \cdot 9$% ($2 \cdot 2$) in the observation group. There was no difference in overall survival between the groups. Grade 3 adverse events occurred in 246 (40%) patients in the interferon group and 60 (10%) in the observation group; grade 4 adverse events occurred in 32 (5%) patients in the interferon group and 14 (2%) in the observation group. In the interferon group, the most common grade 3 or 4 adverse events were fatigue (97 patients, 16%), hepatotoxicity (66, 11%), and depression (39, 6%). Treatment with pegylated interferon alfa-2b was discontinued because of toxicity in 191 (31%) patients.

Interpretation.—Adjuvant pegylated interferon alfa-2b for stage III melanoma has a significant, sustained effect on recurrence-free survival.

▶ The use of interferon alpha in the adjuvant care of patients with melanoma has been confirmed in several randomized controlled trials. The toxicity of the therapy is significant, and as a result many patients will defer the potential benefits in lieu of going on expectant observation. Pegylated interferon alpha is a modified form of interferon alpha-2b and exerts similar immunologic effects with less frequent dosing and less subjective toxicity. In this trial, a regimen of weekly pegylated interferon was compared with expectant observation in patients with an indication for adjuvant interferon therapy. The control arm being observation raises the concern that any modest benefit seen may be inferior to that seen with the standard IV followed by thrice weekly subcutaneous (SC) interferon regimen. In this trial, which included patients with microscopically positive solitary nodes, no difference in overall survival was seen, though an improvement in relapse-free survival was identified. The failure to see an overall survival advantage may be related to similar factors that plagued the most recent interferon-based observational studies. In this regard, inclusion of patients with solitary microscopically positive nodes, who may have a better predicted outcome compared with those patients with macroscopic disease, can preclude the identification of an overall survival advantage. In addition, the availability of standard interferon for those patients who may relapse with local/regional disease may improve their secondary outcome. Toxicity of the pegylated interferon was similar to that of the standard interferon dosing regimen, and similar numbers of patients ultimately discontinued therapy. Comparison of this new regimen with the older intravenous (IV)/SC regimen would be required to determine the relative value of one versus the other.

M. S. Gordon, MD

Bevacizumab Plus Interferon Alfa Compared With Interferon Alfa Monotherapy in Patients With Metastatic Renal Cell Carcinoma: CALGB 90206

Rini BI, Halabi S, Rosenberg JE, et al (Cleveland Clinic Taussig Cancer Inst, OH; Duke Univ Med Ctr, and Cancer and Leukemia Group B Statistical Ctr, Durham, NC; Southeast Cancer Control Consortium Inc, Winston-Salem, NC; et al)

J Clin Oncol 26:5422-5428, 2008

Purpose.—Bevacizumab is an antibody that binds to vascular endothelial growth factor (VEGF) and has activity in metastatic renal cell carcinoma (RCC). Interferon alfa (IFN) is a historic standard first-line treatment for RCC. A prospective, randomized phase III trial of bevacizumab plus IFN versus IFN monotherapy was conducted.

Patients and Methods.—Patients with previously untreated, metastatic clear-cell RCC were randomly assigned to receive either bevacizumab

(10 mg/kg intravenously every 2 weeks) plus IFN (9 million U subcutaneously three times weekly) or the same dose and schedule of IFN monotherapy in a multicenter phase III trial. The primary end point was overall survival (OS). Secondary end points were progression-free survival (PFS), objective response rate (ORR), and safety.

Results.—Between October 2003 and July 2005, 732 patients were enrolled. The prespecified stopping rule for OS has not yet been reached. The median PFS was 8.5 months in patients receiving bevacizumab plus IFN (95% CI, 7.5 to 9.7 months) versus 5.2 months (95% CI, 3.1 to 5.6 months) in patients receiving IFN monotherapy (log-rank $P < .0001$). The adjusted hazard ratio was 0.71 (95% CI, 0.61 to 0.83; $P < .0001$). Bevacizumab plus IFN had a higher ORR as compared with IFN (25.5% [95% CI, 20.9% to 30.6%] v 13.1% [95% CI, 9.5% to 17.3%]; $P < .0001$). Overall toxicity was greater for bevacizumab plus IFN, including significantly more grade 3 hypertension (9% v 0%), anorexia (17% v 8%), fatigue (35% v 28%), and proteinuria (13% v 0%).

Conclusion.—Bevacizumab plus IFN produces a superior PFS and ORR in untreated patients with metastatic RCC as compared with IFN monotherapy. Toxicity is greater in the combination therapy arm.

▶ The treatment of metastatic renal cell cancer (mRCC) has undergone an explosive evolution in the past number of years. The availability of new tyrosine kinase inhibitors targeting vascular endothelial growth factor (VEGF) as well as other kinases has resulted in significantly higher response rates and improved survival. Interferon has long been a recognized standard in mRCC, having demonstrated a significant improvement in survival compared with observation or inactive compounds. Bevacizumab, as a VEGF inhibitor, has been approved by the FDA for numerous indications in combination with chemotherapy, but also demonstrated modest single agent activity in mRCC. The combination of bevacizumab and interferon was explored previously and showed promise, and hence was studied in this randomized controlled trial versus interferon alfa monotherapy. Standard dosing regimens were used for the interferon dosing. The combination of bevacizumab and interferon alfa demonstrated a statistically significant increase in the overall response rate and progression-free survival compared with interferon alfa alone. Adverse events were those typified by VEGF inhibitors and were manageable. Whether these response rates would similarly be seen in the setting of patients who had already progressed on kinase inhibitor therapy is unknown. The regimen of bevacizumab and interferon represents a reasonable combination for front-line therapy of patients with mRCC, and may well be a value for those patients who progress following sunitinib or sorafenib therapy.

M. S. Gordon, MD

Phase III Trial of Consolidation Therapy With Yttrium-90-Ibritumomab Tiuxetan Compared With No Additional Therapy After First Remission in Advanced Follicular Lymphoma

Morschhauser F, Radford J, Van Hoof A, et al (Centre Hospitalier Universitaire, Lille, France; et al)

J Clin Oncol 26:5156-5164, 2008

Purpose.—We conducted an international, randomized, phase III trial to evaluate the efficacy and safety of consolidation with yttrium-90 (^{90}Y)-ibritumomab tiuxetan in patients with advanced-stage follicular lymphoma in first remission.

Patients and Methods.—Patients with CD20$^+$ stage III or IV follicular lymphoma, who achieved a complete response (CR)/unconfirmed CR (CRu) or partial response (PR) after first-line induction treatment, were randomly assigned to receive ^{90}Y-ibritumomab tiuxetan (rituximab 250 mg/m^2 on day –7 and day 0 followed on day 0 by ^{90}Y-ibritumomab tiuxetan 14.8 MBq/kg; maximum of 1,184 MBq) or no further treatment (control). The primary end point was progression-free survival (PFS), which was calculated from the time of random assignment.

Results.—A total of 414 patients (consolidation, n = 208; control, n = 206) were enrolled at 77 centers. ^{90}Y-ibritumomab tiuxetan consolidation significantly prolonged median PFS (after a median observation time of 3.5 years) in all patients (36.5 v 13.3 months in control arm; hazard ratio [HR] = 0.465; $P < .0001$) and regardless of whether patients achieved PR (29.3 v 6.2 months in control arm; HR = 0.304; $P < .0001$) or CR/CRu (53.9 v 29.5 months in control arm; HR = 0.613; $P = .0154$) after induction treatment. Median PFS with consolidation was prolonged in all Follicular Lymphoma International Prognostic Index risk subgroups. After ^{90}Y-ibritumomab tiuxetan consolidation, 77% of patients in PR after induction converted to CR/CRu, resulting in a final CR rate of 87%. The most common toxicity with ^{90}Y-ibritumomab tiuxetan was hematologic, and grade 3 or 4 infections occurred in 8% of patients.

Conclusion.—Consolidation of first remission with ^{90}Y-ibritumomab tiuxetan in advanced-stage follicular lymphoma is highly effective with no unexpected toxicities, prolonging PFS by 2 years and resulting in high PR-to-CR conversion rates regardless of type of first-line induction treatment.

▶ The management of low-grade lymphomas has evolved significantly since the advent of monoclonal antibody therapy targeting the CD20 antigen. Rituximab, the first of these antibodies, produced clinically significant improvements in the progression-free and relapse-free survival of this otherwise incurable disease. Radioimmunoconjugates have demonstrated similar improvements and have single agent activity that may be similar to that of combination chemotherapy.

In this trial the use of the yttrium labeled radioimmunoconjugate antibody ibritumomab was studied as a consolidation therapy after patients had received initial combination therapy. The induction chemotherapy was not dictated, and in some cases included alkylator-based regimens while other regimens included rituximab. Of 502 patients who were screened, 414 who had achieved a partial or complete response to induction therapy were randomized to observation or the investigational arm with the radioimmunoconjugate. The results of the study were strikingly positive with the experimental arm having a statistically significantly prolonged median progression-free survival regardless of the overall response (complete vs partial) to induction therapy. One of the most impressive outcomes was the fact that 77% of the patients in a partial response after induction therapy converted to a complete response after antibody therapy. This study defines a new paradigm for the treatment of patients with follicular nonHodgkin's lymphoma, and the use of the radioimmunoconjugate in the consolidation setting should be considered for patients who achieve a complete or partial response to standard chemotherapy.

M. S. Gordon, MD

Efficacy of everolimus in advanced renal cell carcinoma: a double-blind, randomised, placebo-controlled phase III trial
Motzer RJ, Escudier B, Oudard S, et al (Memorial Sloan-Kettering Cancer Ctr, NY; Institut Gustave Roussy, Villejuif, France; Hôpital Européen Georges Pompidou, Paris, France; et al)
Lancet 372:449-456, 2008

Background.—Everolimus (RAD001) is an orally administered inhibitor of the mammalian target of rapamycin (mTOR), a therapeutic target for metastatic renal cell carcinoma. We did a phase III, randomised, double-blind, placebo-controlled trial of everolimus in patients with metastatic renal cell carcinoma whose disease had progressed on vascular endothelial growth factor-targeted therapy.

Methods.—Patients with metastatic renal cell carcinoma which had progressed on sunitinib, sorafenib, or both, were randomly assigned in a two to one ratio to receive everolimus 10 mg once daily (n=272) or placebo (n=138), in conjunction with best supportive care. Randomisation was done centrally via an interactive voice response system using a validated computer system, and was stratified by Memorial Sloan-Kettering Cancer Center prognostic score and previous anticancer therapy, with a permuted block size of six. The primary endpoint was progression-free survival, assessed via a blinded, independent central review. The study was designed to be terminated after 290 events of progression. Analysis was by intention to treat. This study is registered with ClinicalTrials.gov, number NCT00410124.

Findings.—All randomised patients were included in efficacy analyses. The results of the second interim analysis indicated a significant difference in efficacy between arms and the trial was thus halted early after 191 progression events had been observed (101 [37%] events in the everolimus group, 90 [65%] in the placebo group; hazard ratio 0·30, 95%

CI 0·22–0·40, p<0·0001; median progression-free survival 4·0 [95% CI 3·7–5·5] *vs* 1·9 [1·8–1·9] months). Stomatitis (107 [40%] patients in the everolimus group *vs* 11 [8%] in the placebo group), rash (66 [25%] *vs* six [4%]), and fatigue (53 [20%] *vs* 22 [16%]) were the most commonly reported adverse events, but were mostly mild or moderate in severity. Pneumonitis (any grade) was detected in 22 (8%) patients in the everolimus group, of whom eight had pneumonitis of grade 3 severity.

Interpretation.—Treatment with everolimus prolongs progression-free survival relative to placebo in patients with metastatic renal cell carcinoma that had progressed on other targeted therapies.

▶ Standard front-line therapy for patients with metastatic clear renal cell carcinoma (RCC) has become the use of one of several oral tyrosine kinase inhibitors (TKI). These agents have truly revolutionized the treatment of this disease where previous clinical benefit was modest and improvement in overall survival was limited. Unfortunately, these new agents do not cure patients with metastatic disease, resulting in improved palliation but not eradication of the disease. At some point, all patients become resistant to the effects of sunitinib or sorafenib, and while conversion to the alternate drug has some potential benefit, it is again of limited value. The use of agents directed at the mammalian target of rapamycin (mTOR) has demonstrated antitumor efficacy, in the case of temsirolimus, when compared against standard interferon-alpha therapy in patients with high-risk disease based on the Motzer criteria. Everolimus is an oral mTOR inhibitor that acts in similar fashion and has been studied in patients with metastatic RCC who have progressed on previous TKI therapy. In this randomized trial, patients received either standard doses of everolimus (10 mg once daily) or an identical placebo. All patients had experienced progressive disease on previous TKI therapy. The trial was halted early because of the efficacy seen. Median progression-free survival was 4.0 months in the everolimus group, compared with 1.9 months in the control group. Partial responses were rare, occurring in only 1% of the experimental arm patients with 63% of the everolimus patients experiencing stable disease compared with 32% on the placebo arm. Side effects of the everolimus group were mild to moderate in nature, and included fatigue, stomatitis, and rash. The clinical benefit for everolimus in this patient setting clearly demonstrates that it should become the new standard for patients with TKI resistant or refractory disease, but its limited benefit (median PFS = 4 months) indicates that new agents or combinations are needed.

M. S. Gordon, MD

Warfarin thromboprophylaxis in cancer patients with central venous catheters (WARP): an open-label randomised trial

Young AM, Billingham LJ, Begum G, et al (Univ of Birmingham, UK; et al)
Lancet 373:567-574, 2009

Background.—The role and dose of anticoagulants in thromboprophylaxis for patients with cancer receiving chemotherapy through central venous catheters (CVCs) is controversial. We therefore assessed whether warfarin reduces catheter-related thrombosis compared with no warfarin and whether the dose of warfarin determines the thromboprophylactic effect.

Methods.—In 68 clinical centres in the UK, we randomly assigned 1590 patients aged at least 16 years with cancer who were receiving chemotherapy through CVCs to no warfarin, fixed-dose warfarin 1 mg per day, or dose-adjusted warfarin per day to maintain an international normalised ratio between $1 \cdot 5$ and $2 \cdot 0$. Clinicians who were certain of the benefit of warfarin randomly assigned patients to fixed-dose or dose-adjusted warfarin groups. The primary outcome was the rate of radiologically proven, symptomatic catheter-related thrombosis. Analysis was by intention to treat. This trial is registered as an International Standard Randomised Controlled Trial, number ISRCTN 50312145.

Findings.—Compared with no warfarin (n=404), warfarin (n=408; 324 [79%] on fixed-dose and 84 [21%] on dose-adjusted) did not reduce the rate of catheter-related thromboses (24 [6%] *vs* 24 [6%]; relative risk $0 \cdot 99$, 95% CI $0 \cdot 57$–$1 \cdot 72$, p=$0 \cdot 98$). However, compared with fixed-dose warfarin (n=471), dose-adjusted warfarin (n=473) was superior in the prevention of catheter-related thromboses (13 [3%] *vs* 34 [7%]; $0 \cdot 38$, $0 \cdot 20$–$0 \cdot 71$, p=$0 \cdot 002$). Major bleeding events were rare; an excess was noted with warfarin compared with no warfarin (7 *vs* 1, p=$0 \cdot 07$) and with dose-adjusted warfarin compared with fixed-dose warfarin (16 *vs* 7, p=$0 \cdot 09$). A combined endpoint of thromboses and major bleeding showed no difference between comparisons. We did not note a survival benefit in either comparison.

Interpretation.—The findings show that prophylactic warfarin compared with no warfarin is not associated with a reduction in symptomatic catheter-related or other thromboses in patients with cancer and therefore we should consider newer treatments.

Funding.—Medical Research Council and Cancer Research UK.

▶ This trial evaluates the role of anticoagulation in the prevention of clotting of indwelling intravenous catheters in cancer patients. The study makes 2 significant observations. First, the study design allowed physicians to state whether they were already convinced that warfarin had a role in prevention of catheter clotting. Almost half of the study participants stated a belief in the use of warfarin, and were therefore allowed to randomize their patients to either fixed dose or dose-adjusted warfarin, whereas those uncertain of the benefits of warfarin randomized their patients to the same tow treatment arms or an observation arm. The fact that almost half of the study investigators were already convinced that warfarin was of benefit was surprising, and indicates the degree to which earlier trials had convinced physicians of the validity of this approach. The second noteworthy observation is that warfarin resulted in no benefit in terms of reduction of clotting likelihood (Fig 3A in the original article) and did, to a small extent, increase the likelihood of bleeding episodes. These results corroborate recent studies, which have shown no benefit for warfarin, low-molecular-weight heparin, enoxaparin, and dalteparin. The authors speculate that improvements in catheter technology, placement, and aftercare have reduced the likelihood of clotting or bleeding to the point that prophylaxis is no longer needed; hence, the older observations that prophylaxis might be of some value can no longer be confirmed.

J. T. Thigpen, MD

Steps and Time to Process Clinical Trials at the Cancer Therapy Evaluation Program

Dilts DM, Sandler AB, Cheng SK, et al (Ctr for Management Res in Healthcare, Nashville, TN; Vanderbilt Univ, Nashville, TN; Vanderbilt-Ingram Cancer Ctr, Nashville, TN; et al)
J Clin Oncol 27:1761-1766, 2009

Purpose.—To examine the processes and document the calendar time required for the National Cancer Institute's Cancer Therapy Evaluation Program (CTEP) and Central Institutional Review Board (CIRB) to evaluate and approve phase III clinical trials.

Methods.—Process steps were documented by (1) interviewing CTEP and CIRB staff regarding the steps required to activate a trial from initial concept submission to trial activation by a cooperative group, (2) reviewing standard operating procedures, and (3) inspecting trial records and documents for selected trials to identify any additional steps. Calendar time was collected from initial concept submission to activation using retrospective data from the CTEP Protocol and Information Office.

Results.—At least 296 distinct processes are required for phase III trial activation: at least 239 working steps, 52 major decision points, 20 processing loops, and 11 stopping points. Of the 195 trials activated during the January 1, 2000, to December 31, 2007, study period, a sample of 167 (85.6%) was used for gathering timing data. Median calendar days from initial formal concept submission to CTEP to trial activation by a cooperative group was 602 days (interquartile range, 454 to 861 days). This time has not significantly changed over the past 8 years. There is a high variation in the time required to activate a clinical trial.

Conclusion.—Because of their complexity, the overall development time for phase III clinical trials is lengthy, process laden, and highly variable.

To streamline the process, a solution must be sought that includes all parties involved in developing trials.

▶ This article should be read by all oncologists who are interested in continuing improvement in our therapeutic armamentarium for treating cancer. The primary outlet for performing objective phase III trials in the United States has been the system of cooperative groups funded through the Cancer Therapy and Evaluation Program (CTEP) of the National Cancer Institute. In the last 5 years, this system has been besieged by an ever-increasing bureaucracy that has slowed substantially the development of phase III trials within the cooperative group system. The first added step was a Central Institutional Review Board (CIRB) that added 3 to 4 months to the process by requiring review of all phase III studies sponsored by the National Cancer Institute. Initially billed as a substitute for the review by the local IRB, this quickly became merely another barrier to efficient development of phase III studies because most institutions would not accept the CIRB review since the CIRB refused to indemnify the institutions. This was followed by the development of steering committees to review and approve proposed phase III studies. These steering committees were supposed to take the place of review by CTEP. By disapproval of more than half of submitted proposals, these committees have become yet another barrier to activation of phase III studies by adding another several months to development time for some studies and by blocking others altogether. The steering committees then developed task forces to review the proposals initially. This added yet another layer to the process. Finally, CTEP decided to reinstitute its own review in addition to all of the above, a move that added yet another step to the process. These 4 additional steps, and an ever-increasing complexity of the trials that increase development time and slow accrual, have created major delays in phase III study activation.

Unfortunately, the Dilts study does not reflect the full impact of all of this added complexity. The study covers a period from 2000 through 2007. The full impact of the task forces was not felt until 2008, and the reinstitution of the CTEP review did not occur until later in 2008. The study does, however, point out the unnecessarily long time required to develop a phase III trial, a problem that undoubtedly would be found to be worse if the study were to be repeated today.

In general, the solution of this problem will require a willingness of all parties to unravel much of the complexity of the system by removing unnecessary steps in the process. This will entail decentralizing the process so that we can tap all of the expertise available through the cooperative groups, and not encumber that expertise with unnecessary control from Washington. Hopefully the Dilts study has provided the initial facts that will facilitate the removal of the many barriers to study development that have been erected.

J. T. Thigpen, MD

Consistent Deregulation of Gene Expression between Human and Murine *MLL* Rearrangement Leukemias

Li Z, Luo RT, Mi S, et al (Univ of Chicago, IL; et al)
Cancer Res 69:1109-1116, 2009

Important biological and pathologic properties are often conserved across species. Although several mouse leukemia models have been well established, the genes deregulated in both human and murine leukemia cells have not been studied systematically. We performed a serial analysis of gene expression in both human and murine *MLL-ELL* or *MLL-ENL* leukemia cells and identified 88 genes that seemed to be significantly deregulated in both types of leukemia cells, including 57 genes not reported previously as being deregulated in *MLL*-associated leukemias. These changes were validated by quantitative PCR. The most up-regulated genes include several *HOX* genes (e.g., *HOX A5*, *HOXA9*, and *HOXA10*) and *MEIS1*, which are the typical hallmark of *MLL* rearrangement leukemia. The most down-regulated genes include *LTF*, *LCN2*, *MMP9*, *S100A8*, *S100A9*, *PADI4*, *TGFBI*, and *CYBB*. Notably, the up-regulated genes are enriched in gene ontology terms, such as gene expression and transcription, whereas the down-regulated genes are enriched in signal transduction and apoptosis. We showed that the CpG islands of the down-regulated genes are hypermethylated. We also showed that seven individual microRNAs (miRNA) from the *mir-17-92* cluster, which are overexpressed in human *MLL* rearrangement leukemias, are also consistently overexpressed in mouse *MLL* rearrangement leukemia cells. Nineteen possible targets of these miRNAs were identified, and two of them (i.e., *APP* and *RASSF2*) were confirmed further by luciferase reporter and mutagenesis assays. The identification and validation of consistent changes of gene expression in human and murine *MLL* rearrangement leukemias provide important insights into the genetic base for *MLL*-associated leukemogenesis.

▶ Animal models, including the most widely used mouse systems, for human leukemia have always lived under the cloud of not being relevant to the human disease or predictive of treatment responses observed in humans. However, murine models are becoming more sophisticated and better characterized. A superb example of such advances is the report by Li et al on the characterization of *MLL* rearranged leukemia in the mouse and in humans. A detailed characterization of microarray expression data identified 88 genes that were similarly regulated in both types of leukemia. Of note, these included the *HOX* gene family and *MEIS1*, both of which are classically associated with human *MLL* rearranged leukemia. Even more interesting is the observation of a subset of similarly regulated microRNAs from the *mir-17-92* cluster being expressed in both leukemias. The CpG promoter methylation of genes commonly downregulated in both leukemias provide additional mechanistic similarity between the mouse and human leukemias. These observations should provide a great deal of possible surrogate, molecular markers for testing novel targeted therapy. This type of work is moving us closer to the development of critically needed predictive, preclinical models.

R. J. Arceci, MD, PhD

Change in maximum standardized uptake value on repeat positron emission tomography after chemoradiotherapy in patients with esophageal cancer identifies complete responders
Cerfolio RJ, Bryant AS, Talati AA, et al (Univ of Alabama at Birmingham)
J Thorac Cardiovasc Surg 137:605-609, 2009

Objective.—The objective was to identify whether repeat positron emission tomography scan after neoadjuvant chemoradiotherapy in patients with esophageal cancer predicted a complete response.

Methods.—A retrospective study using a prospective database was performed. Patients had esophageal cancer and underwent neoadjuvant chemoradiotherapy, an initial and repeat positron emission tomography, endoscopic ultrasound with fine-needle aspiration (at the same institution), and Ivor Lewis esophagogastrectomy with lymph node resection.

Results.—There were 221 patients who underwent Ivor Lewis, 86 of whom had their initial and repeat positron emission tomography scans performed at the same center. Of these, 37 patients (43%) were complete responders. The median maximum standardized uptake value of esophageal cancer decreased by 72% in the 37 patients who were complete responders, by 58% in the 31 patients who were partial responders, and by 37% in the 18 patients who had a minimal pathologic response. When the maximum standardized uptake value decreased by more than 64%, the patient was likely to be a complete responder ($P = .003$, area under the curve $= 0.75$).

Conclusion.—When initial and repeat positron emission tomography scans are performed at the same center at least 30 days after the completion of preoperative chemoradiotherapy, the percent change in the maximum standardized uptake value is a predictor of the response to chemoradiotherapy by a patient with esophageal cancer. When the maximum standardized uptake value decreases by 64% or more, it is likely that the patient is a complete responder. These data may help guide neoadjuvant therapy and identify patients for a future randomized study that compares observation with surgical resection in patients with esophageal cancer who appear to be complete responders.

▶ Cerfolio and colleagues are to be commended for another excellent article. In this report they attempt to identify those patients who are complete responders after induction chemoradiotherapy before Ivor Lewis Esophagogastrectomy. Eighty-six of his most recent 221 esophageal resections met the strict entry criteria for analysis. These patients had pretreatment PET scans done at the same facility, and the posttreatment scan done between 30 and 40 days after finishing the last radiation therapy.

They compared maxSUV and its percent decrease to complete pathologic response in the pathology specimen. The area of the tumor was sectioned at 4 mm to ensure complete analysis and identification of viable tumor.

They demonstrated that if the maxSUV decreased more than 64%, the patient was likely to be a complete responder (p = 0.003). 43% of the patients were classified as complete responders. The authors caution that although maxSUV should be identical across facilities, the variables used to calculate it and the timing of injection all affect the maxSUV. However, it is reproducible and reliable within a given facility.

T. L. Bauer II, MD

Understanding Bladder Cancer Death: Tumor Biology Versus Physician Practice
Morris DS, Weizer AZ, Ye Z, et al (Univ of Michigan, Ann Arbor)
Cancer 115:1011-1020, 2009

Background.—To the authors' knowledge, the extent to which death from bladder cancer is attributable to tumor biology or physician practice patterns is unknown, For this reason, the relative importance of broadening indications for aggressive therapy has unclear implications.

Methods.—Patients whose deaths were caused directly by bladder cancer were identified using institutional (n = 126 patients) and administrative (n = 6326 patients) data sources. By using implicit review (clinical data, 2001-2005) and explicit algorithms (Surveillance, Epidemiology, and End Results [SEER]-Medicare, 1992-2002), the authors estimated the proportion of potentially avoidable deaths from bladder cancer.

Results.—After an implicit review of clinical data, 40 of 126 deaths (31.7%) were classified as potentially avoidable. Compared with those patients who were deemed unsalvageable, these patients generally presented with nonmuscle-invasive disease (80% vs 25.6%; $P < .001$), received multiple courses of intravesical therapy (32.5% vs 1.2%; $P < .001$), and had a more protracted course from diagnosis to aggressive treatment (median, 23 months vs 2 months; $P < .001$). An explicit review of claims data indicated that between 31.6% and 46.8% of the 6326 bladder cancer deaths identified in the SEER-Medicare data potentially were avoidable, depending on the survivorship threshold chosen, Patients whose deaths potentially were avoidable more commonly presented with nonmuscle-invasive disease (66.7% vs 24.7%; $P < .0001$) and lower grade disease (35.1% vs 15.1%; $P < .0001$).

Conclusions.—The greatest inroads into reducing death from bladder cancer likely hinge on earlier detection or improvement of systemic therapies, However, changing physician practice may translate into nontrivial reductions in bladder cancer mortality.

▶ We all wrestle with bladder cancer. Unlike prostate and kidney cancer, poor treatment results in death fairly frequently. Also, unlike prostate and kidney cancer, the treatments often have significant morbidity and mortality. This is why many patients and physicians delay aggressive treatment. This article provides strong evidence that these delays have adverse affects. I feel strongly that patients with aggressive noninvasive bladder cancer should be given a shot at bladder preservation with intravesical agents. I feel just as strongly that if these agents fail, the patient should rapidly move to more aggressive treatment. Does this mean that every patient needs a cystectomy? Of course not! But more emphasis on the lethality of the disease needs to be emphasized to the patient. Quality of life is important but so is cure for this deadly disease.

A. S. Kibel, MD

PART FOUR

KIDNEY, WATER, AND ELECTROLYTES

RENEE GARRICK, MD

28 Metabolic Factors and Renal Disease Progression

Introduction

Data generated over the past several years have clearly demonstrated that in both diabetic and nondiabetic kidney disease, angiotensin converting enzyme inhibition (ACEi) and angiotensin receptor blockade (ARB) reduce urinary protein spillage. Several studies have suggested that combination therapy with both ACEi and ARBs is superior to therapy with either agent alone, and a recent meta-analysis suggested that combination therapy results in approximately a 25% greater reduction in proteinuria as compared with monotherapy.[1] As combination therapy has become more commonplace, triple therapy with ACEi, ARBs, and aldactone has also been advocated in certain situations.[2] The meta-analysis by Kunz and colleagues, presented here, evaluated observations gathered from 49 studies involving 6181 participants. This analysis suggested that the effects of ACEi and ARBs are of similar magnitude and that combination therapy results in an additional 18 to 25% lowering of proteinuria. However, as Kunz noted, for the most part the studies were small, of short duration, and typically used proteinuria as a surrogate marker for the progression of chronic kidney disease. In many cases, outcome results of renal function were not available, and information regarding adverse effects was also uncertain.

Prior studies by Kent and colleagues,[3] evaluated data combined from 11 randomized clinical trials of nondiabetic patients with proteinuria. This evaluation suggested that patients with proteinuria less than 500 mg/day do not generally benefit from treatment with angiotensin converting enzyme inhibitors, even when they are at high risk for progression. This year, the IMPROVE trial evaluated the effects of treatment with monotherapy or combination therapy with irbesartan and ramipril in hypertensive patients with underlying cardiovascular disease. Combination therapy with ACEi/ARB resulted in superior blood pressure control. However, the 20-week response of the microalbuminuria to combination therapy of irbesartan plus ramipril versus ramipril alone, was not significantly different. The incidence of adverse effects was similar in both groups.

Other studies this year raised additional questions regarding the safety and efficacy of combination therapy. The ON TARGET trial evaluated the utility of monotherapy with telmisartan, ramipril, or both, in high-risk patients with underlying diabetes or vascular disease. The study demonstrated that telmisartan and ramipril have equivalent effects on protein spillage. In patients at high risk for vascular disease, however, combination therapy was associated with more adverse effects, including an increase in hyperkalemia, hypotensive episodes, and renal impairment.

These results clearly demonstrate that combination therapy with ACEi and ARBs need to be individualized and that outcome data including renal function data are critical.

Other studies this year focused on the role of alternative strategies, other than ACEi and ARB therapy, for the control of proteinuria. The GUARD trial by Bakris and colleagues demonstrated that in patients with hypertensive type 2 diabetes, the addition of a diuretic (hydrochlorothiazide) lowered proteinuria more effectively than monotherapy. Vogt and colleagues evaluated the effect of dietary sodium restriction and hydrochlorothiazide on the antiproteinuric effect of losartan in several types of non-diabetic renal disease. A low sodium diet and hydrochlorothiazide were equally efficacious and superior to losartan alone. Combination therapy with hydrochlorothiazide, salt restriction, and losartan had the greatest anti-proteinuric effect. Thus, it is important for practitioners to specifically address dietary sodium intake with patients, and to stress that dietary modifications are as important as pharmacologic manipulations.

Taken together, especially in view of the data from the ON TARGET trial, it appears that combination ACEi and ARB therapy is likely not appropriate for all patients. The decision to use such therapy must be individualized and the risk carefully weighed against the benefits. Medication complications and renal outcome must be carefully monitored. The use of a diuretic, rather than additional ACEi or ARB therapy, may be preferred for patients with hypertension, microalbuminuria, or proteinuria under 500 mg/day when additional treatment is needed. At this time, triple therapy with ACEi, ARB, and aldosterone blockade is not a considered routine standard of care and such treatment is likely best overseen by a nephrologist.

Also included in this section are the results of the 20-year follow-up of the landmark Modification of Diet in Renal Disease (MDRD) study. The trial, which was initially designed to evaluate the effects of very low dietary protein on the progression of renal disease, has resulted in a number of very important findings, including the development of the MDRD formula for the estimation of glomerular filtration rate (eGFR).

Renee Garrick, MD

References

1. Catapano F, Chiodini P, De Nicola L, et al. Antiproteinuric response to dual blockade of the renin-angiotensin system in primary glomerulonephritis: meta-analysis and meta-regression. *Am J Kidney Dis.* 2008;52:475-485.
2. Navaneethan SD, Nigwekar SU, Sehgal AR, Strippoli GF. Aldosterone antagonist for preventing the progression of chronic kidney disease: a systematic review and meta-analysis. *Clin J Am Soc Nephrol.* 2009;4:542-551.
3. Kent DM, Jafar TH, Hayward RA, et al. Progression risk, urinary protein excretion, and treatment effects of angiotensin-converting enzyme inhibitors in nondiabetic kidney disease. *J Am Soc Nephrol.* 2007;18:1959-1965.

Meta-analysis: Effect of Monotherapy and Combination Therapy with Inhibitors of the Renin–Angiotensin System on Proteinuria in Renal Disease

Kunz R, Friedrich C, Wolbers M, et al (Univ Hosp Basel, Switzerland; Ludwig Maxmilian Univ, Germany)
Ann Intern Med 148:30-48, 2008

Background.—Reduction of proteinuria is associated with delayed progression of chronic kidney disease. Reports suggest that angiotensin-receptor blockers (ARBs) reduce proteinuria, but results are variable. The relative effect of ARBs and angiotensin-converting enzyme (ACE) inhibitors, and their combined administration, remains uncertain.

Purpose.—To establish the effect of ARBs versus placebo and alternative treatments, and the effect of combined treatment with ARBs and ACE inhibitors, on proteinuria.

Data Sources.—English-language studies in MEDLINE and the Cochrane Library Central Register of Controlled Trials (January 1990 to September 2006), reference lists, and expert contacts.

Study Selection.—Randomized trials of ARBs versus placebo, ACE inhibitors, calcium-channel blockers, or the combination of ARBs and ACE inhibitors in patients with or without diabetes and with microalbuminuria or proteinuria for whom data were available on urinary protein excretion at baseline and at 1 to 12 months.

Data Extraction.—Two investigators independently searched and abstracted studies.

Data Synthesis.—Forty-nine studies involving 6181 participants reported results of 72 comparisons with 1 to 4 months of follow-up and 38 comparisons with 5 to 12 months of follow-up. The ARBs reduced proteinuria compared with placebo or calcium-channel blockers over 1 to 4 months (ratio of means, 0.57 [95% CI, 0.47 to 0.68] and 0.69 [CI, 0.62 to 0.77], respectively) and 5 to 12 months (ratio of means, 0.66 [CI, 0.63 to 0.69] and 0.62 [CI, 0.55 to 0.70], respectively). The ARBs and ACE inhibitors reduced proteinuria to a similar degree. The combination of ARBs and ACE inhibitors further reduced proteinuria more than either agent alone: The ratio of means for combination therapy versus ARBs was 0.76 (CI, 0.68 to 0.85) over 1 to 4 months and 0.75 (CI, 0.61 to 0.92) over 5 to 12 months; for combination therapy versus ACE inhibitors, the ratio of means was 0.78 (CI, 0.72 to 0.84) over 1 to 4 months and 0.82 (CI, 0.67 to 1.01) over 5 to 12 months. The antiproteinuric effect was consistent across subgroups.

Limitations.—Most studies were small, varied in quality, and did not provide reliable data on adverse drug reactions. Proteinuria reduction is only a surrogate for important progression of renal failure.

Conclusion.—The ARBs reduce proteinuria, independent of the degree of proteinuria and of underlying disease. The magnitude of effect is similar regardless of whether the comparator is placebo or calcium-channel blocker. Reduction in proteinuria from ARBs and ACE inhibitors is similar, but their combination is more effective than either drug alone. Uncertainty concerning adverse effects and outcomes that are important to patients limits applicability of findings to clinical practice.

▶ I included this study because the use of combinations of angiotensin-converting enzyme inhibitors (ACEi) and angiotensin-receptor blocker (ARB) therapy seems to have become commonplace among many general internal medical practices. These agents are now being used both for the control of hypertension and for the control of proteinuria. This carefully constructed meta analysis used MEDLINE and the Cochrane Library Central Register of Controlled Trials and evaluated studies conducted from January of 1990 through September of 2006. The studies included randomized controlled trials that compared the effect of calcium channel blockers, ACEi or ARB therapy, and combination therapy versus placebo in patients with and without diabetes with micro or macroalbuminuria. The authors identified 49 randomized controlled trials. The longest follow-up period was 12 months. The data suggest that monotherapy with ACEi and ARBs are both effective and have an equivalent effect on proteinuria as compared with placebo. Combination therapy was more effective than monotherapy for patients with higher degrees of proteinuria.

This careful meta analysis raises several questions and cautions. Many studies were done on patients with mild to moderate degrees of renal impairment, and only a few of the combination studies were done on patients with more advanced (stage 3 and 4) kidney disease. None of the studies were long-term, and, therefore, the safety and efficacy of combination therapy cannot be ascertained from the available data. While it is tempting to use a reduction in proteinuria alone as a surrogate marker for preserved renal function, primary studies, which assess renal function itself rather than surrogate markers, are needed. Data on adverse effects were not always carefully documented in the primary studies, however, the authors noted that 86% of the studies listed adverse reactions, and 29 of 49 studies reported episodes of medication discontinuation.

We must realize that there is a limitation to our current knowledge base regarding the long-term use of combination therapy. Based on previous studies,[1,2] it would seem reasonable to reserve combination therapy for patients with high-grade proteinuria to target the proteinuria to the range of approximately 500 mg a day, and to closely monitor the renal function and serum electrolytes. The generalized use, and long-term safety of and efficacy of combination therapy, and the use of such therapy in patients with advanced (stage 4) renal disease, remains to be established.

R. Garrick, MD

References

1. Kent DM, Jafar TH, Hayward R, et al. Progression risk, urinary protein excretion, and treatment effects of angiotensin-converting enzyme inhibitors in nondiabetic kidney disease. *J Am Soc Nephrol.* 2007;18:1959-1965.
2. Jafar TH, Schmid CH, Landa M, et al. Angiotensin-converting enzyme inhibitors and progression of nondiabetic renal disease. a meta-analysis of patient-level data. *Ann Intern Med.* 2001;135:73-78.

Telmisartan, Ramipril, or Both in Patients at High Risk for Vascular Events
The ONTARGET Investigators
N Engl J Med 358:1547-1559, 2008

Background.—In patients who have vascular disease or high-risk diabetes without heart failure, angiotensin-converting–enzyme (ACE) inhibitors reduce mortality and morbidity from cardiovascular causes, but the role of angiotensin-receptor blockers (ARBs) in such patients is unknown. We compared the ACE inhibitor ramipril, the ARB telmisartan, and the combination of the two drugs in patients with vascular disease or high-risk diabetes.

Methods.—After a 3-week, single-blind run-in period, patients underwent double-blind randomization, with 8576 assigned to receive 10 mg of ramipril per day, 8542 assigned to receive 80 mg of telmisartan per day, and 8502 assigned to receive both drugs (combination therapy). The primary composite outcome was death from cardiovascular causes, myocardial infarction, stroke, or hospitalization for heart failure.

Results.—Mean blood pressure was lower in both the telmisartan group (a 0.9/0.6 mm Hg greater reduction) and the combination-therapy group (a 2.4/1.4 mm Hg greater reduction) than in the ramipril group. At a median follow-up of 56 months, the primary outcome had occurred in 1412 patients in the ramipril group (16.5%), as compared with 1423 patients in the telmisartan group (16.7%; relative risk, 1.01; 95% confidence interval [CI], 0.94 to 1.09). As compared with the ramipril group, the telmisartan group had lower rates of cough (1.1% vs. 4.2%, P<0.001) and angioedema (0.1% vs. 0.3%, P = 0.01) and a higher rate of hypotensive symptoms (2.6% vs. 1.7%, P<0.001); the rate of syncope was the same in the two groups (0.2%). In the combination-therapy group, the primary outcome occurred in 1386 patients (16.3%; relative risk, 0.99; 95% CI, 0.92 to 1.07); as compared with the ramipril group, there was an increased risk of hypotensive symptoms (4.8% vs. 1.7%, P<0.001), syncope (0.3% vs. 0.2%, P = 0.03), and renal dysfunction (13.5% vs. 10.2%, P<0.001).

Conclusions.—Telmisartan was equivalent to ramipril in patients with vascular disease or highrisk diabetes and was associated with less angioedema. The combination of the two drugs was associated with more adverse events without an increase in benefit. (ClinicalTrials.gov number, NCT00153101.)

▶ The Renoprotection of Optimal Proteinuric Doses (ROAD) study[1] in patients with nephropathy and chronic kidney disease with and without diabetes demonstrated that high doses of benazepril or losartan reduced proteinuria and were renoprotective. The COOPERATE trial[2] demonstrated that combination therapy with losartan and trandolapril had a greater antiproteinuric effect than did monotherapy. The results of the COOPERATE trial however have been questioned.[3] Other more recent meta-analyses have also suggested that combination therapy with angiotensin-converting enzyme inhibitor (ACEi) and angiotensin receptor blocker (ARB) can be safely used to reduce proteinuria.[4]

The ONTARGET trial was designed to look at the effects of ramapril (10 mg a day), telemisartan, (80 mg a day), or a combination of both agents on primarily vascular outcome events in a high-risk population. A change in protein excretion was not a primary endpoint. This randomized double-blind study evaluated 8576 patients and is one of the largest combination trials performed. The study demonstrated that the agents were equivalent with regard to their prevention of primary outcome events in patients with vascular disease or high-risk diabetes. The incidence of hyperkalemia was significantly higher in patients who received combination therapy. The relative risk of renal impairment (defined as a change in renal function that led an investigator to discontinue the drug), was greater [1.04 (0.96–1.14) vs 1.33 (1.22–1.44)] in the group that received combination therapy.

This study is important because it calls our attention to the fact that combined therapy with ACEi and ARBs must be carefully individualized. The data from the ONTARGET trial suggest that it may be premature for practice guidelines to consider combination ACEi ARB therapy as the routine standard of care, especially for patients with low-grade proteinuria, or for patients with severe vascular disease who are at high risk for hypotensive episodes. The results do suggest that both renal function and serum potassium must be monitored when these agents are used in combination.

R. Garrick, MD

References

1. Hou FF, Xie D, Zhang X, et al. Renoprotection of Optimal Antiproteinuric Doses (ROAD) Study: a randomized controlled study of benazepril and losartan in chronic renal insufficiency. *J Am Soc Nephrol.* 2007;18:1889-1898.
2. Nakao N, Yoshimura A, Morita H, Takada M, Kayano T, Ideura T. Combination treatment of angiotensin-II receptor blocker and angiotensin-converting-enzyme inhibitor in non-diabetic renal disease (COOPERATE): a randomized controlled trial. *Lancet.* 2003;361:117-124.
3. Kunz R, Wolbers M, Glass T, Mann JF. The COOPERATE trial: a letter of concern. *Lancet.* 2008;371:1575-1576.

4. MacKinnon M, Shurraw S, Akbari A, Knoll GA, Jaffey J, Clark HD. Combination therapy with an angiotensin receptor blocker and an ACE inhibitor in proteinuric renal disease: a systematic review of the efficacy and safety data. *Am J Kidney Dis.* 2006;48(1):8-20.

Effects of different ACE inhibitor combinations on albuminuria: results of the GUARD study

Bakris GL, On behalf of the GUARD (Gauging Albuminuria Reduction With Lotrel in Diabetic Patients With Hypertension) Study Investigators (Univ of Chicago, IL; et al)
Kidney Int 73:1303-1309, 2008

Clinical practice guidelines recommend blockers of the renin-angiotensin system alone or in combination with other agents to reduce blood pressure and albuminuria in patients with type 2 diabetes. Dihydropyridine calcium channel blockers, however, may lower blood pressure but not albuminuria in these patients. Here we tested the hypothesis that combining an ACE inhibitor with either a thiazide diuretic or a calcium channel blocker will cause similar reductions in blood pressure and albuminuria in hypertensive type 2 diabetics. We conducted a double blind randomized controlled trial on 332 hypertensive, albuminuric type 2 diabetic patients treated with benazepril with either amlodipine or hydrochlorothiazide for 1 year. The trial employed a non-inferiority design. Both combinations significantly reduced the urinary albumin to creatinine ratio and sitting blood pressure of the entire cohort. The percentage of patients progressing to overt proteinuria was similar for both groups. When we examined patients who had only microalbuminuria and hypertension we found that a larger percentage of the diuretic and ACE inhibitor normalized their albuminuria. We conclude that initial treatment using benzaepril with a diuretic resulted in a greater reduction in albuminuria compared to the group of ACE inhibitor and calcium channel blocker. In contrast, blood pressure reduction, particularly the diastolic component, favored the combination with amilodipine. The dissociation between reductions in blood pressure and albuminuria may be related to factors other than blood pressure.

▶ The presence of hypertension, diabetes, and microalbuminuria are strong prognostic indicators for both mortality and cardiovascular disease in patients with hypertension and diabetes,[1,2] and a variety of treatment strategies and guidelines have been developed in an attempt to reduce cardiovascular risk and preserve renal function.[2-4]

Currently, multiple practice guidelines indicate that initial hypertensive therapy in patients with diabetes or renal disease should include therapy within an angiotensin-converting enzyme inhibitor (ACEi) or an angiotensin receptor blocker (ARB). With regard to additional agents, the findings of the previous Reduction of End points in NIDDM (non-insulin-dependent diabetes mellitus)

With the Angiotensin II Antagonist Losartan (RENAAL) study suggested that when amlodipine was added to losartan for blood pressure control, no significant difference in albumin excretion was detected.[5] At present, when additional therapy is needed, the next best drug class is not specifically delineated in most treatment guidelines. Bakris and colleagues designed the Gauging Albuminuria Reduction With Lotrel in Diabetic Patients With Hypertension (GUARD) trial to test whether combination fixed-dose therapy with an ACE (benazepril/amlodipine), or fixed dose ACEi/diuretic (benazepril/hydrochlorothiazide) was superior with regard to blood pressure control and albumin excretion in hypertensive patients with type II diabetes.

The results demonstrated that both combinations reduced the urinary albumin/creatinine ratio and the sitting blood pressure of the entire cohort, and the percentage of patients progressing to overt proteinuria was similar for both groups. Among patients with only microalbuminuria, normalization of albumin excretion was achieved in a larger percentage of patients treated with hydrochlorothiazide/benazepril than with amlodipine/benazepril. However, blood pressure (especially diastolic blood pressure), was superior with the benazepril/amlodipine combination, and the rate of decline of glomerular filtration rate (GFR) was slower in those randomized to benazepril and amlodipine. The authors note that because urinary sodium excretion was not monitored it is difficult to fully interpret the lower urinary albumin excretion in the benazepril/hydrochlorothiazide cohort.

I included this study because of the recent attention that has been directed toward practice guidelines emanating from "evidence-based medicine" and comparative effectiveness research (CER) and the associated pay-for-performance outcome measurements. Clearly, in what by medical research standards would be described as a very short time span, a number of studies have suggested that varying and distinct combinations of medications may be efficacious under specific circumstances for the treatment of hypertensive, proteinuric, diabetic renal disease. Clearly, these ever-changing data indicate that accurate, individualized clinical decision-making must appropriately consider multiple, nonstatic, patient-specific factors in order to arrive at the best treatment plan for an individual patient. Whether this can be satisfactorily accomplished by applying population-based comparative research techniques and population outcome measurements to the management of the individual patient remains uncertain.

R. Garrick, MD

References

1. Garg JP, Bakris GL. Microalbuminuria: marker of vascular dysfunction, risk factor for cardiovascular disease. *Vasc Med.* 2002;7:35-43.
2. American Diabetes Association. Standards of medical care in diabetes. *Diabetes Care.* 2005;28:S4-S36.
3. KDOQI. KDOQI clinical practice guidelines and clinical practice recommendations for diabetes and chronic kidney disease. *Am J Kidney Dis.* 2007;49: S12-S154.
4. Kidney Disease Outcomes Quality Initiative (K/DOQI). K/DOQI clinical practice guidelines on hypertension and antihypertensive agents in chronic kidney disease. *Am J Kidney Dis.* 2004;43:S1-S290.

5. Bakris GL, Weir MR, Shanifar S, et al. Effects of blood pressure level on progression of diabetic nephropathy: results from the RENAAL Study. *Arch Intern Med.* 2003;163:1555-1565.

Treatment of microalbuminuria in hypertensive subjects with elevated cardiovascular risk: Results of the IMPROVE trial

Bakris GL, Ruilope L, Locatelli F, et al (Univ of Chicago-Pritzker School of Medicine, IL; Hypertension Unit, Madrid, Spain; A Manzoni Hosp, Lecco, Italy; et al)
Kidney Int 72:879-885, 2007

Microalbuminuria independently predicts increased cardiovascular risk in hypertensive patients, especially in those with concomitant diabetes or established cardiovascular disease. Drugs that target the renin–angiotensin–aldosterone system reduce microalbuminuria regardless of diabetic status. The Irbesartan in the Management of PROteinuric patients at high risk for Vascular Events was a multicenter, randomized, double-blind, placebo-controlled paralleled group study in which hypertensive patients with microalbuminuria and increased cardiovascular risk were randomized to 20 weeks treatment with ramipril plus irbesartan or to ramipril plus placebo. Patients discontinued or tapered previous antihypertensive therapy during a 14-day placebo lead-in period. Change in albumin excretion rate from baseline to week 20 was the primary end point. Adjusted week 20 baseline geometric ratios for ramipril plus irbesartan and ramipril plus placebo were not significantly different. Although differences in blood pressure reductions were observed between the two treatments, these changes did not affect microalbuminuria. More patients on dual therapy achieved target blood pressure goals at week 20 than with monotherapy. The incidence of adverse effects and treatment-related adverse effects was similar in both groups. Our results suggest that patients with cardiovascular risk and relatively low albumin excretion rates in early-stage disease may only require monotherapy with renin–angiotensin–aldosterone blocking agents.

▶ I included this study because it adds information as to where we are, or where we are not, in our understanding of combination angiotensin-converting enzyme inhibitors (ACEi) and angiotensin receptor blocker (ARB) therapy in the treatment of proteinuria and hypertension. The Irbesartan in the Management of PROteinuric patients at high risk for Vascular Events (IMPROVE) study was a randomized controlled trial aimed at determining whether combination therapy with ramipril and Irbesartan was more effective than therapy with ramipril alone in reducing albuminuria in hypertensive patients with high cardiovascular risk who had persistent microalbuminuria despite treatment with an ACEi. Major limitations of the study were its length (20 weeks) and the fact that most recipients had microalbuminuria, rather than higher degrees of proteinuria.

With these caveats in mind, this trial demonstrated that while combination therapy improved blood pressure control, it did not improve albumin spillage as compared with ramipril alone. Renal function (creatinine) was not a randomization factor, and kidney outcome measures were not included. The results suggest that for patients with underlying cardiovascular disease and low range proteinuria, monotherapy with angiotensin antagonists will reduce the protein spillage as well as more aggressive combination therapy. If additional antihypertensive control is required, the added agent, with regard to proteinuria, need not be an angiotensin blocker.

R. Garrick, MD

Effects of Dietary Sodium and Hydrochlorothiazide on the Antiproteinuric Efficacy of Losartan

Vogt L, Waanders F, Boomsma F, et al (Univ of Groningen, Netherlands; Erasmus Med Ctr, Rotterdam, Netherlands)
J Am Soc Nephrol 19:999-1007, 2008

There is large interindividual variability in the antiproteinuric response to blockade of the renin-angiotensin-aldosterone system (RAAS). A low-sodium diet or addition of diuretics enhances the effects of RAAS blockade on proteinuria and BP, but the efficacy of the combination of these interventions is unknown. Therefore, this randomized, double-blind, placebo-controlled trial to determine the separate and combined effects of a low-sodium diet and hydrochlorothiazide (HCT) on proteinuria and BP was performed. In 34 proteinuric patients without diabetes, mean baseline proteinuria was 3.8 g/d, and this was reduced by 22% by a low-sodium diet alone. Losartan monotherapy reduced proteinuria by 30%, and the addition of a low-sodium diet led to a total reduction by 55% and the addition of HCT to 56%. The combined addition of HCT and a low-sodium diet reduced proteinuria by 70% from baseline (all $P < 0.05$). Reductions in mean arterial pressure showed a similar pattern (all $P < 0.05$). In addition, individuals who did not demonstrate an antiproteinuric response to losartan monotherapy did respond when a low-sodium diet or a diuretic was added. In conclusion, a low-sodium diet and HCT are equally efficacious in reducing proteinuria and BP when added to a regimen containing losartan and especially seem to benefit individuals who are resistant to RAAS blockade. Combining these interventions in sodium status is an effective method to maximize the antiproteinuric efficacy of RAAS blockade.

▶ Several studies over the last decade have demonstrated the importance of blood pressure control in reducing the rate of decline of renal function. Many of those same trials have also demonstrated that a reduction in protein spillage may also have independent reno-protective effects.[1-3] In addition, it has been suggested that the therapeutic response and individual variation in protein spillage may be predictive of that patient's long-term renal outcome.[4] In this regard, of clinical concern is that an increase in sodium intake can significantly abrogate the antiproteinuric effect of angiotensin blockade.[4] There is a corollary – dietary sodium restriction alone, or in combination with volume depletion induced by diuretics, may enhance the antiproteinuric effects of angiotensin blockade. The present study evaluated this possibility in several types of nondiabetic proteinuric renal disease. The results demonstrate that the combination of losartan and sodium restriction and losartan and diuretic were both superior to losartan alone, and reduced protein spillage in those patients in whom losartan alone had failed. The combination of sodium restriction and a thiazide diuretic more than doubled the reduction in protein spillage. A similar step-wise trend was observed in blood pressure reduction, though by covariate analysis the reduction in proteinuria was independent of the blood pressure response. The low-salt diet and the diuretic both increased the serum creatinine when combined with losartan, and the increase in creatinine was slightly greater when all 3 treatments were combined. The observed change in glomerular filtration rate (GFR) with combined treatment did not account for the change in protein spillage. Hyperkalemia did not develop in any treatment group. Longer term studies will be needed to both establish the stability of the GFR and to determine if the reduction in protein spillage seen with the combined therapy ultimately proves to be renoprotective. The current observation does however suggest that this combination therapy represents a therapeutic alternative in patients with proteinuria that is resistant to angiotensin receptor blocker monotherapy.

R. Garrick, MD

References

1. Brenner BM, Cooper ME, de Zeeuw D, et al. RENAAL Study Investigators. Effects of losartan on renal and cardiovascular outcomes in patients with type 2 diabetes and nephropathy. *N Engl J Med.* 2001;345:861-869.
2. Lewis EJ, Hunsicker LG, Clarke WR, et al. Collaborative Study Group. Renoprotective effect of the angiotensin-receptor antagonist irbesartan in patients with nephropathy due to type 2 diabetes. *N Engl J Med.* 2001;345:851-860.
3. Buter H, Hemmelder MH, Navis G, de Jong PE, de Zeeuw D. The blunting of the antiproteinuric efficacy of ACE inhibition by high sodium intake can be restored by hydrochlorothiazide. *Nephrol Dial Transplant.* 1998;13:1682-1685.
4. Apperloo AJ, de Zeeuw D, de Jong PE. Short-term antiproteinuric response to antihypertensive treatment predicts long-term GFR decline in patients with nondiabetic renal disease. *Kidney Int Suppl.* 1994;45:S174-S178.

Effect of a Very Low-Protein Diet on Outcomes: Long-term Follow-up of the Modification of Diet in Renal Disease (MDRD) Study
Menon V, Kopple JD, Wang X, et al (Tufts Med Ctr, Boston, MA; Los Angeles Biomedical Res Inst at Harbor-UCLA Med Ctr, CA; Cleveland Clinic Found, OH; et al)
Am J Kidney Dis 53:208-217, 2009

Background.—The long-term effect of a very low-protein diet on the progression of kidney disease is unknown. We examined the effect of a very low-protein diet on the development of kidney failure and death during long-term follow-up of the Modification of Diet in Renal Disease (MDRD) Study.

Study Design.—Long-term follow-up of study B of the MDRD Study (1989-1993).

Setting & Participants.—The MDRD Study examined the effects of dietary protein restriction and blood pressure control on progression of kidney disease. This analysis includes 255 trial participants with predominantly stage 4 nondiabetic chronic kidney disease.

Intervention.—A low-protein diet (0.58 g/kg/d) versus a very low-protein diet (0.28 g/kg/d) supplemented with a mixture of essential keto acids and amino acids (0.28 g/kg/d).

Outcomes.—Kidney failure (initiation of dialysis therapy or transplantation) and all-cause mortality until December 31, 2000.

Results.—Kidney failure developed in 227 (89%) participants, 79 (30.9%) died, and 244 (95.7%) reached the composite outcome of either kidney failure or death. Median duration of follow-up until kidney failure, death, or administrative censoring was 3.2 years, and median time to death was 10.6 years. In the low-protein group, 117 (90.7%) participants developed kidney failure, 30 (23.3%) died, and 124 (96.1%) reached the composite outcome. In the very low-protein group, 110 (87.3%) participants developed kidney failure, 49 (38.9%) died, and 120 (95.2%) reached the composite outcome. After adjustment for a priori–specified covariates, hazard ratios were 0.83 (95% confidence interval, 0.62 to 1.12) for kidney failure, 1.92 (95% confidence interval, 1.15 to 3.20) for death, and 0.89 (95% confidence interval, 0.67 to 1.18) for the composite outcome in the very low-protein diet group compared with the low-protein diet group.

Limitations.—Lack of dietary protein measurements during follow-up.

Conclusion.—In long-term follow-up of the MDRD Study, assignment to a very low-protein diet did not delay progression to kidney failure, but appeared to increase the risk of death.

▶ The modification of diet in renal disease (MDRD) study was designed to evaluate the effect of a low-protein diet (LPD) and a very low-protein diet (VLPD) on the progression of renal disease. The study was performed from 1989 and 1993 and was comprised of 2 subgroups: study group A, which involved dietary protein manipulation in patients with a glomerular filtration rate (GFR) of 20 to 55 mls/min/1.73 m^2, and study group B, which included patients with a GFR 13 to 24 mls/min/1.73 m^2. Patients in study group B were randomized to receive either 0.58 g per kilogram per day (LPD) or 0.28 g/kg/day with keto/amino acid supplements (VLPD-KA). Using a factorial design, the groups were randomized to obtain mean blood pressure control of either 107 mmHg or 92 mmHg. The actual protein intakes maintained in the patients in the study B groups were 0.69 and 0.46 g/kg/day. Following completion of the study in 1993, protein intake was assessed once more, 9 months after the end of the study.

The present article presents the long-term effect of dietary protein modification in 255 patients in the B study group of the MDRD study. The results suggest that assignment to a VLPD did not delay progression to kidney failure and may have increased the risk of death.

I included this article because, despite multiple studies, there is still much controversy regarding the potential risks and benefits of dietary protein modification in renal disease. Interpretation of the current study is difficult, and is made more difficult by the fact that dietary follow-up ceased shortly after the conclusion of the study. Therefore, the long-term protein intake of patients in either the LPD or the VLPD-KA groups can only be speculated. In addition, it is important to note that the differences in the death rate largely involve those patients who went on to require dialysis. No data are available regarding the specifics of their dialysis treatment, and those dialysis-related factors may have independently affected patient survival.

However, despite these limitations the study does provide us with remarkable long-term outcome data in a fairly well-defined population. The data suggest that a more complete answer will only be possible through long-term follow-up studies that include both dietary intake and multiple levels of outcome data. Whether such studies will be done remains uncertain. In the meantime, information is readily available in both the scientific and popular press on ways to use an LPD as a means to avoiding or delaying dialysis. Until more definitive data become available, patients who are interested in maintaining a VLPD with appropriate keto/amino supplementation would be best advised to do so only with thorough dietary planning and careful dietitian and clinical follow-up.

R. Garrick, MD

29 Hypertension

Introduction

Several recent exciting developments have occurred in our understanding of hypertension and renal disease. The Multiethnic Study of Atherosclerosis (MESA) study demonstrated that differences in kidney function, as determined by Cystatin C levels, are associated with incident hypertension among individuals without known clinical kidney or cardiovascular disease. While this population-based study does not definitively unravel the "chicken and egg" question of hypertension and renal disease, the data suggest that, in keeping with experimental work, kidney damage may be primary and pivotal in the pathogenesis of essential hypertension.

One of the most exciting findings was the demonstration by Freedman and colleagues that polymorphism in the non-muscle myosin heavy chain nine gene (MYH9) is strongly associated with end-stage renal disease historically attributed to hypertension in African Americans. These results are especially provocative when considered together with the long-term follow-up of the African-American Study of Kidney Disease and Hypertension (AASK trial). The AASK trial demonstrated that renal disease continued to progress despite the blood pressure benefits of renin-angiotensin blockade. The next obvious question is to determine, if possible, the status of the MYH9 gene among the patients in the AASK trial.

The role of allopurinol in hypertension continues to be evaluated. Johnson and colleagues completed a causality trial in which they demonstrated that treatment with allopurinol reduced blood pressure, reduced renin levels, and reduced vascular resistance in adolescents with hypertension, many of whom have the metabolic syndrome. Kumar and colleagues demonstrated that independent of uric acid status, fructose-induced hypertension (which recapitulates many aspects of the metabolic syndrome) may be generated by an increase in salt absorption by the intestine and the kidneys. These are fascinating findings and although the puzzle is not yet untangled, together the results suggest that diet, high-fructose additives (which may increase uric acid as well), and weight control must not be ignored if we are intent on combating the metabolic syndrome and preserving the long-term health of adolescents.

Renee Garrick, MD

243

Differences in Kidney Function and Incident Hypertension: The Multi-Ethnic Study of Atherosclerosis

Kestenbaum B, Rudser KD, de Boer IH, et al (Univ of Washington, Seattle; et al)
Ann Intern Med 148:501-508, 2008

Background.—Kidney disease and hypertension commonly coexist, yet the direction of their association is still debated.

Objective.—To evaluate whether early kidney dysfunction, measured by serum cystatin C levels and urinary albumin excretion, predates hypertension in adults without clinically recognized kidney or cardiovascular disease.

Design.—Observational cohort study using data from 2000 to 2005.

Setting.—The MESA (Multi-Ethnic Study of Atherosclerosis), a community- based study of subclinical cardiovascular disease in adults age 45 to 84 years.

Participants.—2767 MESA participants without prevalent hypertension, cardiovascular disease, or clinically recognized kidney disease (an estimated glomerular filtration rate <60 mL/min per 1.73 m^2 or microalbuminuria).

Measurements.—Cystatin C was measured by using a nephelometer, and urinary albumin and creatinine were measured from a spot morning collection. The primary outcome was incident hypertension, defined as systolic blood pressure of at least 140 mm Hg, diastolic blood pressure of at least 90 mm Hg, or use of an antihypertensive medication.

Results.—During a median follow-up of 3.1 years, 19.7% of the cohort (545 participants) developed hypertension. After adjustment for established hypertension risk factors, each 15-nmol/L increase in cystatin C was associated with a statistically significant 15% greater incidence of hypertension ($P = 0.017$). The highest sex-specific quartile of urinary albumin–creatinine ratio was associated with a statistically insignificant 16% greater incidence of hypertension ($P = 0.192$) compared with the lowest quartile. No statistical evidence suggested a multiplicative interaction.

Limitations.—Unmeasured characteristics may have confounded observed associations of kidney markers with hypertension. Follow-up was relatively short. Hypertension that may have occurred between study visits or hypertension that was not captured by standard cuff measurements may have been missed.

Conclusion.—Differences in kidney function, indicated by cystatin C levels, are associated with incident hypertension among individuals without clinical kidney or cardiovascular disease. These population-based findings complement experimental work implicating early kidney damage in the pathogenesis of essential hypertension.

▶ The multiethnic study of atherosclerosis (MESA) is an ongoing community-based study of subclinical cardiovascular disease among adults aged 45 to 84 years. The original study group recruited between 2000 and 2002, was drawn from 6 diverse communities across the United States. In the current trial, the authors excluded participants if they had any previous diagnosis of cardiovascular disease heart failure, any history of hypertension or borderline hypertension (defined as a blood pressure of 140/90), any history of renal dysfunction defined as a glomerular filtration rate (GFR) of less than 60 mL/min, microalbuminuria defined as a urinary albumin/creatinine of 25 mg/g for women, or 17 mg per gram for men. The remaining 2767 middle-aged adults were followed for approximately 3 years. During this time their GFR was assessed by cystatin C determinations. Overall, approximately 20% of the patients in this multiethnic cohort developed hypertension. Higher baseline cystatin C levels were associated with a higher incidence of hypertension, independent of all other risk factors. Interestingly, measurements of urine albumin/creatinine (obtained on spot samples) were not associated with incident hypertension. Unlike the Framingham Heart Study and the Prevention of Renal and Vascular End Stage Disease (PREVEND) trial, when controlled for confounding factors, the MESA sample did not demonstrate a relationship between urinary albumin and incident hypertension. The findings are of interest because this large multiethnic dataset suggests that early changes in renal dysfunction may be associated with incident hypertension. While the "chicken and egg" story of renal disease and hypertension is extremely difficult to tease out, the findings suggest that, in patients without other markers of renal or cardiovascular disease, renal dysfunction may play a role in the pathogenesis of hypertension. Clinically, this is important, as it suggests that even subtle changes in glomerular filtration rate in the general population may define individuals at risk for hypertension and its subsequent sequelae. They also suggest that patients with reduced nephron number such as those who have undergone nephrectomy may be best monitored via cystatin C determinations. Interestingly, there was no synergistic interaction between the cystatin C level, the urinary albumin to creatinine ratio, and the risk for incident hypertension.

For further reading on this subject I suggest articles by Brantsma et al,[1] and Wang et al.[2]

R. Garrick, MD

References

1. Brantsma AH, Bakker SJ, de Zeeuw D, de Jong PE, Gansevoort RT. Urinary albumin excretion as a predictor of the development of hypertension in the general population. *J Am Soc Nephrol.* 2006;17:331-335.
2. Wang TJ, Evans JC, Meigs JB, et al. Low-grade albuminuria and the risks of hypertension and blood pressure progression. *Circulation.* 2005;111:1370-1376.

Polymorphisms in the non-muscle myosin heavy chain 9 gene (*MYH9*) are strongly associated with end-stage renal disease historically attributed to hypertension in African Americans

Freedman BI, Hicks PJ, Bostrom MA, et al (Wake Forest Univ School of Medicine, Winston-Salem, NC; et al)

Kidney Int 75:736-745, 2009

African Americans have high incidence rates of end-stage renal disease (ESRD) labeled as due to hypertension. As recent studies showed strong association with idiopathic and HIV-related focal segmental glomerulosclerosis and non-muscle myosin heavy chain 9 (*MYH9*) gene polymorphisms in this ethnic group, we tested for *MYH9* associations in a variety of kidney diseases. Fifteen *MYH9* single-nucleotide polymorphisms were evaluated in 175 African Americans with chronic glomerulonephritis-associated ESRD, 696 African Americans reportedly with hypertension-associated ESRD, and 948 control subjects without kidney disease. Significant associations were detected with 14 of the 15 polymorphisms in all 871 non-diabetic patients with ESRD. In hypertension-associated ESRD cases alone, significant associations were found with 13 *MYH9* polymorphisms and the previously reported E1 haplotype. Thus, hypertension-associated ESRD in African Americans is substantially related to *MYH9* gene polymorphisms and this may explain the poor response to blood pressure control in those diagnosed with hypertensive nephrosclerosis. It is possible that many African Americans classified as having hypertension-associated ESRD have occult *MYH9*-associated segmental or global glomerulosclerosis. Our study shows that gene–environment and/or gene–gene interactions may initiate kidney disease in genetically susceptible individuals, because African Americans homozygous for *MYH9* risk alleles do not universally develop kidney disease.

▶ Kidney disease, especially focal segmental glomerulosclerosis (FSGS), is common in African Americans, and, when diabetes is not present, the kidney disease is often attributed to FSGS or to so-called hypertensive nephrosclerosis. However, despite this commonly applied classification, the bioepidemiologic evidence to support the notion that mild to moderate hypertension is actually the underlying primary cause of progressive renal dysfunction is not robust.

Earlier studies[1-3] used admixture linkage disequilibrium to localize genes in admixed ethnic groups, a technique which serves to identify genomic regions with an unusually high contribution from one ancestral population. Studies also showed that genetic variants in nonmuscle myosin heavy chain (*MHY9*) were associated with FSGS in African Americans, and that this association was much more frequent than in European Americans.[1]

This article significantly extends these observations and provides exciting new information regarding the racial disparity seen in patients with nondiabetic kidney disease. The findings suggest that *MYH9* polymorphisms are strongly associated with dialysis dependent renal disease in African Americans. Moreover, the frequency of the *MHY9* gene polymorphism suggested that in many cases so-called hypertension-related renal disease in African Americans may actually be caused by *MYH9* associated focal sclerosis, with the kidney disease, in turn, leading to the development of hypertension.

The underlying mechanism for the kidney disease remains to be established, but it may be linked to the *MYH9* gene product nonmuscle myosin heavy chain type II isoform A. This protein is located on the glomerular podocyte foot process and moves actin filaments into the cell. Alterations on the actin cytoskeleton may disrupt podocyte function and results in alterations in filtration and kidney function. Not all individuals who are homozygote for the *MYH9* allele develop disease. Thus, factors other than *MHY9* gene polymorphism participate in the initiation of the disease process.

More will certainly follow on these exciting new findings.

J. Michaud, MD

References

1. Kopp JB, Smith MW, Nelson GW, et al. MYH9 is a major-effect risk gene for focal segmental glomerulosclerosis. *Nat Genetics*. 2008;40:1175-1184.
2. Kao WH, Klag MJ, Meoni LA, et al. MYH9 is associated with nondiabetic end-stage renal disease in African Americans. *Nat Genetics*. 2008;40:1185-1192.
3. Smith MW, Patterson N, Lautenberger JA, et al. A high-density admixture map for disease gene discovery in African Americans. *Am J Hum Genet*. 2004;74: 1001-1013.

Long-term Effects of Renin-Angiotensin System–Blocking Therapy and a Low Blood Pressure Goal on Progression of Hypertensive Chronic Kidney Disease in African Americans
Appel LJ, for the African American Study of Kidney Disease and Hypertension Collaborative Research Group (The Johns Hopkins insts, Baltimore; et al)
Arch Intern Med 168:832-839, 2008

Background.—Antihypertensive drugs that block the renin-angiotensin system (angiotensin-converting enzyme inhibitors [ACEIs] or angiotensin receptor blockers) are recommended for patients with chronic kidney disease (CKD). A low blood pressure (BP) goal (BP, <130/80 mm Hg) is also recommended. The objective of this study was to determine the long-term effects of currently recommended BP therapy in 1094 African Americans with hypertensive CKD.

Methods.—Multicenter cohort study following a randomized trial. Participants were 1094 African Americans with hypertensive renal disease (glomerular filtration rate, 20-65 mL/min/1.73 m^2). Following a 3 × 2-factorial trial (1995-2001) that tested 3 drugs used as initial antihypertensive therapy (ACEIs, calcium channel blockers, and β-blockers) and 2 levels of BP control (usual and low), we conducted a cohort study (2002-2007) in which participants were treated with ACEIs to a BP lower than 130/80 mm Hg. The outcome measures were a composite of doubling of the serum creatinine level, end-stage renal disease, or death.

Results.—During each year of the cohort study, the annual use of an ACEI or an angiotensin receptor blocker ranged from 83.7% to 89.0% (vs 38.5% to 49.8% during the trial). The mean BP in the cohort study was 133/78 mm Hg (vs 136/82 mm Hg in the trial). Overall, 567 participants experienced the primary outcome; the 10-year cumulative incidence rate was 53.9%. Of 576 participants with at least 7 years of follow-up, 33.5% experienced a slow decline in kidney function (mean annual decline in the estimated glomerular filtration rate, <1 mL/min/1.73 m^2).

Conclusion.—Despite the benefits of renin-angiotensin system–blocking therapy on CKD progression, most African Americans with hypertensive CKD who are treated with currently recommended BP therapy continue to progress during the long term.

▶ The African American Study of Kidney Disease and Hypertension (AASK) Trial concluded that ramipril was more efficacious than metoprolol and amlodipine in reducing the risk of renal endpoints of progression, end-stage renal disease (ESRD), and death in African-American patients with hypertensive renal disease and proteinuria. This study provided follow-up data to determine the long-term effects of renin-angiotensin system (RAS) blockade on progression of renal disease in African-American patients on angiotensin-converting enzyme (ACE) inhibitor or angiotensin receptor blocker (ARB) therapy. Patients were followed for up to 11.5 years. This study supported what is seen clinically in this patient population. Despite aggressive blood pressure control and optimal medical management, African-American patients have progression of chronic kidney disease at a more rapid rate than other patient populations. This study concluded that the 10-year incidence of a renal event (ie, doubling of serum creatinine, progression to ESRD, or death) was 53.9%. Only 33.5% of patients demonstrated a reduction to the targeted annual decline in the eGFR of less than 1 mL/min/1.73 m^2. These long-term follow-up data are troublesome because despite aggressive management of hypertension and proteinuria, renal disease progressed in a majority of patients. This information, along with the new insights provided by the MYH9 polymorphism studies (also reviewed here), suggest that the identification and treatment of African Americans at risk for renal disease and hypertension will require new strategies. Along these lines, if genetic material is available, it would be extremely interesting to evaluate MHY9 genetic polymorphism among the participants of the AASK trial.

J. Michaud, MD

Effect of Allopurinol on Blood Pressure of Adolescents With Newly Diagnosed Essential Hypertension: A Randomized Trial

Feig DI, Soletsky B, Johnson RJ (Baylor College of Medicine, Houston, TX; Univ of Florida School of Medicine, Gainesville)
JAMA 300:924-932, 2008

Context.—Hyperuricemia is a predictor for the development of hypertension and is commonly present in new-onset essential hypertension. Experimentally increasing uric acid levels using a uricase inhibitor causes systemic hypertension in animal models.

Objective.—To determine whether lowering uric acid lowers blood pressure (BP) in hyperuricemic adolescents with newly diagnosed hypertension.

Design, Setting, and Patients.—Randomized, double-blind, placebo-controlled, crossover trial (September 2004-March 2007) involving 30 adolescents (aged 11-17 years) who had newly diagnosed, never-treated stage 1 essential hypertension and serum uric acid levels≥6 mg/dL. Participants were treated at the Pediatric Hypertension Clinic at Texas Children's Hospital in Houston. Patients were excluded if they had stage 2 hypertension or known renal, cardiovascular, gastrointestinal tract, hepatic, or endocrine disease.

Intervention.—Allopurinol, 200 mg twice daily for 4 weeks, and placebo, twice daily for 4 weeks, with a 2-week washout period between treatments. The order of the treatments was randomized.

Main Outcome Measures.—Change in casual and ambulatory blood pressure.

Results.—For casual BP, the mean change in systolic BP for allopurinol was −6.9 mm Hg (95% confidence interval [CI], −4.5 to −9.3 mm Hg) vs −2.0 mm Hg (95% CI, 0.3 to −4.3 mm Hg; $P=.009$) for placebo, and the mean change in diastolic BP for allopurinol was −5.1 mm Hg (95% CI, −2.5 to −7.8 mm Hg) vs −2.4 (95% CI, 0.2 to −4.1; $P=.05$) for placebo. Mean change in mean 24-hour ambulatory systolic BP for allopurinol was −6.3 mm Hg (95% CI, −3.8 to −8.9 mm Hg) vs 0.8 mm Hg (95% CI, 3.4 to −2.9 mm Hg; $P=.001$) for placebo and mean 24-hour ambulatory diastolic BP for allopurinol was −4.6 mm Hg (−2.4 to −6.8 mm Hg) vs −0.3 mm Hg (95% CI, 2.3 to −2.1 mm Hg; $P=.004$) for placebo. Twenty of the 30 participants achieved normal BP by casual and ambulatory criteria while taking allopurinol vs 1 participant while taking placebo ($P<.001$).

Conclusions.—In this short-term, crossover study of adolescents with newly diagnosed hypertension, treatment with allopurinol resulted in reduction of BP. The results represent a new potential therapeutic approach, although not a fully developed therapeutic strategy due to potential adverse effects. These preliminary findings require confirmation in larger clinical trials.

Trial Registration.—clinicaltrials.gov Identifier: NCT00288184.

▶ Although hypertension is commonly associated with hyperuricemia, concomitant factors such as reduced renal function, the use of diuretics, oxidative stress, and alterations in insulin metabolism have made it difficult to establish causality. As such, none of the current guidelines routinely recognize hyperuricemia as a risk factor for hypertension. Several recent studies have demonstrated that hyperuricemia, even in the absence of the metabolic syndrome, can predict the development of hypertension.[1-3] Raising uric acid levels in animals has been demonstrated to induce both hypertension and renal microvascular disease and to increase renin levels. In clinical trials hyperuricemia has been associated with increased levels of renin and reduction of uric acid levels, via xanthine oxidase inhibition with allopurinol, and improves endothelial function.

Johnson and colleagues have previously reported that hyperuricemia is present in up to 90% of adolescents with essential hypertension.[3] This population represents an ideal study model because, unlike their adult counterparts, these children typically do not have multiple underlying comorbid conditions. In the current randomized, double blind, placebo-controlled, crossover trial, Johnson and colleagues demonstrated that allopurinol, as compared with placebo, reduced blood pressure, lowered renin levels, and lowered vascular resistance.

This study was designed as a study of causality, and as such it was very short term, and the results should not be interpreted to suggest that allopurinol is an appropriate therapeutic choice in this group or in others with hypertension. Rather, these extremely intriguing results raise fundamental questions regarding the potential pathogenic mechanisms of hypertension. Of note is that 73% (22/30) of the participants were overweight (≥ 90th percentile body mass index for sex and age), and 30% (9/30) met diagnostic criteria for metabolic syndrome. These results are especially interesting in view of the epidemic of childhood obesity.[4] Larger prospective studies performed in other populations that are designed to control for a possible direct, independent effect of xanthine oxidase itself, should be undertaken. In the mean time, clinicians should be aware of the presence and significance of hyperuricemia in adolescents.

M. Brogan, MD

References

1. Perlstein TS, Gumieniak O, Williams GH, et al. Uric acid and the development of hypertension: the normative aging study. *Hypertension.* 2006;48:1031-1036.
2. Krishnan E, Kwoh CK, Schumacher HR, Kuller L. Hyperuricemia and incidence of hypertension among men without metabolic syndrome. *Hypertension.* 2007;49: 298-303.
3. Feig DI, Johnson RJ. Hyperuricemia in childhood primary hypertension. *Hypertension.* 2003;42:247-252.
4. Johnson RJ, Rideout BA. Uric acid and diet–insights into the epidemic of cardiovascular disease. *N Engl J Med.* 2004;350:1071-1073.

Fructose-induced hypertension: essential role of chloride and fructose absorbing transporters PAT1 and Glut5

Singh AK, Amlal H, Haas PJ, et al (Hannover Med School, Germany; Univ of Cincinnati, OH; et al)
Kidney Int 74:438-447, 2008

Increased dietary fructose in rodents recapitulates many aspects of the Metabolic Syndrome with hypertension, insulin resistance and dyslipidemia. Here we show that fructose increased jejunal NaCl and water absorption which was significantly decreased in mice whose apical chloride/base exchanger Slc26a6 (PAT1, CFEX) was knocked out. Increased dietary fructose intake enhanced expression of this transporter as well as the fructose-absorbing transporter Slc2a5 (Glut5) in the small intestine of wild type mice. Fructose feeding decreased salt excretion by the kidney and resulted in hypertension, a response almost abolished in the knockout mice. In parallel studies, a chloride-free diet blocked fructose-induced hypertension in Sprague Dawley rats. Serum uric acid remained unchanged in animals on increased fructose intake with hypertension. We suggest that fructose-induced hypertension is likely caused by increased salt absorption by the intestine and kidney and the transporters Slc26a6 and Slc2a5 are essential in this process.

▶ Visceral obesity, hypertension, insulin resistance, glucose intolerance, and dyslipidemia are each components of the metabolic syndrome. It has been suggested that fructose intake, primarily as high-fructose corn syrup, has helped spur metabolic syndrome pandemic.[1-4] In addition, changes in urate metabolism induced by high-fructose diets, and related changes in nitric oxide metabolism, have been linked to many of the changes that accompany hypertension and the metabolic syndrome.[2-6]

I included the present study because it offers a unique look at a possible mechanism linking high-fructose intake with reduced urinary chloride excretion, salt overload, and hypertension. Using a knockout mouse model these investigators demonstrated that a high-fructose diet stimulated both the small intestine fructose absorbing transporter (glut 5/Slc2a5) and the small bowel and proximal renal tubule apical chloride transporter Slc26a6. The authors demonstrate that a high-fructose diet both increased intestinal chloride absorption and decreased renal chloride excretion, suggesting a possible pathogenic mechanism for the development of hypertension in the setting of an increased intake of fructose.

The present study did not demonstrate a link between hyperuricemia and hypertension, and the authors suggest that the hyperuricemia that has been associated with a high-fructose diet may be the result of secondary changes and renal function. However, other recent studies[7] have suggested that another well described fructose transporter (Glut 9) is capable of transporting urate, and can affect the serum urate level. Thus, this story is not yet fully told, but given the magnitude of the problem of the metabolic syndrome (especially among the young) it certainly warrants our attention.

R. Garrick, MD

References

1. Grundy SM. Metabolic syndrome: a multiplex cardiovascular risk factor. *J Clin Endocrinol Metab.* 2007;92:399-404.
2. Sinaiko A. Obesity, insulin resistance and the metabolic syndrome. *J Pediatr (Rio J).* 2007;83:3-4.
3. Wassink AM, Olijhoek JK, Visseren FL. The metabolic syndrome: metabolic changes with vascular consequences. *Eur J Clin Invest.* 2007;37:8-17.
4. Reusch JE. Current concepts in insulin resistance, type 2 diabetes mellitus, and the metabolic syndrome. *Am J Cardiol.* 2002;90:19G-26G.
5. Stuhlinger MC, Abbasi F, Chu JW, et al. Relationship between insulin resistance and an endogenous nitric oxide synthase inhibitor. *JAMA.* 2002;287:1420-1426.
6. Cirillo P, Sato W, Reungjui S, et al. Uric Acid, the metabolic syndrome, and renal disease. *J Am Soc Nephrol.* 2006;17:S165-S168.
7. Vitart V, Rudan I, Hayward C, et al. SLC2A9 is a newly identified urate transporter influencing serum urate concentration, urate excretion and gout. *Nat Genet.* 2008;40:437-442.

30 Diabetes

Introduction

Diabetes continues to be an area of intense investigation. New data regarding the use of aliskiren combined with losartan for type 2 diabetic nephropathy has been generated by the AVOID study. The data from this trial suggest that in patients with hypertension and type 2 diabetic nephropathy, aliskiren may have renal protective effects independent of its blood pressure lowering effects. Of note, the comparison groups were designed as losartan/placebo versus losartan/aliskiren, as the investigators believed that an add-on ACEi therapy design, (losartan/ACEi) would have inappropriately suggested that combination therapy (ARB /ACEi) is accepted as the routine "standard therapy" against which to judge.

Studies by Schneider evaluated the effect of pioglitazone on cardiovascular outcomes and diabetes in patients with chronic kidney disease (CKD). This is an important study because it demonstrates that patients with CKD and diabetes treated with pioglitazone were less likely to reach the composite end point of all-cause death, myocardial infarction, and stroke.

A worrisome study emerged from Anthony Bleyer and colleagues. They demonstrated that despite routine access to medical follow-up, the diabetic siblings of diabetics on dialysis have a high prevalence of albuminuria, poor glycemic control and inadequate blood pressure control. Even though practically 80% of these siblings had seen a physician 3 or more times in the last year, routine target goals were not generally being achieved. Given the fact that diabetic siblings of patients with kidney failure are 5 times more likely to develop kidney failure themselves, it is troubling that we are not achieving routine target goals in these high-risk populations.

Renee Garrick, MD

Aliskiren Combined with Losartan in Type 2 Diabetes and Nephropathy

Parving H-H, for the AVOID Study Investigators (Rigshospitalet, Copenhagen, Denmark; et al)

N Engl J Med 358:2433-2446, 2008

Background.—Diabetic nephropathy is the leading cause of end-stage renal disease in developed countries. We evaluated the renoprotective effects of dual blockade of the renin–angiotensin–aldosterone system by adding treatment with aliskiren, an oral direct renin inhibitor, to treatment with the maximal recommended dose of losartan (100 mg daily) and optimal antihypertensive therapy in patients who had hypertension and type 2 diabetes with nephropathy.

Methods.—We enrolled 599 patients in this multinational, randomized, double-blind study. After a 3-month, open-label, run-in period during which patients received 100 mg of losartan daily, patients were randomly assigned to receive 6 months of treatment with aliskiren (150 mg daily for 3 months, followed by an increase in dosage to 300 mg daily for another 3 months) or placebo, in addition to losartan. The primary outcome was a reduction in the ratio of albumin to creatinine, as measured in an early-morning urine sample, at 6 months.

Results.—The baseline characteristics of the two groups were similar. Treatment with 300 mg of aliskiren daily, as compared with placebo, reduced the mean urinary albumin-to-creatinine ratio by 20% (95% confidence interval, 9 to 30; $P < 0.001$), with a reduction of 50% or more in 24.7% of the patients who received aliskiren as compared with 12.5% of those who received placebo ($P < 0.001$). A small difference in blood pressure was seen between the treatment groups by the end of the study period (systolic, 2 mm Hg lower [$P = 0.07$] and diastolic, 1 mm Hg lower [$P = 0.08$] in the aliskiren group). The total numbers of adverse and serious adverse events were similar in the groups.

Conclusions.—Aliskiren may have renoprotective effects that are independent of its blood-pressure–lowering effect in patients with hypertension, type 2 diabetes, and nephropathy who are receiving the recommended renoprotective treatment. (ClinicalTrials.gov number, NCT00097955.)

▶ Blockade with the renin inhibitor Aliskiren has been shown to reduce both systolic and diastolic blood pressure both alone and in combination with angiotensin receptor blockers.[1] Studies using rat models of diabetic nephropathy have demonstrated that aliskiren can reduce albuminuria, interstitial fibrosis, and blood pressure, and may be more effective than angiotensin inhibition.[2] The present study by Parving and colleagues evaluated the effects of aliskiren on urinary protein spillage in hypertensive type II diabetics who had been receiving losartan and other antihypertensive agents. By using this design the investigators were poised to detect if aliskiren, as compared with placebo, was associated with a reduction in albuminuria independent of its antihypertensive effect.

At the conclusion of a 3-month open label run-in period during which patients received 100 mg of losartan daily, patients were randomized to receive either placebo for 6 months, or 3 months treatment with aliskiren at 150 mg daily followed by an additional 3 months treatment of aliskiren at 300 mg daily. At the conclusion of the 6-month period aliskiren therapy reduced the mean urinary albumin to creatinine ratio by 20%, with a reduction of more than 50% in almost 25% of the patients. Blood pressure control was not statistically different between the 2 groups, nor was the incidence of adverse outcomes or serious events.

These findings are interesting and may provide a novel treatment paradigm for diabetic renal disease. Unlike dual therapy with angiotensin-converting enzyme inhibitors (ACEi) and angiotensin receptor blockades (ARBs), treatment with aliskiren may reduce the number of prorenin receptors in the kidney, and thereby may mitigate the activity of profibrotic and apoptotic pathways.[2-4]

With regard to the safety of dual receptor blocker and aliskiren treatment, it is important to note that patients with a glomerular filtration rate (GFR) of < 30 mls/min or a potassium level of greater than 5.1 mEq/L were excluded from the study. Longer-term studies will be required to determine if such dual therapy will provide safe and sustained renoprotective effects.

R. Garrick, MD

References

1. Oparil S, Yarows SA, Patel S, Fang H, Zhang J, Satlin A. Efficacy and safety of combined use of aliskiren and valsartan in patients with hypertension: a randomised, double-blind trial. *Lancet.* 2007;370:221-229.
2. Kelly DJ, Zhang Y, Moe G, Naik G, Gilbert RE. Aliskiren a novel renin inhibitor, is renoprotective in a model of advanced diabetic nephropathy in rats. *Diabetologia.* 2007;50:2398-2404.
3. Feldman DL, Jin L, Xuan H, Miserindino-Molteni R. Effect of the direct rennin inhibitor (DRI) aliskiren on renal gene expression of pro-fibrotic molecules in experimental hypertensive diabetic nephropathy. *J Am Soc Nephrol.* 2007;18: 168A.
4. Nguyen G, Delarue F, Burckle C, Bouzhir L, Giller T, Sraer JD. Pivotal role of the renin/prorenin receptor in angiotensin II production and cellular responses to rennin. *J Clin Invest.* 2002;109:1417-1427.

Effect of Pioglitazone on Cardiovascular Outcome in Diabetes and Chronic Kidney Disease
Schneider CA, Ferrannini E, Defronzo R, et al (Univ of Cologne, Germany; Univ of Pisa, Italy; Univ of Texas Health Science Ctr, San Antonio; et al)
J Am Soc Nephrol 19:182-187, 2008

Patients with diabetes and chronic kidney disease (CKD) are at particularly high risk for cardiovascular disease (CVD). This *post hoc* analysis from the PROspective pioglitAzone Clinical Trial In macroVascular Events (PROactive) investigated the relationship between CKD and incident CVD in a population of patients with diabetes and documented macrovascular disease, as well as the effects of pioglitazone treatment on recurrent CVD. CKD, defined as an estimated GFR <60 ml/min per 1.73m², was present in 597 (11.6%) of 5154 patients. More patients with CKD reached the primary composite end point (all-cause mortality, myocardial infarction (MI), stroke, acute coronary syndrome, coronary/carotid arterial intervention, leg revascularization, or amputation above the ankle) than patients without CKD (27.5 versus 19.6%; $P < 0.0001$). Patients with CKD were also more likely to reach a secondary composite end point (all-cause mortality, MI, and stroke). Patients who had CKD and were treated with pioglitazone were less likely to reach the secondary end point (hazard ratio 0.66; 95% confidence interval 0.45 to 0.98), but this association was not observed among those with better renal function. In addition, there was a greater decline in estimated GFR with pioglitazone (between-group difference 0.8 ml/min per 1.73 m²/yr) than with placebo. In conclusion, CKD is an independent risk factor for cardiovascular events and death among patients with diabetes and preexisting macrovascular disease. Patients who had CKD and were treated with pioglitazone were less likely to reach a composite end point of all-cause death, MI, and stroke, independent of the severity of renal impairment.

▶ Studies involving the peroxisome proliferator-activated receptor gamma (PPARγ) activating thiazolidinedione, rosiglitazone raised questions regarding an increased risk of myocardial infarction and death possibly associated with the use of this agent.[1] The double-blind, randomized, placebo-controlled study PROactive was conducted in high-risk patients with diabetes and macrovascular disease. It investigated several combined vascular end-point effects of Pioglitazone, another PPARγ activating thiazolidinedione. This study demonstrated an approximately 10% (not statistically significant) reduction in the primary endpoint, and a 16% ($P < .027$) reduction in the secondary endpoints of nonfatal myocardial infarction, death, and stroke.[2] The risk reduction seen with Pioglitazone was associated with an increase in edema and nonfatal congestive heart failure, and as such, the possible cardiovascular class effects of these agents continue to be debated.

Treatment randomization in the PROactive trial was not stratified for chronic kidney disease (CKD). Schneider and colleagues retrospectively analyzed the effect of CKD (GFR < 60 ml/min) on the rates of the primary and principal secondary endpoints of the PROactive patients, and they evaluated the effects of Pioglitazone versus placebo on recurrent cardiovascular events in PROactive patients with CKD.

The results demonstrated that the presence of CKD (GFR less than 60 ml/min) was an independent risk factor for cardiovascular events and death among diabetics with macrovascular disease. The results also demonstrated a hazard ratio of 1.51 (95% confidence interval 1.28-1.78 $P < .0001$) for reaching a primary composite endpoint in patients with a GFR of <60 ml/min. Independent of the severity of renal function, diabetics with macrovascular disease with a GFR less than 60 ml/min who were treated with Pioglitazone were less likely to reach the secondary endpoint of all-cause mortality, MI, and stroke.

Multiple previous lines of investigation[3-6] have demonstrated an overlap between the metabolic risk factors believed to promote atherosclerosis in type II diabetes and those present in CKD. For example, abnormalities of risk factors such as oxidative stress, endothelial dysfunction, and dyslipidemia have been demonstrated in both CKD and diabetes.

This post hoc analysis of the PROactive trial by Schneider and colleagues must be carefully interpreted, as it is a retrospective analysis of a data set that included diabetics at high risk for macrovascular complications, and it was not initially stratified for the presence of CKD. Thus, it would be inappropriate to generalize their observation to the population of diabetics with kidney disease as a whole, but nonetheless, their analysis brings important new information regarding CKD and risk stratification to the debate. The exact influence of Pioglitazone on systemic mechanisms of inflammation and atherosclerotic risk, as well as any potentially direct effects it may have on renal function, will clearly require more direct study. This study may help clinicians choose among various therapeutic options as they seek to find the best strategies for risk reduction in high-risk patients with diabetes, CKD, and vascular complications.

R. Garrick, MD

References

1. Nissen SE, Wolski K. Effect of rosiglitazone on the risk of myocardial infarction and death from cardiovascular causes. *N Engl J Med.* 2007;356:2457-2471.
2. Dormandy JA, Charbonnel B, Eckland DJ, et al. Secondary prevention of macrovascular events in patients with type 2 diabetes in the PROactive Study (PROspective pioglitAzone Clinical Trial In macroVascular Events): a randomised controlled trial. *Lancet.* 2005;366:1279-1289.
3. Rahman M, Pressel S, Davis BR, et al. Cardiovascular outcomes in high-risk hypertensive patients stratified by baseline glomerular filtration rate. *Ann Intern Med.* 2006;144:172-180.
4. Berry C, Tardif JC, Bourassa MG. Coronary heart disease in patients with diabetes: parts I and II: recent advances in prevention, noninvasive management, and coronary revascularization. *J Am Coll Cardiol.* 2007;49:631-656.
5. Go AS, Chertow GM, Fan D, McCulloch CE, Hsu CY. Chronic kidney disease and the risks of death, cardiovascular events, and hospitalization. *N Engl J Med.* 2004; 351:1296-1305.
6. Knight EL, Rimm EB, Pai JK, et al. Kidney dysfunction, inflammation, and coronary events: a prospective study. *J Am Soc Nephrol.* 2004;15:1897-1903.

Risk Factors for Development and Progression of Diabetic Kidney Disease and Treatment Patterns Among Diabetic Siblings of Patients With Diabetic Kidney Disease
Bleyer AJ, Sedor JR, Freedman BI, et al (Wake Forest Univ School of Medicine, Winston Salem, NC; Case Western Reserve Univ School of Medicine, Cleveland, OH)
Am J Kidney Dis 51:29-37, 2008

Background.—Diabetic siblings of patients with treated kidney failure from diabetic kidney disease are at a 5-fold increased risk of future kidney failure. The objective of this study is to define risk factors for kidney disease, clinical features, and treatment patterns in diabetic siblings of patients with diabetes with diabetic kidney disease.

Study Design.—Cross-sectional analysis using data collected from diabetic siblings of patients with diabetic kidney disease.

Setting & Participants.—295 diabetic siblings with mean diabetes duration of 15 years from within a 400-mile radius of Cleveland, OH, or Winston-Salem, NC.

Predictors.—Demographic data, diabetes duration, blood pressure (BP), access to health care, and diabetes control.

Outcomes.—Albuminuria (defined as urinary albumin-creatinine ratio ≥ 30 mg/g, with microalbuminuria with albumin of 30 to 300 mg/g and macroalbuminuria with albumin > 300 mg/g), renal function.

Measurements.—BP, urinary albumin-creatinine ratio, serum creatinine, glycosylated hemoglobin (HbA$_{1c}$), estimated glomerular filtration rate.

Results.—Mean diabetes duration was 14.6 ± 10.6 years. Albuminuria was present in 46% of participants. In individuals with diabetes duration of 11 to 15 years, 25% had microalbuminuria and 18.2% had macroalbuminuria. Despite a positive family history and a high prevalence of albuminuria, only 35.3% of participants had a target systolic BP less than 130 mm Hg. HbA$_{1c}$ levels were 7% or greater in 57.4% of patients, and 26.4% of participants were smokers. Only 58% of patients received angiotensin-converting enzyme inhibitors or receptor blockers. In microalbuminuric participants, HbA$_{1c}$ level was greater than 10% in 28.6% versus 13.3% in those without albuminuria ($P = 0.02$).

Limitations.—A control group of diabetic siblings without a family history of diabetic kidney disease was not obtained.

Conclusions.—Diabetic siblings of patients with diabetic kidney disease have a high prevalence of albuminuria and poor glycemic and BP control. Targeting these high-risk individuals for interventions to improve their BP and blood glucose control might prevent or slow the progression of diabetic kidney disease.

▶ The National Institutes of Health (NIH) sponsored Family Investigation of Nephropathy and Diabetes (FIND) study was designed to identify genetic determinants of diabetic nephropathy.[1] This study evaluated the siblings of individuals with diabetes on dialysis. Approximately 64% of the siblings of diabetic dialysis patients identified in the geographic area under investigation agreed to participate. The sibling group was composed of 161 African-Americans, 118 of whom were female–the remainder of the sibling population was Caucasian. It has been well established across every ethnic group that the diabetic siblings of patients with end-stage renal disease are all at increased risk of progression to dialysis.[2] Access to care is clearly an important concern for this high-risk population, and the results demonstrate that approximately 80% of them had seen a physician 3 or more times in the last year, and the vast majority of them (89%) had health insurance.

However, despite access to care, almost 65% of the siblings had a systolic blood pressure greater than 130 mm Hg, 40% of patients were not on angiotensin-converting enzyme inhibitors (ACEi)/angiotensin receptor blocker (ARB) therapy, 40% of the population had a body mass index (BMI) greater than 35, almost 57% of the population had hemoglobin A_{1C} greater than 7%, and almost 25% of this high-risk sibling population were current smokers. Approximately 46% of the sibling group had either micro or macroalbuminuria (greater than 300 mg/day).

The study unfortunately demonstrates that, despite access to care, standard outcome targets are not being routinely achieved in this high-risk sibling population. The results should cause us to focus our efforts on how to better achieve these benchmarks, because by doing so we may ultimately achieve better long-term outcomes for these at-risk patients.

M. Klein, MD, JD

References

1. Knowler WC, Coresh J, Elston RC, et al. The Family Investigation of Nephropathy and Diabetes (FIND): design and methods. *J Diabetes Complications*. 2003;19: 1-9.
2. Quinn M, Angelico MC, Warram JH, Krolewski AS. Familial factors determine the development of diabetic nephropathy in patients with IDDM. *Diabetologia*. 1996;39:940-945.

31 Acute Kidney Injury

Introduction

Bevacizumab is now routinely used to treat a variety of malignancies that are characterized by pathologic angiogenesis. With expanding use, adverse renal effects of this agent have become apparent. Two of the most common are proteinuria and hypertension. Eremina and colleagues have studied these complications by creating an experimental mouse model that selectively targeted the VEGF gene of the glomerular podocyte, which is the major source of glomerular VEGF production. The mice developed hypertension and proteinuria and the biopsy samples demonstrated typical thrombotic microangiopathy. It will be important for clinicians to become familiar with the renal complications of bevacizumab as its clinical use increases.

Contrast induced nephropathy remains among the most common causes of iatrogenic acute kidney injury. An excellent meta-analysis by Kelly and colleagues reviews the current pharmacological manipulations that may help mitigate the risks of contrast administration. Unfortunately, there is no silver bullet. Hydration with saline or bicarbonate remains the therapeutic mainstay. N-acetylcysteine therapy may be beneficial, and while it is reasonably safe, its use should not lull the clinician into having a false sense of security because it does not provide definitive protection.

Postinfectious glomerulonephritis (GN) remains an important cause of acute kidney injury and the current selection provides an update for the "modern era." Several important findings have emerged: the majority of patients have comorbid conditions, especially diabetes; predisposing staphylococcal skin infections have become a more frequent cause of postinfectious GN; and abnormalities of the complement pathway are only detected approximately 70% of the time.

The final selection is important because it demonstrates that an episode of acute kidney injury in elderly individuals, especially those with underlying chronic kidney disease, significantly increases their risk for progression to end-stage renal disease. These findings highlight that there is really no such thing as an insignificant episode of acute renal failure, especially among the elderly.

Renee Garrick, MD

VEGF Inhibition and Renal Thrombotic Microangiopathy

Eremina V, Jefferson JA, Kowalewska J, et al (Univ of Toronto; Univ of Washington, Seattle; et al)
N Engl J Med 358:1129-1136, 2008

The glomerular microvasculature is particularly susceptible to injury in thrombotic microangiopathy, but the mechanisms by which this occurs are unclear. We report the cases of six patients who were treated with bevacizumab, a humanized monoclonal antibody against vascular endothelial growth factor (VEGF), in whom glomerular disease characteristic of thrombotic microangiopathy developed. To show that local reduction of VEGF within the kidney is sufficient to trigger the pathogenesis of thrombotic microangiopathy, we used conditional gene targeting to delete VEGF from renal podocytes in adult mice; this resulted in a profound thrombotic glomerular injury. These observations provide evidence that glomerular injury in patients who are treated with bevacizumab is probably due to direct targeting of VEGF by antiangiogenic therapy.

▶ The discovery that vascular endothelial growth factor (VEGF) is a critical factor in the growth of blood vessels led to the development of VEGF inhibitors, such as bevacizumab, which has been used to treat diseases that are characterized by pathologic angiogenesis, and such cancers as lung, pancreas, breast, liver, and kidney. With the expanding use of bevacizumab and other antiVEGF agents, adverse effects have become apparent. Two of the most common are proteinuria (in 21%-64%) and hypertension (in 3%-36%). This has raised the question as to whether the associated proteinuria is from the underlying disease process or to the inhibition of VGEF.

Quaggin and colleagues demonstrated in 6 cancer patients that following VEGF inhibition renal biopsy samples showed classic pathologic features of thrombotic microangiopathy, and the patients developed proteinuria and hypertension. The renal function, proteinuria, and blood pressure improved after the discontinuation of bevacizumab therapy, suggesting that these processes are transient and can be reversed.

To further explore the association they created an experimental mouse model that only targeted the VEGF gene in podocytes, which are the major source of glomerular VEGF production. The mice developed hypertension and proteinuria, and the renal biopsy samples demonstrated endothelial changes typical of thrombotic microangiopathy.

Of pathogenic interest is that the findings indicate that VEGF production by podocytes is required for health and maintenance of the adjacent glomerular endothelium. Of clinical interest is that the findings indicate that patients treated with VEGF inhibitors should be closely followed for the development of hypertension, proteinuria, and kidney injury.

For further reading on this subject I suggest articles by Zhu et al,[1] Advani et al,[2] and Gurevich et al.[3]

S. Mundra, MD

References

1. Zhu X, Wu S, Dahut WL, Parikh CR. Risks of proteinuria and hypertension with bevacizumab, an antibody against vascular endothelial growth factor: systematic review and meta-analysis. *Am J Kidney Dis.* 2007;49:186-193.
2. Advani A, Kelly DJ, Advani SL, et al. Role of VEGF in maintaining renal structure and function under normotensive and hypertensive conditions. *Proc Natl Acad Sci U S A.* 2007;104:14448-14453.
3. Gurevich F, Perazella MA. Renal effects of anti-angiogenesis therapy: update for the internist. *Am J Med.* 2009;122:322-328.

Meta-analysis: Effectiveness of Drugs for Preventing Contrast-Induced Nephropathy
Kelly AM, Dwamena B, Cronin P, et al (Univ of Michigan, Ann Arbor)
Ann Intern Med 148:284-294, 2008

Background.—N-Acetylcysteine, theophylline, and other agents have shown inconsistent results in reducing contrast-induced nephropathy.

Purpose.—To determine the effect of these agents on preventing nephropathy.

Data Sources.—Relevant randomized, controlled trials were identified by computerized searches in MEDLINE (from 1966 through 3 November 2006), EMBASE (1980 through November 2006), PubMed, Web of Knowledge (Current Contents Connect, Web of Science, BIOSIS Previews, and ISI Proceedings for the latest 5 years), and the Cochrane Library databases (up to November 2006). Databases were searched for studies in English, Spanish, French, Italian, and German.

Study Selection.—Randomized, controlled trials that administered N-acetylcysteine, theophylline, fenoldopam, dopamine, iloprost, statin, furosemide, or mannitol to a treatment group; used intravenous iodinated contrast; defined contrast-induced nephropathy explicitly; and reported sufficient data to construct a 2 × 2 table of the primary effect measure.

Data Extraction.—Abstracted information included patient characteristics, type of contrast media and dose, periprocedural hydration, definition of contrast-induced nephropathy, and prophylactic agent dose and route.

Data Synthesis.—In the 41 studies included, N-acetylcysteine (relative risk, 0.62 [95% CI, 0.44 to 0.88]) and theophylline (relative risk, 0.49 [CI, 0.23 to 1.06]) reduced the risk for contrast-induced nephropathy more than saline alone, whereas furosemide increased it (relative risk, 3.27 [CI, 1.48 to 7.26]). The remaining agents did not significantly affect risk. Significant subgroup heterogeneity was present only for N-acetylcysteine. No publication bias was discerned.

Limitations.—All trials evaluated the surrogate end point of contrastinduced nephropathy as the primary outcome. The lack of a statistically significant renoprotective effect of theophylline may result from insufficient data or study heterogeneity. True study quality remains uncertain.

Conclusion.—N-Acetylcysteine is more renoprotective than hydration alone. Theophylline may also reduce risk for contrast-induced nephropathy, although the detected association was not significant. Our data support the administration of N-acetylcysteine prophylaxis, particularly in high-risk patients, given its low cost, availability, and few side effects.

▶ Kelly and colleagues have provided a meta-analysis of 41 trials involving 6379 patients evaluating the effectiveness of drugs for the prevention of contrast-induced acute kidney injury. Contrast-related kidney injury is typically defined as a 0.5 mg increase in the baseline serum creatinine or a 25% rise in the serum creatinine level 48 hours after contrast exposure. Numerous prophylactic strategies have been studied to determine which, if any, are efficacious in mitigating the risks of renal injury in the setting of contrast exposure. The meta-analysis by Kelly demonstrates that, despite extensive study, the only agent that seems more protective than hydration alone is *N*-acetylcysteine. However, multiple differences in study design and enrollment criteria make definitive recommendations difficult, even for this agent. The meta-analysis supports the prophylactic administration of an acetylcysteine, particularly in high-risk patients such as those with underlying renal disease, congestive heart failure, advanced age, or a combination of diabetes in renal impairment. It should be noted that the strength of the data alone would not support cancellation of the procedure if N-acetylcysteine prophylaxis has not been completed. The recommended dose of acetylcysteine was not definitively established by this meta-analysis. However, other studies[1] have recommended that if *N*-acetylcysteine is to be used, the advised dose is 1200 mg twice daily for 24 hours pre and post-procedure. The authors also note that theophylline administration may prove efficacious, however, at the present time the available data do not support making its use standard practice. However, furosemide treatment increased the risk of contrast nephropathy. Hydration pre and postprocedure with saline or bicarbonate (150 mEq NaHCO3/1000 cc D5W) at 1 to 1.5 mL/kg/hour with a target urine output of 150 mL/hour remains the mainstay prophylactic treatment to mitigate the risk of contrast induced kidney injury.[1,2]

R. Garrick, MD

References

1. Goldfarb S, McCullough PA, McDermott J. Contrast-induced acute kidney injury: specialty-specific protocols for interventional radiology, diagnostic computer tomography, radiology and interventional cardiology. *Mayo Clin Proc.* 2009;84:170-179.
2. McCullough PA. Contrast induced acute kidney injury. *J Am Coll Cardiol.* 2008;51:1419-1428.

Acute Postinfectious Glomerulonephritis in the Modern Era: Experience With 86 Adults and Review of the Literature

Nasr SH, Markowitz GS, Stokes MB, et al (Columbia Univ, NY)
Medicine 87:21-32, 2008

Acute postinfectious glomerulonephritis (APIGN) is uncommon in adults, and its incidence is progressively declining in developed countries. To our knowledge there are no modern North American series addressing epidemiology and outcome. Here we report the clinical and pathologic findings in 86 cases of adult APIGN diagnosed by renal biopsy in a large New York referral center between 1995 and 2005. The male:female ratio was 2:1, and mean age was 56 years, with 33.7% aged older than 64 years. Of the patients, 38.4% had an immunocompromised background, including diabetes (29.1%), malignancy (4.7%), alcoholism (2.3%), acquired immunodeficiency syndrome (AIDS) (2.3%), and intravenous drug use (1.2%). The most common sites of infection were upper respiratory tract (23.3%), skin (17.4%), lung (17.4%), and heart/endocarditis (11.6%). The 2 most frequently identified infectious agents were streptococcus (27.9%) and staphylococcus (24.4%). Hypocomplementemia was present in 73.9% of patients. The most common histologic patterns were diffuse (72.1%), focal (12.8%), and mesangial (8.1%) proliferative glomerulonephritis.

Outcome analysis was performed on the 52 patients with a follow-up of ≥3 months (mean, 25 mo). Among the 41 patients without underlying diabetic glomerulosclerosis, 23 (56.1%) achieved complete remission, 11 (26.8%) had persistent renal dysfunction, and 7 (17.1%) progressed to end-stage renal disease (ESRD). Of the 11 patients with underlying diabetic glomerulosclerosis, 2 (18.2%) had persistent renal dysfunction, and the remaining 9 (81.8%) progressed to ESRD (p<0.001). In patients without underlying diabetic glomerulosclerosis, correlates of complete remission were younger age, female sex, lower serum creatinine at biopsy, and absence of immunocompromised state. By multivariate analysis, age and serum creatinine at biopsy inversely correlated with complete remission, and serum creatinine at biopsy was the only correlate with ESRD. Outcome did not correlate with any pathologic feature (including crescents) or steroid treatment.

Diabetes and aging have emerged as major risk factors for adult APIGN. Full recovery of renal function can be expected in just over half of patients, and prognosis is dismal in those with underlying diabetic glomerulosclerosis.

▶ The incidence of postinfectious glomerulonephritis (GN) has declined considerably over the last 50 years. This study is the largest single modern era report of this important clinical entity. The cases reported here have all been substantiated by renal biopsy. Clinicians should be aware of several important clinical findings regarding the presentation and prognosis of postinfectious GN in the modern era. Previously, most patients had no predisposing comorbid conditions.[1-3] However, in this study almost 30% of the patients had underlying diabetes. The 4 most common sites of infection were upper respiratory, skin, lung (pneumonia), and heart/endocarditis. The infectious agent was identified approximately 60% of the time by culture, or in the case of streptococcal disease by titer change (antistreptolysin O, and anti-DNAaseB antibody). Cases attributable to staphylococcal skin infections have increased in frequency, and two-thirds of the staphylococcal skin infections occurred in diabetics. The latent period between infection and GN range from 4 weeks after upper respiratory infection to 2 weeks after endocarditis. Of significance is that between 7% to 15% of patients had no evidence of infection before the development of renal disease. Complement levels were available in 58 of 86 patients, and C3 or C4 levels were reduced 67.2% of the time. Unlike the optimistic outcome in childhood postinfectious GN, the prognosis in adults is more guarded. Twenty-five percent of adults had persistent renal abnormalities, and nearly 18% eventually went on to dialysis. The prognosis in diabetics is even worse, almost 80% of diabetics with postinfectious GN developed end-stage renal disease. The findings demonstrate that in the modern era postinfectious GN should be included in the differential diagnosis of acute nephritis. Normal serum complements, and the absence of a definitive antecedent infection, especially in the presence of underlying diabetes, do not definitively eliminate the possibility of postinfectious nephritis, and a renal biopsy should be considered.

M. Brogan, MD

References

1. Kushner DS, Armstrong SH, Dubin A, et al. Acute glomerulonephritis in the adult. Longitudinal, clinical, functional and morphologic studies of rates of healing and progression to chronicity. *Medicine (Baltimore)*. 1961;40:203-240.
2. Lien JWK, Mathew TH, Meadows R. Acute poststreptococcal glomerulonephritis in adults: a long-term study. *Q J Med*. 1979;48:99-111.
3. McCluskey RT, Baldwin DS. Natural history of acute glomerulonephritis. *Am J Med*. 1963;35:213-230.

Acute Kidney Injury Increases Risk of ESRD among Elderly

Ishani A, Xue JL, Himmelfarb J, et al (Univ of Minnesota Med School, Minneapolis; Maine Med Ctr, Portland; et al)
J Am Soc Nephrol 20:223-228, 2009

Risk for ESRD among elderly patients with acute kidney injury (AKI) has not been studied in a large, representative sample. This study aimed to determine incidence rates and hazard ratios for developing ESRD in elderly individuals, with and without chronic kidney disease (CKD), who had AKI. In the 2000 5% random sample of Medicare beneficiaries, clinical conditions were identified using Medicare claims; ESRD treatment information was obtained from ESRD registration during 2 yr of follow-up. Our cohort of 233,803 patients were hospitalized in 2000, were aged ≥67 yr on discharge, did not have previous ESRD or AKI, and were

Medicare-entitled for ≥2 yr before discharge. In this cohort, 3.1% survived to discharge with a diagnosis of AKI, and 5.3 per 1000 developed ESRD. Among patients who received treatment for ESRD, 25.2% had a previous history of AKI. After adjustment for age, gender, race, diabetes, and hypertension, the hazard ratio for developing ESRD was 41.2 (95% confidence interval [CI] 34.6 to 49.1) for patients with AKI and CKD relative to those without kidney disease, 13.0 (95% CI 10.6 to 16.0) for patients with AKI and without previous CKD, and 8.4 (95% CI 7.4 to 9.6) for patients with CKD and without AKI. In summary, elderly individuals with AKI, particularly those with previously diagnosed CKD, are at significantly increased risk for ESRD, suggesting that episodes of AKI may accelerate progression of renal disease.

▶ This study is worth our attention because it is the first large sample study aimed at determining the likelihood that an episode of acute kidney injury (AKI) in the elderly will result in the development of dialysis dependent renal failure. Previous studies and studies from single institutions have suggested that between 8% and 10% of patients with AKI will require long-term dialysis.[1] Other studies have suggested that AKI following myocardial infarction is associated with a higher risk of mortality.[2] The current cohort is drawn from a representative sample of 233 800 medicare beneficiaries over the age of 67 who were hospitalized in 2000. In this elderly cohort the incidence of AKI was 3.1%, and baseline chronic kidney disease was present in approximately 12%. Among patients with underlying chronic kidney disease (CKD) an episode of AKI was associated with the development of end-stage renal disease (ESRD) in approximately 10 patients/100. After adjustment for age, gender, race, diabetes, and hypertension, the hazard ratio for developing ESRD after an episode of AKI was 13% in patients without pre-existing kidney disease as compared with 41% for those with a previous history of kidney disease. The results demonstrate that an episode of AKI in patients with underlying CKD is ominous. Patients with CKD who suffered an episode of AKI were 54% more likely to develop dialysis-dependent renal disease than were patients with CKD alone.

The study has limitations because it is a retrospective analysis of the Medicare inpatient claims database and, therefore, the diagnostic accuracy of the severity of the chronic and AKI is dependent upon the accuracy of the coding parameters applied at the time of hospitalization. It is possible that the severity of the underlying CKD may not have been fully appreciated and, therefore, the impact of an episode of AKI on the ultimate occurrence of ESRD would be overestimated. However, even with this limitation in mind, the results indicate that elderly patients with and without underlying CKD who have had an episode of AKI require close follow-up. The data suggest that if an episode of AKI occurs, strategies aimed at controlling the progression of renal injury, such as antiproteinuric and antihypertensive therapy, may be particularly important in this at-risk group.

R. Garrick, MD

References

1. Metcalfe W, Simpson M, Khan IH, et al. On behalf of the Scottish Renal Registry. Acute renal failure requiring renal replacement therapy: incidence and outcome. *Q J Med.* 2002;95:579-583.
2. Parikh CR, Coca SG, Wang Y, Masoudi FA, Krumholz HM. Long-term prognosis of acute kidney injury after acute myocardial infarction. *Arch Intern Med.* 2008; 168:987-995.

32 Chronic Renal Failure and Transplantation

Introduction

Data continue to emerge regarding the cardiovascular burden engendered by the presence of renal disease. The database study of van Domburg and colleagues demonstrates that renal impairment is associated with a graded and independent decrease in the survival of patients with known or suspected coronary artery disease. On a brighter note, the data from Chonchol and colleagues demonstrated that beta-blockade can effectively reduce the incidence of cardiovascular end points in high-risk patients with underlying coronary heart disease regardless of the presence of renal dysfunction. These data suggest that even in patients with renal disease that beta-blockers are cardio-protective and are an effective part of the cardiovascular armamentarium. Reminiscent of the earlier data regarding the siblings of diabetics, data from the Jackson Heart Study demonstrates that despite a high prevalence of chronic kidney disease only a minority of the patients are aware of their diagnosis. These data are troubling as a lack of patient awareness limits the possibilities for early education and intervention. Clearly this is problematic since for therapy to be most effective it must be instituted during the early stages of kidney disease, well before dialysis is needed.

With regard to identified risk factors, the long-term follow-up of data presented by Viske provides strong evidence that preeclampsia is an important risk factor for the development of kidney disease and these women require long-term renal surveillance. Finally, an algorithm containing commonly understood variables has been developed to help clinicians stratify middle-aged and older individuals at high risk for the development of future kidney disease. This algorithm is simple to use and should help clinicians prioritize patients with regard to timing of intervention and education.

Polycystic disease is the most common inherited form of kidney disease. Vasopressin antagonists are in the final stages of clinical study, and the initial finding that they can slow the progression of PKD remains promising. On the experimental side new data have emerged demonstrating that the cystic fibrosis transmembrane conductance regulator can dramatically inhibit cyst number and growth in in vivo and in vitro models of PKD.

The next group of articles deals with the special risk factors faced by patients with chronic renal impairment. Tamura and colleagues have clearly demonstrated that renal disease is associated with cognitive impairment. The accompanying studies focus on preventable medication errors and issues of patient safety both of which have been found to be negatively influenced by the presence of kidney disease. The findings are startling and it is critical that clinicians and patients become educated regarding the special risks posed by kidney disease and that steps be taken to mitigate them. To be successful, these endeavors will require additional resources for intervention and education.

The next 3 selections focus on the area of venous thromboembolism and atrial fibrillation. Data from the LITE trial suggest that kidney disease is a newly identified risk factor for venous thromboembolism. This finding is clinically quite important, and clinicians should likely include renal function when assessing DVT risks and planning prophylactic regimens. Atrial fibrillation is one of the most common arrhythmias in patients with kidney disease and often goes untreated. The next selections focus on the risk-benefit of this decision and the articles by Aronow and Reinecke provide a framework and clinically applicable algorithm for the appropriate management of atrial fibrillation in the setting of advanced kidney disease.

Data continue to emerge regarding the role of phosphorus as an independent risk factor for mortality in patients with chronic kidney disease. The selections by Shoben focus on new information regarding vitamin D balance in patients with chronic kidney disease. The study is important because the findings suggest that oral calcitriol may be one of the few therapeutic manipulations that can potentially alter mortality in this at-risk population. These observational data set the stage for prospective randomized trials. Other new information this year focuses on the role of fibroblast growth factor 23 (FGF23) and mortality among patients undergoing dialysis. This new biomarker may prove to be a clinically important tool to help guide treatment strategies for the management of phosphorus in patients with chronic kidney disease. This may be especially important, given the relationship between abnormal phosphate balance and cardiovascular mortality in patients with chronic kidney disease.

The final selections focus on transplantation outcomes and management. The data by Arichi continue to draw our attention to the need for long-term ongoing cancer surveillance after renal transplantation. This surveillance should be lifelong and should focus on both cutaneous and solid organ malignancies. The data by Ibrahim are very assuring. This long-term donor follow-up study demonstrates that the risk of renal disease in carefully screened donors appears to be similar to that of the general population. The majority of donors have a preserve glomerular filtration rate and normal albumin excretion patterns during long-term post-donation follow-up.

Renee Garrick, MD

Renal Insufficiency and Mortality in Patients with Known or Suspected Coronary Artery Disease

van Domburg RT, Hoeks SE, Welten GMJM, et al (Erasmus Med Ctr, Rotterdam, Netherlands; et al)

J Am Soc Nephrol 19:158-163, 2008

It remains unclear whether mild renal dysfunction is associated with adverse cardiovascular outcome. We investigated whether estimated glomerular filtration rate (eGFR) was associated with mortality and cardiac death among 6447 patients with known or suspected coronary artery disease over a mean follow-up of 7 yr. Cumulative 5- and 10-yr survival rates decreased in a graded fashion from 88% and 70%, respectively, for those with normal renal function to 43% and 33% for those with eGFR <30 ml/min. Compared with patients with normal renal function, the multivariable adjusted hazard ratios for all-cause mortality among patients with mild, moderate, and severe renal impairment were 1.33 (95% confidence interval [CI], 1.21–1.48), 1.67 (95% CI, 1.44–1.93), and 3.38 (95% CI, 2.73–4.19), respectively. Similar relationships between cardiac death and decreasing renal function were found. In conclusion, renal function is a graded and independent predictor of long-term mortality in patients with known or suspected coronary artery disease. Intense treatment and close surveillance of these patients is encouraged.

▶ Using a database of almost 6500 patients, van Domburg and colleagues investigated the relationship between a glomerular filtration rate (GFR), mortality, and cardiac death in patients with known or suspected coronary artery disease (CAD). Using a multivariable adjusted hazard ratio the investigators demonstrated that mild, moderate, and severe renal impairment are associated with a graded and independent decrease in survival in patients with known or suspected CAD (Fig 1 in the original article). Thus, the findings suggest that renal function is an independent predictor of long-term mortality. The findings are similar to those of Wen et al,[1] who evaluated over 460 000 Taiwanese adults who have participated in a medical screening program since 1994. The mean follow-up time was 7.5 years. The risk of death was increased by approximately 80% for individuals with underlying chronic kidney disease (CKD), and the risk of cardiovascular mortality was increased almost 2-fold. In addition to cardiovascular death, studies by Nakayama and colleagues[2] have demonstrated that the presence of CKD (creatinine clearance less than 40 mL/min) results in approximately a 3-fold increased risk for a first symptomatic cerebral vascular accident. The vascular burden in patients with both CKD and dialysis dependent renal disease is substantial. These results are clinically relevant as they help define the need for early intervention. Taken together it seems likely that appropriate interventions (blood pressure control, lipid, weight, and glucose control) during the early stages of CKD are more likely to have a beneficial effect on long-term mortality data than are late-stage interventions.

R. Garrick, MD

References

1. Wen CP, Chang TY, Tsai MK, et al. All cause mortality attributable to chronic kidney disease: a prospective cohort study on 462,293 adults in Taiwan. *Lancet.* 2008;371:2173-2182.
2. Nakayama M, Metoki H, Terawaki H, et al. Kidney dysfunction as a risk factor for first symptomatic stroke events in the general Japanese population: the Ohasama study. *Nephrol Dialysis Transplant.* 2007;22:1910-1915.

Beta-blockers for coronary heart disease in chronic kidney disease
Chonchol M, Benderly M, Goldbourt U (Univ of Colorado Health Sciences Ctr, Denver; Sheba Med Ctr, Israel; et al)
Nephrol Dial Transplant 23:2274-2279, 2008

Background.—Limited data exist on whether the cardioprotective benefit of β-blockers is modified by the presence of chronic kidney disease (CKD).

Methods.—A *post hoc* analysis of the data from the Bezafibrate Infarction Prevention (BIP) study was performed. CKD was defined according to the Modification of Diet in Renal Disease (MDRD) equation as an estimated glomerular filtration rate (GFR)<60 mL/min/1.73 m². The Cox proportional hazard model, including adjustment for propensity score, was used to estimate the hazard ratios (HR) for the composite endpoint combining acute myocardial infarction (AMI) or sudden cardiac death (SCD).

Results.—In this cohort of 3075 coronary heart disease (CHD) patients, 568 (18.5%) had CKD and 1185 (38.5%) were treated with β-blockers. A total of 245 (43.1%) CKD patients received β-blockers at baseline. The mean (± SD) estimated GFR in the CKD and non-CKD subgroups was 55 (±4) and 73 (±9) mL/min/1.73 m², respectively. After a median follow-up of 6.2 years, the crude incidence rates of AMI or SCD/1000 person years (PY) were 25.6, 21.9, 34.6 and 27.5 for the β-blockers−/CKD−, β-blockers+/CKD−, β-blockers−/CKD+ and β-blockers+/CKD+ groups, respectively. Compared to patients with β-blockers−/CKD−, the adjusted HR of AMI or SCD was 0.87 (90% CI 0.71–1.06) for the β-blockers+/CKD−, 1.35 (90% CI 1.05–1.73) for the β-blockers−/CKD+ and 1.06 (90% CI 0.76–1.46) for the β-blockers+/CKD+.

Conclusions.—These analyses suggest that the use of β-blockers is associated with a reduction in event risk in patients with CHD regardless of the presence or absence of CKD.

▶ This post hoc analysis of the Bezafibrate Infarction Prevention (BIP) study stratified participants according to their underlying renal function as defined by the estimated glomerular filtration rate (eGFR) using the Modification of Diet in Renal Disease (MDRD) equation. Of the more than 3000 participants with coronary heart disease, almost 570 had chronic kidney disease (CKD). After a median follow-up of about 6 years, the use of beta-blockers resulted in reduced risk of myocardial infarction or sudden death, and this protective effect was not diminished by the presence of CKD. It is now well documented that patients on dialysis have a high cardiovascular burden and that CKD is associated with a high risk of cardiovascular death. In observational and small randomized trials, beta-blockers have been shown to offer survival benefits in patients on hemodialysis.[1,2] Although the study has limitations because it is a post hoc analysis, the BIP study itself was a placebo controlled secondary prevention trial of lipid control among patients with coronary disease. This retrospective analysis supports the concept that beta-blockers can effectively reduce the incidence of cardiovascular end points in high-risk patients with underlying coronary heart disease regardless of the presence of renal dysfunction. This is an important and clinically relevant observation, especially because so few interventions have been shown to actually improve outcomes in patients with underlying (predialysis) CKD. The potential survival advantage offered by beta-blockers in this at-risk CKD population should be considered when medication regimens are being devised.

R. Garrick, MD

References

1. Foley RN, Herzog CA, Collins AJ. Blood pressure and long-term mortality in United States hemodialysis patients: USRDS waves 3and 4 study. *Kidney Int.* 2002;62:1784-1790.
2. Cice G, Ferrara L, D'Andrea A, et al. Carvedilol increases two-year survival in dialysis patients with dilated cardiomyopathy: a prospective, placebo-controlled trial. *J Am Coll Cardiol.* 2003;41:1438-1444.

Prevalence and Awareness of CKD Among African Americans: The Jackson Heart Study

Flessner MF, Wyatt SB, Akylbekova EL, et al (Univ of Mississippi Med Ctr; et al)
Am J Kidney Dis 53:238-247, 2009

Background.—Chronic kidney disease (CKD) leads to end-stage renal disease and is a growing epidemic throughout the world. In the United States, African Americans have an incidence of end-stage renal disease 4 times that of whites.

Study Design.—Cross-sectional to examine the prevalence and awareness of CKD in African Americans.

Setting & Participants.—Observational cohort in the Jackson Heart Study (JHS).

Predictor.—CKD was defined as an estimated glomerular filtration rate less than $60 \text{ mL/min}/1.73 \text{ m}^2$, the presence of albuminuria, or dialysis therapy.

Outcomes & Measurements.—Data from the JHS were analyzed. Medical history, including disease awareness and drug therapy, anthropometric measurements, and serum and urine samples, were obtained from

JHS participants at the baseline visit. Associations between CKD prevalence and awareness and selected demographic, socioeconomic, health care access, and disease status parameters were assessed by using logistic regression models.

Results.—The prevalence of CKD in the JHS was 20%; CKD awareness was only 15.8%. Older participants had a greater prevalence, but also were more aware of CKD. Hypertension, diabetes, cardiovascular disease, hypercholesterolemia, hypertriglyceridemia, increasing age and waist circumference, and being single or less physically active were associated with CKD. Only advancing CKD stage was associated with awareness.

Limitations.—Cross-sectional assessment, single urine measurement.

Conclusions.—The JHS has a high prevalence and low awareness of CKD, especially in those with less severe disease status. This emphasizes the need for earlier diagnosis and increased education of health care providers and the general population.

▶ In patients with chronic kidney disease (CKD), prevention of complications and delay of progression depend on faithful adherence to a treatment program involving aggressive risk factor modification. Such compliance is impossible if patients are unaware of the nature and extent of their renal disease. This cross-sectional cohort study of African-American adults enrolled in the Jackson Heart Study examined the prevalence and awareness of renal disease in the study population. The study demonstrated similar prevalence of CKD as that noted in the National Health and Nutrition Examination Survey (NHANES) data. Not surprisingly, there was a strong correlation between traditional vascular risk factors and the presence of CKD. However, the awareness of CKD was much lower in African-American patients in younger age brackets and at earlier stages of disease as compared with their awareness of diabetes and hypertension. This was surprising because nearly 86% had health insurance and saw their primary provider within 1 year. This finding highlights the fact that, for various reasons, many African-American patients in this representative cohort seem to lack awareness of their disease, especially in the earlier stages when interventions might be most effective. The findings are interesting because they demonstrate that the main obstacle to adequate prevention is proper education. Because aggressive interventions are needed to minimize the extensive morbidity associated with CKD, specifically hypertension, vascular disease, and the requirement for renal replacement therapy, a new emphasis on education may contribute to improved outcomes.

M. Klein, MD, JD

Preeclampsia and the Risk of End-Stage Renal Disease

Vikse BE, Irgens LM, Leivestad T, et al (Univ of Bergen, Norway; Rikshospitalet, Oslo; et al)

N Engl J Med 359:800-809, 2008

Background.—It is unknown whether preeclampsia is a risk marker for subsequent end-stage renal disease (ESRD).

Methods.—We linked data from the Medical Birth Registry of Norway, which contains data on all births in Norway since 1967, with data from the Norwegian Renal Registry, which contains data on all patients receiving a diagnosis of end-stage renal disease (ESRD) since 1980, to assess the association between preeclampsia in one or more pregnancies and the subsequent development of ESRD. The study population consisted of women who had had a first singleton birth between 1967 and 1991; we included data from up to three pregnancies.

Results.—ESRD developed in 477 of 570,433 women a mean (±SD) of 17 ± 9 years after the first pregnancy (overall rate, 3.7 per 100,000 women per year). Among women who had been pregnant one or more times, preeclampsia during the first pregnancy was associated with a relative risk of ESRD of 4.7 (95% confidence interval [CI], 3.6 to 6.1). Among women who had been pregnant two or more times, preeclampsia during the first pregnancy was associated with a relative risk of ESRD of 3.2 (95% CI, 2.2 to 4.9), preeclampsia during the second pregnancy with a relative risk of 6.7 (95% CI, 4.3 to 10.6), and preeclampsia during both pregnancies with a relative risk of 6.4 (95% CI, 3.0 to 13.5). Among women who had been pregnant three or more times, preeclampsia during one pregnancy was associated with a relative risk of ESRD of 6.3 (95% CI, 4.1 to 9.9), and preeclampsia during two or three pregnancies was associated with a relative risk of 15.5 (95% CI, 7.8 to 30.8). Having a low-birth-weight or preterm infant increased the relative risk of ESRD. The results were similar after adjustment for possible confounders and after exclusion of women who had kidney disease, rheumatic disease, essential hypertension, or diabetes mellitus before pregnancy.

Conclusions.—Although the absolute risk of ESRD in women who have had preeclampsia is low, preeclampsia is a marker for an increased risk of subsequent ESRD.

▶ The ultimate renal effects of preeclampsia have remained elusive. The present study evaluated the long-term (17 ± 9 years followup) incidence of dialysis-dependent renal disease among over 570 000 women with preeclampsia. The overall rate of end-stage renal disease (ESRD) in women with previous preeclampsia was 3.7 per 100 000 women per year. The risk of ESRD varied depending on the number of pregnancies and the number of pregnancies associated with preeclampsia. In women who had more than 3 pregnancies, 1 episode of preeclampsia was associated with a relative risk of ESRD of 6.3, whereas 2 or more episodes of preeclampsia increased the relative risk of ESRD to 15.5. Interestingly, having a low birth weight or a preterm infant was also a risk marker for ESRD, even among women who did not develop clinical preeclampsia. These findings are noteworthy given the possible pathophysiological relationship between intrauterine growth retardation and preeclampsia,[1] and suggest that evidence of placental dysfunction, even in the absence of clinically apparent preeclampsia, may be a marker of future risk.

The results were similar after exclusion of women who had underlying kidney disease and/or other risk factors before pregnancy, and were not affected by possible birth-related confounders such as maternal age at delivery. A weakness of the study is that outcome data were not available on all patients before 1980, and this was addressed by statistical methodology. In addition, the study does not allow evaluation of whether the preeclampsia itself "caused" the renal disease or rather exacerbated some unknown renal-risk factor. The results are nonetheless both interesting and clinically important. Clearly the results suggest that women who have had pregnancies complicated by preeclampsia are at risk for later renal disease and deserve long-term renal surveillance. Renal function, blood pressure, and the presence of microalbuminuria should be serially monitored in this at-risk population. Meanwhile, the fascinating links between endothelial dysfunction, angiogenesis, preeclampsia, and long-term renal outcome deserve further exploration.

R. Garrick, MD

Reference

1. Vikse BE, Irgens LM, Bostad L, Iversen BM. Adverse perinatal outcome and later kidney biopsy in the mother. *J Am Soc Nephrol.* 2006;17:837-845.

A Simple Algorithm to Predict Incident Kidney Disease
Kshirsagar AV, Bang H, Bomback AS, et al (Univ of North Carolina at Chapel Hill; Weill Med College of Cornell Univ, NY)
Arch Intern Med 168:2466-2473, 2008

Background.—Despite the growing burden of chronic kidney disease (CKD), there are no algorithms (to our knowledge) to quantify the effect of concurrent risk factors on the development of incident disease.

Methods.—A combined cohort (N = 14 155) of 2 community-based studies, the Atherosclerosis Risk in Communities Study and the Cardiovascular Health Study, was formed among men and women 45 years or older with an estimated glomerular filtration rate (GFR) exceeding 60 mL/min/1.73 m² at baseline. The primary outcome was the development of a GFR less than 60 mL/min/1.73 m² during a follow-up period of up to 9 years. Three prediction algorithms derived from the development data set were evaluated in the validation data set.

Results.—The 3 prediction algorithms were continuous and categorical best-fitting models with 10 predictors and a simplified categorical model with 8 predictors. All showed discrimination with area under the receiver operating characteristic curve in a range of 0.69 to 0.70. In the simplified

TABLE 2.—Multivariate Models for Chronic Kidney Disease in the Development Data Set Using Categorical Variables[a]

Covariate	β Coefficient (SE)	Odds Ratio (95% Confidence Interval)	P Value	Assigned Score
	Best-Fitting Categorical Model[b]			
Age, y				
50-59	0.60 (0.12)	1.8 (1.4-2.3)	<.001	1
60-69	1.31 (0.12)	3.7 (2.9-4.7)	<.001	2
≥70	1.46 (0.14)	4.3 (3.3-5.6)	<.001	3
White race/ethnicity[c]	0.41 (0.09)	1.5 (1.3-1.8)	<.001	1
Female sex	0.23 (0.07)	1.3 (1.1-1.5)	.001	1
Anemia	0.58 (0.20)	1.8 (1.2-2.7)	.004	1
Hypertension	0.61 (0.07)	1.8 (1.6-2.1)	<.001	1
Diabetes mellitus	0.32 (0.10)	1.4 (1.1-1.7)	.001	1
History of cardiovascular disease	0.25 (0.10)	1.3 (1.0-1.5)	.03	1
History of heart failure[d]	0.51 (0.25)	1.7 (1.0-2.7)	.04	1
Low high-density lipoprotein cholesterol level[e]	0.28 (0.08)	1.3 (1.1-1.6)	<.001	1
Peripheral vascular disease (circulation problem in legs)	0.42 (0.13)	1.5 (1.2-2.0)	.001	1
	Simplified Categorical Model[f]			
Age, y				
50-59	0.63 (0.12)	1.9 (1.5-2.4)	<.001	1
60-69	1.33 (0.12)	3.8 (3.0-4.8)	<.001	2
≥70	1.46 (0.14)	4.3 (3.3-5.6)	<.001	3
Female sex	0.13 (0.07)	1.1 (1.0-1.3)	.05	1
Anemia	0.48 (0.20)	1.6 (1.1-2.4)	.02	1
Hypertension	0.55 (0.07)	1.7 (1.5-2.0)	<.001	1
Diabetes mellitus	0.33 (0.10)	1.4 (1.2-1.7)	<.001	1
History of cardiovascular disease	0.26 (0.10)	1.3 (1.1-1.6)	.009	1
History of heart failure[d]	0.50 (0.25)	1.6 (1.0-2.7)	.04	1
Peripheral vascular disease (circulation problem in legs)	0.41 (0.13)	1.5 (1.2-1.9)	.002	1

[a]The total sample comprised 9470 subjects. The development data set was formed with two-thirds randomly selected from the Atherosclerosis Risk in Communities Study and with two-thirds randomly selected from the Cardiovascular Health Study.

[b]Area under the receiver operating characteristic curve, 0.70; Akaike information criterion, 6262; and Bayesian information criterion, 6355. Smaller Akaike and Bayesian information criteria indicate a better model fit.

[c]In the Cardiovascular Health Study, white subjects (on average) had a longer follow-up period than black subjects.

[d]Because status for only the past 2 weeks was ascertained, decreased power is expected.

[e]High-density lipoprotein cholesterol level of 40 mg/dL or less (to convert cholesterol level to millimoles per liter, multiply by 0.0259).

[f]Area under the receiver operating characteristic curve, 0.69; Akaike information criterion, 6295; and Bayesian information criterion, 6374.

(Reprinted from Kshirsagar AV, Bang H, Bomback AS et al. A simple algorithm to predict incident kidney disease. *Arch Intern Med.* 2008;168:2466-2473. Copyright 2008, American Medical Association. All rights reserved.)

model, age, anemia, female sex, hypertension, diabetes mellitus, peripheral vascular disease, and history of congestive heart failure or cardiovascular disease were associated with the development of a GFR less than 60 mL/min/1.73 m². A numeric score of at least 3 using the simplified algorithm captured approximately 70% of incident cases (sensitivity) and accurately predicted a 17% risk of developing CKD (positive predictive value).

Conclusions.—An algorithm containing commonly understood variables helps to stratify middle-aged and older individuals at high risk for future CKD. The model can be used to guide population-level prevention

TABLE 3.—Diagnostic Characteristics of the Screening Rules in the Validation Data Set[a]

Screening Rule	Identified, %[b]	Sensitivity	Specificity	Positive Predictive Value	Negative Predictive Value
Probability of chronic kidney disease categorical[c]					
≥0.17	20	42	83	24	92
≥0.13	30	60	70	20	93
≥0.12	40	68	62	19	94
≥0.09	50	75	53	17	94
Total score (best-fitting) categorical[d]					
≥6	10	25	93	29	91
≥5	24	49	80	23	92
≥4	46	71	57	17	94
≥3	74	91	28	14	96
Total score simplified categorical[e]					
≥5	8	20	93	28	90
≥4	23	45	80	22	92
≥3	45	69	58	17	94
≥2	73	89	29	14	96

[a]The total sample comprised 4624 subjects. The validation data set was formed with the remaining one-third from the Atherosclerosis Risk in Communities Study and with the remaining one-third from the Cardiovascular Health Study.
[b]Percentage of participants who met the condition specified in the first column.
[c]Estimated probability from logistic regression model. Area under the receiver operating characteristic curve, 0.70; Akaike information criterion, 3002; and Bayesian information criterion, 3015.
[d]Area under the receiver operating characteristic curve, 0.70; Akaike information criterion, 3013; and Bayesian information criterion, 3026.
[e]Area under the receiver operating characteristic curve, 0.68; Akaike information criterion, 3053; and Bayesian information criterion, 3066.

(Reprinted from Kshirsagar AV, Bang H, Bomback AS et al. A simple algorithm to predict incident kidney disease. *Arch Intern Med.* 2008;168:2466-2473. Copyright 2008, American Medical Association. All rights reserved.)

efforts and to initiate discussions between practitioners and patients about risk for kidney disease (Tables 2 and 3).

▶ Using 2 nonconcurrent cohorts, the Atherosclerosis Risk in Communities (ARIC) and the Cardiovascular Health Study (CHS), August and colleagues have developed and validated a mathematical algorithm with which to predict the likelihood that an individual patient with identified risk factors will develop clinically significant kidney disease (defined as a glomerular filtration rate [GFR] of less than 60 mL/min/1.73 m^2) over the ensuing 9 years. As shown in Tables 2 and 3, the investigators developed 2 models. The simplified model uses 9 commonly available clinical characteristics. In this model, a numeric score of at least 3 properly predicts approximately 70% of the incident cases of renal disease, and accurately predicts a 17% risk of developing chronic kidney disease (CKD). The best-fit model uses 10 clinical variables, including race/ethnicity and high-density lipoprotein (HDL)-cholesterol. Using this model, the investigators were able to predict incident renal disease with a sensitivity of 93%, and accurately predicted a 29% risk of developing CKD.

The investigators point out that because the data were drawn from population studies, certain clinical characteristics that are known to be risk factors for kidney disease, such as hematuria, microalbuminuria, proteinuria, and family history are not included in the algorithm. Going forward, additional factors may be included that might change the predictive model.

Even with these caveats in mind, this algorithm has great clinical potential. This first-of-its-kind algorithm incorporates a variety of concomitant risk factors and can serve as a guideline to allow clinicians to stratify a middle-age patient's individual risk of developing kidney disease. In addition, this tool may help identify patients at greatest risk and most risk and thereby foster appropriate clinical intervention and education.

R. Garrick, MD

Small-Molecule CFTR Inhibitors Slow Cyst Growth in Polycystic Kidney Disease
Yang B, Sonawane ND, Zhao D, et al (Univ of California, San Francisco; et al)
J Am Soc Nephrol 19:1300-1310, 2008

Cyst expansion in polycystic kidney disease (PKD) involves progressive fluid accumulation, which is believed to require chloride transport by the cystic fibrosis transmembrane conductance regulator (CFTR) protein. Herein is reported that small-molecule CFTR inhibitors of the thiazolidinone and glycine hydrazide classes slow cyst expansion in *in vitro* and *in vivo* models of PKD. More than 30 CFTR inhibitor analogs were screened in an MDCK cell model, and near-complete suppression of cyst growth was found by tetrazolo-$CFTR_{inh}$-172, a tetrazolo-derived thiazolidinone, and Ph-GlyH-101, a phenyl-derived glycine hydrazide, without an effect on cell proliferation. These compounds also inhibited cyst number and growth by >80% in an embryonic kidney cyst model involving 4-d organ culture of embryonic day 13.5 mouse kidneys in 8-Br-cAMP–containing medium. Subcutaneous delivery of tetrazolo-$CFTR_{inh}$-172 and Ph-GlyH-101 to neonatal, kidney-specific PKD1 knockout mice produced stable, therapeutic inhibitor concentrations of >3 μM in urine and kidney tissue. Treatment of mice for up to 7 d remarkably slowed kidney enlargement and cyst expansion and preserved renal function. These results implicate CFTR in renal cyst growth and suggest that CFTR inhibitors may hold therapeutic potential to reduce cyst growth in PKD.

▶ Polycystic kidney disease (PCKD) is the most common inherited renal disorder leading to end-stage renal disease. Autosomal dominant PCKD is caused by mutation in 1 of 2 genes that code for the proteins polycystin and polycystin 2. The cyst growth in PCKD is accompanied by fluid secretion into the lumen of the cyst and hyperplasia of the surrounding epithelial cells. Recent breakthroughs in genetics and transport physiology have demonstrated that the cystic fibrosis transmembrane conductance regulator (CFTR) protein, a cyclic AMP regulated chloride channel, may be important for regulating chloride entry into the renal cysts. Verkman and colleagues have previously shown that inhibition of CFTR can slow cyst growth in a cell culture model of PCKD.[1] The present study demonstrates in both in vivo and in vitro models of PCKD that various thiazolidinone and glycine hydrazide agents remarkably slowed cyst and renal enlargement, and preserved renal function. These are the same agents that have been suggested to be efficacious in the treatment of chloride secretory diarrhea.[2] This exciting discovery deserves our attention, and additional translational research may demonstrate a possible new therapeutic approach for patients of PCKD.

R. Garrick, MD

References

1. Ma T, Thiagarajah JR, Yang H, et al. Thiazolidinone CFTR inhibitor identified by high throughput screening blocks cholera toxin-induced intestinal fluid secretion. *J Clin Invest.* 2002;110:1651-1658.
2. Sonawane ND, Verkman AS. Thiazolidinone CFTR inhibitors with improved water solubility identified by structure–activity analysis. *Bioorg Med Chem.* 2008;16:8187-8195.

Vasopressin Directly Regulates Cyst Growth in Polycystic Kidney Disease
Wang X, Wu Y, Ward CJ, et al (Mayo Clinic College of Medicine, Rochester, MN)
J Am Soc Nephrol 19:102-108, 2008

The polycystic kidney diseases (PKD) are a group of genetic disorders causing renal failure and death from infancy to adulthood. Arginine vasopressin (AVP) V2 receptor antagonists inhibit cystogenesis in animal models of cystic kidney diseases, presumably by downregulating cAMP signaling, cell proliferation, and chloride-driven fluid secretion. For confirmation that the protective effect of these drugs is due to antagonism of AVP, PCK ($Pkhd1^{-/-}$) and Brattleboro ($AVP^{-/-}$) rats were crossed to generate rats with PKD and varying amounts of AVP. At 10 and 20 weeks of age, PCK $AVP^{-/-}$ rats had lower renal cAMP and almost complete inhibition of cystogenesis compared with PCK $AVP^{+/+}$ and PCK $AVP^{+/-}$ rats. The V2 receptor agonist 1-deamino-8-D-arginine vasopressin increased renal cAMP and recovered the full cystic phenotype of PCK $AVP^{-/-}$ rats and aggravated the cystic disease of PCK $AVP^{+/+}$ rats but did not induce cystic changes in wild-type rats. These observations indicate that AVP is a powerful modulator of cystogenesis and provide further support for clinical trials of V2 receptor antagonists in PKD.

▶ Autosomal dominant polycystic kidney disease (ADPKD) is the most common of the inherited cystic renal diseases. While a variety of genetic mutations have been described (mis-sense, frameshift, deletion, etc) in the vast majority of cases, ADPKD is caused by mutations in either of 2 distinct genes that encode polycystic[1] (ADPKD1; chromosome 16) and polycystic[2] (ADPKD 2; chromosome 4). Although the exact cause of cyst growth has not been fully elucidated, the downstream signaling pathways of the proteins encoded for by polycystin 1 and polycystin 2 represent possible therapeutic targets for ADPKD.[1,2] Along these lines, it has long been suggested that via the V2 receptor arginine vasopressin antagonists can reduce cyst formation and growth by down-regulating cAMP signaling.[3,4] This study is the first study to definitively demonstrate a direct relationship between vasopressin V2 signaling and cyst growth.

In these elegant studies, the authors bred Brattleboro rats, which completely lack vasopressin to rats with polycystic disease to produce rats with varying amounts of vasopressin and polycystic kidney diseases (PKD). At 10 and 20 weeks of age PKD rats with no vasopressin had lower levels of cAMP, and almost no cyst growth as compared with PKD rats with vasopressin. The administration of the V2 receptor agonist 1-deamino-8-D-arginine vasopressin (dDAVP) increased renal cAMP and aggravated cyst formation in the PKD rats but not the wild-type controls.

This study represents an important breakthrough in our understanding of cyst growth. The results are especially exciting in view of the ongoing stage III human trials, which are using the vasopressin antagonist tolvaptan to reduce cyst growth in patients with ADPKD.

R. Garrick, MD

References

1. Grantham JJ. Lillian Jean Kaplan International Prize for advancement in the understanding of polycystic kidney disease. Understanding polycystic kidney disease: a systems biology approach. *Kidney Int.* 2003;64:1157-1162.
2. Grantham JJ. Clinical practice. autosomal dominant polycystic kidney disease. *N Engl J Med.* 2008;359:1477.
3. Torres VE, Harris PC. Mechanisms of disease: Autosomal dominant and recessive polycystic kidney diseases. *Nat Clin Pract Nephrol.* 2006;2:40-54.
4. Gattone VH, Wang X, Harris PC, Torres VE. Inhibition of renal cystic disease development and progression by a vasopressin V2 receptor antagonist. *Nat Med.* 2003;9:1323-1326.

Kidney Function and Cognitive Impairment in US Adults: The Reasons for Geographic and Racial Differences in Stroke (REGARDS) Study
Kurella Tamura M, Wadley V, Yaffe K, et al (Univ of California San Francisco; Univ of Alabama at Birmingham; et al)
Am J Kidney Dis 52:227-234, 2008

Background.—The association between kidney function and cognitive impairment has not been assessed in a national sample with a wide spectrum of kidney disease severity.

Study Design.—Cross-sectional.

Setting & Participants.—23,405 participants (mean age, 64.9 ± 9.6 years) with baseline measurements of creatinine and cognitive function participating in the REasons for Geographic And Racial Differences in Stroke (REGARDS) Study, a study of stroke risk factors in a large national sample.

Predictor.—Estimated glomerular filtration rate (eGFR).

Outcome.—Cognitive impairment.

Measurements.—Chronic kidney disease (CKD) was defined as eGFR less than 60 mL/min/1.73 m^2. Kidney function was analyzed in 10-mL/min/1.73 m^2 increments in those with CKD, and in exploratory analyses, across the range of kidney function. Cognitive function was assessed using the 6-Item Screener, and participants with a score of 4 or less were considered to have cognitive impairment.

Results.—CKD was associated with an increased prevalence of cognitive impairment independent of confounding factors (odds ratio, 1.23; 95% confidence interval, 1.06 to 1.43). In patients with CKD, each 10-mL/min/1.73 m^2 decrease in eGFR less than 60 mL/min/1.73 m^2 was associated with an 11% increased prevalence of impairment (odds ratio, 1.11; 95% confidence interval, 1.04 to 1.19). Exploratory analyses showed a nonlinear association between eGFR and prevalence of cognitive impairment, with a significant increased prevalence of impairment in those with eGFR less than 50 and 100 mL/min/1.73 m^2 or greater.

Limitations.—Longitudinal measures of cognitive function were not available.

Conclusions.—In US adults, lower levels of kidney function are associated with an increased prevalence of cognitive impairment. The prevalence of impairment appears to increase early in the course of kidney disease; therefore, screening for impairment should be considered in all adults with CKD.

▶ Previous studies have suggested that cognitive impairment accompanies renal disease. While the findings have been most marked in patients on dialysis, evidence of cognitive dysfunction has been noted in patients with moderate degrees of renal impairment.[1-3] The Reasons for Geographic and Racial Differences in Stroke (REGARDS) study was a large cross-sectional national nationwide study that involved patients with a wide variety of underlying kidney disease of varying degrees of severity; 23 405 disciplines were evaluated using a 6-item test of global cognitive function. The large sample size allowed investigators to evaluate the association between cognitive impairment and renal disease across a wide spectrum of kidney function, as defined by the Modification of Diet in Renal Disease (MDRD) equation.

The patients with chronic kidney disease tended to be older and had a greater prevalence of concomitant vascular disease, left ventricular dysfunction, and hypertension. However independent of these comorbidities, chronic kidney disease itself was associated with impaired cognition. Alterations in cognitive function were present in patients with an estimated glomerular filtration rate (eGFR) of less than 50 mL/min/ 1.73m^2, and became more profound as renal disease progressed. Impaired cognition was about 60% more likely in patients with an eGFR of 20 to 29 mL/min/1.73m^2 as compared with patients with a GFR of over 80 mL/min/1.73 m^2. Although the reasons for the cognitive impairment and longitudinal measurements of cognitive function are not available from this study, the results are clinically important. The fact that cognitive dysfunction can be detected with relatively mild degrees of renal impairment is especially important. These patients often have concomitant comorbidities such as diabetes and cardiac disease, which necessitate the routine use of complex medication and dietary regimens. Practitioners, family members, and pharmacists must be aware of these potential cognitive issues in order for these regimens to be safely and effectively administered.

R. Garrick, MD

References

1. Murray AM, Pederson SL, Tupper DE. Variation in cognitive functioning hemodialysis patients: a cohort study with repeated measures. *Am J Kidney Dis.* 2007;50:270-278.
2. Kurella M, Yaffe K, Shlipak MG, et al. Chronic kidney disease and cognitive impairment in menopausal women. *Am J Kidney Dis.* 2005;45:66-76.
3. Seliger SL, Siscovick DS, Stehman-Breen CO, et al. Moderate renal impairment and risk of dementia among older adults: the cardiovascular health cognition study. *J Am Soc Nephrol.* 2004;15:1904-1911.

Frequency of and Risk Factors for Preventable Medication-Related Hospital Admissions in the Netherlands

Leendertse AJ, for the HARM Study Group (Utrecht Univ, the Netherlands; et al)
Arch Intern Med 168:1890-1896, 2008

Background.—Medication-related problems that lead to hospitalization have been the subject of many studies, many of which were limited to 1 hospital or lacked patient follow-up. Furthermore, little information exists on potential risk factors associated with preventable medication-related hospitalizations.

Methods.—A prospective multicenter study was conducted to determine the frequency and patient outcomes of medication-related hospital admissions. A case-control design was used to determine risk factors for potentially preventable admissions. All unplanned admissions in 21 hospitals were assessed during 40 days. Controls were patients admitted for elective surgery. Cases and controls were followed up until hospital discharge. The frequency of medication-related hospital admissions, potential preventability, and outcomes were assessed. For potentially preventable medication-related admissions, risk factors were identified in the case-control study.

Results.—Almost 13 000 unplanned admissions were screened, of which 714 (5.6%) were medication related. Almost half (46.5%) of these admissions were potentially preventable, resulting in 332 case patients matched with 332 controls. Outcomes were favorable in most patients. The main determinants of preventable medication-related hospital admissions were impaired cognition (odds ratio, 11.9; 95% confidence interval, 3.9-36.3), 4 or more comorbidities (8.1; 3.1-21.7), dependent living situation

(3.0; 1.4-6.5), impaired renal function (2.6; 1.6-4.2), nonadherence to medication regimen (2.3; 1.4-3.8), and polypharmacy (2.7; 1.6-4.4).

Conclusions.—Adverse drug events are an important cause of hospitalizations, and almost half are potentially preventable. The identified risk factors provide a starting point for preventing medication-related hospital admissions.

▶ Multiple lines of investigation from the Institute of Medicine, The Joint Commission, and other quality improvement organizations have demonstrated that medication errors represent one of the most common causes of hospital readmission and that often these errors were preventable. The Observational Hospital Admissions Related to Medication (HARM) study was conducted between 2005 and 2006 in the Netherlands. The findings indicated that about 6% of the 13 000 unplanned readmissions were related to medication issues. Of great importance was the finding that impaired renal function per se was an important risk factor for medication-related unplanned readmission (odds ratio=2.6). Impaired cognition, the number of different prescribers, and the numbers of medications used represented additional risk factors. This constellation of risks is especially worrisome for patients with underlying renal disease as this population typically consumes more than 10 medications, is known to have abnormalities of cognition (see article by Kurella also reviewed here), and typically receives medication for multiple prescribers. In this study among the risk factors identified, polypharmacy (defined as ≥ 5 drugs) was the most important risk factor, and this mediation number is exceeded by almost every patient with renal disease.

One limitation of the study is that the case-control design may have resulted in control patients who may have been less ill than the study group. However, the strengths of the HARM trial are the prospective multicenter design, with careful follow-up and a focus on well-defined risk factors. Overall, it is quite clear that it is imperative that the patient and the involved practitioners each be aware of all of the medications used, their dosages, and the intended length of the prescription. It is especially important that practitioners understand the need to use extra caution in patients with renal disease where cognitive impairment may also be present.

R. Garrick, MD

Chronic Kidney Disease Adversely Influences Patient Safety
Seliger SL, Zhan M, Hsu VD, et al (Univ of Maryland School of Medicine, Baltimore; Univ of Maryland School of Pharmacy, Baltimore, MD)
J Am Soc Nephrol 19:2414-2419, 2008

Reducing medical errors and improving patient safety have become a national priority. Patients with chronic kidney disease (CKD) may be at higher risk for adverse consequences of medical care, but few studies have evaluated this question. Here, data for patients hospitalized in the

TABLE 2.—Rates of PSI among Hospitalized Patients with and without CKD[a]

PSI	PSI Description	No. of Events	Rate in CKD[b]	Rate in Non-CKD[b]	aIRR (95% CI)[c]	P
	Complications of surgical care					
1	Complications of anesthesia	58	0.12	0.08	1.60 (1.07 to 2.37)	0.020
8	Postoperative hip fracture	17	0.11	0.02	4.89 (2.79 to 8.57)	<0.001
9	Postoperative hemorrhage or hematoma	170	0.30	0.26	0.96 (0.72 to 1.29)	0.800
10	Postoperative physiological/ metabolic derangement	239	0.96	0.20	4.00 (3.18 to 5.02)	<0.001
11	Postoperative respiratory failure	1086	4.01	1.97	1.37 (1.19 to 1.57)	<0.001
12	Postoperative PE or DVT	645	1.23	0.96	1.04 (0.88 to 1.22)	0.700
13	Postoperative sepsis	407	2.47	1.33	1.39 (1.14 to 1.71)	0.001
14	Postoperative wound dehiscence	80	0.90	0.59	1.12 (0.74 to 1.70)	0.600
	Complications of any acute hospitalization					
2	Death in low-mortality DRG	107	0.47	0.18	1.53 (1.14 to 2.05)	0.005
3	Decubitus ulcer	1176	1.64	1.20	0.95 (0.84 to 1.08)	0.500
4	Failure to rescue	1491	11.0	11.2	0.95 (0.85 to 1.05)	0.300
7	Infection as a result of medical care	359	0.34	0.16	2.33 (1.92 to 2.82)	<0.001

[a]DRG, diagnosis-related group; DVT, deep vein thrombosis; PE, pulmonary embolism.
[b]Events per 100 hospitalizations.
[c]Adjusted for age, gender, race, diabetes, CVD, and cancer.
(Reprinted from Seliger SL, Zhan M, Van Hsu D, et al. Chronic kidney disease adversely influences patient safety. *J Am Soc Nephrol.* 2008;19:2414-2419.)

Veteran's Health Administration during 2004 to 2005 was analyzed to conduct a cross-sectional study of CKD and adverse safety events. Outcomes included 13 patient safety indicators (PSI) defined by the Agency for Healthcare Research and Quality and six experimental PSI relevant to CKD. The 71,666 (29%) hospitalized veterans with CKD had a higher risk for several PSI, even after case-mix adjustment. Among surgical hospitalizations, CKD was associated with increased risk for hip fracture, physiologic/metabolic derangements, and complications of anesthesia. Among all acute hospitalizations, the PSI with the highest risk in patients with CKD were infection as a result of medical care and death among those in diagnosis-related groups normally associated with low mortality. Furthermore, as preadmission estimated GFR decreased, a significant trend of increasing risk for all PSI was observed ($P = 0.001$). In conclusion, hospitalized patients with CKD are at increased risk for adverse safety events, measured by established PSI. Further investigation is needed to develop and test interventions to reduce this risk (Tables 2 and 3).

▶ These data are drawn from patients hospitalized in the Veterans Administration (VA) system during 2004-2005. They demonstrate that approximately 29% of hospitalized veterans had chronic kidney disease (CKD) and that when compared with all acute hospitalizations, patient safety indicators suggest

TABLE 3.—Rates of Additional PSI among Hospitalized Patients with and without CKD[a]

PSI	No. of Events	Rate in CKD[b]	Rate in Non-CKD[b]	aIRR (95% CI)[c]	P
Technical difficulty with procedure	1535	0.51	0.66	0.91 (0.80 to 1.03)	0.100
Physiological derangement, medical and surgical admissions	29,628	15.70	10.80	1.36 (1.30 to 1.41)	<0.001
Aspiration pneumonia	376	0.77	0.57	0.91 (0.74 to 1.11)	0.400
CABG after PTCA	32	0.69	0.64	0.83 (0.45 to 1.50)	0.500
Postoperative in-hospital MI	665	2.14	0.83	1.18 (1.05 to 1.34)	0.007
Postoperative cardiogenic iatrogenic complications	1505	3.31	2.10	1.11 (0.99 to 1.25)	0.060

[a]CABG, coronary artery bypass grafting; PTCA, percutaneous coronary angioplasty; MI, myocardial infarction.
[b]Events per 100 hospitalizations.
[c]Adjusted for age, gender, race, diabetes, CVD, and cancer.
(Reprinted from Seliger SL, Zhan M, Van Hsu D, et al. Chronic kidney disease adversely influences patient safety. *J Am Soc Nephrol.* 2008;19:2414-2419.)

that patients with CKD are at increased risk for adverse safety events. These data are startling. They demonstrate, for the first time, that when patients with CKD are admitted to the hospital they are more likely to have an adverse outcome due to a lapse of patient safety than are other patients. Many of the adverse events noted were cardiovascular in nature, and it is uncertain whether this excess risk was related to adverse consequence of health care, or to something unique and specific about underlying cardiovascular disease in the setting of CKD. However, patients with CKD had other adverse outcomes as well, such as hip fractures and complications of anesthesia.

Clearly, patients with CKD present a complex physiology in the setting of complex underlying medical problems. Typically, one might anticipate that this would cause health care providers to be even more vigilant when caring for this at-risk population. However, the data suggest that CKD patients are at high risk for potentially avoidable adverse clinical outcomes. Given the magnitude of these findings (Tables 2 and 3) and the rising incidence of CKD in the general population, the data from the VA system should be extended and the risk on the general population better defined. In addition, steps should be taken to educate caregivers about the unique needs of patients with CKD.

R. Garrick, MD

Chronic Kidney Disease Increases Risk for Venous Thromboembolism
Wattanakit K, Cushman M, Stehman-Breen C, et al (Univ of Minnesota, Minneapolis; Univ of Vermont, Burlington; Amgen, Thousand Oaks, CA; et al)
J Am Soc Nephrol 19:135-140, 2008

Chronic kidney disease (CKD) is associated with increased risk for cardiovascular disease morbidity and mortality, but its association with incident venous thromboembolism (VTE) in non–dialysis-dependent patients has not been evaluated in a community-based population. With the use of data from the Longitudinal Investigation of Thromboembolism Etiology (LITE) study, 19,073 middle-aged and elderly adults were categorized on the basis of estimated GFR, and cystatin C (available in 4734 participants) was divided into quintiles. During a mean follow-up time of 11.8 yr, 413 participants developed VTE. Compared with participants with normal kidney function, relative risk for VTE was 1.28 (95% confidence interval [CI] 1.02 to 1.59) for those with mildly decreased kidney function and 2.09 (95% CI 1.47 to 2.96) for those with stage 3/4 CKD, when adjusted for age, gender, race, and center. After additional adjustment for cardiovascular disease risk factors, an increased risk for VTE was still observed in participants with stage 3/4 CKD, with a multivariable adjusted relative risk of 1.71 (95% CI 1.18 to 2.49). There was no significant association between cystatin C and VTE. In conclusion, middle-aged and elderly patients with CKD (stages 3 through 4) are at increased risk for incident VTE, suggesting that VTE prophylaxis may be particularly important in this population.

▶ Using the Longitudinal Investigation of Thromboembolism Etiology (LITE) study the authors have demonstrated over a mean follow-up time of almost 12 years that patients with chronic kidney disease (CKD) have risk of incidence venous thromboembolism. Regression analysis suggests that the risk of venous embolism begins to increase when the estimated glomerular filtration rate (eGFR) is as high as 75 mL/min/1.73m^2. Patients with this stage 3 and 4 CKD (eGFR 15-59 mL/min/1.73 m^2) had an almost 2-fold increased risk for venous thromboembolism compared with those with normal renal function. This appears to be a newly identified association that has potential clinical importance. Currently, The American College of Chest Physicians guidelines[1] do not include CKD as a risk factor, and many clinicians are reluctant to use prophylactic anticoagulation in this population. Further studies will be required to determine whether or not a "threshold GFR" exists for the initiation of routine prophylaxis for venous thromboembolism during hospitalization. In the meantime, the findings suggest that clinicians must approach patients with CKD with a heightened awareness for the risk of venous thromboembolism.

R. Garrick, MD

Reference

1. Geerts WH, Pineo GF, Heit JA, et al. Prevention of venous thromboembolism: the seventh ACCP conference on antithrombotic and thrombolytic therapy. *Chest.* 2004;126:338S-400S.

Dilemmas in the Management of Atrial Fibrillation in Chronic Kidney Disease

Reinecke H, Brand E, Mesters R, et al (Univ Hosp of Muenster, Germany; et al)
J Am Soc Nephrol 20:705-711, 2009

Patients with chronic kidney disease (CKD) have an increased risk for cardiovascular morbidity and mortality. Little attention has been paid to the problem of atrial fibrillation, although this arrhythmia is very frequent with a prevalence of 13 to 27% in patients on long-term hemodialysis. Because of the large number of pathophysiologic mechanisms involved, these patients have a high risk for both thromboembolic events and hemorrhagic complications. Stroke is a frequent complication in CKD: The US Renal Data System reports an incidence of 15.1% in hemodialysis patients compared with 9.6% in patients with other stages of CKD and 2.6% in a control cohort without CKD. The 2-yr mortality rates after stroke in these subgroups were 74, 55, and 28%, respectively. Although oral coumadin is the treatment of choice for atrial fibrillation, its use in patients with CKD is reported only in limited studies, all in hemodialysis patients, and is associated with a markedly increased rate of bleeding compared with patients without CKD. With regard to the high risk for stroke and the conflicting data about oral anticoagulation, an individualized stratification algorithm is presented based on relevant studies.

▶ Within the general population, hazard ratios and practice guidelines have been established for the treatment of atrial fibrillation. The guidelines are intended to reduce the occurrence of complications of atrial fibrillation, including the major complication of ischemic stroke.[1] The applicability of these guidelines to patients with various stages of chronic kidney disease (CKD) and to patients with end-stage renal disease (ESRD) has remained uncertain. Single-center studies of hemodialysis patients with atrial fibrillation have demonstrated that the risk of thromboembolic events is increased approximately 4.5 times the rate seen in dialysis patients in normal sinus rhythm. The United States Renal Data System (USRDS) demonstrates that ESRD patients with atrial fibrillation have a 1.6-fold higher rate of ischemic stroke than those without fibrillation. This was largely due to an increased risk of ischemic rather than hemorrhagic stroke.[2] The treatment of atrial fibrillation in dialysis patients is further complicated by the fact that dialysis patients are prothrombotic, but also simultaneously have an increased risk of bleeding.[3-6]

Drawing from several resources, including the Cardiac Failure Hypertension Age Diabetes Stroke (CHADS$_2$) score,[7] Reincke and colleagues have devised a unique algorithm with which to approach anticoagulation in patients with atrial fibrillation and CKD. The authors correctly point out that the bleeding risk in patients with renal disease is complex and, therefore, cannot be calculated by a simple scoring system. Rather, appropriate implementation of the algorithm requires the input of a qualified physician who is both knowledgeable about patient specific factors (dementia, fall risk, etc) and also understands both contradictions and complexities of hemostasis in the setting of kidney disease. Longitudinal prospective studies evaluating this individualized ratification algorithm should prove clinically useful.

R. Garrick, MD

References

1. Fuster V, Ryden LE, Cannom DS, et al. ACC/AHA/ESC 2006 guidelines for the management of patients with atrial fibrillation: Executive summary—A report of the American College of Cardiology/American Heart Association Task Force on Practice Guidelines and the European Society of Cardiology Committee for Practice Guidelines. *J Am Coll Cardiol.* 2006;48:854-906.
2. US Renal Data System: USRDS 2006 Annual Data Report. *Atlas of End-Stage Renal Disease in the United States, Bethesda, National Institutes of Health, National Institute of Diabetes and Digestive and Kidney Diseases.* 2006; 2006.
3. Vazquez E, Sanchez-Perales C, Lozano C, et al. Comparison of prognostic value of atrial fibrillation versus sinus rhythm in patients on long-term hemodialysis. *Am J Cardiol.* 2003;92:868-871.
4. Boccardo P, Remuzzi G, Galbusera M. Platelet dysfunction in renal failure. *Semin Thromb Haemost.* 2004;30:579-589.
5. Tveit DP, Hypolite IO, Hshieh P, Cruess D, et al. Chronic dialysis patients have high risk for pulmonary embolism. *Am J Kidney Dis.* 2002;39:1011-1017.
6. Gangji AS, Sohal AS, Treleaven D. Bleeding in patients with renal insufficiency: a practical guide to clinical management. *Thromb Res.* 2006;118:423-428.
7. Lo DS, Rabbat CG, Clase CM. Thromboembolism and anticoagulant management in hemodialysis patients: a practical guide to clinical management. *Thromb Res.* 2006;118:385-395.

Acute and Chronic Management of Atrial Fibrillation in Patients With Late-Stage CKD
Aronow WS (New York Med College, Valhalla)
Am J Kidney Dis 53:701-710, 2009

A 76-year-old white woman with stage 5 chronic kidney disease (CKD) receiving hemodialysis for the past 3 months develops atrial fibrillation with a ventricular rate of 170 beats/min, precipitating left-sided heart failure and pulmonary congestion. Her blood pressure is 140/90 mm Hg. Her medical history is notable for type 2 diabetes mellitus (hemoglobin A_{1c} level of 6.8%) and transient cerebral ischemic attack 6 months prior. Her left ventricular ejection fraction (LVEF) was 35%, as assessed 2 months earlier. Her serum low-density lipoprotein (LDL) cholesterol is 70 mg/dL (1.81 mmol/L). Medications include 5 mg glipizide and 40 mg simvastatin daily. How should her atrial fibrillation (AF) with rapid ventricular response be treated?

▶ As noted in the study of Reinecke and colleagues, atrial fibrillation likely contributes to the increased cardiovascular morbidity and mortality associated with chronic kidney disease (CKD). This article reviews the available data regarding the incidence and prevalence of atrial fibrillation and its complications in patients with late-stage kidney disease. Of special interest is the fact that long-term (50-month) follow-up mortality rates in patients with atrial fibrillation and CKD were increased by almost 50% compared with similar patients without atrial fibrillation.[1,2] This study demonstrates that the lack of available prospective data involving a well matched population hampers definitive conclusions regarding the use of warfarin in this population. The importance of these types of data is demonstrated by the observational study[3] drawn from the United States renal data service, which found that among dialysis patients hospitalized for atrial fibrillation, only warfarin use and systolic blood pressure were associated with increased survival. The analysis presented by Aronow suggests that warfarin can be safely used in patients with CKD, especially if approached on an individualized basis. Until additional prospective studies are available, the risk stratification approach suggested by Reinecke and colleagues (reviewed elsewhere here) will likely help clinicians determine patient-specific strategies for the management of atrial fibrillation in patients with CKD.

Aronow also reviews the medications available for ventricular rate control and their safety and applicability in patients with CKD. This offers a useful management guide for this patient population.

R. Garrick, MD

References

1. Vazquez E, Sanchez-Perales C, Lozano C, et al. Comparison of prognostic value of atrial fibrillation versus sinus rhythm in patients on long-term hemodialysis. *Am J Cardiol.* 2003;92:868-871.
2. Vazquez-Ruiz de Castroviejoa E, Sanchez-Perales C, Lozano-Cabezas C, et al. Incidence of atrial fibrillation in hemodialysis patients. A prospective long-term follow-up study. *Rev Esp Cardiol.* 2006;59:779-784.
3. Abbott KC, Trespalacios FC, Taylor AJ, Agodoa LY. Atrial fibrillation in chronic dialysis patients in the United States: risk factors for hospitalization and mortality. *BMC Nephrol.* 2003;4:1.

Fibroblast Growth Factor 23 and Mortality among Patients Undergoing Hemodialysis
Gutiérrez OM, Mannstadt M, Isakova T, et al (Massachusetts General Hosp and Harvard Med School, Boston)
N Engl J Med 359:584-592, 2008

Background.—Fibroblast growth factor 23 (FGF-23) is a hormone that increases the rate of urinary excretion of phosphate and inhibits renal production of 1,25-dihydroxyvitamin D, thus helping to mitigate hyperphosphatemia in patients with kidney disease. Hyperphosphatemia and low 1,25-dihydroxyvitamin D levels are associated with mortality among patients with chronic kidney disease, but the effect of the level of FGF-23 on mortality is unknown.

Methods.—We examined mortality according to serum phosphate levels in a prospective cohort of 10,044 patients who were beginning hemodialysis treatment and then analyzed FGF-23 levels and mortality in a nested case–control sample of 200 subjects who died and 200 who survived during the first year of hemodialysis treatment. We hypothesized that increased FGF-23 levels at the initiation of hemodialysis would be associated with increased mortality.

Results.—Serum phosphate levels in the highest quartile (>5.5 mg per deciliter [1.8 mmol per liter]) were associated with a 20% increase in the multivariable adjusted risk of death, as compared with normal levels (3.5 to 4.5 mg per deciliter [1.1 to 1.4 mmol per liter]) (hazard ratio, 1.2; 95% confidence interval [CI], 1.1 to 1.4). Median C-terminal FGF-23 (cFGF-23) levels were significantly higher in case subjects than in controls (2260 vs. 1406 reference units per milliliter, P<0.001). Multivariable adjusted analyses showed that increasing FGF-23 levels were associated with a monotonically increasing risk of death when examined either on a continuous scale (odds ratio per unit increase in log-transformed cFGF-23 values, 1.8; 95% CI, 1.4 to 2.4) or in quartiles, with quartile 1 as the reference category (odds ratio for quartile 2, 1.6 [95% CI, 0.8 to 3.3]; for quartile 3, 4.5 [95% CI, 2.2 to 9.4]; and for quartile 4, 5.7 [95% CI, 2.6 to 12.6]).

Conclusions.—Increased FGF-23 levels appear to be independently associated with mortality among patients who are beginning hemodialysis treatment. Future studies might investigate whether FGF-23 is a potential biomarker that can be used to guide strategies for the management of phosphorus balance in patients with chronic kidney disease.

▶ Fibroblast growth factor 23 (FGF-23), a hormone that is secreted by osteoblasts, is an important regulator of phosphorus and vitamin D metabolism. FGF-23 downregulates the activity of type IIa sodium phosphate co-transporter in the kidney, leading to phosphate excretion, and also suppresses 1{alpha} hydroxylase, leading to reduced levels of active 1.25 vitamin D3.

In patients with kidney disease, normal serum phosphate levels are maintained despite a declining nephron mass, in part by a progressive "secondary" increase in the FGF-23 level, which stimulates greater excretion of phosphate through the remaining nephrons and limits the absorption of dietary phosphorus by inhibiting the synthesis of 1,25-dihydroxyvitamin D. It has been shown that increased serum phosphate levels and decreased 1,25-dihydroxyvitamin D levels are associated with increased mortality, but its effect on the compensatory increase in FGF-23 secretion on mortality is unknown.

In this prospective cohort study of 10 044 United States patients who initiated hemodialysis between 2004 and 2005, patients in the highest quartile of serum phosphate level (> 1.8 mmol/l) had a 1.2-fold greater risk of death than those in the quartile with normal serum phosphate levels (1.1-1.5 mmol/l). FGF-23 levels and mortality were then analyzed in a nested case-control sample of 200 subjects who died (cases) and 200 who survived (controls) during the first year of hemodialysis treatment. The median plasma level of C-terminal FGF-23 fragments (cFGF-23) was lower among survivors than among nonsurvivors (1406 U/ml vs. 2,260 U/ml; *P* < .001). This trend persisted when each quartile of serum phosphate level was examined separately, apart from the highest quartile, in which the difference was not significant. After adjustment for case-mix factors and laboratory variables, each unit increase in the natural log-transformed cFGF-23 level was associated with a 1.8-fold increase in mortality risk. Patients in the highest quartile of cFGF-23 had a 5.7-fold greater risk of death than those in the lowest quartile. The data also showed that FGF-23 levels tended to be lower among black and Hispanic patients. Black patients with the lowest FGF-23 levels had an even lower risk of death than did white patients with similar levels, which echoes previous observations of a reduced mortality rate among black dialysis patients.

Because it is an observational study, the results do not indicate whether increased FGF-23 is itself toxic, or if it is a surrogate marker of other factors. Nonetheless, the study is of interest because so few interventions have been shown to alter mortality in patients with renal failure. This observational study raises the interesting possibility that reducing serum phosphate to levels lower than the now-current "normal range" might reduce FGF-23 secretion, potentially reducing mortality. Prospective, controlled studies involving patients with normal phosphate levels, but high FGF-23 levels, may be useful to test the possibilities raised here.

For further reading on this subject I suggest articles by Danziger,[1] Gutierrez et al,[2] Hsu,[3] and Zoccali.[4]

S. Mundra, MD

References

1. Danziger J. The bone-renal axis in early chronic kidney disease: an emerging paradigm. *Nephrol Dial Transplant.* 2008;23:2733-2737.
2. Gutierrez O, Isakova T, Rhee E, et al. Fibroblast growth factor-23 mitigates hyperphosphatemia but accentuates calcitriol deficiency in chronic kidney disease. *J Am Soc Nephrol.* 2005;16:2205-2215.
3. Hsu C-Y. FGF-23 and Outcomes Research—when physiology meets epidemiology. *N Engl J Med.* 2008;359:640-642.
4. Zoccali C. FGF-23 in dialysis patients: ready for prime time? *Nephrol Dial Transplant.* 2009;24:1078-1081.

Association of Oral Calcitriol with Improved Survival in Nondialyzed CKD

Shoben AB, Rudser KD, de Boer IH, et al (Puget Sound Veterans' Affairs Med Ctr)
J Am Soc Nephrol 19:1613-1619, 2008

Parenteral vitamin D is associated with improved survival among long-term hemodialysis patients. Among nondialyzed patients with chronic kidney disease (CKD), oral activated vitamin D reduces parathyroid hormone levels, but the impact on clinical outcomes is unknown. We evaluated associations of oral calcitriol use with mortality and dialysis dependence in 1418 nondialysis patients with CKD and hyperparathyroidism in the Veterans' Affairs Consumer Health Information and Performance Sets database. Incident calcitriol users and nonusers were selected on the basis of stages 3 to 4 CKD, hyperparathyroidism, and the absence of hypercalcemia before calcitriol use and then were matched by age and estimated kidney function. During a median follow-up of 1.9 yr, 408 (29%) patients died and 217 (16%) initiated long-term dialysis. After adjustment for demographics; comorbidities; estimated kidney function; medications; and baseline levels of parathyroid hormone, calcium, and phosphorous, oral calcitriol use was associated with a 26% lower risk for death (95% confidence interval 5 to 42% lower; $P=0.016$) and a 20% lower risk for death or dialysis (95% confidence interval 1 to 35% lower; $P=0.038$). The association of calcitriol with improved survival was not statistically different across baseline parathyroid hormone levels. Calcitriol use was associated with a greater risk for hypercalcemia. In conclusion, oral calcitriol use is associated with lower mortality in nondialysis patients with CKD.

▶ The kidneys are responsible for the conversion of 25-hydroxyvitamin D to 1, 25-dihydroxyvitamin D (calcitriol), the most biologically potent form of vitamin D. Intravenous administration of active analogues of 1,25 vitamin D3, has been associated with a reduction in mortality among dialysis patients.[1,2] Previous meta-analyses[3] in patients with predialysis and dialysis dependent kidney disease suggested that therapy with activated vitamin D compounds was associated with higher levels of calcium and phosphate treatment, but was not associated with reduced mortality. This study evaluated the association of oral calcitriol use with mortality and dialysis dependence in 1418 patients with stages 3 to 4 chronic kidney disease (CKD) and hyperparathyroidism. After adjustment for demographics, comorbidities, and appropriate laboratory values, the authors demonstrated during a 1.9-year follow-up that patients who received oral therapy with calcitriol had lower rates of death and deaths plus progression to dialysis. This was an observational study, and although the authors did take several steps to control for confounding by indication, it is possible that differences in unmeasured comorbidities may have influenced the results. With this in mind, it is noteworthy that these are among the first data to demonstrate that therapy with oral calcitriol may significantly affect outcomes in patients with stages 3 and 4 CKD. The study is important because the findings suggest that oral calcitriol may be one of the few therapeutic manipulations that can potentially alter mortality in this at-risk population. These observational data set the stage for prospective randomized trials.

M. Brogan, MD

References

1. Teng M, Wolf M, Ofsthun MN, et al. Activated injectable vitamin D and hemodialysis survival: a historical cohort study. *J Am Soc Nephrol.* 2005;16:1115-1125.
2. Tentori F, Hunt WC, Stidley CA, et al. Mortality risk among hemodialysis patients receiving different vitamin D analogs. *Kidney Int.* 2006;70:1858-1865.
3. Palmer SC, McGregor DO, Macaskill P, Craig JC, Elder GJ, Strippoli GF. Meta-analysis: Vitamin D compounds in chronic kidney disease. *Ann Intern Med.* 2007;147:840-853.

Malignancy Following Kidney Transplantation

Arichi N, Kishikawa H, Nishimura K, et al (Hyogo Prefectural Nishinomiya Hosp, Japan; et al)
Transplant Proc 40:2400-2402, 2008

A cohort of 429 patients who received kidney grafts between 1973 and 2007 at our hospital was studied for the incidence and sites of malignancy. Sixty-two malignant diseases developed in 57 of 429 patients (13.3%). The cumulative incidences of malignancy increased markedly in the second and third posttransplantation decades. The overall rates were 1.8% at 5 years, 6.7% at 10 years, 12.5% at 15 years, 17.3% at 20 years, and 25.6% at 25 years. In the second and third posttransplantation decades, patients without malignancy showed significantly superior survival versus than those with cancer ($P = .0002$). Their survival rates were 83.4% versus 86.9% at 10 years and 63.1% versus 80.3% at 20 years, respectively. Skin cancer, renal cell carcinoma of the native kidney, hepatocellular carcinoma, posttransplantation lymphoproliferative disease, uterine cancer, and colorectal cancer were common in our series. The 5-year survival rates after the treatment of malignancy were better for skin cancer and renal cell carcinoma of the native kidney. Concerning the effects of immunosuppression, the tacrolimus-based group displayed a higher incidence among 3 groups ($P = .0044$).

▶ It is well known that transplant immunosuppression increases the risk of de novo malignancy. This article confirms this fact and goes on to categorize the types of malignancies and the relevant timeframes during which we could expect to detect them. In 429 recipients, skin cancer, hepatocellular carcinoma, native kidney renal cell carcinoma, lymphoma, uterine, and colorectal cancers were among the most common malignancies noted. Survival rates of patients with skin and renal cell carcinoma appeared somewhat better than others. With regard to surveillance, it is important for clinicians to be aware that most of the malignancies appeared after the second decade posttransplant, and negatively impacted survival in those decades. In addition, patient age at time of transplant and the use of tacrolimus appeared to influence the risk of later malignancy. This study serves as a reminder that even though the history of transplantation may be remote, long-term vigilance for malignancy must be maintained and screening protocols must be strictly followed.

M. Klein, MD, JD

Long-Term Consequences of Kidney Donation

Ibrahim HN, Foley R, Tan L, et al (Univ of Minnesota, Minneapolis; Chronic Disease Res Group, Minneapolis)
N Engl J Med 360:459-469, 2009

Background.—The long-term renal consequences of kidney donation by a living donor are attracting increased appropriate interest. The overall evidence suggests that living kidney donors have survival similar to that of nondonors and that their risk of end-stage renal disease (ESRD) is not increased. Previous studies have included relatively small numbers of donors and a brief follow-up period.

Methods.—We ascertained the vital status and lifetime risk of ESRD in 3698 kidney donors who donated kidneys during the period from 1963 through 2007; from 2003 through 2007, we also measured the glomerular filtration rate (GFR) and urinary albumin excretion and assessed the prevalence of hypertension, general health status, and quality of life in 255 donors.

Results.—The survival of kidney donors was similar to that of controls who were matched for age, sex, and race or ethnic group. ESRD developed in 11 donors, a rate of 180 cases per million persons per year, as compared with a rate of 268 per million per year in the general population. At a mean ($\pm$SD) of 12.2 ± 9.2 years after donation, 85.5% of the subgroup of 255 donors had a GFR of 60 ml per minute per 1.73 m^2 of body-surface area or higher, 32.1% had hypertension, and 12.7% had albuminuria. Older age and higher body-mass index, but not a longer time since donation, were associated with both a GFR that was lower than 60 ml per minute per 1.73 m^2 and hypertension. A longer time since donation, however, was independently associated with albuminuria. Most donors had quality-of-life scores that were better than population norms, and the prevalence of coexisting conditions was similar to that among controls from the National Health and Nutrition Examination Survey (NHANES) who were matched for age, sex, race or ethnic group, and body-mass index.

Conclusions.—Survival and the risk of ESRD in carefully screened kidney donors appear to be similar to those in the general population. Most donors who were studied had a preserved GFR, normal albumin excretion, and an excellent quality of life.

▶ The long-term impact of unilateral nephrectomy on health status was previously based on observations of veterans with traumatic nephrectomy, and on children with acongenital decrease in renal mass.[1-3] None of these subgroups gives us confidence in counseling potential kidney donors as to the real risks inherent in their gift. This study was designed to assess the long-term effects 20 years after donation. Based on interview data from 2199 donors, the authors concluded that kidney donation has no adverse effects on renal survival, the incidence of hypertension, or the development of albuminuria. For most donors the overall quality of life score was better than the population norm.

The statistical analysis is limited due to varied techniques for measurement of glomerular filtration rate (GFR) over time and the inherent censoring of those donors no longer living, but it is the best evidence to date that long-term exposure to elective unilateral nephrectomy has no adverse effects on the donor.

These data provide clinicians with the empiric evidence necessary to reassure potential donors as to the long-term safety of their contemplated donation. This, in turn, may help secure more living donors, and minimize the waiting time for cadaveric transplantation.

M. Klein, MD, JD

References

1. Thorner PS, Arbus GS, Celermajer DS, Baumal R. Focal segmental glomerulosclerosis and progressive renal failure associated with a unilateral kidney. *Pediatrics.* 1984;3:806-810.
2. Baudoin P, Provoost A, Molenaar J. Renal function up to 50 years after unilateralphrectomy in childhood. *Am J Kidney Dis.* 1993;21:603-611.
3. Narkun-Burgess DM, Nolan CR, Norman JE, Page WF, Miller PL, Meyer TW. Forty-five year follow-up after uninephrectomy. *Kidney Int.* 1993;43:1110-1115.

PART FIVE

PULMONARY DISEASE

JAMES A. BARKER, MD

Introduction

Welcome to the 2009 edition of the YEAR BOOK OF MEDICINE. I would encourage all of you to look at the entire 2009 YEAR BOOK OF PULMONARY DISEASE because it really is chock full of great articles.

We have picked some of the very best ones to go into this edition of YEAR BOOK OF MEDICINE. For example, in the chapter on lung cancer by Dr Tanoue, there is a great article about chronic obstructive pulmonary disease (COPD) and lung cancer mortality in patients who have never smoked. This is a follow-up to some previous articles and again strengthens the somewhat previous weak connection between COPD and lung cancer. Dr Tanoue has some insightful discussion about this. In addition, there is an excellent review of early stage non–small cell lung cancer again, which is important baseline knowledge for all of us pulmonologists.

Dr Maurer has some equally insightful articles discussed in regard to lung transplantation as well as COPD. There is a very nice discussion of anastomotic airway complications after transplant from Murthy and others at Cleveland Clinic. This is a major problem in lung transplant. In addition, there is another article about tacrolimus versus cyclosporine (Hachem et al) that I found extremely helpful. Cyclosporine, of course, has been a fantastic mainstay drug for transplantation of many organs. However, it has many drug interactions. Progressive essential hypertension and renal insufficiency are common side effects. Tacrolimus is replacing cyclosporine in the armamentarium. This article adds further evidence to that. The COPD articles likewise are bread and butter important articles. For example, I had no idea that there are geographic variations in COPD exacerbation rates. The impact of COPD on results after myocardial infarction makes sense but is newly in print.

Dr Ali Raza has likewise found some wonderful articles to discuss. The article by Stawikisp et al is particularly pertinent. They did a nice study looking at how useful transthoracic echocardiography is when looking for pulmonary embolism in the ICU. This is one of those areas where the more you look the more you find. A caveat from this study is that baseline echocardiograms are particularly helpful for showing new significant changes later. One of the more useful things, of course, was that they had already found DVT by duplex ultrasonography. The most common finding is tricuspid regurgitation. I encourage you to read this article and all the rest here outlined from Dr Raza. We as pulmonary/critical care physicians have no choice but to become more and more adept at doing our own ultrasounds. We must understand this great technology that this offers as well as its limits. I also love another of his that we have listed here by Anderson et al. This is a randomized control trial of computerized pulmonary angiography versus VQ scans. Despite our current acceptance of CT angiography as the gold standard, there really has not been excellent literature demonstration of efficiency. In general, this modality seems to outpace the literature as far as technical expertise occurs.

King et al did us a great service in publishing Build-1. This trial uses bosentan in idiopathic pulmonary fibrosis. I found this a very exciting study. Unfortunately, it does not have a positive result. There is a great deal of interest in trying to treat the pulmonary hypertension associated with pulmonary fibrosis and also in the agents for possibly slowing the primary disease. Unfortunately, this is a negative result study but certainly should not keep us from moving forward in this area. Further study is definitely indicated.

Dr Shirley F. Jones has found a number of great sleep articles to share with us as well. Again, I would encourage the reader to pick up the YEAR BOOK OF PULMONARY DISEASE to be able to read her entire chapter. She has adroitly reviewed the article about adaptive servoventilation (ASV) by Allam et al at the Mayo Clinic. I think this is a really important article since many of us now consider this the treatment of choice for Cheyne-Stokes associated sleep-disordered breathing (SDB), yet it is not a truly easy modality to use. Another great study by Hwang et al in regard to associated SDB with postoperative complications is a must-read in my opinion. It has been my bias that sleep apnea definitely increases perioperative complications for quite some time. This study confirms that bias. In addition, Dr Jones has nicely discussed the issues at play here.

Finally, the Critical Care chapter of this year's YEAR BOOK OF PULMONARY DISEASE has many fascinating articles and I would encourage you to read all of these. There is just a taste here in the YEAR BOOK OF MEDICINE. First of all, I would direct you to the work of Dr Wes Ely and cohorts in the evaluation of acute brain dysfunction with different medications, the MENDS Trial. I completely agree with these investigators that delirium in the ICU is a much more major problem then we've often paid attention to. Another fun article is by Kory et al. In this study, the authors looked at whether simulation training really does add over traditional training in basic critical care skills such as airway management. All of us are moving to simulator training, so it is nice to know that it works. This article shows that it is definitely the case. "See one," "do one," "teach one" is dead. Let us bury it! There are more fantastic articles on critical care, pulmonary infections, asthma, and so on. Please dig in and enjoy!

James A. Barker, MD

33 Lung Cancer

Treatment of Non-small Cell Lung Cancer Stage I and Stage II: ACCP Evidence-Based Clinical Practice Guidelines (2nd Edition)
Scott WJ, Howington J, Feigenberg S, et al (Fox Chase Cancer Ctr, Philadelphia, PA; Univ of Cincinnati Medical Ctr, Cincinnati, OH; et al)
Chest 132:234S-242S, 2007

Background.—The surgical treatment of stage I and II non-small cell lung cancer (NSCLC) continues to evolve in the areas of intraoperative lymph node staging (specifically the issue of lymph node dissection vs sampling), the role of sublobar resections instead of lobectomy for treatment of smaller tumors, and the use of video-assisted techniques to perform anatomic lobectomy. Adjuvant therapy (both chemotherapy and radiation therapy) and the use of larger fractions of radiotherapy delivered to a smaller area for nonoperative treatment of early stage NSCLC have shown promising results.

Methods.—The panel selected the following areas for review based on clinical relevance and the amount and quality of data available for analysis: surgical approaches to resecting early stage NSCLC, methods of lymph node staging at the time of surgical resection, adjuvant chemotherapy in the treatment of early stage NSCLC, and the use of radiation therapy for primary treatment of early stage NSCLC as well as in the adjuvant setting. Recommendations by the multidisciplinary writing committee were based on literature review using established methods.

Results and Conclusions.—Surgical resection remains the treatment of choice for stage I and II NSCLC, although surgical methods continue to evolve. Adjuvant chemotherapy for patients with stage II, but not stage I, NSCLC is well established. Radiotherapy remains an important treatment for either cases of early stage NSCLC that are medically inoperable or patients who refuse surgery.

► Pulmonologists are typically involved with lung cancer patients at the front end of their care, directing the process of diagnosis and staging. Although few of us participate directly in treatment, it is important to be cognizant of current state of the art treatment practices, as we often serve as the point of reference for patient referral to appropriate other specialties.

Non-small cell lung cancer (NSCLC) treatment is increasingly multidisciplinary, as optimal treatment even for early stage patients is likely to involve multiple modalities. Care of lung cancer patients through a multidisciplinary thoracic oncology team ensures that all relevant subspecialists will be involved in decisions related to treatment. In situations where such a team is not readily available, it may be the diagnosing pulmonologist who will decide on referral to thoracic surgery, medical oncology, radiation therapy, and/or palliative services. Because there are an ever-increasing number of effective therapies available to lung cancer patients, treatment referrals should be made with as little nihilism as possible to allow the patient access to new therapies and clinical trials.

This report by Scott and colleagues summarizes the current spectrum of treatment for stage I and II NSCLC, and is part of the American College of Chest Physician Evidence-Based Guidelines for the Diagnosis and Management of Lung Cancer. The outcomes of surgical approaches to early stage NSCLC, including adjuvant therapy, as well as alternatives to surgery for patients medically unfit for resection were critically examined in an extensive review of the medical literature. Companion articles by Robinson and colleagues, Jett and colleagues, and Socinski and colleagues in these guidelines summarize the evidence and current practices for treatment of Stage IIIA, Stage IIIB, and Stage IV NSCLC, respectively.[1-3] The recommendations in this group of articles provide a concise summary of state-of-the-art treatment for patients with NSCLC.

L. T. Tanoue, MD

References

1. Socinski MA, Crowell R, Hensing TE, et al. Treatment of non-small cell lung cancer, stage IV: ACCP evidence-based clinical practice guidelines (2nd edition). *Chest*. 2007;132:277S-289S.
2. Robinson LA, Ruckdeschel JC, Wagner H Jr, Stevens CW. Treatment of non-small cell lung cancer-stage IIIA: ACCP evidence-based clinical practice guidelines (2nd edition). *Chest*. 2007;132:243S-265S.
3. Jett JR, Schild SE, Keith RL, Kesler KA. Treatment of non-small cell lung cancer, stage IIIB: ACCP evidence-based clinical practice guidelines (2nd edition). *Chest*. 2007;132:266S-276S.

Risk factors for 30-day mortality after resection of lung cancer and prediction of their magnitude

Strand TE, Rostad H, Damhuis RAM, et al (Cancer Registry of Norway; Rotterdam Cancer Registry, The Netherlands; et al)
Thorax 62:991-997, 2007

Background.—There is considerable variability in reported postoperative mortality and risk factors for mortality after surgery for lung cancer. Population-based data provide unbiased estimates and may aid in treatment selection.

Methods.—All patients diagnosed with lung cancer in Norway from 1993 to the end of 2005 were reported to the Cancer Registry of Norway (n = 26 665). A total of 4395 patients underwent surgical resection and were included in the analysis. Data on demographics, tumour characteristics and treatment were registered. A subset of 1844 patients was scored according to the Charlson co-morbidity index. Potential factors influencing 30-day mortality were analysed by logistic regression.

Results.—The overall postoperative mortality rate was 4.4% within 30 days with a declining trend in the period. Male sex (OR 1.76), older age (OR 3.38 for age band 70–79 years), right-sided tumours (OR 1.73) and extensive procedures (OR 4.54 for pneumonectomy) were identified as risk factors for postoperative mortality in multivariate analysis. Postoperative mortality at high-volume hospitals (≥20 procedures/year) was lower (OR 0.76, p = 0.076). Adjusted ORs for postoperative mortality at individual hospitals ranged from 0.32 to 2.28. The Charlson co-morbidity index was identified as an independent risk factor for postoperative mortality (p = 0.017). A prediction model for postoperative mortality is presented.

Conclusions.—Even though improvements in postoperative mortality have been observed in recent years, these findings indicate a further potential to optimise the surgical treatment of lung cancer. Hospital treatment results varied but a significant volume effect was not observed. Prognostic models may identify patients requiring intensive postoperative care.

▶ Surgery remains the cornerstone of treatment for patients with early stage lung cancer. Unfortunately, individuals with lung cancer are typically older and often have comorbid medical conditions that are tobacco-related. Risk assessment in patients with lung cancer being considered for surgical resection remains a challenging aspect of their care.

In this report by Strand and colleagues, preoperative risks and postsurgical outcomes were assessed for all patients in Norway who underwent surgical resection for lung cancer from 1993 to 2005. This was a very large study, including over 4000 patients. Multivariate analysis identified male sex, older age (> 70 years), right-sided tumors, and more extensive procedures (pneumonectomy > bilobectomy > lower lobectomy > upper lobectomy) as risk factors for postoperative mortality, defined as death within 30 days of surgery. Higher hospital volume (> 20 operations/year) was associated with a decreased risk of postoperative mortality, but was not statistically significant in the multivariate analysis. The impact of the Charlson comorbidity index (CCI) was evaluated in a subset of 1844 patients. Postoperative mortality in patients without comorbidity (CCI score 0) was 3.8%, compared with patients with CCI scores of 1-2, 3-4, or > 5, in whom postoperative mortality was 5.8%, 10.3%, and 15.4%, respectively.

Risk assessment is a crucial part of evaluation for all patients being considered for lung cancer resection. Because surgery still offers the best opportunity for long-term survival, denying a patient resection on the basis of risk can only be done after careful consideration.[1] For patients identified as high-risk for surgery, consideration should be given to preparing the patient by optimizing any comorbid medical conditions, planning for intensive postoperative care, and possibly referral to a high-volume institution for resection.

L. T. Tanoue, MD

Reference

1. Colice GL, Shafazand S, Griffin JP, Keenan R, Bolliger CT. Physiologic evaluation of the patient with lung cancer being considered for resectional surgery: ACCP evidenced-based clinical practice guidelines (2nd edition). *Chest.* 2007;132: 161S-177S.

Evaluation of Patients with Pulmonary Nodules: When is it Lung Cancer?: ACCP Evidence-Based Clinical Practice Guidelines (2nd Edition)
Gould MK, Fletcher J, Iannettoni MD, et al (Stanford School of Medicine, CA; Indiana Univ School of Medicine, Indianapolis, IN; Univ of Iowa Carver College of Medicine, Iowa City, IA; et al)
Chest 132:108S-130S, 2007

Background.—Pulmonary nodules are spherical radiographic opacities that measure up to 30 mm in diameter. Nodules are extremely common in clinical practice and challenging to manage, especially small, "subcentimeter" nodules. Identification of malignant nodules is important because they represent a potentially curable form of lung cancer.

Methods.—We developed evidence-based clinical practice guidelines based on a systematic literature review and discussion with a large, multidisciplinary group of clinical experts and other stakeholders.

Results.—We generated a list of 29 recommendations for managing the solitary pulmonary nodule (SPN) that measures at least 8 to 10 mm in diameter; small, subcentimeter nodules that measure < 8 mm to 10 mm in diameter; and multiple nodules when they are detected incidentally during evaluation of the SPN. Recommendations stress the value of risk factor assessment, the utility of imaging tests (especially old films), the need to weigh the risks and benefits of various management strategies (biopsy, surgery, and observation with serial imaging tests), and the importance of eliciting patient preferences.

Conclusion.—Patients with pulmonary nodules should be evaluated by estimation of the probability of malignancy, performance of imaging tests to characterize the lesion(s) better, evaluation of the risks associated with various management alternatives, and elicitation of patient preferences for treatment.

▶ The solitary pulmonary nodule (SPN) is one of the most common reasons that patients are referred for pulmonary evaluation. Older studies estimated that approximately 150 000 such nodules are identified in the community annually, but these estimates were based on identification of nodules by plain chest radiography.[1,2] Based on the number of computed tomography (CT) scans done annually in the nation (approaching 30 million body CTs per year according to Brenner and Hall[3]), the reported 12% to 46% prevalence of pulmonary nodules found in studies evaluating low-dose CT for screening purposes,[4] and the knowledge that approximately 40 million Americans are current or former smokers who would match the entry criteria for those studies, the actual prevalence of pulmonary nodules found on CT scans annually is almost certainly substantially higher than those previous estimates.

The obvious goals in the evaluation of SPNs are to identify those nodules that are malignant, as they potentially represent curable lung cancers, and to avoid as much as possible interventions on nodules that are benign. This report by Gould and colleagues was prepared for the American College of Chest Physicians Evidence-Based Guidelines on the Diagnosis and Management of Lung Cancer. It presents 29 recommendations for SPN evaluation based on an extensive systematic literature review. The first of these recommendations states, "In every patient with a SPN, we recommend that clinicians estimate the pretest probability of malignancy either qualitatively by using clinical judgment or quantitatively by using a validated model." This summarizes the first important step of lung cancer risk assessment based on patient clinical features and the radiographic appearance of the nodule. The assessment made in this initial evaluation drives the decision process of whether to pursue a more extensive evaluation incorporating further imaging studies, biopsy, or resection. The process is outlined in algorithmic form in Fig 1 for SPNs measuring > 8 mm in diameter, and in Fig 2 for those measuring < 8 mm in diameter.

This report comprehensively discusses the nuances of SPN evaluation, including a discussion of cancer risk assessment, including clinical and radiographic features and mathematical models. The report also evaluates the performance characteristics of CT scanning and positron emission tomography (PET), as well as the efficacy of various invasive techniques. Importantly, the recommendations made regarding the accuracy and limitations of these interventions are evidence-based, and thus should serve as a reliable source of guidance for the practicing clinician.

L. T. Tanoue, MD

References

1. Holin SM, Dwork RE, Glaser S, Rikli AE, Stocklen JB. Solitary pulmonary nodules found in a community-wide chest roentgenographic survey; a five-year follow-up study. *Am Rev Tuberc.* 1959;79:427-439.
2. Ost D, Fein AM, Feinsilver SH. Clinical practice. The solitary pulmonary nodule. *N Engl J Med.* 2003;348:2535-2542.
3. Brenner DJ, Hall EJ. Computed tomography–an increasing source of radiation exposure. *N Engl J Med.* 2007;357:2277-2284.
4. Mulshine JL, Sullivan DC. Clinical practice. Lung cancer screening. *N Engl J Med.* 2005;352:2714-2720.

Chronic Obstructive Pulmonary Disease is Associated with Lung Cancer Mortality in a Prospective Study of Never Smokers
Turner MC, Chen Y, Krewski D, et al (Univ of Ottawa, Canada; et al)
Am J Respir Crit Care Med 176:285-290, 2007

Rationale.—Several studies have suggested that previous lung disease may increase the risk of lung cancer. It is important to clarify the association between previous lung disease and lung cancer risk in the general population.

Objectives.—The association between self-reported physician-diagnosed chronic bronchitis and emphysema and lung cancer mortality was examined in a U.S. prospective study of 448,600 lifelong nonsmokers who were cancer-free at baseline.

Methods.—During the 20-year follow-up period from 1982 to 2002, 1,759 lung cancer deaths occurred. Cox proportional hazards models were used to obtain adjusted hazard ratios (HRs) for lung cancer mortality associated with chronic bronchitis and emphysema as well as for both of these diseases together.

Measurements and Main Results.—Lung cancer mortality was significantly associated with both emphysema (HR, 1.66; 95% confidence interval [CI], 1.06, 2.59) and with the combined endpoint of emphysema and chronic bronchitis (HR, 2.44; 95% CI, 1.22, 4.90) in analyses that combined men and women. No association was observed with chronic bronchitis alone (HR, 0.96; 95% CI, 0.72, 1.28) in the overall analysis, although the association was stronger in men (HR, 1.59; 95% CI, 0.95, 2.66) than women (HR, 0.82; 95% CI, 0.58, 1.16; p for interaction, 0.04). The association between emphysema and lung cancer was stronger in analyses that excluded early years of follow-up.

Conclusions.—This large prospective study strengthens the evidence that increased lung cancer risk is associated with nonmalignant pulmonary conditions, especially emphysema, even in lifelong nonsmokers (Table 2).

▶ Approximately 15% of lung cancers in women and 5% of lung cancers in men occur in nonsmokers in the United States. Whether chronic obstructive pulmonary disease (COPD) is an independent risk factor for lung cancer has been an area of some controversy, as an association of COPD with lung cancer may be biased by confounding from smoking itself. In other countries, COPD may be more likely to be the result of noncigarette exposures, such as indoor air pollution from cooking oil fumes and burning of coal.[1,2] This has been observed in Asia, where a substantially larger percentage of lung cancers occur in nonsmokers, particularly women, than in western countries. To address the question of whether COPD, specifically chronic bronchitis and emphysema, is independently associated with lung cancer in the United States, Turner and colleagues evaluated lung cancer mortality in lifelong nonsmokers in the Cancer Prevention Study II (CPS II) cohort. Among the nearly 1.2 million participants originally enrolled starting in 1982, 448 600 were never smokers, among whom 1759 lung cancer deaths occurred. This represents the largest reported prospective cohort of nonsmokers in whom an association between COPD and lung cancer could be examined. Physician-diagnosed chronic bronchitis and emphysema were reported by 2.7% and 0.5% of lifelong nonsmokers, respectively. The study is limited in that physician-diagnosed COPD was self-reported and not validated. Accepting that limitation, lung cancer mortality was significantly associated with combined emphysema and chronic bronchitis, but not with chronic bronchitis alone, as outlined in Table 2. These findings support an

TABLE 2.—Relation of Lung Cancer Mortality to Chronic Obstructive Pulmonary Disease Among Never Smokers in the Cancer Prevention Study II Cohort, United States, 1982–2002

Previous Lung Disease	No. of Lung Cancer Deaths	Person-Years	Death Rate*	Minimally Adjusted Hazard Ratio† (95% CI)	Fully Adjusted Hazard Ratio‡ (95% CI)
Chronic bronchitis					
Yes	48	210,569	19.0	0.96 (0.72, 1.28)	0.96 (0.72, 1.28)
No	1,711	7,932,210	21.1	1.00	1.00
Emphysema					
Yes	20	35,418	42.0	1.71 (1.10, 2.66)	1.66 (1.06, 2.59)
No	1,739	8,107,361	21.0	1.00	1.00
Chronic bronchitis and emphysema					
Yes	8	10,585	52.6	2.50 (1.24, 5.02)	2.44 (1.22, 4.90)
No	1,751	7,907,377	21.1	1.00	1.00

Definition of abbreviation: CI = confidence interval.
*Per 100,000 person-years, age-standardized to the age distribution of the entire Cancer Prevention Study II cohort.
†Age, sex, and race stratified.
‡Age, sex, and race stratified, and adjusted for education, marital status, body mass index, occupational exposures, beer, wine, and liquor consumption, vegetable/fruit/fiber intake, fat intake, and passive smoking.
(Reprinted from Turner MC, Chen Y, Krewski D, et al. Chronic obstructive pulmonary disease is associated with lung cancer mortality in a prospective study of never smokers. *Am J Respir Crit Care Med.* 2007;176:285-290. Official Journal of the American Thoracic Society © American Thoracic Society.)

association of COPD, particularly emphysema, with lung cancer in lifelong nonsmokers. This suggests that addressing the toll of lung cancer in nonsmokers should include evaluation for symptoms and signs of underlying lung dysfunction, including diseases such as emphysema, for which they might not typically be considered at risk.

L. T. Tanoue, MD

References

1. Kleinerman RA, Wang Z, Wang L, et al. Lung cancer and indoor exposure to coal and biomass in rural China. *J Occup Environ Med.* 2002;44:338-344.
2. Brenner AV, Wang Z, Kleinerman RA, et al. Previous pulmonary diseases and risk of lung cancer in Gansu Province, China. *Int J Epidemiol.* 2001;30:118-124.

Long-Term Use of Supplemental Multivitamins, Vitamin C, Vitamin E, and Folate Does Not Reduce the Risk of Lung Cancer

Slatore CG, Littman AJ, Au DH, et al (Univ of Washington, Seattle; et al)(Yale University)
Am J Respir Crit Care Med 177:524-530, 2008

Rationale.—Lung cancer is the leading cause of cancer-related mortality in the United States. Although supplements are used by half the population, limited information is available about their specific effect on lung cancer risk.

Objectives.—To explore the association of supplemental multivitamins, vitamin C, vitamin E, and folate with incident lung cancer.

Methods.—Prospective cohort of 77,721 men and women aged 50–76 years from Washington State in the VITAL (VITamins And Lifestyle) study. Cases were identified through the Seattle–Puget Sound SEER (Surveillance, Epidemiology, and End Results) cancer registry.

Measurements and Main Results.—Hazard ratios (HRs) for incident lung cancer according to 10-year average daily use of supplemental multi-vitamins, vitamin C, vitamin E, and folate. A total of 521 cases of lung cancer were identified. Adjusting for smoking, age, and sex, there was no inverse association with any supplement. Supplemental vitamin E was associated with a small increased risk of lung cancer (HR, 1.05 for every 100-mg/d increase in dose; 95% confidence interval [CI], 1.00–1.09; $P = 0.033$). This risk of supplemental vitamin E was largely confined to current smokers (HR, 1.11 for every 100-mg/d increase; 95% CI, 1.03–1.19; $P < 0.01$) and was greatest for non-small cell lung cancer (HR, 1.07 for every 100-mg/d increase; 95% CI, 1.02–1.12; $P = 0.004$).

Conclusions.—Supplemental multivitamins, vitamin C, vitamin E, and folate were not associated with a decreased risk of lung cancer. Supplemental vitamin E was associated with a small increased risk. Patients should be counseled against using these supplements to prevent lung cancer.

▶ An estimated 90 million persons in the United States are ever smokers, defined as having smoked > 100 cigarettes during their lifetime.[1] Approximately 44.5 million United States' adults are current smokers, and another 45.6 million persons are former smokers.[1] Although the likelihood of lung cancer diminishes progressively with years of smoking cessation, all of these persons are at increased risk, even those with many years of abstinence. Interventions that could decrease cancer risk for these individuals, such as chemoprevention, would clearly have enormous potential benefit.

There has long been interest in the use of supplemental vitamins as chemo-preventive agents. Dietary studies have demonstrated an association of increased intake of certain fruits and vegetables with a lower incidence of lung cancer.[2,3] However, there is little evidence that supplementation with vitamins decreases cancer risk, and at least one supplement, β-carotene, has been associated with increased risk of lung cancer and cardiovascular disease in an at-risk population.[4] Nonetheless, over half of adult Americans use some type of vitamin supplementation with the intent of improving their health.[5]

This report by Slatore and colleagues comes from the VITAL (VITamins And Lifestyle) study, which is a prospective cohort study of dietary supplements and cancer risk. Recruitment of the study population was targeted to supplement users, and so supplement use by participants was typically high and of long duration. Over 77 000 persons aged 50 to 76 years were enrolled and prospectively followed. At a mean follow-up of 4.05 years, 521 persons had developed lung cancer. After adjusting for tobacco exposure, age, and sex, there was no evidence that use of multivitamins, vitamin C, vitamin E, or folate was associated with any reduction in incidence of lung cancer. Of concern, intake of higher doses of supplemental vitamin E was associated with a small increase in lung cancer incidence that was most evident in current smokers and those persons with nonsmall cell lung cancer. Similar trends toward an increased risk of lung cancer associated with vitamin E supplementation have been noted previously by other groups.[6,7]

These results reinforce the conclusion of other studies that the use of supplemental multivitamins, vitamin C, vitamin E, folate, vitamin A, and β-carotene does not decrease lung cancer incidence. Although increased dietary consumption of certain foods containing these vitamins may be associated with an apparent decrease in lung cancer risk, taking vitamin supplements does not appear to recreate that benefit. Furthermore, the association of β-carotene with increased lung cancer incidence and the trend toward a similar association with vitamin E are concerning in light of the wide prevalence of vitamin supplementation use.

L. T. Tanoue, MD

References

1. Maurice E, Trosclair A, Merritt R, et al. Cigarette smoking among adults: United States, 2004. *Morbidity and Mortality Weekly Report.* 2005;54:1121-1124.
2. Smith-Warner SA, Spiegelman D, Yaun SS. Fruits, vegetables and lung cancer: a pooled analysis of cohort studies. *Int J Cancer.* 2003;107:1001-1011.
3. Linseisen J, Rohrmann S, Miller AB, et al. Fruit and vegetable consumption and lung cancer risk: updated information from the European Prospective Investigation into Cancer and Nutrition (EPIC). *Int J Cancer.* 2007;121:1103-1114.
4. Omenn GS, Goodman GE, Thornquist MD, et al. Effects of a combination of beta carotene and vitamin A on lung cancer and cardiovascular disease. *N Engl J Med.* 1996;334:1150-1155.
5. Radimer K, Bindewald B, Hughes J, Ervin B, Swanson C, Picciano MF. Dietary supplement use by US adults: data from the National Health and Nutrition Examination Survey, 1999–2000. *Am J Epidemiol.* 2004;160:339-349.
6. Lee IM, Cook NR, Gaziano JM, et al. Vitamin E in the primary prevention of cardiovascular disease and cancer: the Women's Health Study: a randomized controlled trial. *Jama.* 2005;294:56-65.
7. MRC/BHF Heart Protection Study of antioxidant vitamin supplementation in 20,536 high-risk individuals: a randomised placebo-controlled trial. *Lancet.* 2002;360:23-33.

34 Lung Transplantation

Impact of Anastomotic Airway Complications After Lung Transplantation
Murthy SC, for the Members of Cleveland Clinic's Pulmonary Transplant Team
(Cleveland Clinic, OH)
Ann Thorac Surg 84:401-409, 2007

Background.—Because improper airway healing continues as a source of morbidity after lung transplantation, we determined prevalence and risk factors for anastomotic complications and examined their impact on survival.

Methods.—From January 1997 to January 2004, 272 patients undergoing pulmonary transplantation were studied for anastomotic airway complications. Complications were categorized as necrosis or obstruction and treatment as none, endoscopic (stenting, bronchoplasty, ablation), or open repair. Survival impact was assessed by follow-up (mean, 3.0 ± 2.2 years) using competing-risks nonproportional hazards methodology in the context of repeated events.

Results.—By 24 months, 94 anastomotic airway complications (26 necrotic, 67 obstructive, 1 torsion) had developed in 48 patients (18%), and 23 (8.5% overall; 48% of affected patients) underwent intervention. Risk of necrotic complications preceded obstruction. Risk factors were telescoping anastomosis $(p < 0.0001)$, more recent transplant $(p < 0.0001)$, donor–recipient size mismatch $(p = 0.008)$, and previously treated anastomotic airway complication $(p < 0.0001)$. Seventy-eight interventions were performed for 60 of the 94 complications. Compared with patients experiencing no anastomotic airway complications, those with treated complications had equivalent early survival (82% versus 80% at 12 months, $p = 0.9$) but worse late survival (60% versus 27% at 48 months, $p = 0.03$), and those with untreated complications had worse early survival (82% versus 62% at 12 months, $p = 0.004$) but equivalent late survival $(p = 0.4)$.

Conclusions.—Anastomotic airway complications occur in about one fifth of patients after lung transplantation and are formidable and persistent problems. Early complications are necrosis, followed by obstruction. Few risk factors are modifiable. Because these complications importantly affect survival, improving efficacy of intervention strategies should improve outcome.

▶ Anastomotic complications have been reported since the beginning of lung transplantation. With improvements in surgical technique, the risk of this type of complication and early deaths, as a result, have decreased in number in some reports; however, little has been reported on the long-term outcomes of patients with compromised airways. The data reported in this study is sobering. It suggests that the long-term survival is markedly reduced in those patients; at 4 years, the survival is less than half that of patients without airway complications. The study highlights the need for ongoing surgical technique refinement, but also the need to develop better approaches to early and late management of anastomotic complications. Clearly, patients with airway problems require ongoing close surveillance. What is not reported in this study are the causes of death in the patients with anastomotic complications. More information about causes of death could inform the best approach to long-term surveillance.

J. R. Maurer, MD, MBA

A Randomized Controlled Trial of Tacrolimus Versus Cyclosporine After Lung Transplantation
Hachem RR, Yusen RD, Chakinala MM, et al (Washington Univ, St Louis)
J Heart Lung Transplant 26:1012-1018, 2007

Background.—The optimal maintenance immunosuppressive regimen after lung transplantation is uncertain.

Methods.—We conducted a randomized controlled trial of tacrolimus versus cyclosporine in combination with azathioprine and prednisone after lung transplantation. Ninety adults were randomized to tacrolimus (n = 44) or cyclosporine (n = 46). The primary end point was a composite of a cumulative acute rejection A score of 3 or higher, a cumulative lymphocytic bronchitis B score of 4 or higher, or the onset of bronchiolitis obliterans syndrome (BOS) stage 0-p.

Results.—Recipients randomized to cyclosporine were significantly more likely to develop the primary end point than those randomized to tacrolimus. During the study period, the primary end point developed in 39 of 46 cyclosporine subjects compared with 24 of 44 tacrolimus subjects ($p = 0.002$); acute rejection or lymphocytic bronchitis end points developed in 29 of 46 cyclosporine subjects compared with 18 of 44 tacrolimus subjects ($p = 0.036$). Furthermore, BOS stage 0-p was more likely to develop in the cyclosporine group than in the tacrolimus group, but this was not statistically significant (log-rank $p = 0.1$). In addition, there was a trend to a higher incidence of diabetes among those in the tacrolimus group, but there was no significant difference in graft survival or the total number of infections, or in the incidence of hypertension, chronic kidney disease, or cancer between the 2 groups.

Conclusions.—Tacrolimus is associated with a lower burden of acute rejection and lymphocytic bronchitis and a trend to a greater freedom from BOS stage 0-p than cyclosporine after lung transplantation.

▶ This is an important study because randomized prospective studies, of any type, are rare in lung transplantation. Randomized controlled trials often require multiple centers to complete, since the number of transplants in any one center is usually inadequate to complete randomized studies in a timely manner. One previous single center study comparing the same 2 immunosuppressants concluded that they were not different in terms of acute rejection or survival.[1] The current study is also a single center study and, therefore, has a relatively small number of patients in it (though the authors calculated and reached the number of participants needed to have a power of 80% to detect a 30% reduction in the composite endpoint described in the abstract—with tacrolimus). Although this study seems to indicate that tacrolimus is a better immunosuppressant than cyclosporine, a close look at the outcomes make that implication less clear. In fact, though there is an unusually high rate of acute rejection in the cyclosporine patients, this does not translate into higher rates of clinically important bronchiolitis obliterans syndrome or reduced graft survival. There are also significant complications, including a high rate of diabetes with tacrolimus. Hopefully, this study will be extended a few more years so we can get a better feel for the long-term outcome parameters.

J. R. Maurer, MD, MBA

Reference

1. Keenan RJ, Konishi H, Kawai A, et al. Clinical trial of tacrolimus versus cyclosporine in lung transplantation. *Ann Thorac Surg.* 1995;60:580-585.

35 Chronic Obstructive Pulmonary Disease

Geographic Variation in Chronic Obstructive Pulmonary Disease Exacerbation Rates
Joo MJ, Lee TA, Weiss KB (Hines VA Hosp, IL; Northwestern Univ, Chicago; Univ of Illinois, Chicago)
J Gen Intern Med 22:1560-1565, 2007

Background.—Exacerbations are important disease events for patients with chronic obstructive pulmonary disease (COPD) as they are relatively frequent, result in significant resource use and can indicate worsening disease. Little is known about variation in COPD exacerbation rates across a health system in various geographic regions.

Objective.—To compare COPD exacerbation rates by regional service networks called Veterans Integrated Service Network (VISN) in the Veterans Health Administration (VA) system.

Design.—Retrospective, observational study.

Subjects.—Patients with a COPD diagnosis from October 1999 to September 2000 with follow-up to September 2002.

Measurements.—Acute exacerbations of COPD during the baseline and follow-up periods.

Results.—A total of 198,981 patients were identified. Average exacerbation rate at baseline was 0.503 events per person per year. In the follow-up period, there were 187,686 exacerbations experienced by 87,494 persons (44.0% of cohort). During follow-up, the average adjusted exacerbation rate was 0.589 per person per year and varied from 0.335 (95% CI, 0.328–0.342) in VISN 1 to 0.749 (95% CI, 0.735–0.0763) in VISN 9. Using the median rate of exacerbation during the baseline period as the referent, 9 VISNs had lower adjusted rate ratios and 12 VISNs had higher adjusted rate ratios in the follow-up period.

Conclusions.—Geographic variation in the VA VISN system supports evidence that the medical care system including provider factors, and less so, patient factors affect COPD exacerbations. Understanding the reasons underlying this variation in COPD exacerbation rates may lead to improvements in future care and outcomes.

▶ This review of a large Veterans Health Administration (VA) database presents some very interesting information about variation of exacerbations in patients with chronic obstuctive pulmonary disease (COPD) in different parts of the United States. It is important to note that this variation was present, despite adjustments for baseline exacerbation rates, race, age, comorbidities, health care utilization, and climate. From the lowest exacerbation rate areas (New England) to the highest exacerbation rate areas (Kentucky and Tennessee), there was more than a 2-fold difference. The obvious question: Does this represent variations in the baseline care of these patients? This question must be asked because the number of studies now suggest that the use of inhaled corticosteroids and/or long-acting bronchodilators, and possibly influenza and pneumococcal vaccination, reduce the risk of exacerbations. Previously published reports from other areas of medicine—for example, care of patients with MI—have suggested that variation in care provider in different geographic areas impacts outcomes.[1] Whether or not this is the underlying cause of the difference, the exacerbation rate in this report requires further study. This investigation has several obvious faults. Not only is it a retrospective study, but it also focuses on a select delivery system, the VA and affiliated networks, and therefore may not reflect the broader practice in the various geographic areas. A similar study in the Medicare population, for which large databases also exist, may give a more representative picture of variations in practice in management of COPD if they exist. If they do, we can start to probe into the reasons for these geographic variations in care.

J. R. Maurer, MD, MBA

Reference

1. Krumholz HM, Chen J, Rathore SS, Wang Y, Radford MJ. Regional variation in the treatment and outcomes of myocardial infarction: investigating New England's advantage. *Am Heart J*. 2003;146:242-249.

Impact of Chronic Obstructive Pulmonary Disease on Post-Myocardial Infarction Outcomes

Salisbury AC, Reid KJ, Spertus JA (Mayo Graduate School of Medicine, Rochester, MN; Saint Luke's Hosp, Kansas City, MO; Univ of Missouri-Kansas City)
Am J Cardiol 99:636-641, 2007

Although chronic obstructive pulmonary disease (COPD) is common in patients with myocardial infarction (MI), its association with long-term mortality after MI is controversial and little is known about its influence on patients' health status (symptoms, function, and quality of life). We prospectively enrolled 2,481 patients presenting with MI at 19 United States centers to examine the relations between COPD and patients' long-term mortality, rehospitalization rates, and health status after MI. Patients were administered the disease-specific Seattle Angina Questionnaire and the generic Short Form 12 at baseline and 1 year later. COPD was common (15.6% of patients) and was associated with a substantially greater risk of

1-year mortality (15.8% vs 5.7%, p <0.001) and rehospitalization (48.7% vs 38.6%, p <0.001). After extensive adjustment for baseline differences, patients with COPD had a twofold greater 1-year mortality rate (hazard ratio 2.00, 95% confidence interval [CI] 1.44 to 2.79) and higher rehospitalization rates (hazard ratio 1.22, 95% CI 1.01 to 1.48). Similarly, adjusted 1-year health status was worse in patients with COPD, with lower 1-year Seattle Angina Questionnaire quality-of-life score (−2.53 points, 95% CI −0.25 to −4.81) and Short Form 12 physical component score (−1.83 points, 95% CI −0.43 to −3.24). In addition, COPD was associated with a trend toward a greater prevalence of angina at 1 year (risk ratio 1.12, 95% CI 0.89 to 1.41). In conclusion, patients with COPD have greater mortality, higher rehospitalization rates, and poorer health status 1 year after a MI. Although additional research is needed, clinicians should recognize that patients with COPD are at high risk for poor outcomes after MI.

▶ Although it is generally accepted (and often written about) that comorbidities affect outcomes in patients with chronic illness, specific data are often hard to come by. Thus, this multicenter, prospective observational study designed to assess the impact of a pre-existing diagnosis of chronic obstructive pulmonary disease (COPD) on outcomes of patients suffering a myocardial infarction is welcome and intriguing. The major weakness of the study is that there was no documentation of the COPD diagnosis by spirometry or other means, and no attempts were made to verify historical data documenting the diagnosis so we do not know the severity of disease or even if it was present in all cases. Those shortcomings may not matter because it appears "as if" treating physicians acted on that historical information. In particular, COPD patients were significantly less likely to get percutaneous coronary intervention, have beta blockers started (despite the low risk of exacerbation), less likely to be put on aspirin at discharge, and less likely to be referred for cardiac rehabilitation. Death rates and rehospitalization were significantly higher in the COPD patients. Was it because of their COPD comorbidity, or was it because these patients did not get the same care? Perhaps it was a combination of both. This is an unanswered question that needs more investigation, but treating physicians should be vigilant to ensure that effective care is not withheld simply because a patient has a comorbidity.

J. R. Maurer, MD, MBA

Arterial Stiffness and Osteoporosis in Chronic Obstructive Pulmonary Disease
Sabit R, Bolton CE, Edwards PH, et al (Cardiff Univ, England; Univ Hosp of Wales, Heath Park, Cardiff, England; Univ of Cambridge, England)
Am J Respir Crit Care Med 175:1259-1265, 2007

Rationale.—Chronic obstructive pulmonary disease (COPD) is associated with an increased risk of cardiovascular events and osteoporosis.

Increased arterial stiffness is an independent predictor of cardiovascular disease.

Objectives.—We tested the hypothesis that patients with COPD would have increased arterial stiffness, which would be associated with osteoporosis and systemic inflammation.

Methods.—We studied 75 clinically stable patients with a range of severity of airway obstruction and 42 healthy smoker or ex-smoker control subjects, free of cardiovascular disease. All subjects underwent spirometry, measurement of aortic pulse wave velocity (PWV) and augmentation index, dual-energy X-ray absorptiometry, and blood sampling for inflammatory mediators.

Measurements and Main Results.—Mean (SD) aortic PWV was greater in patients, 11.4 (2.7) m/s, than in control subjects, 8.95 (1.7) m/s, $p < 0.0001$. Inflammatory mediators and augmentation index were also greater in patients. Patients with osteoporosis at the hip had a greater aortic PWV, 13.1 (1.8) m/s, than those without, 11.2 (2.7) m/s, $p < 0.05$. In patients, aortic PWV was related to age ($r = 0.63$, $p < 0.0001$) and $\log_{10}$ IL-6 ($r = 0.31$, $p < 0.01$), and inversely to FEV_1 ($r = -0.34$, $p < 0.01$). The strongest predictors of aortic PWV in all subjects were age ($p < 0.0001$), percent predicted FEV_1 ($p < 0.05$), mean arterial pressure ($p < 0.05$), and $\log_{10}$ IL-6 ($p < 0.05$).

Conclusions.—Increased arterial stiffness was related to the severity of airflow obstruction and may be a factor in the excess risk for cardiovascular disease in COPD. The increased aortic PWV in patients with osteoporosis and the association with systemic inflammation suggest that age-related bone and vascular changes occur prematurely in COPD.

▶ Patients with chronic obstructive pulmonary disease (COPD) are at increased risk of multiple other chronic problems including, for example, cardiovascular disease, osteoporosis, nonpulmonary cancers. These comorbidities are likely related, in part, to the systemic nature of COPD in recent years, confirmed by the high levels of inflammatory markers found in these patients. The exact mechanism involved in the development of comorbid conditions, however, generally remains unknown. This study, performed in stable patients with confirmed COPD, is an attempt to shed some light on why COPD patients have increased rates of atherosclerotic disease. The authors were able to show that even in early disease, there is stiffening of arterial walls and that this was particularly true in patients with osteoporosis and high levels of IL-6, a regulator of C-reactive protein. Although this study still does not shed light on the mechanism of the development of these comorbidities, it does suggest a likely early event in the premature onset of cardiovascular disease is arterial wall stiffening. The authors had a control group of healthy nonsmokers and exsmokers who were shown to have significantly more pliant arterial walls. The next step is to define the mechanism of these changes so they can be addressed early in the disease.

J. R. Maurer, MD, MBA

Determinants of airflow obstruction in severe alpha-1-antitrypsin deficiency
DeMeo DL, Sandhaus RA, Barker AF, et al (Brigham and Women's Hosp, Boston; Natl Jewish Med and Research Ctr, Denver; Oregon Health and Science Univ, Portland; et al)
Thorax 62:806-813, 2007

Background.—Severe α_1-antitrypsin (AAT) deficiency is an autosomal recessive genetic condition associated with an increased, but variable, risk for chronic obstructive pulmonary disease (COPD). A study was undertaken to assess the impact of chronic bronchitis, pneumonia, asthma and sex on the development of COPD in individuals with severe AAT deficiency.

Methods.—The AAT Genetic Modifier Study is a multicentre family-based cohort study designed to study the genetic and epidemiological determinants of COPD in AAT deficiency. 378 individuals (age range 33–80 years), confirmed to be homozygous for the SERPINA1 Z mutation, were included in the analyses. The primary outcomes of interest were a quantitative outcome, forced expiratory volume in 1 s (FEV_1) percentage predicted, and a qualitative outcome, severe airflow obstruction (FEV_1 <50% predicted).

Results.—In multivariate analysis of the overall cohort, cigarette smoking, sex, asthma, chronic bronchitis and pneumonia were risk factors for reduced FEV_1 percentage predicted and severe airflow obstruction ($p<0.01$). Index cases had lower FEV_1 values, higher smoking histories and more reports of adult asthma, pneumonia and asthma before age 16 than non-index cases ($p<0.01$). Men had lower pre- and post-bronchodilator FEV_1 percentage predicted than women ($p<0.0001$); the lowest FEV_1 values were observed in men reporting a history of childhood asthma (26.9%). This trend for more severe obstruction in men remained when index and non-index groups were examined separately, with men representing the majority of non-index individuals with airflow obstruction (71%). Chronic bronchitis (OR 3.8, CI 1.8 to 12.0) and a physician's report of asthma (OR 4.2, CI 1.4 to 13.1) were predictors of severe airflow obstruction in multivariate analysis of non-index men but not women.

Conclusion.—In individuals with severe AAT deficiency, sex, asthma, chronic bronchitis and pneumonia are risk factors for severe COPD, in addition to cigarette smoking. These results suggest that, in subjects severely deficient in AAT, men, individuals with symptoms of chronic bronchitis and/or a past diagnosis of asthma or pneumonia may benefit from closer monitoring and potentially earlier treatment.

▶ Patients who are homozygous for the Z allele (PI ZZ) of the α_1-antitrypsin gene have very low levels of the enzyme, yet there is significant variability in the development of emphysema. The authors of this study looked at a relatively large population of homozygous individuals to try and better understand other risk factors for development of clinical disease. All study subjects were identified as relatives of a known patient with PI ZZ disease. Men, whether they had ever smoked or not, had more severe disease than women, and patients with a history of asthma before age 16 also had more severe disease. A history of pneumonia or chronic bronchitis was also predictive of worse disease. This study is important for a couple of reasons. All individuals included had confirmed PI ZZ disease and, to minimize testing variability, spirometry across participating centers was standardized. The limitations are that diagnoses of asthma and pneumonia were by report only and not verified. The study should encourage physicians who care for PI ZZ patients to be aware of the environmental factors other than smoking that appear to precipitate more severe and more rapid loss of lung function.

J. R. Maurer, MD, MBA

36 Pleural, Interstitial Lung, and Pulmonary Vascular Disease

Transthoracic Echocardiography for Pulmonary Embolism in the ICU: Finding the "Right" Findings
Stawicki SP, Seamon MJ, Kim PK, et al (Univ of Pennsylvania School of Medicine, PA)
J Am Coll Surg 206:42-47, 2008

Background.—Use of transthoracic echocardiography (TTE) in documenting cardiac disorders is well accepted. This study reviews institutional experience with TTE in the clinical setting of pulmonary embolism (PE).

Study Design.—Retrospective review of surgical ICU patients who underwent TTE within 72 hours of diagnosis of PE, from January 2005 to March 2007. Collected data included symptoms, clinical suspicion of PE, preexisting conditions, operative procedures, TTE findings, presence of deep venous thrombosis, and treatments used for PE. Preexisting TTEs, when available, were compared with those obtained after acute PE. TTEs subsequent to the first post-PE study were analyzed for change in severity of findings.

Results.—Thirty-one patients (12 men, 19 women, mean age 66 years, APACHE II 18.1) were included. Twenty-two had high, and nine had moderate, clinical suspicion for PE. Radiographic diagnosis of PE was made by computed tomography (25 of 31) and by ventilation-perfusion scans (6 of 31). Twelve of 31 patients had extremity deep venous thrombosis by duplex ultrasonography. Tricuspid regurgitation was the most common TTE finding (28 of 31), followed by pulmonary hypertension (24), dilated right ventricle (23), right heart strain (19), and underfilled, hyperdynamic left ventricle (17). Seventeen patients had previous or "baseline" echocardiograms, and when compared with the post-PE TTE, all patients demonstrated worsening in at least one TTE finding.

Conclusions.—This study identified findings that can be used in prospective evaluation of TTE for suspected PE. The importance of baseline TTE has also been emphasized. Additional prospective evaluation of TTE in diagnosis of suspected PE in the ICU is warranted.

▶ The above study identifies Echo findings in pulmonary embolism (PE) in acute cases and then compares it with subsequent echo after a period of time. Tricuspid regurgitation, pulmonary hypertension, dilated RV, right heart strain, and underfilled LV are the most common initial findings of PE. All the patients who had baseline PE showed worsening of at least 1 or 2 transthoracic echocardiography (TTE) findings.

M. Ali Raza, MD

Computed Tomographic Pulmonary Angiography vs Ventilation-Perfusion Lung Scanning in Patients With Suspected Pulmonary Embolism: A Randomized Controlled Trial
Anderson DR, Kahn SR, Rodger MA, et al (Dalhousie Univ Halifax, Canada; McGill Univ, Montreal, Quebec, Canada; Ottawa Univ, Ottawa, Ontario; et al)
JAMA 298:2743-2753, 2007

Context.—Ventilation-perfusion $\dot{V}/\dot{Q}$ lung scanning and computed tomographic pulmonary angiography (CTPA) are widely used imaging procedures for the evaluation of patients with suspected pulmonary embolism. Ventilation-perfusion scanning has been largely replaced by CTPA in many centers despite limited comparative formal evaluations and concerns about CTPA's low sensitivity (ie, chance of missing clinically important pulmonary embuli).

Objectives.—To determine whether CTPA may be relied upon as a safe alternative to $\dot{V}/\dot{Q}$ scanning as the initial pulmonary imaging procedure for excluding the diagnosis of pulmonary embolism in acutely symptomatic patients.

Design, Setting, and Participants.—Randomized, single-blinded noninferiority clinical trial performed at 4 Canadian and 1 US tertiary care centers between May 2001 and April 2005 and involving 1417 patients considered likely to have acute pulmonary embolism based on a Wells clinical model score of 4.5 or greater or a positive D-dimer assay result.

Intervention.—Patients were randomized to undergo either $\dot{V}/\dot{Q}$ scanning or CTPA. Patients in whom pulmonary embolism was considered excluded did not receive antithrombotic therapy and were followed up for a 3-month period.

Main Outcome Measure.—The primary outcome was the subsequent development of symptomatic pulmonary embolism or proximal deep vein thrombosis in patients in whom pulmonary embolism had initially been excluded.

Results.—Seven hundred one patients were randomized to CTPA and 716 to $\dot{V}/\dot{Q}$ scanning. Of these, 133 patients (19.2%) in the CTPA group vs 101 (14.2%) in the $\dot{V}/\dot{Q}$ scan group were diagnosed as having pulmonary embolism in the initial evaluation period (difference, 5.0%; 95% confidence interval [CI], 1.1% to 8.9%) and were treated with anticoagulant therapy. Of those in whom pulmonary embolism was considered excluded, 2 of 561 patients (0.4%) randomized to CTPA vs 6 of 611 patients (1.0%) undergoing V̇/Q̇ scanning developed venous thromboembolism in follow-up (difference, −0.6%; 95% CI, −1.6% to 0.3%) including one patient with fatal pulmonary embolism in the V̇/Q̇ group.

Conclusions.—In this study, CTPA was not inferior to V̇/Q̇ scanning in ruling out pulmonary embolism. However, significantly more patients were diagnosed with pulmonary embolism using the CTPA approach. Further research is required to determine whether all pulmonary emboli detected by CTPA should be managed with anticoagulant therapy.

Trial Registration.—isrctn.org Identifier: ISRCTN65486961.

▶ Pulmonary embolism (PE) needs timely and definite evaluation. The dilemma is the chance that we are going to miss it in patients who have PE and go on to have life-threatening complications. The study referenced above is tackling the question of are we better now with mostly doing computed tomographic pulmonary angiography (CTPA) versus old school ventilation-perfusion V̇/Q̇ scan. The results are encouraging and would mean that for acute venous thromboembolism (VTE) CTPA is as good as or even better in some ways to find PE.

There are problems and relative benefits for both the tests. First off, if we are dealing with chronic PE it is likely that CTPA will miss it more often than not. I have seen patients with chronic PE in our pulmonary hypertension center who have "normal" CTPA scans and are found to have large segmental defects found on the V̇/Q̇ scan. Renal failure is another relative contraindication for CTPA. On the other hand, if patient is in respiratory distress V̇/Q̇ scan does take a long time and would be hard to interpret in cases of chronic interstitial lung disease (ILD) and acute pneumonitis. Interpreter experience also matters a lot in both cases.

I believe these tools should be used to our advantage and should complement each other as in the study patients crossed over, but it is good to know that CTPA is as good or better than V̇/Q̇ scan.

M. Ali Raza, MD

BUILD-1: A Randomized Placebo-Controlled Trial of Bosentan in Idiopathic Pulmonary Fibrosis
King TE Jr, Behr J, Brown KK, et al (Univ of California, San Francisco, CA; Medizinische Klinik I, Klinikum Grosshadern der Universität, Munich, Germany; Natl Jewish Med and Res Ctr, Denver, CO; et al)
Am J Respir Crit Care Med 177:75-81, 2008

Rationale.—Idiopathic pulmonary fibrosis (IPF) is a progressive, fatal lung disease lacking effective treatment.

Objectives.—To determine the effects of bosentan on exercise capacity and time to disease progression in patients with IPF.

Methods.—In a double-blind, multicenter trial, patients with IPF were randomized to receive oral bosentan 62.5 mg twice daily for 4 weeks, increased to 125 mg twice daily thereafter, or placebo, for 12 months or longer. The primary efficacy endpoint was change from baseline up to Month 12 in exercise capacity, as measured by a modified six-minute-walk test. Secondary endpoints were time to death or disease progression (worsening pulmonary function tests [PFTs] or acute decompensation), change in PFT scores, and quality of life (QOL) assessed using Short-Form36 and St. George's Respiratory Questionnaire.

Measurements and Main Results.—A total of 158 patients randomly received bosentan (n = 74) or placebo (n = 84). Bosentan showed no superiority over placebo in six-minute-walk distance (6MWD) up to Month 12, the primary efficacy endpoint. A trend in favor of bosentanwas observed in the secondary endpoint of time to death or disease progression (hazard ratio [HR], 0.613; 95% confidence interval [CI], 0.328–1.144; $P = 0.119$), which was more pronounced in a patient subgroup diagnosed using surgical lung biopsy (*post hoc* analysis; HR, 0.315; 95% CI, 0.126–0.789; $P = 0.009$). Changes from baseline up to Month 12 in assessments of dyspnea and QOL favored treatment with bosentan. No unexpected adverse events were reported.

Conclusions.—Bosentan treatment in patients with IPF did not show superiority over placebo on 6MWD. A trend in delayed time to death or disease progression, and improvement in QOL, was observed with bosentan. The more pronounced treatment effect in patients with biopsy-proven IPF warrants further investigation.

Clinical trial registered with www.clinicaltrials.gov (NCT 00071461).

▶ We do not have any proven treatments for idiopathic pulmonary fibrosis (IPF) to improve mortality. There have been many studies trying to look at steroids, γ-interferon, and many more treatment modalities to find any viable treatment, and they have all met the same fate. Bosentan, an endothelin receptor blocker, has been approved for pulmonary arterial hypertension and has been known to have anti-inflammatory properties. In this study, a well-designed trial was done to see the efficacy of bosentan in IPF. I think it comes down to whether you see it from optimistic versus pessimistic point of view. Because the outlook for this particular disease is poor it seems likely that bosentan has a positive effect on quality of life (QOL) in 6 weeks but got insignificant in 12 months. A trend toward lower mortality and decreased disease progression were seen ($P = .009$) in patients with proven diagnosis by open lung biopsy. Six-minute-walk distance increase was less impressive. I believe that IPF is a progressive disease and anything that halts the progression is a viable option and that's why we need to look for the results of bosentan use in interstitial lung disease (BUILD)-3 trial, a large randomized controlled trial (RCT) coming soon.

M. Ali Raza, MD

Prevalence of HIV-related Pulmonary Arterial Hypertension in the Current Antiretroviral Therapy Era

Sitbon O, Lascoux-Combe C, Delfraissy J-F, et al (Hôpital Antoine Béclère, Clamart, France; Hôpital Saint Louis, Paris, France; Hôpital Bicêtre, Le Kremlin Bicêtre, France; et al)
Am J Respir Crit Care Med 177:108-113, 2008

Rationale.—The prevalence of HIV-associated pulmonary arterial hypertension (PAH) has not been evaluated since introduction of combined, highly active antiretroviral treatments.

Objectives.—To establish the current prevalence of PAH in a large HIV-positive population.

Methods.—Prospective study conducted in 7,648 consecutive HIV-positive adults in 14 HIV clinics in France. PAH was identified through screening with a predefined algorithm. Patients with dyspnea unexplained by other causes underwent transthoracic Doppler echocardiography. PAH was suspected if peak velocity of tricuspid regurgitation was greater than 2.5 m/second and was confirmed by right heart catheterization.

Measurements and Main Results.—PAH was diagnosed if mean pulmonary arterial pressure at rest was 25 mm Hg or greater (with pulmonary capillary wedge pressure $\leq$ 15 mm Hg) or 30 mm Hg or greater on exercise. A total of 739 patients had dyspnea, of which 312 met exclusion criteria and 150 refused to participate. Among the remaining 277, 30 had known PAH and 247 had unexplained dyspnea and underwent echocardiography; PAH was suspected in 18 and confirmed in 5, to give a total of 35 cases. The prevalence was thus 0.46% (95% confidence interval, 0.32–0.64%). All new cases had relatively milder PAH.

Conclusions.—The prevalence of HIV-associated PAH is about the same as it was in the early 1990s. Given the current good long-term prognosis of patients with HIV, the severity of PAH in HIV-infected patients, and the absence of predictive factors, careful screening for PAH is warranted for patients with unexplained dyspnea.

▶ It is known that HIV is a risk factor for pulmonary arterial hypertension (PAH). HIV has the highest mortality associated with PAH compared with all the other diseases, including idiopathic PAH, scleroderma, and sickle cell disease.

It is also postulated that viral load has a linear relationship with severity of the pulmonary hypertension and mortality. The above study is showing that even with better diagnostic tools and timely treatment of HIV in these patients, the prevalence of PAH is still the same as it was in the 1990s. It means a lot of things, including aggressive early treatment of PAH in this patient population so we can change the high mortality associated with these 2 diseases.

M. Ali Raza, MD

Clinical Outcome of Patients With Upper-Extremity Deep Vein Thrombosis: Results From the RIETE Registry

Muñoz FJ, Mismetti P, Poggio R, et al (Hosp de Mollet, Barcelona, Spain; Hosp Bellevue, Saint-Etienne, France; Hosp Galliera, Genoa, Italy; et al)
Chest 133:143-148, 2008

Background.—There is little information on the clinical outcome of patients with upper-extremity deep vein thrombosis (DVT).

Methods.—RIETE is an ongoing registry of consecutive patients with objectively confirmed, symptomatic, acute DVT or pulmonary embolism (PE). In this analysis, we analyzed the demographic characteristics, treatment, and 3-month outcome of all patients with DVT in the arm.

Results.—Of the 11,564 DVT patients enrolled, 512 patients (4.4%) had arm DVT. They presented less often with clinically overt PE (9.0% vs 29%; odds ratio, 0.24; 95% confidence interval [CI], 0.18 to 0.33) than those with lower-limb DVT, but their 3-month outcome was similar. Of the 512 patients with arm DVT, 196 patients (38%) had cancer and 228 patients (45%) had catheter-related DVT. During follow-up, those with cancer DVT had an increased incidence of major bleeding (4.1% vs 0.9%; odds ratio, 4.4; 95% CI, 1.2 to 21), recurrent venous thromboembolism (6.1% vs 2.8%; odds ratio, 2.2; 95% CI, 0.91 to 5.6; $p = 0.04$), and death (22% vs 3.5%; odds ratio, 7.8; 95% CI, 4.0 to 16). Thirty patients had the composite event of recurrent DVT, symptomatic PE, or major bleeding. They were significantly older, more often had cancer, and presented more frequently with symptomatic PE on hospital admission. On multivariate analysis, only cancer patients with arm DVT had an increased risk for the composite event (odds ratio, 3.0; 95% CI, 1.4 to 6.4).

Conclusions.—At presentation, patients with arm DVT have less often clinically overt PE than those with lower-limb DVT, but their 3-month outcome is similar. Among patients with arm DVT, those with cancer have the worse outcome.

▶ RIETE registry includes more than 11 500 patients with deep vein thrombosis (DVT). Upper extremity DVT is considered to have very low incidence and not usually seen as a main cause of morbidity. An interesting observation seen in the above study is that almost half (45%) of the upper extremity DVT was associated with central venous catheter insertion, a relatively preventable cause.

We would expect the incidence to be low, but 9% vs 29% is not negligible as an incidence. In patients with cancer, the incidence is higher with increased morbidity. The fact that 3-month outcome for recurrence and symptomatic PE being similar, could be related to the general medical and functional condition of the patient.

There have been studies on upper extremity DVTs and the largest I know is including > 500 patients but no outcome data is available. The above-mentioned study has flaws that every registry observational study is susceptible to but makes a good point.

We should see central venous catheters as a cause of major morbidity like pulmonary embolism (PE)/DVT and try to prevent it. The outcome of symptomatic PE and recurrent PE is the same with cancer patients having upper extremity DVT, so needs to be respected.

M. Ali Raza, MD

Assessment of the pulmonary embolism rule-out criteria rule for evaluation of suspected pulmonary embolism in the emergency department
Wolf SJ, McCubbin TR, Nordenholz KE, et al (Denver Health Med Ctr, CO; Kaiser Permanente/Exempla St Joseph Hosp, Denver, CO; Univ of Colorado Health Sciences Ctr, Denver, CO)
Am J Emerg Med 26:181-185, 2008

Background.—Overuse of resources when evaluating pulmonary embolism (PE) is a concern if the D-dimer assay is improperly used in the evaluation of emergency department patients with suspected PE. The pulmonary embolism rule-out criteria (PERC) rule was derived to prevent unnecessary diagnostic testing in this patient population. The objective of this study was to assess the PERC rule's performance in an external population.

Methods.—This was a secondary analysis of a prospectively collected database comparing PERC rule variables to diagnosis of PE in consecutive patients with suspicion for PE. Bivariate analysis on individual variables and the overall accuracy of the PERC rule were performed.

Results.—Patients on 120 randomly assigned shifts were enrolled with a PE prevalence of 12%. The sensitivity, specificity, positive predictive, and negative predictive values of the PERC rule were 100% (95% confidence interval [CI], 79%-100%), 16% (95% CI, 10%-24%), 14% (95% CI, 8%-14%), and 100% (95% CI, 80%-100%), respectively, for the total patient population, and 100% (95% CI, 25%-100%), 33% (95% CI, 12%-35%), 2% (95% CI, 0%-11%), and 100% (95% CI, 75%-100%), respectively, for the low pretest probability population. Bivariate analysis showed unilateral leg swelling, recent surgery, and a history of venous thromboembolic event to be predictive of the diagnosis of PE.

Conclusions.—The PERC rule may identify a cohort of patients with suspected PE for whom diagnostic testing beyond history and physical examination is not indicated.

▶ We spend a major portion of money in health care on laboratory and radiological tests that are highly unlikely to make the diagnosis of certain diseases. In fact, they are there most of the time to rule out diseases. One of the major examples is computed tomographic (CT) chest with contrast to rule out pulmonary embolism (PE). In addition to the adverse effect rendered by the IVP dye and 250 chest X-ray equivalent radiations to the patient, it is a test that could be avoided easily if certain algorithms are followed. One of those criteria is pulmonary embolism rule-out criteria (PERC) rule that helps rule out PE in patients with suspected PE and prevents them from unnecessary testing. D-dimer as a test with high negative predictive value can also supplement the clinical picture and clinical suspicion of PE. The high sensitivity and low specificity of the PERC rule suggests that we are not going to be missing very many PE/venous thromboembolisms (VTE), but there are a few cases, 7% in one series and 2% in other case reports, showing that nothing is perfect. In the authors' view this rule when applied with a low clinical suspicion and normal D-dimer has a significant role in ruling out PE/VTE. The thought that we may still miss some PE that was there, is priceless.

M. Ali Raza, MD

Computed Tomography Findings in Pathological Usual Interstitial Pneumonia: Relationship to Survival
Sumikawa H, Johkoh T, Colby TV, et al (Osaka Univ Graduate School of Medicine, Japan; Mayo Clinic, Arizona; et al)
Am J Respir Crit Care Med 177:433-439, 2008

Rationale.—Patients with a clinicopathological diagnosis of idiopathic pulmonary fibrosis (IPF) may have typical findings of usual interstitial pneumonia (UIP) on computed tomography (CT) or nonspecific or atypical findings, including those often seen in nonspecific interstitial pneumonia.

Objectives.—The aims of this study were to revisit the high-resolution CT findings of IPF and to clarify the correlation between the CT findings and mortality.

Methods.—The study included 98 patients with a histologic diagnosis of UIP and a clinical diagnosis of IPF. Two observers evaluated the CT findings independently and classified each case into one of the following three categories: (*1*) definite UIP, (*2*) consistent with UIP, or (*3*) suggestive of alternative diagnosis. The correlation between the CT categories and mortality was evaluated using the Kaplan-Meier method and the log-rank test, as well as Cox proportional hazards regression models.

Measurements and Main Results.—Thirty-three of the 98 CT scans were classified as definite UIP, 36 as consistent with UIP, 29 as suggestive of an alternative diagnosis. The mean survival was 45.7, 57.9, and 76.9 months, respectively. There was no significant difference in survival among the three categories (all $P > 0.05$). Traction bronchiectasis and fibrosis scores were significant predictors of outcome (hazard ratios: 1.30 and 1.10, respectively; 95% confidence intervals: 1.18–14.2 and 1.03–1.19, respectively).

Conclusions.—In patients with IPF and UIP pattern on the biopsy, the pattern of abnormality on thin-section CT, whether characteristic of UIP or suggestive of alternative diagnosis, does not influence prognosis. Prognosis is influenced by traction bronchiectasis and fibrosis scores.

▶ Diagnosis of usual interstitial pneumonia (UIP) and trying to isolate it from nonspecific interstitial pneumonia (NSIP) and other interstitial lung diseases is difficult and is fraught with controversy. There are cases with UIP and NSIP or BOOP seen in the same biopsy specimen. Some experts have suggested that it is a continuum rather than single isolated disease, but we know that when we have idiopathic pulmonary fibrosis (IPF) still with the worst prognosis than all the others.

The above retrospective study from Japan is making a few very important points. The fibrotic scores and traction bronchiectasis are the 2 independent factors that will influence mortality regardless of the actual consensus on the diagnosis. This may be related to the lack of interobserver agreement in the other diagnostic criteria, like presence of nodules or thickening of bronchovascular bundles. There is a definite trend toward improved prognosis when the diagnosis is not definite or alternate to IPF.

M. Ali Raza, MD

37 Asthma and Cystic Fibrosis

Clinical Use of Ibuprofen Is Associated with Slower FEV₁ Decline in Children with Cystic Fibrosis

Konstan MW, Schluchter MD, Xue W, et al (Univ School of Medicine, Cleveland, OH)

Am J Respir Crit Care Med 176:1084-1089, 2007

Rationale.—High-dose ibuprofen in a 4-year controlled trial slowed FEV_1 decline in young subjects with cystic fibrosis, but the effectiveness of ibuprofen has not been assessed in a large group of patients treated clinically with this therapy.

Objectives.—To assess the effect of ibuprofen therapy on FEV_1 decline in children and adolescents with cystic fibrosis, using observational data from the Cystic Fibrosis Foundation Patient Registry.

Methods.—The rate of decline in FEV_1 percent predicted over 2–7 years among patients age 6–17 years with $FEV_1 > 60\%$ predicted, and who were treated with ibuprofen (1,365), was compared with patients of similar age and disease severity who were not treated with this therapy (8,960). Multi-level repeated-measures mixed-regression models were used to estimate rates of decline, adjusting for characteristics and therapies that influenced FEV_1 decline. Adverse effects were compared among those treated versus not treated with ibuprofen.

Measurements and Main Results.—FEV_1 declined less rapidly among patients treated with ibuprofen (difference, 0.60% predicted per year; 95% confidence interval, 0.31 to 0.89; $P < 0.0001$); a 29% reduction in slope based on an average decline of 2.08% predicted per year for patients not treated. Those treated with ibuprofen were more likely to have an episode of gastrointestinal bleeding requiring hospitalization, but the occurrence was rare in both groups (annual incidence, 0.37 vs. 0.14%; relative risk, 2.72; $P < 0.001$).

Conclusions.—Slower rates of FEV_1 decline are seen in children and adolescents with cystic fibrosis who are treated with ibuprofen. The apparent benefits of ibuprofen therapy outweigh the small risk of gastrointestinal bleeding.

▶ In cystic fibrosis, FEV_1 decline predicts survival. Hence measures to limit lung destruction and progressive FEV_1 decline are important goals in treatment. In an article published by Konstan and colleagues, high dose ibuprofen slowed the decline in FEV_1 in subjects with cystic fibrosis. However, since its publication newer drugs have developed for cystic fibrosis treatment, and hence the current effect of ibuprofen on FEV_1 decline is not well understood. Using the Cystic Fibrosis Foundation Registry, data was obtained from over 17 000 patients ages 6 to 17 years old with moderate or better airflow obstruction from multiple CF centers from 1996 to 2002. The use of ibuprofen was associated with a significantly slower decline in FEV_1 compared with the nontreated group after adjusting for confounders. Although gastrointestinal bleeding was significantly higher (a 2-fold increased risk) in the treated group, overall incidence was quite low. An interesting finding was the faster FEV_1 decline in children with CF treated with inhaled tobramycin and/or dornase alfa, which may represent a bias as those who are sicker are more likely to receive these drugs. Several points not addressed are inherent limitations when using registry data. What is the ideal dose of ibuprofen? What was the adherence to therapy? Causality to the findings of decline in FEV_1 with use of inhaled tobramycin and/or dornase alfa nor increased risk of gastrointestinal bleeding cannot be established. Overall, this study favors the use of ibuprofen in children with CF with mild-moderate disease with a benefit of slower FEV_1 decline with a small risk of gastrointestinal bleeding.

S. F. Jones, MD

Randomised placebo controlled trial of non-invasive ventilation for hypercapnia in cystic fibrosis

Young AC, Wilson JW, Kotsimbos TC, et al (Alfred Hosp, Melbourne, Australia; et al)
Thorax 63:72-77, 2008

Background.—The clinical benefits of domiciliary non-invasive positive pressure ventilation (NIV) have not been established in cystic fibrosis (CF). We studied the effects of nocturnal NIV on quality of life (QoL), functional and physiological outcomes in CF subjects with awake hypercapnia (arterial carbon dioxide pressure Pa_{CO_2}>45 mm Hg).

Methods.—In a randomised, placebo controlled, crossover study, eight subjects with CF, mean (SD) age 37 (8) years, body mass index 21.1 (2.6) kg/m², forced expiratory volume in 1 s 35 (8)% predicted and $PaCO_2$ 52 (4) mm Hg received 6 weeks of nocturnal (1) air (placebo), (2) oxygen and (3) NIV. The primary outcome measures were CF specific QoL, daytime sleepiness and exertional dyspnoea. Secondary outcome measures were awake and asleep gas exchange, sleep architecture, lung function and peak exercise capacity.

Results.—Compared with air, NIV improved the chest symptom score in the CF QoL Questionnaire (mean difference 10; 95% CI 5 to 16; p = 0.002) and the transitional dyspnoea index score (mean difference 3.1; 95% CI 1.2-5.0; p = 0.01). It reduced maximum nocturnal pressure of transcutaneous CO_2 ($PtcCO_2$ mean difference -17 mm Hg; 95% CI

-7 to -28 mm Hg; $p = 0.005$) and increased exercise performance on the Modified Shuttle Test (mean difference 83 m; 95% CI 21 to 144 m; $p = 0.02$). NIV did not improve sleep architecture, lung function or awake $PaCO_2$.

Conclusion.—6 weeks of nocturnal NIV improves chest symptoms, exertional dyspnoea, nocturnal hypoventilation and peak exercise capacity in adult patients with stable CF with awake hypercapnia. Further studies are required to determine whether or not NIV can improve survival.

▶ Noninvasive ventilation (NIV) has been used in a number of settings. In the acute setting, such as exacerbation of chronic obstructive pulmonary disease (COPD) complicated by respiratory acidosis and hypercarbia, studies have shown positive outcomes with reduction in mortality and length of hospital stay. However, nocturnal noninvasive ventilation in stable COPD has not been as promising. The investigators in this study have attempted to address similar issues in 8 stable hypercarbic cystic fibrosis patients. By using a randomized placebo-controlled crossover design, investigators aim to identify improvements in exercise tolerance, dyspnea, quality of life, blood gas analysis, and sleep parameters while comparing air versus oxygen versus noninvasive ventilation.

Although the study is very small (7/8 subjects were able to complete all arms), the findings are interesting. NIV improved dyspnea and exercise measures and nocturnal transcutaneous CO_2 with an average of 4.3 hours of use per night. Daytime hypercarbia was not affected. One plausible reason in improvement is the reduction in work of breathing that NIV may provide, but this study was not designed to determine causality.

My concern in this study is the lack of sham or placebo NIV. Before NIV is recommended in stable CF, further research needs to be conducted with a larger sample and same clinical measures to include survival and even exacerbation rate.

S. F. Jones, MD

Adherence to treatment by patients with asthma or COPD: Comparison between inhaled drugs and transdermal patch

Tamura G, Ohta K (Airway Inst in Sendai, Japan; Teikyo Univ, Tokyo)
Respir Med 101:1895-1902, 2007

An Internet-based questionnaire study involving patients with asthma and chronic obstructive pulmonary disease (COPD) and parents of children with asthma was conducted to evaluate adherence to treatment and convenience of inhalation and transdermal formulations. Valid responses were obtained from 1470 patients. Among asthmatic patients, the percentage of those who selected "taking as prescribed" was 52.7% for inhalant users and 83.2% for transdermal users. Among patients with COPD, the corresponding values were 54.7% and 86.6%. There was a significant difference $(p < 0.01)$ in treatment compliance between inhalation and transdermal formulations in both groups. The most common reason for poor adherence was "frequency of administration", and 83.2% of the patients preferred a once-daily administration. In addition, patients who had used both types of formulations preferred the transdermal ones. In conclusion, health care professionals should further educate their patients about the importance of treatment with inhalants, since poor adherence to treatment with inhalation formulations significantly hinders achievement of optimal efficacy. In addition, transdermal tulobuterol patch, which is administered once daily as a long-acting, β_2-agonist, appeared to be useful for long-term control of both asthma and COPD.

▶ The authors conducted an Internet based questionnaire and received results from a large number of asthmatic and chronic obstructive pulmonary disease (COPD) patients who were receiving either inhaled beta agonists or trans-dermal long acting beta agonists (LABA). A significant difference was noted between the adherence of subjects using transdermal LABA (83.2% asthmatics; 86.6% COPD), versus inhaled beta agonists (57.7% asthmatics; 54.7% COPD), $P < 0.01$ for both. Reasons cited most often for nonadherence to medical therapy by surveyed subjects included method of administration, frequency of administration, and timing of administration. Practitioners must educate patients about the need for adherence to therapy for asthma and COPD. In the event that optimal adherence cannot be achieved, and particularly when disease control is faltering, consideration may be given to the use of transder-mally applied agents, keeping in mind that certain transdermally applied agents may be difficult to tolerate.

S. K. Willsie, DO

The Use of Household Cleaning Sprays and Adult Asthma: An International Longitudinal Study

Zock J-P, Plana E, Jarvis D, et al (Municipal Inst of Med Research, Barcelona; Imperial College, London; Pompeu Fabra Univ, Barcelona; et al)
Am J Respir Crit Care Med 176:735-741, 2007

Rationale.—Cleaning work and professional use of certain cleaning products have been associated with asthma, but respiratory effects of nonprofessional home cleaning have rarely been studied.

Objectives.—To investigate the risk of new-onset asthma in relation to the use of common household cleaners.

Methods.—Within the follow-up of the European Community Respiratory Health Survey in 10 countries, we identified 3,503 persons doing the cleaning in their homes and who were free of asthma at baseline. Frequency of use of 15 types of cleaning products was obtained in a face-to-face interview at follow-up. We studied the incidence of asthma defined as physician diagnosis and as symptoms or medication usage at

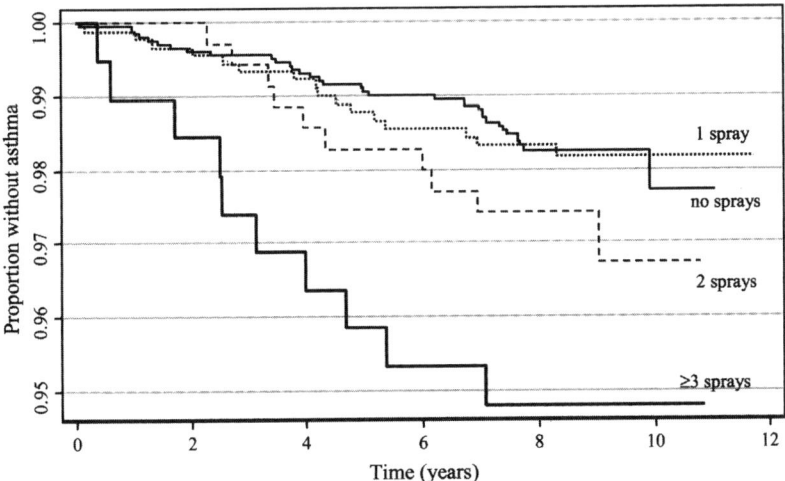

FIGURE 1.—Kaplan-Meier survival curve for physician-diagnosed asthma according to the number of sprays used at least weekly. Onset of disease was defined as date of first attack of asthma. (Reprinted from Zock J-P, Plana E, Jarvis D, et al. The use of household cleaning sprays and adult asthma: an international longitudinal study. *Am J Respir Crit Care Med.* 2007;176:735-741, Official Journal of the American Thoracic Society © American Thoracic Society.)

follow-up. Associations between asthma and the use of cleaning products were evaluated using multivariable Cox proportional hazards or log-binomial regression analysis.

Measurements and Main Results.—The use of cleaning sprays at least weekly (42% of participants) was associated with the incidence of asthma symptoms or medication (relative risk [RR], 1.49; 95% confidence interval [CI], 1.12–1.99) and wheeze (RR, 1.39; 95% CI, 1.06–1.80). The incidence of physician-diagnosed asthma was higher among those using sprays at least 4 days per week (RR, 2.11; 95% CI, 1.15–3.89). These associations were consistent for subgroups and not modified by atopy. Dose–response relationships ($P < 0.05$) were apparent for the frequency of use and the number of different sprays. Risks were predominantly found for the commonly used glass-cleaning, furniture, and air-refreshing sprays. Cleaning products not applied in spray form were not associated with asthma.

Conclusions.—Frequent use of common household cleaning sprays may be an important risk factor for adult asthma (Fig 1).

▶ This is an international cohort of 3503 participants from the European Community Respiratory Health Survey who were free of asthma at the time of the original survey but who were responsible for cleaning their homes. A face-to-face interview was conducted with each subject to determine the frequency of use of 15 different types of cleaning products, as well as physician-diagnosis of asthma and symptoms of asthma at follow-up. Increased risk of development of asthma was found for commonly used glass-cleaning, and furniture and air-freshner sprays. Use of nonspray cleaners did not increase the risk of development of asthma. This is the first known study showing that the use of household cleaning products in spray form by nonprofessionals is associated with new-onset asthma in adults. Precautions should be taken by the public when using these items, and health care providers should begin to educate their patients of the attendant risks of the use of spray cleaners.

S. K. Willsie, DO

A Comprehensive Analysis of Adverse Obstetric and Pediatric Complications in Women with Asthma

Tata LJ, Lewis SA, McKeever TM, et al (Univ of Nottingham, England; London School of Hygiene and Tropical Medicine, London)
Am J Respir Crit Care Med 175:991-997, 2007

Rationale.—Previous studies have raised concern that women with asthma have increased risks of adverse obstetric and pediatric complications, but these have generally been underpowered.

Objectives.—To quantify risks of major adverse pregnancy outcomes and obstetric complications in women with and without asthma.

Methods.—We extracted information on 281,019 pregnancies from the Health Improvement Network database between 1988 and 2004. We analyzed the data using logistic regression.

Measurements and Main Results.—In 37,585 pregnancies of women with asthma compared with 243,434 pregnancies of women without asthma, risks of stillbirth and therapeutic abortion were similar; however, the risk of miscarriage was slightly higher (odds ratio [OR], 1.10; 95% confidence interval [CI], 1.06–1.13). Risks of most obstetric complications (placental abruption, placental insufficiency, placenta previa, preeclampsia, hypertension, gestational diabetes, thyroid disorders in pregnancy, and assisted delivery) were not higher in pregnancies of women with asthma compared with those without asthma, with the exception of increases in antepartum (OR, 1.20; 95% CI, 1.08–1.34) or postpartum (OR, 1.38; 95% CI, 1.21–1.57) hemorrhage, anemia (OR, 1.06; 95% CI, 1.01–1.12), depression (OR, 1.52; 95% CI, 1.36–1.69), and caesarean section (OR, 1.11; 95% CI, 1.07–1.16). Risks of miscarriage, depression, and caesarean section increased moderately in women with more severe asthma and previous asthma exacerbations.

Conclusions.—We found some increased risks in women with asthma that need to be considered in the future; however, our results indicate that women with asthma have similar reproductive risks compared with women without asthma in the general population for most of the range of outcomes studied (Tables 4 and 5).

▶ This study involved extraction of data on 281 019 pregnancies from the Health Improvement Network database; 37 585 represented pregnancies of asthmatics. Results for pregnant asthmatics were compared with 243 434

TABLE 4.—Association of Asthma Severity and Exacerbations in the Year Before Pregnancy with Pregnancy Outcomes

Pregnancy Outcome	Unmedicated Asthma ($n = 23,898$)	SABA-Medicated Asthma ($n = 4,838$)	ICS/LABA-Medicated Asthma ($n = 8,849$)	No Exacerbations ($n = 34,990$)	≥ 1 Exacerbation ($n = 2,595$)
			Adjusted Odds Ratio* (95% CI) for Pregnancy Outcomes		
Live birth	1.03 (1.00–1.06)	0.87† (0.81–0.93)	0.90† (0.86–0.95)	0.99 (0.97–1.02)	0.78† (0.72–0.85)
Stillbirth	0.98 (0.78–1.23)	1.17 (0.75–1.82)	1.10 (0.79–1.55)	1.02 (0.84–1.23)	1.28 (0.72–2.28)
Miscarriage	1.03 (0.99–1.08)	1.14† (1.05–1.24)	1.24† (1.17–1.32)	1.08† (1.05–1.12)	1.28† (1.15–1.43)
Therapeutic abortion	0.93† (0.89–0.96)	1.10† (1.02–1.20)	0.95 (0.89–1.01)	0.94† (0.91–0.97)	1.16†(1.04–1.30)

Definition of abbreviations: CI = confidence interval; ICS/LABA = inhaled corticosteroid with or without long-acting β-agonist therapy; SABA = short-acting β-agonist therapy.
*Reference group is pregnancies in women with no asthma (n = 243,434). Odds ratios adjusted for maternal age, smoking habit, and body mass index.
†p < 0.05.
(Reprinted from Tata LJ, Lewis SA, McKeever TM, et al. A comprehensive analysis of adverse obstetric and pediatric complications in women with asthma. *Am J Respir Crit Care Med.* 2007;175:991-997. Official Journal of the American Thoracic Society © American Thoracic Society.)

TABLE 5.—Association of Asthma Severity and Exacerbations in the Year Before Pregnancy with Obstetric Complications

| | Adjusted Odds Ratios* (95% CI) for Obstetric Complications | | | | |
| | Pregnancies by Asthma Severity | | | Pregnancies by Exacerbation | |
Obstetric Complication	Unmedicated Asthma (n = 17,604)	SABA-Medicated Asthma (n = 3,409)	ICS/LABA-Medicated Asthma (n = 6,305)	No Exacerbations (n = 25,541)	≥ 1 Exacerbation (n = 1,777)
Antepartum hemorrhage	1.17† (1.02–1.33)	1.22 (0.93–1.60)	1.27† (1.04–1.55)	1.19† (1.06–1.33)	1.33 (0.93–1.91)
Postpartum hemorrhage	1.47† (1.27–1.71)	1.56† (1.13–2.16)	1.01 (0.75–1.35)	1.42† (1.24–1.62)	0.83 (0.46–1.52)
Placental abruption	1.00 (0.60–1.67)	1.26 (0.47–3.41)	1.21 (0.56–2.60)	0.99 (0.64–1.52)	2.44 (0.89–6.66)
Placenta previa	0.85 (0.49–1.45)	2.02 (1.00–4.10)	1.18 (0.61–2.28)	0.92 (0.60–1.39)	3.24† (1.53–6.88)
Preeclampsia or eclampsia	1.19 (0.96–1.48)	0.96 (0.58–1.60)	1.00 (0.69–1.45)	1.15 (0.96–1.39)	0.58 (0.24–1.41)
Hypertension during pregnancy	1.04 (0.88–1.22)	0.96 (0.68–1.37)	0.95 (0.73–1.23)	1.00 (0.88–1.15)	1.04 (0.66–1.62)
Diabetes during pregnancy	1.08 (0.87–1.33)	0.63 (0.36–1.11)	1.05 (0.79–1.41)	1.00 (0.84–1.18)	1.22 (0.74–2.01)
Anemia during pregnancy	1.07 (1.00–1.14)	1.04 (0.91–1.19)	1.08 (0.97–1.19)	1.07† (1.01–1.12)	1.04 (0.86–1.25)
Thyroid disorder during pregnancy	0.92 (0.69–1.24)	1.19 (0.68–2.07)	2.03† (1.46–2.81)	1.19 (0.95–1.48)	1.79 (0.98–3.27)
Depression during pregnancy	1.47† (1.29–1.68)	1.49† (1.15–1.94)	1.64† (1.36–1.97)	1.47† (1.32–1.64)	2.06† (1.53–2.78)
Caesarean section pregnancy	1.09† (1.03–1.14)	1.03 (0.93–1.14)	1.24† (1.15–1.33)	1.10† (1.06–1.14)	1.37† (1.22–1.55)
Assisted delivery	1.03 (0.97–1.10)	1.14 (1.00–1.31)	1.06 (0.96–1.18)	1.05 (0.99–1.10)	1.13 (0.94–1.36)

Definition of abbreviations: CI = confidence interval; ICA/LABA = inhaled corticosteroid with or without long-acting β-agonist therapy; SABA = short-acting β-agonist therapy.
*Reference group is pregnancies in women with no asthma (n = 180,325). Odds ratios adjusted for maternal age, smoking habit, and body mass index.
†p < 0.05.
(Reprinted from Tata LJ, Lewis SA, McKeever TM, et al. A comprehensive analysis of adverse obstetric and pediatric complications in women with asthma. *Am J Respir Crit Care Med.* 2007;175:991-997, Official Journal of the American Thoracic Society © American Thoracic Society.)

pregnancies not complicated by asthma. As opposed to previous smaller studies reported in the literature, this analysis showed that the risks of stillbirth and therapeutic abortion were similar between asthmatics and nonasthmatics; the risk of miscarriage was slightly higher for asthmatic pregnancies (OR: 1.10; 95% CI 1.06-1.13). Risks of antepartum and postpartum depression were higher in pregnant asthmatics versus controls, as was the incidence of cesarean section (primarily increased in women with more severe asthma or previous asthma exacerbations). This study provides some reassurance for asthmatics considering pregnancy and for the health care providers who will care for them.

S. K. Willsie, DO

Treating Asthma and Comorbid Allergic Rhinitis in Pregnancy
Yawn B, Knudtson M (Univ of Minnesota, Rochester; Univ of California at Irvine)
J Am Board Fam Med 20:289-298, 2007

Women with severe or uncontrolled asthma are at higher risk for pregnancy complications and adverse fetal outcomes than women with well-controlled asthma. Recent evidence-based guidelines have concluded that it is safer for pregnant women with asthma to be treated pharmacologically than to continue to have asthma symptoms and exacerbations. According to the Asthma and Pregnancy Working Group (APWG) of the National Asthma Education and Prevention Program, optimal treatment of asthma during pregnancy includes treatment of comorbid allergic rhinitis (AR), which can trigger or aggravate asthma symptoms. In general, treatment of both asthma and AR during pregnancy should follow the same stepwise approach that is used in the general population. This article presents the specific recommendations from the most recent APWG report and from other systematic reviews about which asthma and allergic rhinitis drugs should be preferred during pregnancy. Of the corticosteroids, budesonide has the most data and is listed as Pregnancy Category B (no evidence of risk in humans). Other inhaled and intranasal corticosteroids have less data and are listed as Pregnancy Category C but may be continued during pregnancy if the patient's asthma was well controlled with the medication before pregnancy. Family physicians should help their patients control allergic rhinitis and asthma during pregnancy, encouraging adherence to needed medications.

▶ This is a review of recently published evidence-based guidelines related to the treatment of asthma and comorbid allergic rhinitis (AR) during pregnancy. Drug classification for asthma and AR are presented. As noted by others, when a patient is well-controlled and in pre-pregnancy on asthma or AR drugs without known teratogenic effects, it might be wisest to maintain asthma control/previous medicines after the diagnosis of pregnancy.

S. K. Willsie, DO

A Study to Evaluate Safety And Efficacy of Mepolizumab in Patients With Moderate Persistent Asthma

Flood-Page P, Swenson C, Faiferman I, et al (Royal Gwent Hosp, Newport, UK; Univ of Wisconsin-Madison, WI; Respiratory and Inflammation Discovery Medicine, Greenford, UK; et al)

Am J Respir Crit Care Med 176:1062-1071, 2007

Rationale.—Accumulation of eosinophils in the bronchial mucosa of individuals with asthma is considered to be a central event in the pathogenesis of asthma. In animal models, airway eosinophil recruitment and airway hyperresponsiveness in response to allergen challenge are reduced by specific targeting of interleukin-5. A previous small dose-finding study found that mepolizumab, a humanized anti-interleukin-5 monoclonal antibody, had no effect on allergen challenge in humans.

Objectives.—To investigate the effect of three intravenous infusions of mepolizumab, 250 or 750 mg at monthly intervals, on clinical outcome measures in 362 patients with asthma experiencing persistent symptoms despite inhaled corticosteroid therapy (400–1,000 µg of beclomethasone or equivalent).

Methods.—Multicenter, randomized, double-blind, placebo-controlled study.

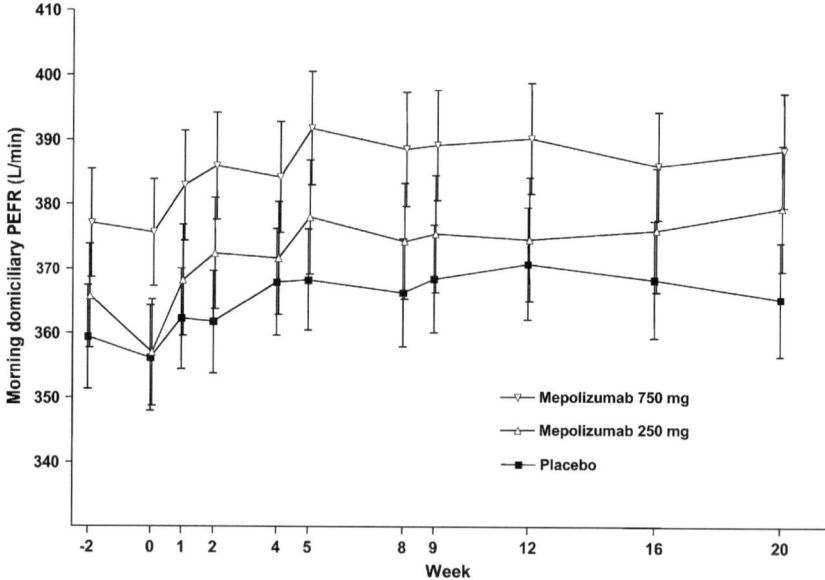

FIGURE 3.—Mean (SEM) values for morning domiciliary peak expiratory flow rate (PEFR; L/min). (Reprinted from Flood-Page P, Swenson C, Faiferman I, et al. A study to evaluate safety and efficacy of mepolizumab in patients with moderate persistent asthma. *Am J Respir Crit Care Med.* 2007;176:1062-1071. Official Journal of the American Thoracic Society © American Thoracic Society.)

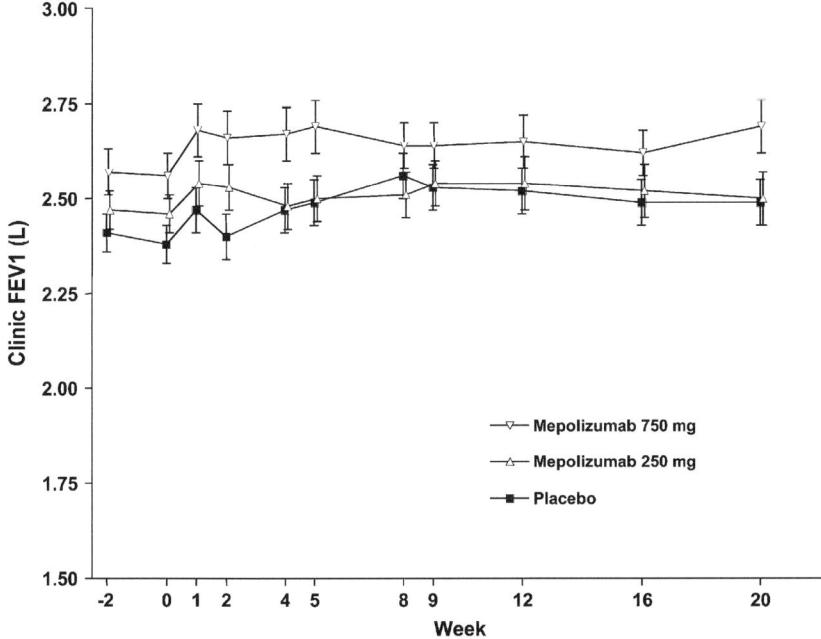

FIGURE 4.—Mean (SEM) values for clinic FEV_1 (L). (Reprinted from Flood-Page P, Swenson C, Faiferman I, et al. A study to evaluate safety and efficacy of mepolizumab in patients with moderate persistent asthma. *Am J Respir Crit Care Med.* 2007;176:1062-1071. Official Journal of the American Thoracic Society © American Thoracic Society.)

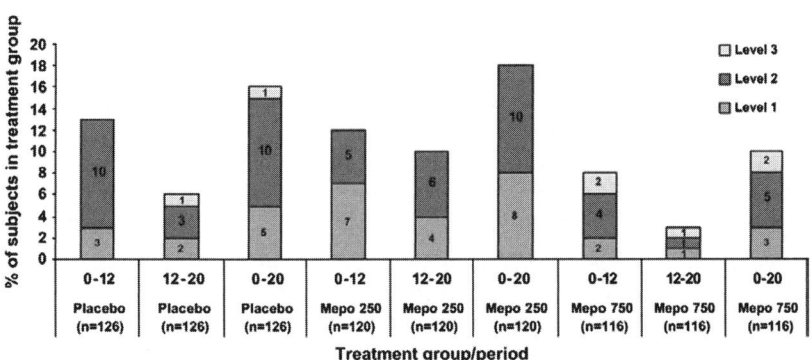

FIGURE 6.—Percentage of exacerbations by level of severity, within each treatment group, by period in the study (each subject was counted only once, at the highest level of severity). Mepo = mepolizumab. (Reprinted from Flood-Page P, Swenson C, Faiferman I, et al. A study to evaluate safety and efficacy of mepolizumab in patients with moderate persistent asthma. *Am J Respir Crit Care Med.* 2007;176:1062-1071. Official Journal of the American Thoracic Society © American Thoracic Society.)

Measurements and Main Results.—Morning peak expiratory flow, forced expiratory volume in 1 second, daily β_2-agonist use, symptom scores, exacerbation rates, and quality of life measures. Sputum eosinophil levels were also measured in a subgroup of 37 individuals. Mepolizumab was associatedwith a significant reduction in blood and sputum eosinophils in both treatment groups (blood, $P < 0.001$ for both doses; sputum, $P = 0.006$ for 250 mg and $P = 0.004$ for 750 mg). There were no statistically significant changes in any of the clinical end points measured. There was a nonsignificant trend for decrease in exacerbation rates in themepolizumab 750-mg treatment group ($P = 0.065$).

Conclusions.—Mepolizumab treatment does not appear to add significant clinical benefit in patients with asthma with persistent symptoms despite inhaled corticosteroid therapy. Further studies are needed to investigate the effect of mepolizumab on exacerbation rates, using protocols specifically tailored to patients with asthma with persistent airway eosinophilia (Figs 3, 4 and 6).

▶ This is a randomized, double-blind, placebo controlled study of 3 doses of 250 mg and 750 mg of mepolizumab compared with placebo. All subjects received inhaled corticosteroids (ICS). Despite statistically significant reductions in eosinophils in both blood and sputum, no significant differences were noted in endpoints (pulmonary function; symptom scores). In the group receiving the 750 mg dosing of M, there was a trend toward reduced exacerbations versus placebo ($P = 0.065$) (study was underpowered). No significant benefit was observed in administration of this selective IL-5 monoclonal antibody to asthmatics receiving ICS. Application of this therapy to all comers of asthmatics on ICS is not indicated. Only additional research will determine whether or not a subset of asthma (eg, those with persistent airway eosinophilia) may benefit from this therapy.

S. K. Willsie, DO

Body mass index and asthma severity in the National Asthma Survey
Taylor B, Mannino D, Brown C, et al (Emory Univ, Atlanta, GA; Univ of Kentucky, Lexington; Ctrs for Disease Control and Prevention, Atlanta, GA)
Thorax 63:14-20, 2008

Background.—The association between obesity and asthma severity remains controversial and limited to small studies.

Methods.—We determined the association of body mass index (BMI) and asthma severity in the National Asthma Survey. We included adults (age ≥18 years) who self-reported symptoms of asthma in the past 5 years. A total of 3095 patients were divided into the following BMI categories: 1080 (35%) non-overweight (BMI <25), 993 (32%) overweight (BMI ≥25 and <30) and 1022 (33%) obese (BMI ≥30). Asthma severity measures included respiratory symptoms, healthcare utilisation, medication use, missed work days and the Global Initiative for Asthma (GINA) severity classification. Models were adjusted for: gender, race, age, education, income, employment status, smoking status, family history of asthma, state of residence and residence in a metropolitan statistical area.

Results.—Compared with non-overweight subjects, obese subjects with asthma were more likely to report continuous symptoms (OR 1.66, 95% CI 1.09 to 2.54), miss more work days (OR 1.35, 95% CI 1.01 to 1.81), use short acting beta agonists (OR 1.36, 95% CI 1.06 to 1.75), use inhaled corticosteroids (OR 1.34, 95% CI 1.01 to 1.79) and use any controller medication according to GINA guidelines (OR 1.37, 95% CI 1.01 to 1.85). Also, obese respondents were less likely to be in asthma remission (OR 0.56, 95% CI 0.38 to 0.82) and were more likely to have severe persistent asthma (GINA IV) (OR 1.42, 95% CI 1.05 to 1.90).

Conclusions.—In a large, diverse sample of adults with asthma, obesity was associated with measures of asthma severity after adjusting for potential confounders.

▶ This database study, using the National Asthma Survey, evaluates adults with symptoms of asthma for > 5 years. Nonoverweight, overweight (BMI > 25 but < 30), and obese (≥30) were compared using reported asthma symptoms, health care use/events, missed work days, and Global Initiative for Asthma (GINA) severity classification. Contribution of race, gender, education, income, employment status, smoking history, and family history were evaluated. Obese asthmatics more commonly reported continuous symptoms, were less likely to experience asthma remission, and more likely to have severe persistent asthma according to GINA guidelines. These results persisted even after adjusting for potential confounders/comorbid conditions. The investigators rightfully conclude that obese asthmatics deserve mandatory weight control counseling/efforts in addition to appropriate asthma therapy.

S. K. Willsie, DO

38 Sleep Disorders

Efficacy of Adaptive Servoventilation in Treatment of Complex and Central Sleep Apnea Syndromes

Allam JS, Olson EJ, Gay PC, et al (Mayo Clinic, Rochester, MN; et al)

Chest 132:1839-1846, 2007

Background.—Complex sleep apnea syndrome (CompSAS) is recognized by the concurrence of mixed or obstructive events with central apneas, the latter predominating on exposure to continuous positive airway pressure (CPAP). Treatment of CompSAS or central sleep apnea (CSA) syndrome with adaptive servoventilation (ASV) is now an option, but no large series exist describing the application and effectiveness of ASV.

Methods.—Retrospective chart review of the first 100 patients who underwent polysomnography using ASV at Mayo Clinic Sleep Center.

Results.—ASV titration was performed for CompSAS (63%), CSA (22%), or CSA/Cheyne Stokes breathing patterns (15%). The median diagnostic sleep apnea hypopnea index (AHI) was 48 events per hour (range, 24 to 62). With CPAP, obstructive apneas decreased, but the appearance of central apneas maintained the AHI at 31 events per hour (range, 17 to 47) [p = 0.02]. With bilevel positive airway pressure (BPAP) in spontaneous mode, AHI trended toward worsening vs baseline, with a median of 75 events per hour (range, 46 to 111) [p = 0.055]. BPAP with a backup rate improved the AHI to 15 events per hour (range, 11 to 31) [p = 0.002]. Use of ASV dramatically improved the AHI to a mean of 5 events per hour (range, 1 to 11) vs baseline and vs CPAP (p < 0.0001). ASV also resulted in an increase in rapid eye movement sleep vs baseline and CPAP (18% vs 12% and 10%, respectively; p < 0.0001). Overall, 64 patients responded to the ASV treatment with a mean AHI < 10 events per hour. Of the 44 successful survey follow-up patients contacted, 32 patients reported some improvement in sleep quality.

Conclusion.—The ASV device appears to be an effective treatment of both CompSAS and CSA syndromes that are resistant to CPAP.

▶ The authors describe their findings in the first 100 subjects that used adaptive servo ventilation in the treatment of central sleep apnea (CSA), CSA with Cheyne-Stokes respirations (CSA/CSR), and complex apnea. Although the retrospective nature weakens the study, adaptive servo ventilation seemed to fare better than bilevel positive airway pressure (BPAP), bilevel positive airway pressure spontaneous and timed mode (BPAP-S/T), and continuous positive airway pressure (CPAP) with oxygen in treatment of complex apnea. What is

345

an interesting finding in this study is that only 53% of patients who had a successful adaptive servoventilation (ASV) trial actually received ASV. The authors did not comment on potential explanations to this finding. Perhaps, it is because the modality is not widely accepted as useful, the expense, or the availability to the patient. What would also be interesting is speculation on the lack of success of this device. The median end expiratory pressure of 8 (range 5-10) was noted in this study. In my opinion, some patients need a higher end expiratory pressure to control the obstructive events. Further investigation in the use of ASV is needed.

S. F. Jones, MD

Long-term Effect of Continuous Positive Airway Pressure on BP in Patients With Hypertension and Sleep Apnea
Campos-Rodriguez F, Perez-Ronchel J, Grilo-Reina A, et al(Valme Univ Hosp, Sevilla, Spain)
Chest 132:1847-1852, 2007

Objective.—To analyze the long-term effect of continuous positive airway pressure (CPAP) on ambulatory BP in patients with obstructive sleep apnea (OSA) and hypertension, and to identify subgroups of patients for whom CPAP could be more effective.

Methods.—We conducted a prospective, long-term follow-up trial (24 months) in 55 patients with OSA and hypertension (mean CPAP use, 5.3 ± 1.9 h/d [$\pm$ SD]). Twenty-four-hour ambulatory BP monitoring (ABPM) was measured at baseline and after intervention with CPAP on an intention-to-treat basis. In addition, the correlation between the changes in 24-h mean arterial pressure (24hMAP) and CPAP compliance, OSA severity, and baseline ABPM was assessed.

Results.—At the end of follow-up, a significant decrease was shown only in diastolic BP (− 2.2 mm Hg; 95% confidence interval [CI], − 4.2 to − 0.1; $p = 0.03$) but not in 24hMAP or other ABPM parameters. However, a correlation between changes in 24hMAP and baseline systolic BP ($r = -0.43$, $p = 0.001$), diastolic BP ($r = -0.38$, $p = 0.004$), and hours of use of CPAP ($r = -0.30$, $p = 0.02$) was observed. A significant decrease in the 24hMAP was achieved in a subgroup of patients with incompletely controlled hypertension at entry (− 4.4 mm Hg; 95% CI, − 7.9 to − 0.9 mm Hg; $p = 0.01$), as well as in those with CPAP compliance > 5.3 h/d (− 5.3 mm Hg; 95% CI, − 9.5 to − 1.2 mm Hg; $p = 0.01$). Linear regression analysis showed that baseline systolic BP and hours of CPAP were independent predictors of reductions in BP with CPAP.

Conclusion.—Long-term CPAP reduced BP modestly in the whole sample. However, patients with higher BP at entry and good CPAP compliance achieved significant reductions in BP.

▶ The effect of continuous positive airway pressure (CPAP) on blood pressure has been evaluated in previous studies showing mixed results and has been criticized based on small sample size and length of follow-up. The investigators in this study examined the long-term effect (24 months) of CPAP on ambulatory blood pressure in patients with obstructive sleep apnea and hypertension. They also aimed to identify subgroups of patients who received the most benefit from CPAP. Although the findings do show modest improvement in diastolic BP for all subjects, the investigators were able to identify that those subjects with incompletely controlled hypertension and those with greater than 5.3 hours of CPAP use received the most improvement in mean, systolic, diastolic, daytime, and nighttime blood pressure with the use of CPAP. The numbers of subjects were smaller in these subsets and the study was not powered with these specific aims in mind. However, a signal was certainly detected. Another study powered specifically to address these particular subsets is needed to confirm the investigators' findings.

S. F. Jones, MD

Slow-wave sleep and the risk of type 2 diabetes in humans
Tasali E, Leproult R, Ehrmann DA, et al (Univ of Chicago, IL)
Proc Natl Acad Sci U S A 105:1044-1049, 2008

There is convincing evidence that, in humans, discrete sleep stages are important for daytime brain function, but whether any particular sleep stage has functional significance for the rest of the body is not known. Deep non-rapid eye movement (NREM) sleep, also known as slow-wave sleep (SWS), is thought to be the most "restorative" sleep stage, but beneficial effects of SWS for physical well being have not been demonstrated. The initiation of SWS coincides with hormonal changes that affect glucose regulation, suggesting that SWS may be important for normal glucose tolerance. If this were so, selective suppression of SWS should adversely affect glucose homeostasis and increase the risk of type 2 diabetes. Here we show that, in young healthy adults, all-night selective suppression of SWS, without any change in total sleep time, results in marked decreases in insulin sensitivity without adequate compensatory increase in insulin release, leading to reduced glucose tolerance and increased diabetes risk. SWS suppression reduced delta spectral power, the dominant EEG frequency range in SWS, and left other EEG frequency bands unchanged. Importantly, the magnitude of the decrease in insulin sensitivity was strongly correlated with the magnitude of the reduction in SWS. These findings demonstrate a clear role for SWS in the maintenance of normal glucose homeostasis. Furthermore, our data suggest that reduced sleep quality with low levels of SWS, as occurs in aging and in many obese individuals, may contribute to increase the risk of type 2 diabetes.

▶ Slow-wave sleep (SWS) may have a role in memory processing, but its role in metabolic function and glucose regulation is unknown. The investigators examined the role of SWS suppression and its effect on glucose regulation. After suppression of SWS for 3 days, insulin sensitivity was decreased by about 25% and insulin response was blunted. These effects were independent of increases in the arousal index or change in total sleep time.

It is known that normal age-related changes in sleep include a reduction in the amount of SWS. In addition, patients with sleep-disordered breathing (SDB) experience frequent arousals and fragmentation, leading to disruption in the normal sleep architecture and less amounts of SWS. In addition, those with SDB are likely to be overweight or obese, a finding linked with the development of diabetes. Could these "normal" age-related changes combined with the increasing prevalence of obesity actually increase risk or predispose patients to diabetes? Could sleep be the causal link? The findings necessitate additional investigation.

S. F. Jones, MD

Prognosis of Patients With Heart Failure and Obstructive Sleep Apnea Treated With Continuous Positive Airway Pressure
Kasai T, Narui K, Dohi T, et al (Toranomon Hosp, Tokyo, Japan; et al)
Chest 133:690-696, 2008

Background.—Therapy with continuous positive airway pressure (CPAP) provides several benefits for patients with heart failure (HF) complicated by obstructive sleep apnea (OSA). However, the effect on the prognosis of such patients remains unknown.

Aims.—To determine whether CPAP therapy and compliance affects the prognosis of HF patients with OSA.

Methods.—We classified 88 patients with HF and moderate-to-severe OSA into a CPAP-treated group (n = 65) and an untreated group (n = 23), and then those treated with CPAP were further subclassified according to CPAP therapy compliance. The frequency of death and hospitalization was analyzed using multivariate analysis.

Results.—During a mean (± SD) period of 25.3 ± 15.3 months, 44.3% of the patients died or were hospitalized. Multivariate analysis showed that the risk for death and hospitalization was increased in the untreated group (hazard ratio [HR], 2.03; 95% confidence interval [CI], 1.07 to 3.68; p = 0.030) and in less compliant CPAP-treated patients (HR, 4.02; 95% CI, 1.33 to 12.2; p = 0.014).

Conclusion.—Therapy with CPAP significantly reduced the risk of death and hospitalization among patients with HF and OSA. However, reduced compliance with CPAP therapy was significantly associated with an increased risk of death and hospitalization.

▶ This was an interesting hypothesis generating analysis. It showed a relationship between the use of continuous positive airway pressure (CPAP) in patients with congestive heart failure (CHF) and a composite of death and hospitalizations, as well as a relationship between compliance with CPAP treatment and noncompliance. Unfortunately, because of the nature of a prospective observational study and the small number of events, no definitive answer has been reached. A larger study is needed to confirm the findings. Further research into the mechanisms to explain this are needed, but may be related to hypoxia-induced inflammation and sympathetic activity.

If the treatment group had 1 more death or if the nontreated group had 1 more survival a mortality benefit could not have been reached.

S. F. Jones, MD

Association of Sleep-Disordered Breathing With Postoperative Complications
Hwang D, Shakir N, Limann B, et al (North Shore Long Island Jewish Health Systems, Mahasset, NY)
Chest 133:1128-1134, 2008

Background.—Obstructive sleep apnea (OSA) is associated with increased perioperative risk, but the incidence of postoperative complications and the severity of OSA associated with increased risk have not been established. We investigated the relationship between intermittent hypoxemia measured by home nocturnal oximetry with the occurrence of postoperative complications in patients with clinical signs of OSA identified during preoperative assessment for elective surgery.

Methods.—This study was performed at a tertiary care hospital. Home nocturnal oximetry was performed on elective surgical patients with clinical features of OSA. The number of episodes per hour of oxygen desaturation (or oxygen desaturation index) of $\geq 4\%$ (ODI4%) was determined. Subjects with five or more desaturations per hour (ODI4% ≥ 5) were compared to those with less than five desaturations per hour (ODI4% < 5). Hospital records were reviewed to assess the incidence and type of postoperative complications.

Results.—A total of 172 patients were investigated as part of this study. No significant differences were observed between groups in terms of age, body mass index, number of medical comorbidities, or smoking history. Patients with an ODI4% ≥ 5 had a significantly higher rate of postoperative complications than those with ODI4% < 5 (15.3% vs 2.7%, respectively [$p < 0.01$; adjusted odds ratio, 7.2; 95% confidence interval, 1.5 to 33.3 [$p = 0.012$]). The complication rate also increased with increasing ODI severity (patients with an ODI4% of 5 to 15 events per hour, 13.8%; patients with an ODI4% of ≥ 15 events per hour, 17.5%; $p = 0.01$) Complications were respiratory (nine patients), cardiovascular (five patients), GI (one patient), and bleeding (two patients). The hospital length of stay was similar in both groups.

Conclusion.—An ODI4% ≥ 5, determined by home nocturnal oximetry, in patients with clinical features of OSA is associated with an increased rate of postoperative complications.

▶ I like this study because it addresses a simple question: Is there a relationship between intermittent hypoxemia and postoperative complications? The answer is, yes. Investigators used a simple screening protocol that included assessment of obstructive sleep apnea signs and symptoms, followed by home nocturnal oximetry to identify patients who are at increased risk of perioperative complications. The number of episodes per hour of oxygen desaturation of $\geq 5;4\%$ (ODI4%), a surrogate marker for sleep-disordered breathing, were measured and subjects were classified as ODI4% ≥ 5 or ODI4% < 5. Most of the complications occurred in the first group. Complications varied across organ systems (atelectasis to bleeding to cardiac arrythmias). Overall, an ODI4% ≥ 5 was associated with an increased rate of postoperative complications (adjusted hazard ratio 7.2), compared with subjects with ODI4% < 5. If we can identify those patients who, based on their history, are likely to have sleep apnea, and use a simple assessment tool (eg, nocturnal pulse oximetry) on them, we may be able to target a population that may benefit from perioperative therapy for sleep-disordered breathing to prevent complication. Of course, a randomized controlled trial is necessary to answer this question.

S. F. Jones, MD

39 Critical Care Medicine

Effect of Sedation With Dexmedetomidine vs Lorazepam on Acute Brain Dysfunction in Mechanically Ventilated Patients: The MENDS Randomized Controlled Trial
Pandharipande PP, Pun BT, Herr DL, et al (Vanderbilt Univ Schools of Medicine and Nursing, Nashville, TN; Washington Hosp Ctr, WA; et al)
J Am Med Assoc 298:2644-2653, 2007

Context.—Lorazepam is currently recommended for sustained sedation of mechanically ventilated intensive care unit (ICU) patients, but this and other benzodiazepine drugs may contribute to acute brain dysfunction, ie, delirium and coma, associated with prolonged hospital stays, costs, and increased mortality. Dexmedetomidine induces sedation via different central nervous system receptors than the benzodiazepine drugs and may lower the risk of acute brain dysfunction.

Objective.—To determine whether dexmedetomidine reduces the duration of delirium and coma in mechanically ventilated ICU patients while providing adequate sedation as compared with lorazepam.

Design, Setting, Patients, and Intervention.—Double-blind, randomized controlled trial of 106 adult mechanically ventilated medical and surgical ICU patients at 2 tertiary care centers between August 2004 and April 2006. Patients were sedated with dexmedetomidine or lorazepam for as many as 120 hours. Study drugs were titrated to achieve the desired level of sedation, measured using the Richmond Agitation-Sedation Scale (RASS). Patients were monitored twice daily for delirium using the Confusion Assessment Method for the ICU (CAM-ICU).

Main Outcome Measures.—Days alive without delirium or coma and percentage of days spent within 1 RASS point of the sedation goal.

Results.—Sedation with dexmedetomidine resulted in more days alive without delirium or coma (median days, 7.0 vs 3.0; $P = .01$) and a lower prevalence of coma (63% vs 92%; $P < .001$) than sedation with lorazepam. Patients sedated with dexmedetomidine spent more time within 1 RASS point of their sedation goal compared with patients sedated with lorazepam (median percentage of days, 80% vs 67%; $P = .04$). The 28-day mortality in the dexmedetomidine group was 17% vs 27% in the lorazepam group ($P = .18$) and cost of care was similar between groups. More patients in the dexmedetomidine group (42% vs 31%;

$P = .61$) were able to complete post-ICU neuropsychological testing, with similar scores in the tests evaluating global cognitive, motor speed, and attention functions. The 12-month time to death was 363 days in the dexmedetomidine group vs 188 days in the lorazepam group ($P = .48$).

Conclusion.—In mechanically ventilated ICU patients managed with individualized targeted sedation, use of a dexmedetomidine infusion resulted in more days alive without delirium or coma and more time at the targeted level of sedation than with a lorazepam infusion.

Trial Registration.—clinicaltrials.gov Identifier: NCT00095251.

▶ Confusion and frank delirium are extremely common in ICU patients. The consequences are severe as well: self extubation or removal of important tubes such as Foley catheters, chest tubes, and central lines can lead to increases in both morbidity and mortality. Thus, it is common to deeply sedate patients who are on ventilators and demonstrate confusional behavior. We no longer use paralytic agents routinely in such patients because of the significant side effects of prolonged paralysis, prolonged weakness, and myopathies that have been frequently reported. Yet there is mounting evidence that common sedating medications such as lorazepam, fentanyl, morphine, or propofol may themselves worsen confusional states and change sleep patterns in deleterious ways. Dexmedetomidine (DEX) is a central alpha agent that appears to be minimally sedating compared with the others; yet, does affect delirium in positive ways. The concerns with using it have been of increased cost and of the current FDA approval for only 24-hour usage. In addition, some concerns of cardiac suppression have been voiced as well. This study appears to put all those concerns to rest. The DEX-treated group achieved their target Richmond Agitation-Sedation Scale (RASS) scores more often than the lorazepam group, were awake significantly more often, came close to improved survival statistically, and no worse cardiovascular outcomes than seen with lorazepam. Perhaps, this will become the drug of choice for ICU sedation. (Especially if costs drop to equivalent levels to the other medications in common use.)

J. A. Barker, MD

Initial Airway Management Skills of Senior Residents: Simulation Training Compared With Traditional Training
Kory PD, Eisen LA, Adachi M, et al (Beth Israel Med Ctr, NY; William W. Backus Hosp, Norwich, CT; et al)
Chest 132:1927-1931, 2007

Background.—Scenario-based training (SBT) with a computerized patient simulator (CPS) is effective in teaching physicians to manage high-risk, low-frequency events that are typical of critical care medicine. This study compares the initial airway management skills of a group of senior internal medicine residents trained using SBT with CPS during their first year of postgraduate training (PGY) with a group of senior internal medicine residents trained using the traditional experiential method.

Methods.—This was a prospective, controlled trial that compared two groups of PGY3 internal medicine residents at an urban teaching hospital. One group (n = 32) received training in initial airway management skills using SBT with CPS in their PGY1 (*ie*, the simulation-trained [ST] group). The second group (n = 30) received traditional residency training (*ie*, the traditionally trained [TT] group). Each group was then tested during PGY3 in initial airway management skills using a standardized respiratory arrest scenario.

Results.—The ST group performed significantly better than the TT group in 8 of the 11 steps of the respiratory arrest scenario. Notable differences were found in the ability to attach a bag-valve mask (BVM) to high-flow oxygen (ST group, 69%; TT group, 17%; p < 0.001), correct insertion of oral airway (ST group, 88%; TT group, 20%; p < 0.001), and achieving an effective BVM seal (ST group, 97%; TT group, 20%; p < 0.001).

Conclusions.—Traditional training consisting of 2 years of clinical experience was not sufficient to achieve proficiency in initial airway management skills, mostly due to inadequate equipment usage. This suggests that SBT with CPS is more effective in training medical residents than the traditional experiential method.

▶ There is no question that we need to throw the "see one, do one, teach one" sequence out with the bath water. Internal medicine residents now have as few as 3 months of critical care and cannot have more than 6. They may or may not intubate during code conditions. Thus, the traditional training on the fly style we all grew up with is just not practical. Even the most facile young physicians will not be competent without adequate training, opportunities, and feedback followed by repetition. Simulator systems have much to offer: There is no risk to a live patient. Failed attempts can actually provide important feedback. There are countless opportunities for repetition. Feedback can be immediate and, often, can be as a video debriefing, which may actually be more effective (since the physician can view and critique herself).

J. A. Barker, MD

Efficacy and safety of a paired sedation and ventilator weaning protocol for mechanically ventilated patients in intensive care (Awakening and Breathing Controlled trial): a randomised controlled trial
Girard TD, Kress JP, Fuchs BD, et al (Ctr for Health Services Res; Univ of Chicago, IL, USA; Univ of Pennsylvania School of Medicine, PA; et al)
Lancet 371:126-134, 2008

Background.—Approaches to removal of sedation and mechanical ventilation for critically ill patients vary widely. Our aim was to assess a protocol that paired spontaneous awakening trials (SATs)—ie, daily interruption of sedatives—with spontaneous breathing trials (SBTs).

Methods.—In four tertiary-care hospitals, we randomly assigned 336 mechanically ventilated patients in intensive care to management with a daily SAT followed by an SBT (intervention group; n=168) or with sedation per usual care plus a daily SBT (control group; n=168). The primary endpoint was time breathing without assistance. Data were analysed by intention to treat. This study is registered with ClinicalTrials.gov, number NCT00097630.

Findings.—One patient in the intervention group did not begin their assigned treatment protocol because of withdrawal of consent and thus was excluded from analyses and lost to follow-up. Seven patients in the control group discontinued their assigned protocol, and two of these patients were lost to follow-up. Patients in the intervention group spent more days breathing without assistance during the 28-day study period than did those in the control group (14·7 days *vs* 11·6 days; mean difference 3·1 days, 95% CI 0·7 to 5·6; p=0·02) and were discharged from intensive care (median time in intensive care 9·1 days *vs* 12·9 days; p=0·01) and the hospital earlier (median time in the hospital 14·9 days *vs* 19·2 days; p=0·04). More patients in the intervention group self-extubated than in the control group (16 patients *vs* six patients; 6·0% difference, 95% CI 0·6% to 11·8%; p=0·03), but the number of patients who required reintubation after self-extubation was similar (five patients *vs* three patients; 1·2% difference, 95% CI −5·2% to 2·5%; p=0·47), as were total reintubation rates (13·8% *vs* 12·5%; 1·3% difference, 95% CI −8·6% to 6·1%; p=0·73). At any instant during the year after enrolment, patients in the intervention group were less likely to die than were patients in the control group (HR 0·68, 95% CI 0·50 to 0·92; p=0·01). For every seven patients treated with the intervention, one life was saved (number needed to treat was 7·4, 95% CI 4·2 to 35·5).

Interpretation.—Our results suggest that a wake up and breathe protocol that pairs daily spontaneous awakening trials (ie, interruption of sedatives) with daily spontaneous breathing trials results in better outcomes for mechanically ventilated patients in intensive care than current standard approaches and should become routine practice.

▶ I am surprised at this article. This really should be the standard-of-care. That is, every ICU patient should have sedatives lifted once a day. This serves multiple important purposes: the neurologic status can be assessed more accurately, the family can interact with the patient, pain can be monitored, and probably most importantly, the pharmacologic agents can be pulled back to allow them to clear. I have been reminded (painfully) many times just how long some patients may take to clear drugs that have been given by infusion. Midazolam can accumulate as can propofol, for example. It makes perfect sense to pair the sedation hold protocol with the automatic ventilator weaning protocol. In fact, we have done this in our ICU for over 4 years now. The intervention group used lower medication total amounts. They also had much less ventilator time and shorter overall hospital length of stay.

J. A. Barker, MD

Burnout in a surgical ICU team

Verdon M, Merlani P, Perneger T, et al (Service of Intensive Care, Dept of Anaesthesiology, Geneva; Univ Hosp of Geneva)
Intensive Care Med 34:152-156, 2008

Objective.—Psychologically stressful situations, a physically demanding workload and a high requirement for technological skills can lead ICU caregivers to burnout. The aim of our study was to evaluate their level of burnout as well as the related factors.

Design.—A self-administered anonymous questionnaire.

Setting.—A 20-bed surgical ICU in a university hospital.

Patients and Participants.—Nurse assistants and nurses.

Interventions.—None.

Measurements and Results.—Ninety-seven of 107 questionnaires (91%) were returned. Of the members of ICU nursing team, 28% showed a high level of burnout. They reported a number of concerns, and they felt discomfort and suffering. There was a discrepancy between the factors felt to be important by them and those statistically related to the burnout. Among the reported concerns, only the lack of patients' cooperation, the organization of the service and the rapid patient turnover were independently associated with a high level of burnout. As many as 49% of the nursing team felt stressed.

Conclusions.—Almost a third of the ICU nursing team showed a high level of burnout. The factors felt to be important may not be those related to burnout. Since the well-being of the nursing team is important for the quality of care, corrective actions against the related factors should be sought out in order to alleviate the suffering.

▶ This fairly simple survey study documents what many of us fear: burnout is real and is often just around the corner. With a significant nursing and intensivist shortage present now, and predicted to be worse in the future, this is a problem worthy of study. What I note in this unit is that the nurses appear to have good patient care ratios and staffing; however, 8 hour shifts result in 5 days a week that may deepen the immersion and therefore hasten the burnout process. In addition, these nurses must also work weekends. Of interest is the finding that rapid patient turnover is thought to lead to burnout. I have always held the opposite opinion, namely that those lingering, long-term patients worsen the strain on staff. My own experience is that it is unusual for nurses to go beyond 15 years in a single ICU unless they move into management (and, in fact, the stay is often much shorter). Is this a natural cycle or is it preventable? Most of the nurses leaving ICU seem to use their skills well in related, but less intense, jobs such as postoperative recovery rooms, telemetry units, and cardiopulmonary rehabilitation. Perhaps we should, again, look at other industries (such as the airlines) to learn other ways to prevent burnout. I suspect the results will be straightforward—lots of time off, regular debriefing, rotation of tasks or even assignments, and regular rest and exercise.

J. A. Barker, MD

Heparinized solution vs. saline solution in the maintenance of arterial catheters: A double blind randomized clinical trial

Del Cotillo M, Grané N, Llavoré M, et al (Intensive Care Unit (ICU), Hosp Mútua de Terrassa)
Intensive Care Med 34:339-343, 2008

Objectives.—The objectives were to analyze the effectiveness of heparinized solution vs. saline solution for the maintenance of arterial catheters and to detect changes in the activated partial thromboplastin time (aPTT) and platelet count in the samples extracted from both groups of arterial catheters.

Design.—Randomized, double blind, placebo-controlled clinical trial.

Setting.—Intensive Care Unit of a third-level hospital in Terrassa, Barcelona, Spain.

Patients.—One hundred and thirty-three patients were included in the trial. The selection criteria were: adults, informed consent, not receiving either full-dose anticoagulant or fibrinolytic treatment, and no thrombocytopenia.

Interventions.—Sixty-five patients received heparinized solution (1 IU/ml) and 68 received saline solution. Measurements: Arterial catheter functionality was compared in the groups every 8 h and at catheter removal. Patency, reliability of arterial pressure, and curve quality were used to evaluate the functionality of the catheters. Blood was drawn, discarding 7.5 ml, from the arterial catheter and from the venouscatheter simultaneously for coagulation tests.

Results.—The median duration of catheters being in place was 5.1 days (IQR = 8.1) in the heparin group, and 5.4 (IQR = 7.3) in the saline group ($p = 0.7$). Kaplan–Meier curves showed no differences between groups ($p = 0.6$). The number of manipulations required to maintain the patency of the arterial catheters was 35% vs. 40% ($p = 0.5$). The heparin group had a significantly longer aPTT (2.1 ± 1.3 vs. 1.25 ± 0.3, $p = 0.001$).

Conclusions.—The use of heparinized solution for arterial catheter maintenance does not appear to be justified. It did not increase the duration of the catheters, nor did it improve their functionality significantly. On the other hand, heparin Na altered aPTT significantly.

▶ This is a study I had planned doing, but I am glad Del Cotillo et al did it. Like so many other things we do in medicine, the routine usage of heparin to flush lines in ICUs and ORs really has little proof of efficacy. Now there is a swing back away from this practice, primarily because of fear of heparin-induced thrombocytopenia (HIT). At Palmetto Richland Hospital we have used saline only for line flushes for well over 2 years. Note in this article that there was no difference of platelet counts in either group. Perhaps HIT is not the concern we think it is. I was surprised at the length of time these arterial lines were left in (over 5 days). As catheters are left in longer, there is perhaps less clotting in the heparin flush group—although it did not reach a *P* value < .05. Likewise, only about 80% of catheters are still functional at 5 days. A surprise finding to me was that the measured partial thromboplastin times (PTTs) were prolonged in the heparin flush group. Clearly, these patients get more heparin than we realize. The take-home message is clear: Saline is just as good as heparin for flushing arterial lines. The other take-home message should be to take the lines out quickly—certainly before the fourth day of usage.

J. A. Barker, MD

Should etomidate be used for rapid-sequence intubation induction in critically ill septic patients?

Fengler BT (Univ of Virginia School of Medicine, Charlottesville, VA)
Am J Emerg Med 26:229-232, 2008

Etomidate is an agent often used by emergency medicine physicians for rapid-sequence intubation induction of critically ill patients because of its reliable pharmacokinetics and cardiovascular stability. Etomidate is known to inhibit endogenous cortisol production through inhibition of 11β-hydroxylase. Previous studies in undifferentiated emergency department patients and healthy, elective surgical patients have shown this effect to be only transient and not clinically significant. Recent retrospective studies in the pediatric and adult intensive care literature have shown an association between a single induction dose of etomidate in critically ill septic patients and sustained suppression of the adrenal axis with an increase in mortality. It is unknown at this time if any increase in mortality associated with etomidate-induced adrenal suppression would be offset by concomitant corticosteroid administration. Aggressive resuscitation of septic patients with fluids, antibiotics, and vasopressors has been shown to significantly reduce mortality and may allow for the use of alternative agents that had previously been discouraged because of concern for hemodynamic collapse during intubation. A prospective randomized trial in septic patients of etomidate induction with early corticotropin stimulation testing or corticosteroid supplementation vs the use of alternative induction agents with enough power to detect differences in mortality is needed to further address this clinical dilemma.

▶ Etomidate is a fantastic drug for intubation. It has minimal side effects, rapid onset, and does not paralyze the patient. For those of us who fear the side effects and risks of using neuromuscular blockers in the process of endotracheal intubation, this drug has been a godsend. The concern about adrenal suppression is a real one. However, a careful review of previous literature has led me to conclude that using etomidate as a continuous infusion clearly renders many patients adrenal insufficient. Yet there is little evidence that patients given small doses to facilitate intubation become significantly adrenal insufficient. The jury is still out. In the meanwhile, I agree with the authors: If a question of adrenal insufficiency arises, measure cortisol and give the patient coverage with intravenous steroids. The story is not yet over.

J. A. Barker, MD

The Current Status of Traumatic Diaphragmatic Injury: Lessons Learned From 105 Patients Over 13 Years

Hanna WC, Ferri LE, Fata P, et al (McGill Univ Health Ctr, Montréal, Québec, Canada)
Ann Thorac Surg 85:1044-1048, 2008

Background.—Our understanding of traumatic diaphragmatic injury (TDI) is based primarily on outdated retrospective series. We sought to reexamine present day patterns of diagnosis, associated injuries, predictors of mortality, and long-term outcomes of this condition.

Methods.—A prospectively entered trauma database from the Montréal General Hospital was reviewed for patients admitted with a TDI from 1993 to 2006. Hospital charts were reviewed, and patient characteristics, mechanism of injury, associated injuries, operative management, and post-operative outcomes were recorded. Logistic regression was used to identify predictors for mortality.

Results.—Identified were 105 patients with TDI consisting of blunt in 37% and penetrating in 63%. Only 23% of TDI were diagnosed on initial chest roentgenogram. External wounds in penetrating TDI cases were found in the abdomen alone in 19%, in the chest alone in 46%, and in both in 35%, which was associated with intraabdominal organ injury in 83%, 55%, and 87%, respectively. Less than half of patients had a dia-phragmatic hernia. Lung, chest wall, and thoracic organ injuries were more common in blunt trauma, but there was no significant difference between abdominal injuries in both mechanisms. Overall mortality from TDI was 18%, and there was no difference between blunt and penetrating injury. In blunt trauma, brain injury and an Injury Severity Score (ISS) exceeding 15 were independently associated with increased death. In pene-trating trauma, only an ISS exceeding 15 predicted death.

TABLE 1.—Injuries Associated With Traumatic Diaphragmatic Injury

Patients Reviewed	Total	Blunt	Penetrating	*p* Value
Patients, No.	24,703	20,748	3955	
TDI-associated injury, No.	105	39	66	
Any associated injuries	105	39	66	N/A
Head	20	20	0	<0.001[a]
Thorax	47	27	20	0.003[a]
Heart/aorta	6	0	6	N/A
Solid organ (abdomen)	62	25	37	0.50
Hollow viscus (abdomen)	39	13	26	0.64
Pelvis	18	18	0	<0.001[a]

N/A = not applicable
TDI = traumatic diaphragmatic injury.
[a]Statistically significant.

Conclusions.—Traumatic diaphragmatic injury remains a challenge to diagnose and treat, primarily due to the presence of associated injuries. The high incidence of intraabdominal organ injury, irrespective of the site of penetrating wound, dictates a transabdominal approach for exploration and repair. Severity of associated injuries (ISS) predicts death (Table 1).

▶ Fortunately, pulmonary/intensivists rarely care acutely for trauma patients. However, this particular question of whether a traumatic diaphragm injury is present comes up often. Diaphragm paralysis is a relatively common office consult question, but probably more frequently we are looking for reasons for weaning failure in the intubated hospital patient. I was neither aware of the high frequency of other organ involvement (Table 1) nor realized that trauma surgeons usually diagnose and treat it so acutely (over 90% in this article). Finally, it is useful for us to know – in case our surgical colleague is not a traumatologist – that an abdominal approach is mandatory since abdominal injuries are so common and so severe.

J. A. Barker, MD

40 Miscellaneous

Efficacy of Short-Course Antibiotic Regimens for Community-Acquired Pneumonia: A Meta-analysis
Li JZ, Winston LG, Moore DH, et al (Univ of California, San Francisco)
Am J Med 120:783-790, 2007

Purpose.—There is little consensus on the most appropriate duration of antibiotic treatment for community-acquired pneumonia. The goal of this study is to systematically review randomized controlled trials comparing short-course and extended-course antibiotic regimens for community-acquired pneumonia.

Methods.—We searched MEDLINE, Embase, and CENTRAL, and reviewed reference lists from 1980 through June 2006. Studies were included if they were randomized controlled trials that compared short-course (7 days or less) versus extended-course (>7 days) antibiotic mono-therapy for community-acquired pneumonia in adults. The primary outcome measure was failure to achieve clinical improvement.

Results.—We found 15 randomized controlled trials matching our inclusion and exclusion criteria comprising 2796 total subjects. Short-course regimens primarily studied the use of azithromycin (n = 10), but trials examining beta-lactams (n = 2), fluoroquinolones (n = 2), and keto-lides (n = 1) were found as well. Of the extended-course regimens, 3 studies utilized the same antibiotic, whereas 9 involved an antibiotic of the same class. Overall, there was no difference in the risk of clinical failure between the short-course and extended-course regimens (0.89, 95% confidence interval [CI], 0.78-1.02). In addition, there were no differences in the risk of mortality (0.81, 95% CI, 0.46-1.43) or bacteriologic eradication (1.11, 95% CI, 0.76-1.62). In subgroup analyses, there was a trend toward favorable clinical efficacy for the short-course regimens in all antibiotic classes (range of relative risk, 0.88-0.94).

Conclusions.—The available studies suggest that adults with mild to moderate community-acquired pneumonia can be safely and effectively treated with an antibiotic regimen of 7 days or less. Reduction in patient exposure to antibiotics may limit the increasing rates of antimicrobial drug resistance, decrease cost, and improve patient adherence and tolerability (Fig 3).

▶ Community-acquired pneumonia is both a very common and expensive medical problem throughout the world. Recently, a number of clinical trials have investigated new approaches to community-acquired pneumonia,

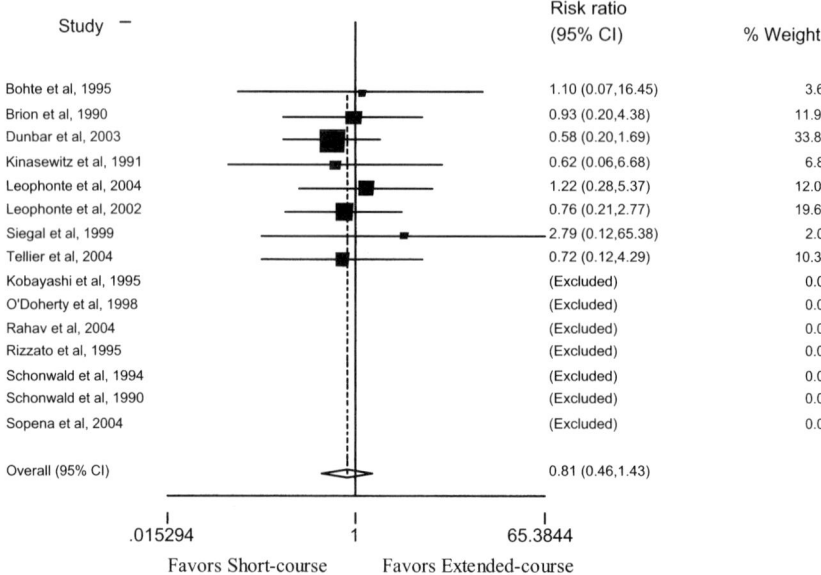

FIGURE 3.—Relative risk mortality with short-course versus extended-course antibiotic regimens. (The relative risk of mortality could not be calculated in 7 studies due to the lack of deaths in both arms). (Reprinted from Li JZ, Winston LG, Moore DH, et al. Efficacy of short-course antibiotic regimens for community-acquired pneumonia: a meta-analysis. *Am J Med.* 2007;120:783-790. Copyright 2007, with permission from Elsevier.)

including rapid changes from IV to oral antibiotics when temperatures return to normal, increased home management, and shorter courses of antibiotics. All of these approaches are aimed to both reduce antibiotic side effects and to contain health care costs. To date, the "right" approach to management of this very common cause of morbidity and mortality is not definitive. The authors of this meta-analysis on short-course regimens were hampered by the variability of the antibiotics used in different trials; however, on balance they found no differences between antibiotic courses < 7 and those > 7 days in terms of major outcome parameters. This was true across a wide range of analyses including both intention-to-treat and per-protocol populations, high quality studies, and individual antibiotic classes. It appears safe to use a short course approach in patients with mild or moderately severe community-acquired pneumonia, particularly with azithromycin, which was used in 10 of the 15 trials included.

J. R. Maurer, MD, MBA

Treatment Outcomes of Patients with HIV and Tuberculosis

Nahid P, Gonzalez LC, Rudoy I, et al (Univ of California, San Francisco; et al)
Am J Respir Crit Care Med 175:1199-1206, 2007

Rationale.—The optimal length of tuberculosis treatment in patients coinfected with HIV is unknown.

Objectives.—To evaluate treatment outcomes for HIV-infected patients stratified by duration of rifamycin-based tuberculosis therapy.

Methods.—We retrospectively reviewed data on all patients with tuberculosis reported to the San Francisco Tuberculosis Control Program from 1990 through 2001. Patients were followed for up to 12 months after treatment completion.

Measurements and Main Results.—Of 700 patients, 264 (38%) were HIV infected, 315 (45%) were not infected, and 121 (17%) were not tested. Mean duration of treatment was extended to 10.2 months for HIV-infected patients versus 8.4 months for uninfected/unknown patients (p < 0.001). Seventeen percent of the HIV-infected and 37% of the HIV uninfected/unknown patients received 6 months of rifamycin-based therapy. The relapse rate among HIV-infected was 9.3 per 100 person-years versus 1.0 in HIV-uninfected/unknown patients (p < 0.001). HIV-infected individuals who received a standard 6-month rifamycin-based regimen were more likely to relapse than those treated longer (adjusted hazard ratio, 4.33; p = 0.02). HIV-infected individuals who received intermittent therapy were also more likely to relapse than those treated on daily basis (adjusted hazard ratio, 4.12; p = 0.04). The use of highly active antiretroviral therapy was associated with more rapid conversion of smears and cultures and with improved survival.

Conclusions.—HIV-infected patients who received a 6-month rifamycin-based course of tuberculosis treatment or who received intermittent therapy had a higher relapse rate than HIV-infected subjects who received longer therapy or daily therapy, respectively. Standard 6-month therapy may be insufficient to prevent relapse in patients with HIV.

▶ The current standard therapy for drug-susceptible tuberculosis (TB) in non-HIV infected persons is a 6-month rifamycin-based regimen (typically rifampin and isoniazid) with pyrazinamide during the initial 2 months of treatment. Treatment failure rates in this setting are very low. This regimen is also recommended for HIV-infected patients with drug-susceptible TB.[1] However, whether this represents an adequate treatment course for these patients is an area of some controversy, as concern has been raised that the duration of treatment should be longer based on observations of higher recurrence rates with the standard regimen.

This retrospective study by Nahid and colleagues evaluated a very large number of patients with TB and specifically examined the outcomes of patients with and without HIV infection treated for the standard 6 months with a rifamycin-based regimen. Some patients were treated daily (5-7 days/week) and others were treated intermittently (once-, twice-, or thrice-weekly). Access to resources was not a limiting factor, and most patients received directly observed therapy. Recurrence rates were higher in the HIV-infected group (6.6%) compared with the non-HIV-infected group (0.8%). Multivariate analysis demonstrated 2 factors that were significantly associated with relapse: 1) treatment for 6 months compared with longer durations of treatment (Hazard Ratio [HR] 4.33 [95% CI, 1.26-14.8]); and 2) intermittent compared with daily treatment (HR 4.12 [95% CI, 1.09-15.6]).

Other studies have not demonstrated such a difference in outcomes between HIV-infected and non-HIV-infected patients with drug-susceptible TB.[2] The official recommendation of the Centers for Disease Control and Prevention, American Thoracic Society, and the Infectious Diseases Society of America is that 6 months of treatment suffices for both groups.[1] Based on the results of this study, treatment for HIV-infected patients should be given as daily therapy, and re-evaluation at the end of the 6-month treatment period is probably warranted to at least consider whether a longer duration of treatment might be of benefit.

L. T. Tanoue, MD

References

1. Blumberg HM, Burman WJ, Chaisson RE, et al. American Thoracic Society/Centers for Disease Control and Prevention/Infectious Diseases Society of America: treatment of tuberculosis. *Am J Respir Crit Care Med.* 2003;167:603-662.
2. Sterling TR, Alwood K, Gachuhi R, et al. Relapse rates after short-course (6-month) treatment of tuberculosis in HIV-infected and uninfected persons. *AIDS.* 1999;13:1899-1904.

PART SIX

HEART AND CARDIOVASCULAR DISEASE

BERNARD J. GERSH, MB, CHB, D.PHIL, FRCP

41 Cardiac Arrhythmias, Conduction Disturbances, and Electrophysiology

---

Ablation for longstanding permanent atrial fibrillation: Results from a randomized study comparing three different strategies
Elayi CS, Verma A, Di Biase L, et al (Ambroise Pare Hospital, Neuilly sur Seine, France; Southlake Regional Health Ctr, ON, Canada; Univ of Foggia, Italy; et al)
Heart Rhythm 5:1658-1664, 2008

Background.—This prospective multicenter randomized study aimed to compare the efficacy of 3 common ablation methods used for longstanding permanent atrial fibrillation (AF).

Methods.—A total of 144 patients with longstanding permanent AF (median duration 28 months) were randomly assigned to circumferential pulmonary vein ablation (CPVA, group 1, n = 47), to pulmonary vein antrum isolation (PVAI, group 2, n = 48) or to a hybrid strategy combining ablation of complex fractionated or rapid atrial electrograms (CFAE) in both atria followed by a pulmonary vein antrum isolation (CFAE + PVAI, group 3, n = 49).

Results.—Scarring in the left atrium and structural heart disease/hypertension were present in most patients (65%). After a mean follow-up of 16 months, 11% of patients in group 1, 40% of patients in group 2 and 61% of patients in group 3 were in sinus rhythm after one procedure and with no antiarrhythmic drugs ($P < .001$). Sinus rhythm maintenance would increase respectively to 28% (group 1), 83% (group 2), and 94% (group 3) after 2 procedures and with antiarrhythmic drugs (AADs, $P < .001$). The AF terminated during ablation, either by conversion to sinus rhythm or organization into an atrial tachyarrhythmia, in 13% of patients (group 1), 44% (group 2), and 74% (group 3) respectively. CFAE alone, performed as the first step of the ablation in group 3, organized AF in only 1 patient.

Conclusion.—In this study, the hybrid AF ablation strategy including antrum isolation and CFAE ablation had the highest likelihood of maintaining sinus rhythm in patients with longstanding permanent AF. Electrical isolation of the PVs, although inadequate if performed alone, is relevant to achieve long-term sinus rhythm maintenance after ablation. Bi-atrial CFAE ablation had a minimal impact on AF termination during ablation.

▶ Once again, this study points to the empiric approach (ie, ablation of atrial fibrillation). It also demonstrates once again that bi-atrial complex fractionated atrial electrogram ablation as a stand-alone strategy has a minimal impact on the success of atrial fibrillation ablation.

A. L. Waldo, MD

Atrial fibrillation after cardiac surgery: Risk factors and their temporal relationship in prophylactic drug strategy decision
Mariscalco G, Engström KG (Univ of Insubria, Varese, Italy; Umeå Univ Hosp, Sweden)
Int J Cardiol 129:354-362, 2008

Objective.—Postoperative atrial fibrillation (AF) is a vexing problem in cardiac surgery. Our aim was to identify risk factors between surgical procedures, all having cardiopulmonary bypass (CPB) in common, and how AF contributes to early and late mortality.

Methods.—Patients were reviewed during a 10-year period, comprising coronary artery bypass grafting (CABG, $n=7056$), aortic valve replacement (AVR, $n=690$) and their combination (COMB, $n=688$). The study assessed 43 variables of which pre-/intraoperative data were evaluated for uni/multivariate analysis in relation to AF and type of surgery. Data were reviewed versus hospital and 1-year mortality; the latter being obtained from the Swedish population registry.

Results.—The surgery subgroups exhibited obvious differences. The overall incidence of AF was 25.6%, ranging from 22.7% for CABG to 44.0% for COMB procedures. Numerous interaction patterns were seen among the analyzed parameters. In multivariate fashion, age was encountered in all groups, whereas coronary disease superimposed risk factors with reference to myocardial conditions at CPB weaning. Postoperative AF increased the length of hospitalization, whereas it did not affect hospital mortality. In CABG patients only, AF gave rise to increased 1-year mortality ($p < 0.001$).

Conclusions.—In addition to the accepted risk factors of AF, primarily age, we emphasize the importance of considering details at CPB weaning, a correlation that was coronary specific. The weaning period hides valuable information that can be useful for more specific AF-prophylactic strategies. The AF-related increase in late mortality after CABG but not after valve procedures is intriguing, and draws attention to possible AF recurrence during patient follow-up and management.

▶ Postoperative atrial fibrillation following cardiac surgery is a very common problem with a reported incidence between 16% to over 40% in various reports.[1-4] It has been shown in these studies that atrial fibrillation is associated with important consequences including an increase in hospital stay and expenses along with increased early and late mortality. Various investigations have suggested that pharmacologic prophylaxis including amiodarone and beta blockade may be beneficial.[5-7] Investigations have been aimed at determining the preoperative characteristics of patients at highest risk to ensure that prophylactic therapies are directed toward these populations. To this end, the authors sought to broaden the search for predictors of atrial fibrillation by including intraoperative variables.

Drs Mariscalco and Engström retrospectively reviewed the records of patients during a 10-year period, including 7056 individuals undergoing coronary artery bypass grafting (CABG), 690 having aortic valve replacement, and a combination group undergoing both of these procedures in 688. The analysis included 43 variables, including pre/intraoperative data.

The authors found that the overall incidence of atrial fibrillation was 25.6%, which was lowest in the CABG group (22.7%) and the highest in the combination group (44%). They performed various modeling techniques and commented on the interaction between variables in the models. Independent predictors of atrial fibrillation in the CABG group included age > 70 years of age, inotropic support, advanced New York Heart Association (NYHA) functional class, temporary pacing, and the need for defibrillation. In the aortic valve replacement group, older age was the single independent predictor of postoperative atrial fibrillation. In the combination group, age > 70 years, complicated weaning from cardiopulmonary bypass, and stroke were all identified as significant. They found that postoperative atrial fibrillation increased the length of hospitalization but did not affect mortality. It is noteworthy that atrial fibrillation predicted an increased one-year mortality in the CABG group.

This is an interesting study in that it extends previous work, which largely focused on preoperative factors predicting postoperative atrial fibrillation. It is particularly useful to surgeons to consider that intraoperative factors, including postoperative pacing, may influence postoperative arrhythmias and potentially may guide prophylaxis strategy. Once high-risk patients are identified, initiating an early amiodarone-loading protocol, for instance, might be an appropriate modification to standard postoperative management protocols. Although this study is a retrospective review, it would be interesting to use the data to construct a prospective randomized study in an effort to tease out truly independent factors and to determine the success of a selective approach for postoperative prophylaxis based on the introduction of intraoperative data.

R. Suri, MD, DPhil

References

1. Villareal RP, Hariharan R, Liu BC, et al. Postoperative atrial fibrillation and mortality after coronary artery bypass grafting surgery. *J Am Coll Cardiol.* 2004;43:742-748.
2. Aranki SF, Shaw DP, Adams DH, et al. Predictors of atrial fibrillation after coronary artery bypass grafting surgery. Current trends and impact on hospital resources. *Circulation.* 1996;94:390-397.
3. Almass GH, Schowalter T, Nicolosi AC, et al. Atrial fibrillation after cardiac surgery: a major morbid event? *Ann Surg.* 1997;226:501-511.
4. Crewell LL, Schuessler RB, Rosenbloom M, Cox JL. Hazards of postoperative atrial arrhythmias. *Ann Thorac Surg.* 1993;56:539-549.
5. Matthew JP, Fontes ML, Tudor IC, et al. A multicenter risk index for atrial fibrillation after cardiac surgery. *JAMA.* 2004;291:1720-1729.
6. Burgess DC, Kilborn MJ, Keech AC. Interventions for prevention of postoperative atrial fibrillation and its complications after cardiac surgery: a meta-analysis. *Eur Heart J.* 2006;27:2846-2857.
7. Sanjuan R, Blasco M, Carbonell N, et al. Preoperative use of sotalol versus atenolol for atrial fibrillation after cardiac surgery. *Ann Thorac Surg.* 2004;77:838-843.

Atrial fibrillation in stroke-free patients is associated with memory impairment and hippocampal atrophy

Knecht S, Oelschläger C, Duning T, et al (Univ of Münster, Germany)
Eur Heart J 29:2125-2132, 2008

Aims.—To determine whether atrial fibrillation (AF) in stroke-free patients is associated with impaired cognition and structural abnormalities of the brain. AF contributes to stroke and secondary cognitive decline. In the absence of manifest stroke, AF can activate coagulation and cause cerebral microembolism which could damage the brain.

Methods and Results.—We cross-sectionally evaluated 122 stroke-free individuals with AF recruited locally within the German Competence Network on AF. As comparator, we recruited 563 individuals aged 37–84 years without AF from the same community. Subjects underwent 3 T magnetic resonance imaging to assess covert territorial brain infarction, white matter lesions, and brain volume measures. Subjects with evidence for stroke, dementia, or depression were excluded. Cognitive function was assessed by an extensive neuropsychological test battery covering the domains learning and memory, attention and executive functions, working memory, and visuospatial skills. Cognitive scores and radiographic measures were compared across individuals with and without AF by stepwise multiple regression models. Stroke-free individuals with AF performed significantly worse in tasks of learning and memory ($\beta = -0.115$, $P < 0.01$) as well as attention and executive functions ($\beta = -0.105$, $P < 0.01$) compared with subjects without AF. There was also a trend ($P = 0.062$) towards worse performance in learning and memory tasks in patients with chronic as compared with paroxysmal AF. Corresponding to the memory impairment, hippocampal volume was reduced in patients with AF. Other radiographic measures did not differ between groups.

Conclusion.—Even in the absence of manifest stroke, AF is a risk factor for cognitive impairment and hippocampal atrophy. Therefore, cognition and measures of structural brain integrity should be considered in the evaluation of novel treatments for AF.

▶ This subject has interested this editor for many years. There are a long series of articles that indicate deterioration of mental status is associated with atrial fibrillation. We are aware that multiple small strokes are associated with serious mental problems, particularly Alzheimer-like syndromes. We are also aware that many ischemic strokes have neither motor nor sensory manifestations, in part because many of these strokes are caused by emboli that are pencil-point sized. It speaks again to one of the putative advantages of sinus rhythm, namely, that patients in sinus rhythm are significantly less prone to embolic stroke. Importantly, there is well-known difficulty in maintaining patients' INRs in the therapeutic range on oral anticoagulants presently available, so that from time-to-time, patients' INRs are subtherapeutic. When the INR falls below 2, there is a steep rise in the odds ratio for stroke and embolic phenomena. Perhaps, there is the rub.

A. L. Waldo, MD

Delayed rhythm control of atrial fibrillation may be a cause of failure to prevent recurrences: reasons for change to active antiarrhythmic treatment at the time of the first detected episode
Cosio FG, Aliot E, Botto GL, et al (Hospital Universitario de Getafe, Madrid, Spain; Hôpital de Brabois, Nancy, France; Sant'Anna Hospital, Como, Italy; et al)
Europace 10:21-27, 2008

Atrial fibrillation (AF) is associated with impaired functional capacity and quality of life and significant morbidity and mortality. The current management approach fails to maintain stable sinus rhythm (SR) in the majority of patients. For many years, guidelines have recommended antiarrhythmic treatment of a first AF episode only if the AF is poorly tolerated, a position that has been reinforced by studies showing no mortality or morbidity advantage of rhythm control over rate control. During the last decade, research has shown mechanisms of self-perpetuation of AF based on electrophysiological and structural remodelling induced by AF itself. There is mounting evidence that '*lone*' AF is because of a host of factors, some of which may be easily treatable, such as hypertension, sleep apnoea, and obesity, thus allowing secondary prevention at the time of the first episode of AF. According to these concepts, lack of early intervention could be one of the reasons for long-term failure of maintenance of SR. In this position paper, we propose testing the working hypothesis that if an SR maintenance strategy is selected, treatment of AF should commence at the first-detected episode and should be based on a double strategy of SR restoration and aggressive treatment of associated conditions that promote atrial remodelling.

▶ This is a thoughtful review and position statement issued by a working group from the European Society of Cardiology. They make a persuasive case that if one is intent on following an arrhythmia control strategy, prompt restoration of sinus rhythm and a vigorous attempt to maintain sinus rhythm is the appropriate management paradigm. This is worth a read.

A. L. Waldo, MD

Heart Rate Control in Patients With Atrial Fibrillation Referred for Exercise Testing
Hilliard AA, Miller TD, Hodge DO, et al (Mayo Foundation, Rochester, MN)
Am J Cardiol 102:704-708, 2008

Clinical practice guidelines for patients with atrial fibrillation (AF) recommended a heart rate (HR) of 60 to 80 beats/min at rest and 90 to 115 at moderate exercise. The degree to which HR control at rest and with exercise in patients with AF complies with these recommendations is unknown. HR at rest and at peak exercise was retrospectively examined in 1,097 consecutive patients with AF referred for exercise myocardial perfusion imaging. In a subgroup of 195 patients, HR was also measured at an intermediate "moderate" level. Median HR at rest was 80 beats/min, at the upper end of the recommended range of 60 to 80. Only patients administered a β blocker (BB; 31%) had lower (p <0.001) median HRs at rest. Median HR at moderate exercise was 128 beats/min, higher than the range of 90 to 115 recommended by the guidelines. Only patients administered a BB had significantly reduced HRs (p <0.003) at moderate exercise. Median peak exercise HR was 147 beats/min. Forty-five percent of patients exceeded their age-predicted maximal HR. Patients administered BBs were significantly less likely (p <0.01) to exceed their age-predicted maximal HR. In conclusion, in patients with AF, HR control at rest and during exercise often did not comply with guideline recommendations. Regimens including a BB were more effective in achieving HR control.

▶ This study indicates that heart rate control at rest, at moderate exercise, and at maximal exercise was suboptimal in most patients with atrial fibrillation referred for exercise single-photon emission computer tomography. It is this editor's observation that this is a major problem for patients who remain symptomatic with atrial fibrillation whether one attempts a rate or a rhythm control strategy. Attention to rate control during activities of daily living is a good index of efficacy of rate control. The 24-hour ambulatory electrocardiogram (ECG [Holter]) monitor examination should be most helpful. Using the Atrial Fibrillation Follow-up Investigation of Rhythm Management (AFFIRM) guidelines, a resting rate below 80 beats/min and a rate during activities of daily living < 110 beats/min seems a pretty good goal. The RACE investigators suggest that resting rates below 100 beats/min might also serve that purpose, but when one looks at their data carefully, the mean resting rate in the RACE trial was 84 beats/min, not far more than the mean resting rate in the AFFIRM trial of 78 beats/min.

A. L. Waldo, MD

Long-term survival in patients undergoing cardiac resynchronization therapy: the importance of performing atrio-ventricular junction ablation in patients with permanent atrial fibrillation

Gasparini M, for the Multicentre Longitudinal Observational Study (MILOS) Group (IRCCS Istituto Clinico Humanitas Rozzano-Milano, Italy; et al)

Eur Heart J 29:1644-1652, 2008

Aims.—To investigate the effects of cardiac resynchronization therapy (CRT) on survival in heart failure (HF) patients with permanent atrial fibrillation (AF) and the role of atrio-ventricular junction (AVJ) ablation in these patients.

Methods and Results.—Data from 1285 consecutive patients implanted with CRT devices are presented: 1042 patients were in sinus rhythm (SR) and 243 (19%) in AF. Rate control in AF was achieved by either ablating the AVJ in 118 patients (AVJ-abl) or prescribing negative chronotropic drugs (AF-Drugs). Compared with SR, patients with AF were significantly older, more likely to be non-ischaemic, with higher ejection fraction, shorter QRS duration, and less often received ICD back-up. During a median follow-up of 34 months, 170/1042 patients in SR and 39/243 in AF died (mortality: 8.4 and 8.9 per 100 person-year, respectively). Adjusted hazard ratios were similar for all-cause and cardiac mortality [0.9 (0.57–1.42), $P = 0.64$ and 1.00 (0.60–1.66) $P = 0.99$, respectively]. Among AF patients, only 11/118 AVJ-abl patients died vs. 28/125 AF-Drugs patients (mortality: 4.3 and 15.2 per 100 person-year, respectively, $P < 0.001$). Adjusted hazard ratios of AVJ-abl vs. AF-Drugs was 0.26 [95% confidence interval (CI) 0.09–0.73, $P = 0.010$] for all-cause mortality, 0.31 (95% CI 0.10–0.99, $P = 0.048$) for cardiac mortality, and 0.15 (95% CI 0.03–0.70, $P = 0.016$) for HF mortality.

Conclusion.—Patients with HF and AF treated with CRT have similar mortality compared with patients in SR. In AF, AVJ ablation in addition to CRT significantly improves overall survival compared with CRT alone, primarily by reducing HF death.

▶ Once again, a nonrandomized registry study, but nevertheless, it provides useful information to support the notion that atrioventricular junctional ablation is important for cardiac resynchronization therapy (CRT) to be effective in patients with atrial fibrillation.

A. L. Waldo, MD

Does Microvolt T-Wave Alternans Testing Predict Ventricular Tachyarrhythmias in Patients With Ischemic Cardiomyopathy and Prophylactic Defibrillators? The MASTER (Microvolt T Wave Alternans Testing for Risk Stratification of Post-Myocardial Infarction Patients) Trial
Chow T, on behalf of the MASTER Trial Investigators (The Lindner Clinical Trial Ctr, Cincinnati, OH; et al)
J Am Coll Cardiol 52:1607-1615, 2008

Objectives.—The purpose of this trial was to determine whether microvolt T-wave alternans (MTWA) predicts ventricular tachyarrhythmic events (VTEs) in post-myocardial infarction patients with left ventricular ejection fraction (LVEF) ≤30%.

Background.—Previous studies have established MTWA as a predictor for total and arrhythmic mortality, but its ability to identify prophylactic implantable cardioverter-defibrillator (ICD) recipients most likely to experience VTEs remains uncertain.

Methods.—This prospective trial was conducted at 50 U.S. centers. Patients were eligible if they met MADIT-II (Multicenter Automatic Defibrillator Implantation Trial II) indications for device implant. All patients underwent MTWA testing followed by ICD implantation, with pre-specified programming to minimize the likelihood of therapies for non–life-threatening VTE. Minimum follow-up was 2 years with annual MTWA testing. Initially indeterminate MTWA tests were repeated.

Results.—Analyses were conducted on 575 patients (84% male; average age ± SD = 65 ± 11 years; average LVEF ± SD = 0.24 ± 0.05). The final distribution of MTWA results were: MTWA positive in 293 (51%), MTWA negative in 214 (37%), and indeterminate in 68 patients (12%). Over an average follow-up of 2.1 ± 0.9 years, there were 70 VTEs. A VTE occurred in 48 of 361 (13%, 6.3%/year) MTWA non-negative and 22 of 214 (10%, 5.0%/year) MTWA negative patients. A non-negative MTWA test result was not associated with VTE (hazard ratio: 1.26; 95% confidence interval: 0.76 to 2.09; p = 0.37), although total mortality was significantly increased (hazard ratio: 2.04; 95% confidence interval: 1.10 to 3.78; p = 0.02).

Conclusions.—In MADIT-II–indicated ICD-treated patients, the risk of VTE does not differ according to MTWA classification, despite differences

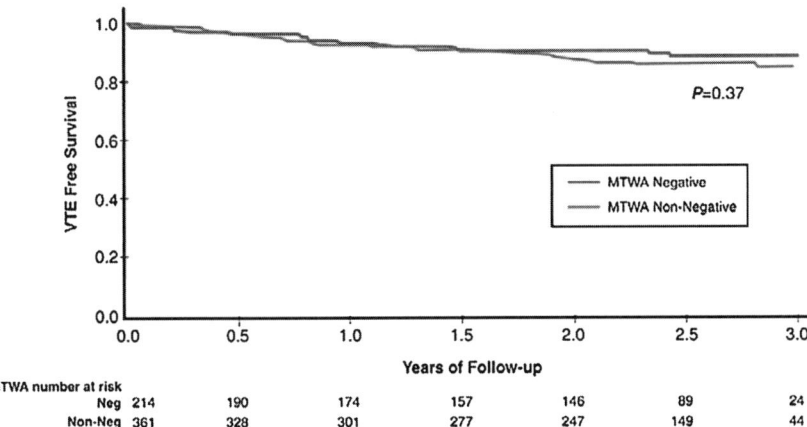

FIGURE 1.—Kaplan-Meier Survival Curves for VTE Free Survival. MTWA = microvolt T-wave alternans; VTE = ventricular tachyarrhythmic event (primary end point). (Reprinted from Chow T, on behalf of the MASTER Trial Investigators. Does microvolt T-wave alternans testing predict ventricular tachyarrhythmias in patients with ischemic cardiomyopathy and prophylactic defibrillators? The MASTER (Microvolt T Wave Alternans Testing for Risk Stratification of Post-Myocardial Infarction Patients) trial. *J Am Coll Cardiol.* 2008;52:1607-1615, with permission from the American College of Cardiology.)

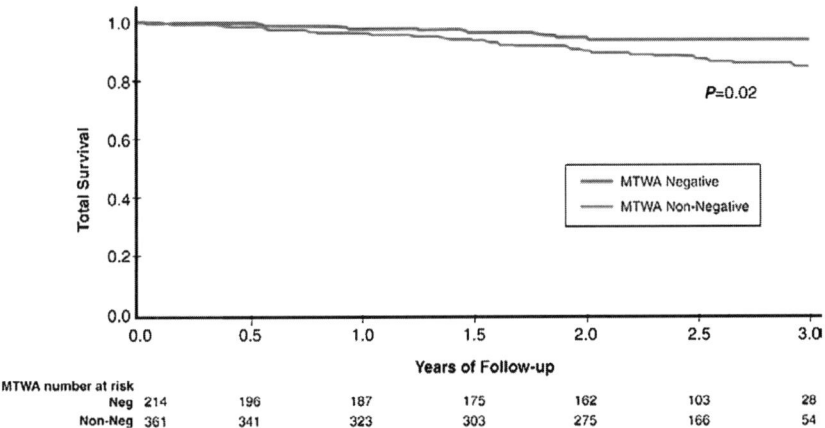

FIGURE 2.—Kaplan-Meier Survival Curves for Total Mortality. MTWA = microvolt T-wave alternans. (Reprinted from Chow T, on behalf of the MASTER Trial Investigators. Does microvolt T-wave alternans testing predict ventricular tachyarrhythmias in patients with ischemic cardiomyopathy and prophylactic defibrillators? The MASTER (Microvolt T Wave Alternans Testing for Risk Stratification of Post-Myocardial Infarction Patients) trial. *J Am Coll Cardiol.* 2008;52:1607-1615, with permission from the American College of Cardiology.)

in total mortality. (MASTER I–Microvolt T Wave Alternans Testing for Risk Stratification of Post MI Patients; NCT00305240) (Figs 1 and 2).

▶ The search to find better predictors of malignant ventricular arrhythmias (MVA) and sudden cardiac death in postmyocardial infarction (PMI) patients than left ventricular ejection fraction (LVEF) is important to limit implantable cardioverter-defibrillator (ICD) implantation to those who will benefit most. Finding a way of identifying the patients at highest risk is especially compelling in a financially overburdened health care system where ICDs are implanted in patients at low risk for MVA. Detection of microvolt T-wave alternans (MTWA) during controlled heart rate elevation has been reported to be a potential predictor of MVA and mortality[1] in PMI patients,[2] in those with ischemic cardiomyopathy[3] or heart failure.[4] The Microvolt T-Wave Alternans Testing for Risk Stratification of Post-Myocardial Infarction Patients (MASTERS) trial is a prospective, multihospital trial of patients meeting the Multicenter Automatic Defibrillator Implantation Trial II (MADIT II) indications for ICD implantation: LVEF ≤ 30% in patients ≥1 month PMI (with many exclusions) where MTWA was done. In the minimal follow-up time of 2 years, with MTWA done annually, there was no observed correlation between MTWA results and MVA and sudden death. There was a significant if very small difference in total mortality, with the MTWA non-negative group having a slightly lower survival. With subgroup analyses, including those on β-blockers, with cardiac synchronization therapy, and by the New York Heart Association (NYHA) class, MTWA prediction did not achieve statistical significance. These findings are consistent with several recently published prospective studies of MTWA testing in low-LVEF patients, including the Sudden Cardiac Death in Heart Failure Trial (SCD-HeFT) (MTWA substudy) and the Cardiac Arrhythmias and Risk Stratification after Myocardial Infarction (CARISMA) study. Although it is possible that, bundled with other known risk factors for MVA or in a more differentiated subgroup of patients, MTWA will add predictive value for identifying patients at high risk of MVA, at present it appears that MTWA, at least in the PMI patients with low LVEF, does not identify the patients at high-risk for MVA.

M. D. Cheitlin, MD

References

1. Gehi AK, Stein RH, Metz LD, Gomes JA. Microvolt T-wave alternans for the risk stratification of ventricular tachyarrhythmic events: a meta-analysis. *J Am Coll Cardiol.* 2005;46:75-82.
2. Ikeda T, Saito H, Tanno K, et al. T-wave alternans as a predictor for sudden cardiac death after myocardial infarction. *Am J Cardiol.* 2002;89:79-82.
3. Chow T, Kereiakes DJ, Bartone C, et al. Prognostic utility of microvolt T-wave alternans in risk stratification of patients with ischemic cardiomyopathy. *J Am Coll Cardiol.* 2006;47:1820-1827.
4. Bloomfield DM, Bigger JT, Steinman RC, et al. Microvolt T-wave alternans and the risk of death or sustained ventricular arrhythmias in patients with left ventricular dysfunction. *J Am Coll Cardiol.* 2006;47:456-463.

Randomized Trial of Cardiac Resynchronization in Mildly Symptomatic Heart Failure Patients and in Asymptomatic Patients With Left Ventricular Dysfunction and Previous Heart Failure Symptoms

Linde C, Abraham WT, Gold MR, et al (Karolinska Univ Hosp, Stockholm, Sweden; Ohio State Univ, Columbus; Med Univ of South Carolina, Charleston; et al)
J Am Coll Cardiol 52:1834-1843, 2008

Objectives.—We sought to determine the effects of cardiac resynchronization therapy (CRT) in New York Heart Association (NYHA) functional class II heart failure (HF) and NYHA functional class I (American College of Cardiology/American Heart Association stage C) patients with previous HF symptoms.

Background.—Cardiac resynchronization therapy improves left ventricular (LV) structure and function and clinical outcomes in NYHA functional class III and IV HF with prolonged QRS.

Methods.—Six hundred ten patients with NYHA functional class I or II heart failure with a QRS $\geq$120 ms and a LV ejection fraction $\leq$40% received a CRT device ($\pm$defibrillator) and were randomly assigned to active CRT (CRT-ON; n = 419) or control (CRT-OFF; n = 191) for 12 months. The primary end point was the HF clinical composite response, which scores patients as improved, unchanged, or worsened. The prospectively powered secondary end point was LV end-systolic volume index. Hospitalization for worsening HF was evaluated in a prospective secondary analysis of health care use.

Results.—The HF clinical composite response end point, which compared only the percent worsened, indicated 16% worsened in CRT-ON compared with 21% in CRT-OFF (p = 0.10). Patients assigned to CRT-ON experienced a greater improvement in LV end-systolic volume index (-18.4 ± 29.5 ml/m^2 vs. -1.3 ± 23.4 ml/m^2, p < 0.0001) and other measures of LV remodeling. Time-to-first HF hospitalization was significantly delayed in CRT-ON (hazard ratio: 0.47, p = 0.03).

Conclusions.—The REVERSE (REsynchronization reVErses Remodeling in Systolic left vEntricular dysfunction) trial demonstrates that CRT, in combination with optimal medical therapy ($\pm$defibrillator), reduces the risk for heart failure hospitalization and improves ventricular structure and function in NYHA functional class II and NYHA functional class I (American College of Cardiology/American Heart Association stage C) patients with previous HF symptoms. (REsynchronization reVErses Remodeling in Systolic Left vEntricular Dysfunction [REVERSE]; NCT00271154).

▶ The REsynchronization reVErses Remodeling in Systolic left vEntricular dysfunction (REVERSE) trial shows for the first time in a large multicenter, randomized, double blind study that cardiac resynchronization therapy (CRT) improves ventricular structure and function in patients with asymptomatic and mildly symptomatic heart failure. In addition, the trial demonstrates a significant reduction in heart failure morbidity defined as the need for hospitalization for worsening heart failure. And finally, REVERSE found no significant improvement in quality of life or exercise capacity with CRT. The number of deaths in the study was so small that it was very hard to say anything about mortality. Thus, what would have happened with cardiac resynchronization therapy-defibrillator (CRT-D)? For this patient population, that therapy doesn't seem appropriate, but data do seem to support CRT-D for patients with more severe heart failure.

A. L. Waldo, MD

42 Cardiac Surgery

Aortic Root Operations for Marfan Syndrome: A Comparison of the Bentall and Valve-Sparing Procedures

Patel ND, Weiss ES, Alejo DE, et al (The Johns Hopkins Med Insts, Baltimore, MD)
Ann Thorac Surg 85:2003-2011, 2008

Background.—We compared results of the Bentall procedure with valve-sparing aortic root replacement (VSRR) for aortic root aneurysm in Marfan syndrome.

Methods.—Marfan syndrome patients who had the Bentall procedure or VSRR at our institution between April 1997 and September 2006 were identified. Follow-up information was obtained from hospital charts and contact with patients or their physicians. Kaplan-Meier survival and propensity score analyses were performed.

Results.—One hundred forty Marfan syndrome patients had either the Bentall procedure (n = 56) or VSRR (n = 84; 40 remodeling and 44 reimplantation). Bentall patients were older than VSRR patients (38 versus 29 years; $p = 0.0001$) and had more aortic dissections (16% versus 1%; $p = 0.0012$); more urgent/emergent surgery (20% versus 2%; $p = 0.0008$); larger preoperative sinus diameter (5.7 versus 5.1 cm; $p = 0.0004$); and more preoperative 3+/4+ aortic insufficiency (59% versus 10%; $p < 0.0001$). There were no operative deaths. Postoperatively, 9% Bentall patients (5 of 56) and 1% of VSRR patients (1 of 84) suffered thromboembolic events ($p = 0.03$). Two percent (1 of 56) of Bentall patients required reoperation on the aortic root versus 6% of VSRR patients (5 of 84; $p = 0.40$). Eight-year freedom from aortic valve replacement was 90% for VSRR patients. Eight-year survival was 90% for Bentall and 100% for VSRR patients ($p = 0.01$). Propensity-adjusted regression showed that the Bentall procedure did not predict mortality ($p = 1.00$) and did not protect from reoperation (odds ratio = 0.28; 95% confidence interval: 0.01 to 4.33; $p = 0.36$).

Conclusions.—The Bentall procedure and VSRR have similar operative results in Marfan syndrome. The procedures are distinguished by higher rates of thromboembolism among Bentall patients and higher rates of reoperation among VSRR patients. Lower late survival among Bentall patients probably reflects the preferential use of the Bentall procedure for higher risk patients.

▶ Marfan syndrome is an autosomal dominant connective tissue disorder caused by mutations in the fibrillin-1 gene leading to abnormalities, including aortic root aneurysms and aortic dissection. Cardiac care professionals are charged with the responsibility of diagnosing, following, and intervening on these patients at an appropriate time to avoid these disastrous outcomes. The traditional surgical standard has been the Bentall procedure as shown by Gott et al.[1] Although the Bentall procedure has excellent short- and long-term results, implanting a mechanical aortic valve prosthesis as a combined valve graft conduit is associated with a significant risk of anticoagulation-related morbidity and mortality. It is for this reason that valve-sparing root operations have evolved which replace the abnormal aortic sinuses but spare normal aortic valve cusps. Valve-sparing operations were initially introduced by Yacoub[2] and David.[3] The difficulty with these early iterations was the increased rate of mid- to long-term valvular incompetence leading to aortic valve reoperation. Subsequent versions of the operation have evolved that stabilize the aortic annulus inside a tunnel of Dacron tubing, preventing annular dilatation as a cause of aortic valve regurgitation. The creation of aortic neo-sinuses also theoretically prevents cusp abrasion on the edge of the Dacron conduit and creates more normal sinus flow dynamics. The latest iterations have typically been referred to as versions of the "David V" operation.[4] Dr Cameron and colleagues from Johns Hopkins University have championed a specific modification of the "David V" operation that uses a preformed sinus of Valsalva graft. Importantly, Dr Cameron cites that he determines the optimal size of the graft by estimating the ideal sinotubular junction diameter and then selecting a graft that is 2 to 3 mm larger. He states that most patients have an optimal diameter of 28 to 30 mm, which translates into a usual graft size of 30 to 32 mm.

The authors have retrospectively analyzed their impressive series of Bentall and valve-sparing root operations in treating Marfan syndrome patients with aortic root aneurysms. Between 1997 to 2006, all patients who underwent such operations were included. The authors stated that they selected against a valve-sparing operation if the annular diameter was greater than 34, the leaflets were fenestrated or asymmetrical, acute aortic dissection existed, the patient was unstable, or a "giant" aortic root was present. The aortic cusp anatomy was also involved in the subjective selection criteria as abnormal tissue quality, including calcification, prolapse, thickening, or fenestrations, were not selected for preservation. A total of 140 patients were studied; 56 had the Bentall operation, and 84 had a valve-sparing root replacement. Bentall patients were significantly older and were more likely to have an aortic dissection, bicuspid aortic valves, urgent/emergent operations, a larger preoperative sinus dimension, and more frequently preoperative 3+/4+ aortic insufficiency. Mean cross-clamp times were significantly longer in the Bentall group. More of these patients had concomitant mitral valve replacement and coronary artery bypass grafting. There were no early deaths. Late survival at 8 years was 90.1% for Bentall patients and 100% for the valve-sparing patients. In-hospital complications were similar in both groups; however, thromboembolic events were more frequent after the Bentall operation than after valve-sparing root replacement (Bentall—8.9% vs valve-sparing root replacement—1.2%, $P < .03$). Aortic root reoperation was required in one Bentall patient (thrombosed aortic valve) and 5 valve-sparing root patients. All 5 valve-sparing patients who required reoperation had significant aortic valve incompetence owing to annular dilatation following treatment with an early iteration of the valve-sparing root operation without annular stabilization. Of interest, the authors are clear to point out that no patient who had a reimplantation operation ("later version") including annular stabilization with the Valsalva graft required reoperation for valve failure. Freedom from re-operation on the aortic root was 95.8% in the Bentall group and 90.4% for the valve-sparing group at 8 years. The authors performed propensity score analysis to control for the effects of self-stated selection bias. Propensity score regression modeling demonstrated that the Bentall procedure was not a predictor of late mortality nor did it predict reoperation.

The presented series by Dr Cameron's group is an important contribution to the literature. They have transitioned away from the Bentall procedure as a default gold standard operation for aortic root aneurysms in Marfan syndrome–a trend that is supported by clear data in the article. In order to prevent differential lengths of follow-up, they analyzed the data from a more recent era (1997-2006) when both the Bentall operation and valve-sparing root procedures were performed. The early and late results are excellent, as would be expected with increasing familiarity performing this technically challenging operation. The authors also report in their subgroup analysis that no patient who had reimplantation with the Valsalva graft (including annular stabilization) had greater than 2+ aortic valve insufficiency and none required operation—both of which are impressive findings. The authors state that their current recommendation is to offer surgery for aortic root aneurysms in Marfan syndrome when the aortic root diameter is greater than 5 cm, when the sinus diameter increases more then 1 cm per year, or when aortic valve insufficiency is progressive. The ideal next step in comparing the outcomes of these two platforms would be to perform a randomized control trial. However, as the authors admit, there is substantial surgical bias within the field that likely precludes the ability to perform such a trial. Nonetheless, the current series is one of the most impressive in the literature and does justify the referral of patients with aortic root aneurysms because of Marfan disease or diseases of abnormal connective tissue but with normal cusp anatomy where aortic valve-sparing root operation can reliably be safely performed with excellent long-term durability.

R. Suri, MD, DPhil

References

1. Gott VL, Greene PS, Alejo DE, et al. Replacement of the aortic root in patients with Marfan's syndrome. *N Engl J Med.* 1999;340:1307-1313.
2. Sarsan MAI, Yacoub M. Remodeling of the aortic valve annulus. *J Thorac Cardiovasc Surg.* 1993;105:435-438.
3. David TE, Feindel CM. An aortic valve-sparing operation for patients with aortic incompetence and aneurysm of the ascending aorta. *J Thorac Cardiovasc Surg.* 1992;103:617-620.
4. Miller DC. Valve-sparing aortic root replacement in patients with Marfan's syndrome. *J Thorac Cardiovasc Surg.* 2003;25:773-778.

Aortic Valve Replacement for Low-Flow/Low-Gradient Aortic Stenosis: Operative Risk Stratification and Long-Term Outcome: A European Multicenter Study

Levy F, Laurent M, Monin JL, et al (Univ Hosp, Amiens, France; Univ Hosp, Rennes, France; Henri Mondor Hosp, Créteil, France; et al)

J Am Coll Cardiol 51:1466-1472, 2008

Objectives.—We evaluated a large multicenter series of patients operated on for low-flow/low-gradient aortic stenosis (LF/LGAS) to stratify the operative risk, assess whether perioperative mortality has decreased over recent years, and analyze the post-operative outcome.

Background.—Although LF/LGAS is classically associated with a high operative risk, few data are available concerning the results of surgery in this setting.

Methods.—A total of 217 consecutive patients (168 men, 77%) with severe aortic stenosis (area <1 cm^2), low ejection fraction (EF) ($\leq$35%), and low mean gradient (MG) ($\leq$30 mm Hg) who underwent aortic valve replacement (AVR) between 1990 and 2005 were included.

Results.—Perioperative mortality was 16% and decreased dramatically from 20% in the 1990 to 1999 period to 10% in the 2000 to 2005 period. Higher European System for Cardiac Operative Risk Evaluation score (EuroSCORE), very low MG and EF, New York Heart Association functional class III or IV, history of congestive heart failure, and multivessel coronary artery disease (MVD) were associated with perioperative mortality. On multivariate analysis, very low pre-operative MG and MVD were predictors of excess perioperative mortality. In the subgroup of patients with dobutamine stress echocardiography, the absence of contractile reserve was a strong predictor of perioperative mortality. Overall 5-year survival rate was 49 ± 4%. Lower MG, higher EuroSCORE, prior atrial fibrillation, and MVD were identified as independent predictors of overall long-term mortality.

Conclusions.—In view of the very poor prognosis of unoperated patients, the current operative risk, and the long-term outcome after surgery, AVR is the treatment of choice in the majority of cases of LF/LGAS.

▶ Aortic valve stenosis in the setting of left ventricular dysfunction is a difficult clinical problem, as patients do poorly without surgery; yet, operative mortality has been reported to be quite high.[1,2] The subset of patients with a diminished ejection fraction and a low mean gradient has been particularly identified as problematic in the past.[3] The definition of "low-gradient" aortic stenosis encompasses those with aortic valve stenosis and a gradient of less than 30 mm Hg in the setting of left ventricular dysfunction.[4] The authors sought to determine the postsurgical outcome of a series of 217 patients with severe aortic valve stenosis defined by a valve area of less than 1 cm^2 with an ejection fraction of less than 35% and a mean gradient of less than 30 mm Hg who underwent aortic valve replacement between 1990 and 2005.

The authors observed an operative mortality of 60%, which decreased over the study period from 20% early on to 10% between 2000 and 2005. Independent predictors of poor outcome were very low preoperative mean gradient and multivessel disease. They further analyzed a subset of 38% of patients who underwent dobutamine stress echo finding that the absence of contractile reserve was a strong predictor of early mortality. Mid-term survival at 5 years was 49%, and independent predictors of poor outcome were lower mean gradient, higher EuroSCORE, atrial fibrillation, and multivessel disease. The authors make the point that more than half of the late deaths were because of noncardiac causes and underline that significant coronary artery disease and very low mean gradient (less than 20 mm Hg) are predictive of increased early and late mortality.

This is an impressive study analyzing a large series of patients from multiple centers affected by a challenging disease. The lack of uniformity in obtaining a dobutamine stress echo is perhaps a limiting factor; however, the authors are to be congratulated for their ability to identify influential prognostic indicators. It is likely that the increased use of dobutamine stress echo in the future will help better stratify risk in this patient population. In summary, the study indicates that the early surgical survival of aortic valve replacement for low-gradient aortic valve stenosis in the current era is now acceptable— approximately 90%. Preoperative dobutamine stress echocardiography, coronary angiography, and symptoms are very helpful in stratifying risk in patients and will be helpful to cardiologist and surgeon alike in helping to determine which patients should undergo surgical intervention.

R. Suri, MD, DPhil

References

1. Vaquette B, Corbineau H, Laurent M, et al. Valve replacement in patients with critical aortic stenosis and depressed left ventricular function: predictors of operative risk, left ventricular recovery, and long-term outcome. *Heart.* 2005;91: 1324-1329.
2. Connolly H, Oh J, Orszulak TA, et al. Aortic valve replacement for aortic stenosis with left ventricular dysfunction. Prognostic indicators. *Circulation.* 1997;95: 2395-2400.
3. Connolly H, Oh J, Schaff HV, et al. Severe aortic stenosis with low transvalvular gradient and severe left ventricular dysfunction: result of aortic valve replacement in 52 patients. *Circulation.* 2000;101:1940-1946.
4. Bonow RO, Carabello B, Chatterjee K, et al. ACC/AHA 2006 practice guidelines for the management of patients with valvular heart disease–executive summary: a report of the American College of Cardiology/American Heart Association Task Force on Practice Guidelines (Writing Committee to Revise the 1998 guidelines for the Management of Patients with Valvular Heart Disease). *J Am Coll Cardiol.* 2006;48:598-675.

Aortic valve replacement in patients aged 50 to 70 years: Improved outcome with mechanical versus biologic prostheses
Brown ML, Schaff HV, Lahr BD, et al (Mayo Clinic, Rochester, Minn)
J Thorac Cardiovasc Surg 135:878-884, 2008

Objective.—Improved durability of bioprostheses has led some surgeons to recommend biologic rather than mechanical prostheses for patients younger than 65 years. We compared late results of contemporary bioprostheses and bileaflet mechanical prostheses in patients who underwent aortic valve replacement between 50 and 70 years old.

Methods.—In this retrospective study, patients received either St Jude bileaflet valves or Carpentier–Edwards bioprostheses. Operations were performed between January 1991 and December 2000, and groups were matched one-to-one according to age, sex, need for coronary artery bypass grafting, and valve size.

Results.—Four hundred forty patients were matched, and follow-up was 92% complete, with median durations of 9.1 years for patients who received mechanical valves and 6.2 years for patients who received bioprostheses. The 5- and 10-year unadjusted survivals were 87% and 68% for mechanical valves and 72% and 50% for bioprostheses, respectively ($P < .01$). Freedoms from reoperation at 10 years were 98% for mechanical valves and 91% for bioprostheses ($P = .06$). Rates of late stroke or other embolic events and of endocarditis were similar between groups. Hemorrhagic complications necessitating hospitalization occurred in 15% of patients with mechanical valves and 7% of patients with bioprostheses ($P = .01$). Notably, 19% of patients with bioprostheses were receiving warfarin sodium at last follow-up. After adjustment for unmatched variables, including diabetes, renal failure, lung disease, New York Heart Association functional class, ejection fraction, and stroke, the use of a mechanical valve was protective against late mortality (hazard ratio 0.46, $P < .01$).

Conclusion.—In this study, patients aged 50 to 70 years who underwent aortic valve replacement with mechanical valves had a survival advantage relative to matched patients who received bioprostheses. These findings question recommendations of bioprostheses for younger patients and suggest that a randomized trial may be warranted.

▶ The current ACC/AHA guidelines suggest that mechanical valve replacement should be considered in those younger than age 65 to minimize the subsequent need for reoperation.[1] There has been recent debate among clinicians whether this age should be lowered because of the suggestion by medical device companies that current-generation bioprostheses offer improved device durability. The debate largely focuses around patients between the ages of 50 to 70 years. The literature lacks a large and robust study addressing the issue of valve superiority in this patient population. Brown and colleagues from Mayo Clinic studied patients undergoing aortic valve replacement (AVR) with either the St. Jude bileaflet mechanical valve or the Carpentier-Edwards bovine bioprosthesis between 1991 and 2000. Four hundred and forty patients were matched, and follow-up was 92% complete with a mean duration of 9.1 years for mechanical valves and 6.2 years for bioprostheses. Ten-year survival was 68% for mechanical and 50% for bioprosthetic valves, which was significantly different. Freedom from reoperation at 10 years was 98% for mechanical and 91% for bioprostheses ($P = 0.06$). The rates of late thromboembolic events and endocarditis were similar between the two groups. Hemorrhagic complications necessitating hospitalization occurred in 15% of those with mechanical valves and 7% with bioprosthesis. Nineteen percent of patients with bioprostheses were being treated with warfarin at the time of last follow-up. Multiple variable analysis identified the use of a mechanical valve as protective against late mortality.

This is an important study addressing a very topical subject, which is debated daily in clinics and operating rooms worldwide. The suggestion that the increased risk of reoperation following implantation of a bioprosthetic valve might somehow not be an important item of consideration because of the potential evolution of future nonsurgical strategies is speculative and dangerous. Previous data have shown superior survival for patients with a mechanical valve compared with biological prostheses.[2-4] The reported freedom from structural biological valve deterioration ranges between 54% at 15 years to 96% at 12 years.[5,6] Of importance is the fact that implantation of biological prostheses in those younger than 70 years of age will likely necessitate a reoperation after the age of 80, which often is associated with an increased risk of mortality—as high as 17.4% in reported series.[7] Some argue that freedom from warfarin anticoagulation following implantation of a biological prosthesis justifies the widespread use of these devices at a younger age. However, as this series shows, patients often acquire an indication for anticoagulation as they age, which is often not prosthesis-related. Moreover, with the widespread availability of home INR monitoring patient compliance and safety of anticoagulation will likely be increased. This issue is currently being investigated in randomized control trials worldwide. Another important finding in this study was the fact that there was no difference in late thromboembolism between the two prosthetic types. The higher rate of death in the bioprosthetic group may have been due to the effect of senescent biological valves in patients who were too ill or have refused reoperation. In summary, the current improved survival of patients receiving mechanical prostheses between the ages of 50 to 70 years warrants careful consideration. This important study suggests that recommending a bioprosthetic aortic valve for those younger than 65 years of age should be weighed against the consequences of increased reoperation risk and decreased long-term survival. It is important that these data are shared objectively with the patient during preoperative consultation previous to aortic valve replacement.

R. Suri, MD, DPhil

References

1. American College of Cardiology/American Heart association Task Force on Practice Guidelines, Society of Cardiovascular Anesthesiologists, Society for Cardiovascular Angiography and Interventions, Society of Thoracic Surgeons, Bonow RO, Carbello BA, Kanu C, et al. ACC/AHA 2006 practice guidelines for the management of patients with valvular heart disease–executive summary: a report of the American College of Cardiology/American Heart Association Task Force on Practice Guidelines (Writing Committee to Revise the 1998 guidelines for the Management of Patients with Valvular Heart Disease): developed in collaboration with the Society of Cardiovascular Anesthesiologists: endorsed by the Society for Cardiovascular Angiography and Interventions and the Society of Thoracic Surgeons. *Circulation.* 2006;114:e84-e231.
2. Hammermeister K, Sethi GK, Henderson WG, Grover FL, Oprian C, Rahimtoola SH. Outcomes 15 years after valve replacement with a mechanical versus a bioprosthetic valve: final report of the Veterans Affairs randomized trial. *J Am Coll Cardiol.* 2000;36:1152-1158.
3. Oxenham H, Bloomfield P, Wheatley DJ, et al. Twenty year comparison of a Bjork-Shiley mechanical heart valve with porcine bioprostheses. *Heart.* 2003;89: 715-721.
4. Hanania G, Michel PL, Montely JM, et al. Outcomes 15 years after valve replacement with a mechanical versus a bioprosthetic valve in patients between 60 and 70 years of age. *J Am Coll Cardiol.* 2002;39:423A.
5. Jamieson WR, Lemieus MD, Sullivan JA, Munro IA, Métras J, Cartier PC. Medtronic Intact porcine bioprosthesis experience to twelve years. *Ann Thorac Surg.* 2001;7:S278-S281.
6. Cohn LH, Collins JJ Jr, Rizzo RJ, Adams DH, Couper GS, Aranki SF. Twenty-year follow-up of the Hancock modified orifice porcine aortic valve. *Ann Thorac Surg.* 1998;66:S30-S34.
7. Eitz T, Fritsche D, Kleikamp G, Zittermann A, Horstkotte D, Körfer R. Reoperation of the aortic valve in octogenarians. *Ann Thorac Surg.* 2006;82:1385-1391.

A Blocking Anti-CD28-Specific Antibody Induces Long-Term Heart Allograft Survival by Suppression of the PKCθ-JNK Signal Pathway

Jang M-S, Pan F, Erickson LM, et al (Astellas Res Inst of America, Skokie, IL)
Transplantation 85:1051-1055, 2008

This study investigated the effects of a blocking anti-CD28 antibody (Anti-CD28-PV1-IgG3) in vitro and in vivo. Anti-CD28-PV1-IgG3, a hamster-mouse chimeric antibody against murine CD28, which does not provide CD28-positive signaling during TCR-driven T cell activation, enabled long-term survival of heart allografts across a complete mismatch of the MHC in rats. Among the T cell signaling proteins tested in the spleens from recipients, we found that recipients treated with anti-CD28-PV1-IgG3 exhibited suppression of alloantigen-initiated proximal TCR signaling events, including Lck, Zap70, Vav, and PI3K expression, and their PKCθ- and JNK-regulated expression/activation. This leads to attenuation of intragraft T cell infiltration and expression of T cell effector molecules. These results indicate that targeting the CD28 receptor with a blocking antibody leads to long-term allograft survival by reducing activation of alloantigen-mediated key signaling events in T cells that might be crucial for full T cell activation.

▶ The authors sought to investigate the effects of a novel blocking anti-CD28 antibody (anti-CD28-PV1-IgG3) in vitro and in vivo. They investigated the effects of a novel chimeric antibody against murine CD28, which blocks CD28-signaling during T cell activation. The authors explain that previous attempts in earlier anti-CD28 models failed because of positive adjuvant-like signaling of the antibody, which overcame the attempt at costimulatory blockade.[1,2]

The first in vitro tests were basic mixed leukocyte reaction MLR assays comparing 2 allogeneic mouse subsets. CD28 blockage resulted in a decrease in T cell proliferation and IL-2 elaboration. A subsequent in vivo model demonstrated the ability of the anti-CD28 antibody to block the CD3-dependent stimulation, resulting in decrease in splenocyte proliferation and IL-2 mRNA expression by PCR. The authors then performed an in vivo transplant survival study in which the LEW recipients of BN hearts were treated with anti-CD28. The endpoints were rat survival, detection of intragraft T cell infiltration, and gene expression. Anti-CD28 resulted in significantly prolonged allograft survival from 7 days in controls to a median of 23 days. The effect was dose dependent. Moreover, cotreatment with tacrolimus (TAC) resulted in further prolongation of allograft survival. Finally, hearts from animals that had a prolonged survival and were explanted had profound reduction in CD25 T cell infiltration as proportion total CD6[+] T cells.

The study presents interesting incremental evidence that a true in vivo effect of CD28 costimulatory blockade is possible and is capable of altering T cell responses significantly enough to influence allograft survival. The findings of this study will have implications in devising regimens aimed at modifying pathologic immune responses both in clinical transplantation and autoimmune disease.[3] Finally, the authors did find an interesting correlation between the mechanism of graft prolongation and PKCθ/JNK pathway alteration that will need to be investigated further in future studies.

R. Suri, MD, DPhil

References

1. Yu XZ, Bidwell SJ, Martin PJ, et al. CD28-specific antibody prevents graft-versus-host disease in mice. *J Immunol*. 2000;164:4564.
2. Dengler TJ, Szabo G, Sido B, et al. Prolonged allograft survival but no tolerance induction by modulating CD28 antibody JJ319 after high-responder rat heart transplantation. *Transplantation*. 1999;67:392.
3. Larsen CP, Elwood ET, Alexander DZ, et al. Long-term acceptance of skin and cardiac allografts after blocking CD40 and CD28 pathways. *Nature*. 1996;381: 434.

A Prospective, Multicenter Trial of the VentrAssist Left Ventricular Assist Device for Bridge to Transplant: Safety and Efficacy

Esmore D, Kaye D, Spratt P, et al (The Alfred Hosp Melbourne, Australia; St Vincent's Hosp, Sydney, Australia; et al)
J Heart Lung Transplant 27:579-588, 2008

Background.—The increasing prevalence of chronic heart failure has stimulated the ongoing development of left ventricular assist devices (LVADs) for both bridge-to-transplant (BTT) and destination therapy (DT). The aim of this prospective, multicenter clinical trial was to determine the efficacy and safety of a third-generation LVAD, the VentrAssist, in a BTT cohort.

Methods.—Patients (n = 33) with end-stage chronic heart failure who required circulatory support as BTT therapy were implanted with a VentrAssist device. The primary outcome was survival until transplant or transplant eligibility with the device in situ at trial end-point (Day 154 after implant). The secondary outcomes were pump flow index and end-organ function. Safety, patient functional status and resource use were also assessed.

Results.—At trial end-point, the success rate was 82% (39.4% transplanted, 42.4% transplant-eligible). The LVAD pump flow index (median ≥ 2.7 liters/min/m^2) was sufficient to maintain an adequate circulation and significantly improve end-organ function. Of the 77 protocol-defined serious adverse events, most occurred within 30 days of implantation. No patients died as a direct result of pump failure or malfunction. After implantation, patient functional status improved, with 70% of patients achieving hospital discharge, and resource use was reduced.

Conclusions.—This trial demonstrated a favorable efficacy and safety profile for use of the VentrAssist LVAD in BTT patients.

▶ It is well known that chronic heart failure is a significant problem in current medicine, and the lack of a sufficient supply of donor hearts limits cardiac allotransplantation as a universal solution. The advent of third-generation left ventricular assist devices (LVADs) for bridge-to-transplant purposes (BTT) may impact patient survival and increase the survival rates until an appropriate organ substitute is found. The third-generation devices are continuous-flow machines with modifications addressing previous earlier generation LVAD limitations including bulky size, noise, diminished reliability, and mechanical failure.

This study by Dr Esmore and colleagues reports on the results of a prospective, multicenter clinical trial examining the safety and efficacy of a third-generation LVAD, the VentrAssist device as a bridge to transplantation (BTT). Thirty-three individuals underwent implantation of the device and survival and transplant eligibility with the device in place were the primary end points. Secondary end points were pump flow index, end-organ function, safety, functional status, and resource use. The authors reported that out of 43 screened patients, 33 underwent implantation with the VentrAssist. The reasons for exclusion included septicemia, right heart failure, death, and inflammatory valve disease. Mean device implant time was 197 days, and 39.4% were successfully bridged to transplant although 42.4% remain transplant eligible. The causes of death for those who did not survive to transplantation include sepsis, ischemic valve disease, multiple organ failure, and elective treatment withdrawal because of poor prognosis. Mean pump flow index was 2.7 liters. The device provided adequate hemodynamic support to restore end-organ function as determined by improvements in kidney and liver indices. Device-related adverse events were highest in the first 30 days following implant (68%). The authors state that of all device-related adverse events only 6 were caused by LVAD malfunction. There were no catastrophic pump failures. Early right ventricular failure was seen in patients with marginal right ventricular function, which numbered 4 in the first 30 days following implantation. Significant improvement was found in the quality of life questionnaire score with 81% attaining New York Heart Association Class 1 or 2 status by postoperative day 154. The use of cardiac medication, including inotropes and diuretics, was decreased and 70% were dismissed from hospital. Importantly, 74% required readmission.

The study is a clear confirmation that third-generation LVADs are a viable mechanism to increase patient stability while allowing clinical improvement in a difficult population of patients awaiting cardiac transplantation. The results demonstrate significant progress from trials of previous generations of LVAD.[1] One year following VentrAssist implantation, 80% of patients were either transplanted or remained transplant eligible, and adverse events were similar to other LVADs.[1-3] In a previous trial of the HeartMate II device, 75% obtained this endpoint.[1] The authors suggest that even better results may have been obtained if the device had been implanted in earlier stage heart failure patients. As reported in other trials, common adverse events included infectious, hemorrhagic, thromboembolic, neurologic, and cardiovascular complications. It is interesting that the favorable results were obtained even in centers with limited LVAD experience, causing the authors to propose that the learning curve for implantation of the device might be short.

In summary, this is a very interesting study demonstrating the clinical utility of third-generation LVAD devices in improving patient quality of life, decreasing resource utilization, and allowing successful bridge to transplantation in a complex and heterogeneous group of patients. Subsequent studies, including the European BRACE Study, will examine this.

R. Suri, MD, DPhil

References

1. Miller LW, Pagani FD, Russell SD, et al. Use of a continuous-flow device in patients awaiting heart transplantation. *N Engl J Med.* 2007;357:895-896.
2. Deng MC, Edwards LB, Hertz MI, et al. Mechanical circulatory support device database of the International Society for Heart and Lung Transplantation. Third annual report—2005. *J Heart Lung Transplant.* 2005;24:1182-1187.
3. Sharples LD, Cafferty F, Demitis N, et al. Evaluation of the clinical effectiveness of the Ventricular Assist Device Program in the United Kingdom (EVAD UK). *J Heart Lung Transplant.* 2007;26:9-15.

Absence of Cognitive Decline One Year After Coronary Bypass Surgery: Comparison to Nonsurgical and Healthy Controls

Sweet JJ, Finnin E, Wolfe PL, et al (Evanston Northwestern Healthcare, IL; Northwestern Univ Feinberg School of Med, Chicago, IL; National Rehabilitation Hosp, Washington, DC)
Ann Thorac Surg 85:1571-1578, 2008

Background.—Cognitive decline after open-heart surgery has been the subject of a number of conflicting reports in recent years. Determination of possible cognitive impairment due to surgery or use of cardiopulmonary bypass is complicated by numerous factors, including use of appropriate comparison groups and consideration of practice effects in cognitive testing.

Methods.—Neuropsychological data were gathered from 46 healthy controls, 42 cardiac patients referred for percutaneous coronary intervention (PCI), and 43 cardiac patients referred for coronary artery bypass grafting (CABG). Fourteen cognitive function tests were utilized at baseline and at three time points after surgery (3 weeks, 4 months, 1 year). Measures showing acceptable test-retest reliability based on intraclass correlations were compared using regression-based reliable change indices.

Results.—No clear pattern of group differences or change at follow-up emerged. A greater percentage of CABG patients than controls worsened in seven tests (three at 1 year), but a greater percentage of PCI patients than controls also worsened in seven tests (three at 1 year). Generalized estimating equations showed only two tests (Wechsler Adult Intelligence Scale, Third Edition, Digit Symbol, and Hopkins Verbal Learning Test, Revised, Total Recall) to be significantly different between groups from baseline to 1 year. Interestingly, compared with healthy controls, more PCI patients than CABG patients worsened in the former of those two tests, whereas more PCI and CABG patients improved on the latter.

Conclusions.—Using healthy controls and a relevant nonsurgical comparison group to contend with important methodological considerations, current CABG procedure does not appear to create cognitive decline.

▶ Alterations in cognitive performance following coronary artery bypass grafting have been reported in the past; however, recent data suggest that there may be no significant change as compared with similarly matched populations not undergoing cardiac surgery.[1-3] This study was unique in that the authors sought to determine the extent of cognitive decline using neuropsychological data from 14 cognitive function tests. All tests were applied in a group of 43 surgical patients undergoing coronary artery bypass grafting along with 46 healthy controls and 42 cardiac patients referred for percutaneous coronary intervention (PCI). All tests were administered at baseline and subsequently at 3 designated time points after surgery/intervention—3 weeks, 4 months, and 1 year. The authors found that no clear differences at follow-up. Although more coronary artery bypass graft (CABG) patients than controls had diminished performance in 7 tests, a greater portion of PCI patients also deteriorated in performance following intervention. A statistical method known as the generalized estimating equation suggested that 2 tests—the Wechsler Adult Intelligence Scale and Hopkins Verbal Learning were significantly different between groups from baseline to 1 year; however, compared with healthy controls more PCI patients than CABG patients worsened in the former test. Of interest, coronary artery bypass graft surgery was performed using cardiopulmonary bypass, moderate hypothermia, epi-aortic ultrasonographic analysis of the ascending aorta before cannulation, and maintenance of a mean perfusion pressure of greater than 60 mm Hg during cardiopulmonary bypass time.

The results of this study are interesting in that they confirm recent data suggesting that no significant decline in cognitive function occurs following bypass surgery beyond that expected in a similarly risk matched population.[1-3] The authors have attempted to use "neurocognitive best practice" employing consensus-recommended neurocognitive testing. What is clear is that no clear trend in postprocedural cognitive function could be detected between healthy controls and the intervention groups. Recent studies have also suggested that there are no significant differences between on- and off-pump strategies during coronary revascularization.[4] This study will likely be an important reference article setting the standard for future meaningful comparisons of cognitive changes following intervention, particularly because of the strategic use of healthy controls and baseline measures.

R. Suri, MD, DPhil

References

1. Newman MF, Kirchner JL, Phillips-Bute B, et al. Longitudinal assessment of neurocognitive function after coronary artery bypass grafting surgery. *N Engl J Med*. 2001;344:395-402.
2. Roach GW, Kanchuger M, Mangano CM, et al. Adverse cerebral outcomes after coronary artery bypass grafting surgery. *N Engl J Med*. 1996;335:1857-1863.
3. Moody DM, Brown WR, Chalia VR, Stump DA, Reboussin DM, Legault C. Brain microemboli associated with cardiopulmonary bypass: a histologic and magnetic resonance imaging study. *Ann Thor Surg*. 1995;59:1304-1307.
4. Rankin K, Kochamba G, Boone K, Petitti DB, Buckwalter JG. Presurgical cognitive deficits in patients receiving coronary artery bypass grafting surgery. *J Int Neuropsych Soc*. 2003;9:913-924.

43 Coronary Heart Disease

Comparison of Thrombolysis Followed by Broad Use of Percutaneous Coronary Intervention with Primary Percutaneous Coronary Intervention for ST-Segment–Elevation Acute Myocardial Infarction: Data From the French Registry on Acute ST-Elevation Myocardial Infarction (FAST-MI)

Danchin N, for the FAST-MI Investigators (Hôpital Européen Georges Pompidou, Paris, France; et al)

Circulation 118:219-222, 2008

Background.—Intravenous thrombolysis remains a widely used treatment for ST-elevation myocardial infarction; however, it carries a higher risk of reinfarction than primary PCI (PPCI). There are few data comparing PPCI with thrombolysis followed by routine angiography and PCI. The purpose of the present study was to assess contemporary outcomes in ST-elevation myocardial infarction patients, with specific emphasis on comparing a pharmacoinvasive strategy (thrombolysis followed by routine angiography) with PPCI.

Methods and Results.—This nationwide registry in France included 223 centers and 1714 patients over a 1-month period at the end of 2005, with 1-year follow-up. Sixty percent of the patients underwent reperfusion therapy, 33% with PPCI and 29% with intravenous thrombolysis (18% prehospital). At baseline, the Global Registry of Acute Coronary Events score was similar in thrombolysis and PPCI patients. Time to initiation of reperfusion therapy was significantly shorter in thrombolysis than in PPCI (median 130 versus 300 minutes). After thrombolysis, 96% of patients had coronary angiography, and 84% had subsequent PCI (58% within 24 hours). In-hospital mortality was 4.3% for thrombolysis and 5.0% for PPCI. In patients with thrombolysis, 30-day mortality was 9.2% when PCI was not used and 3.9% when PCI was subsequently performed (4.0% if PCI was performed in the same hospital and 3.3% if performed after transfer to another facility). One-year survival was 94% for thrombolysis and 92% for PPCI (*P*=0.31). After propensity score matching, 1-year survival was 94% and 93%, respectively.

Conclusions.—When used early after the onset of symptoms, a pharma-coinvasive strategy that combines thrombolysis with a liberal use of PCI yields early and 1-year survival rates that are comparable to those of PPCI.

▶ This registry study from France describes the management and outcome of consecutive patients admitted to intensive care units with a definite diagnosis of myocardial infarction in 223 centers during a 1-month period in 2005. The analysis was confined to 1714 patients with ST-segment myocardial infarction (STEMI), of whom 60% underwent reperfusion therapy.

Primary percutaneous coronary intervention (PPCI) was the most frequently used form of reperfusion therapy (33%), with thrombolysis used in 29% (79% of whom received prehospital therapy). A key component of the thrombolytic strategy was the performance of coronary angiography and percutaneous coronary intervention (PCI) if necessary before discharge and within 24 hours in 75%.

As expected, patients without reperfusion therapy presented later and were a much sicker population with poor outcomes. This large registry study makes a strong case for a pharmacoinvasive strategy in patients presenting in the community, among which the strategy of primary PCI (PPCI) might entail a significant treatment delay. From first call to reperfusion therapy averaged 130 minutes in patients treated with thrombolysis versus 300 minutes with PPCI, and this was 85 minutes less in patients receiving prehospital lytic therapy. Thirty-day and 1-year mortality rates were similar in the 2 groups, but among the thrombolytic-treated patients, subsequent PCI was associated with a significant reduction in mortality. Consistent with previous data, mortality with PPCI tended to be lower than that with thrombolysis with increasing time from symptoms,[1,2] and these data also support the strategy of prehospital thrombolysis.[3]

The slope of the curve relating the duration of symptoms before reperfusion to the extent of myocardial salvage and reduction in mortality is consistent with the results of this registry study.[4] Few would dispute the superiority of PPCI given equal times to therapy, but the incremental delay in the performance of PCI is a key issue, particularly during the critical window of opportunity within the first 3 hours. A key component of this strategy is the liberal use of coronary angiography and PCI, if appropriate, after the administration of lytics with the option of either rescue or routine angiography within 24 to 48 hours.[5]

B. J. Gersh, MB, ChB, DPhil, FRCP

References

1. Kalla K, Christ G, Karnik R, et al. Implementation of guidelines improves the standard of care: the Viennese registry on reperfusion strategies in ST-elevation myocardial infarction (Vienna STEMI registry). *Circulation.* 2006;113: 2398-2405.
2. Steg PG, Bonnefoy E, Chabaud S, et al. Impact of time to treatment on mortality after prehospital fibrinolysis or primary angioplasty: data from the CAPTIM randomized clinical trial. *Circulation.* 2003;108:2851-2856.
3. Welsh RC, Travers AS, Senaratne M, Williams R, Armstrong PW. Feasibility and applicability of paramedic-based prehospital fibrinolysis in a large North American center. *Am Heart J.* 2006;152:1007-1014.

4. Gersh BJ, Stone GW, White HD, Holmes DR Jr. Pharmacological facilitation of primary percutaneous coronary intervention for acute myocardial infarction; is the slope of the curve the shape of the future? *JAMA.* 2005;293:979-986.
5. Ting HH, Rihal CS, Gersh BJ, et al. Regional systems of care to optimize timeliness of reperfusion therapy for ST-elevation myocardial infarction; the Mayo Clinic STEMI Protocol. *Circulation.* 2007;116:729-736.

Long-Term Benefit of Postconditioning

Thibault H, Piot C, Staat P, et al (Université Claude Bernard Lyon 1, France; Hôpital Arnaud de Villeneuve, Montpellier, France; et al)
Circulation 117:1037-1044, 2008

Background.—We previously demonstrated that ischemic postconditioning decreases creatine kinase release, a surrogate marker for infarct size, in patients with acute myocardial infarction. Our objective was to determine whether ischemic postconditioning could afford (1) a persistent infarct size limitation and (2) an improved recovery of myocardial contractile function several months after infarction.

Methods and Results.—Patients presenting within 6 hours of the onset of chest pain, with suspicion for a first ST-segment–elevation myocardial infarction, and for whom the clinical decision was made to treat with percutaneous coronary intervention, were eligible for enrollment. After reperfusion by direct stenting, 38 patients were randomly assigned to a control (no intervention; n=21) or postconditioned group (repeated inflation and deflation of the angioplasty balloon; n=17). Infarct size was assessed both by cardiac enzyme release during early reperfusion and by ^{201}thallium single photon emission computed tomography at 6 months after acute myocardial infarction. At 1 year, global and regional contractile function was evaluated by echocardiography. At 6 months after acute myocardial infarction, single photon emission computed tomography rest-redistribution index (a surrogate for infarct size) averaged 11.8 ± 10.3% versus 19.5 ± 13.3% in the postconditioned versus control group (*P*=0.04), in agreement with the significant reduction in creatine kinase and troponin I release observed in the postconditioned versus control group (−40% and −47%, respectively). At 1 year, the postconditioned group exhibited a 7% increase in left ventricular ejection fraction compared with control (*P*=0.04).

Conclusions.—Postconditioning affords persistent infarct size reduction and improves long-term functional recovery in patients with acute myocardial infarction.

▶ The history of reperfusion therapy for ST-segment elevation myocardial infarction (STEMI) and, in particular, the use of primary percutaneous coronary intervention (PPCI) has been characterized by a high success rate in terms of achieving patency of the infarct-related artery and consequent benefit with regard to myocardial salvage and mortality. The new frontier of reperfusion therapy is the achievement of optimal myocardial perfusion—a much more elusive target. Microvascular dysfunction and the more controversial entity of reperfusion injury are possibly the final common denominators of a number of pathophysiologic processes as yet not clearly defined,[1] but which nonetheless appear to result in the no-reflow phenomenon and impaired perfusion of the myocardium.[2] Moreover, it appears that surrogates of myocardial perfusion (eg, ST-segment resolution and myocardial blush grade) are also very important determinants of long-term prognosis.

In the experimental model of occlusion and reperfusion, a host of pharmacologic agents and other approaches have yielded positive results. In contrast, the results in the clinical setting have been extremely disappointing, and this area of investigation has been the graveyard of multiple clinical trials. For these reasons, the demonstration that the use of postconditioning results in long-term benefits on the infarct size and left ventricular function, when performed at the time of PPCI for STEMI, is indeed encouraging. The beneficial impact of ischemic preconditioning upon myocardial salvage is well documented in the experimental laboratory.[3] Several clinical studies have suggested an early effect on infarct size as assessed by the extent of the early rise in cardiac enzymes such as CK and troponin I.[4] This study takes matters a step further by demonstrating a reduction in sestamibi-determined infarct size at 6 months and as one would logically expect improved left ventricular function at 12 months. Although the study is small and there are no clinical outcome data, the results are most encouraging and support the initiation of larger randomized trials.

Although the phenomenon of ischemic preconditioning appears to be cardioprotective, its role in clinical medicine is very limited by the fact that one has to precondition before the onset of myocardial infarction—an impractical situation. Postconditioning, however, has the attraction in that this is performed at the time of PPCI, and it is also easy to do. This is a developing area to which we should stay tuned.

B. J. Gersh, MB, ChB, DPhil, FRCP

References

1. Kloner RA. Does reperfusion injury exist in humans? *J Am Coll Cardiol.* 1993;21: 537-545.
2. Kloner RA, Jennings RB. Consequences of brief ischemia: stunning, preconditioning, and their clinical implications: part 2. *Circulation.* 2001;104:3158-3167.
3. Zhao ZQ, Corvera JS, Halkos ME, et al. Inhibition of myocardial injury by ischemic postconditioning during reperfusion: comparison with ischemic preconditioning. *Am J Physiol.* 2003;285:H579-H588.
4. Staat P, Rioufol G, Piot C, et al. Postconditioning the human heart. *Circulation.* 2005;112:2143-2148.

Systems of Care to Improve Timeliness of Reperfusion Therapy for ST-Segement Elevation Myocardial Infraction During Off Hours: The Mayo Clinic STEMI Protocol

Holmes DR Jr, Bell MR, Gersh BJ, et al (Mayo Clinic, Rochester, MN)
J Am Coll Cardiol Intv 1:88-96, 2008

Objectives.—We implemented the Mayo Clinic ST-segment elevation myocardial infarction (STEMI) protocol and evaluated the timeliness of reperfusion therapy during off hours versus regular hours.

Background.—Patients with STEMI who present during off hours have longer door-to-balloon times and door-to-needle times.

Methods.—The Mayo STEMI protocol was implemented in May 2004 to optimize timeliness of reperfusion therapy for STEMI patients presenting to Saint Marys Hospital, a tertiary facility with on-site percutaneous coronary intervention (PCI), and for those presenting to 28 regional hospitals located up to 150 miles away from Saint Marys Hospital. We compared door-to-balloon times and door-to-needle times for 597 consecutive patients who presented during off hours (weekdays from 5 PM to 7 AM and any time on weekends or holidays) versus regular hours (weekdays from 7 AM to 5 PM). In 2003, prior to implementing the protocol, median door-to-balloon time at Saint Marys Hospital was 85 min during regular hours and 98 min during off hours.

Results.—Among 258 patients who presented to Saint Marys Hospital, median door-to-balloon time was 65 min during regular hours versus 74 min during off hours (p = 0.085). Among 105 patients transferred from regional hospitals for primary PCI, median door-to-balloon time was 118 min during regular hours versus 114 min during off hours (p = 0.15). Among 131 patients treated with fibrinolytic therapy at regional hospitals, median door-to-needle time was 21 min during regular hours versus 26 min during off hours (p = 0.067).

Conclusions.—The Mayo Clinic STEMI protocol demonstrates the rapid times that can be achieved through coordinated systems of care for STEMI patients presenting during off hours and regular hours.

▶ This study based upon the Mayo Clinic ST-segment elevation myocardial infarction (STEMI) regional protocol, covering 28 hospitals, highlights rapidly developing trends in the management of STEMI. It is generally accepted that many of the clinical issues regarding the optimal therapeutic approaches to acute myocardial infarction have been answered.[1] The current focus has shifted to developing systems of care that deliver the most appropriate strategy as quickly and to as many eligible patients as possible.[2]

This study is reassuring that it demonstrates rapid times to treatment can be achieved by coordinated systems of care, 7 days per week and 24 hours per day. This is an essential component of management because different therapeutic strategies based upon the time of presentation will lead to confusion and additional delays to treatment. During off hours, patients presenting to the referral hospital (Saint Marys Hospital, Rochester, MN) incurred slightly longer door-to-balloon times because of a longer time from catheterization laboratory activation and laboratory arrival. In contrast, among patients who are transferred from the regional hospitals, the transfer time created a buffer, which provided sufficient time for the on-call catheterization team to be activated and respond during off hours. Whether the additional 9-minute delay in patients presenting to Saint Marys Hospital would justify placing a catheterization team in-house 24 hours per day is debatable.

A national campaign organized by the American College of Cardiology in partnership with the American Heart Association and 37 other organizations is the subject of another article in the same issue of this journal.[3] The D2B Alliance has enrolled approximately 1000 hospitals with a goal of achieving D2B times of less than or equal to 19 minutes for at least 75% of transferred patients. Strategies have been identified and one is optimistic that the lessons to be learned from creating and implementing this alliance will ensure rapid, effective, and widespread application of newly proven therapies and enhance the efficiency with which our healthcare systems can treat patients with acute myocardial infarction.

B. J. Gersh, MB, ChB, DPhil, FRCP

References

1. Gersh BJ, Stone BW, White HD, Holmes DR Jr. Pharmacological facilitation of primary percutaneous coronary intervention for acute myocardial infarction; is the slope of the curve the shape of the future? *JAMA*. 2005;293:979-986.
2. Ting HH, Rihal CS, Gersh BJ, et al. Regional systems of care to optimize timeliness of reperfusion therapy for ST-elevation myocardial infarction: the Mayo Clinic STEMI protocol. *Circulation*. 2007;116:729-736.
3. Krumholz HM, Bradley EH, Nallamothu BK, et al. A campaign to improve the timeliness of primary percutaneous coronary intervention–door-to-balloon: an alliance for quality. *J Am Coll Cardiol Intv*. 2008;1:97-104.

Treatment and outcomes of acute coronary syndromes in India (CREATE): a prospective analysis of registry data
Xavier D, on behalf of the CREATE registry investigators (St John's Med College and St John's Res Inst, Bangalore, India; et al)
Lancet 371:1435-1442, 2008

Background.—India has the highest burden of acute coronary syndromes in the world, yet little is known about the treatments and outcomes of these diseases. We aimed to document the characteristics, treatments, and outcomes of patients with acute coronary syndromes who were admitted to hospitals in India.

Methods.—We did a prospective registry study in 89 centres from 10 regions and 50 cities in India. Eligible patients had suspected acute myocardial infarction with definite electrocardiograph changes (whether elevated ST [STEMI] or non-STEMI or unstable angina), or had suspected myocardial infarction without ECG changes but with prior evidence of ischaemic heart disease. We recorded a range of clinical outcomes, and all-cause mortality at 30 days.

Findings.—We enrolled 20 937 patients. Of the 20 468 patients who were given a definite diagnosis, 12 405 (60·6%) had STEMI. The mean age of these patients was 57·5 (SD 12·1) years; patients with STEMI were younger (56·3 [12·1] years) than were those with non-STEMI or unstable angina (59·3 [11·8] years). Most patients were from lower middle 10 737 (52·5%) and poor 3999 (19·6%) social classes. The median time from symptoms to hospital was 360 (IQR 123–1317) min, with 50 (25–68) min from hospital to thrombolysis. 6226 (30·4%) patients had diabetes; 7720 (37·7%) had hypertension; and 8242 (40·2%) were smokers. Treatments for STEMI differed from those for non-STEMI or unstable angina. More patients with STEMI than with non-STEMI were given anti-platelet drugs (98·2% *vs* 97·4%); angiotensin-converting enzyme (ACE) inhibitors or angiotensin receptor blockers (ARB) (60·5% *vs* 51·2%); and percutaneous coronary interventions (8·0% *vs* 6·7%, p<0·0001 for all comparisons). Thrombolytics (96·3% streptokinase) were used for 58·5% of patients with STEMI. Conversely, fewer patients with STEMI than those with non-STEMI or unstable angina were given beta blockers (57·5% *vs* 61·9%); lipid-lowering drugs (50·8% *vs* 53·9%); and coronary bypass graft surgery (1·9% *vs* 4·4%, p<0·0001 for all comparisons). The 30-day outcomes for patients with STEMI were death (8·6%), reinfarction (2·3%), and stroke (0·7%). Outcomes for those with non-STEMI or unstable angina were better: death (3·7%), reinfarction (1·2%), and stroke (0·3%, p<0·0001 for all comparisons). Use of key treatments also differed by socioeconomic status: more rich patients than poor patients were given thrombolytics (60·6% *vs* 52·3%), beta blockers (58·8% *vs* 49·6%), lipid-lowering drugs (61·2% *vs* 36·0%), ACE inhibitors or ARB (63·2% *vs* 54·1%), percutaneous coronary intervention (15·3% *vs* 2·0%), and coronary artery bypass graft surgery (7·5% *vs* 0·7%, p<0·0001 for all comparisons). Mortality was higher for poor patients than for rich patients (8·2% *vs* 5·5%, p<0·0001). Adjustment for treatments (but not risk factors and baseline characteristics) eliminated this difference in mortality.

Interpretation.—Patients in India who have acute coronary syndromes have a higher rate of STEMI than do patients in developed countries. Since most of these patients were poor, less likely to get evidence-based treatments, and had greater 30-day mortality, reduction of delays in access to hospital and provision of affordable treatments could reduce morbidity and mortality.

▶ This large registry study from India provides a useful insight into the major differences in the presentation and management of cardiovascular disease in the developed and developing worlds. In 2001, ischemic heart disease accounted for 7.1 million deaths worldwide,[1] and 80% of these occurred in the developing world.[2] These proportions applied to cardiovascular disease in general, including stroke. By 2010, 60% of the world's heart disease is expected to occur in India. Moreover, in the developing world, the disease occurs at an earlier age with a consequent larger impact upon the workforce and gross national product.

This registry focuses upon the acute coronary syndromes and illustrates the younger age of patients in India in comparison with other registries consisting primarily of patients in North America and Europe. In addition, most Indian patients presented with an ST-segment elevation myocardial infarction (STEMI), whereas the opposite occurs in the developed worlds. The reasons for this discordance are unclear, but perhaps the greater implementation of primary prevention and the previous use of treatments such as β-blockers, aspirin, and revascularization in addition to the older age of patients in developed countries might be contributory factors.

Although Indian patients were younger, their mortality appears higher than that expected from registry data in developed countries. There are also striking differences in the use of angiography, although the use of appropriate drugs is similar to that in other registries—there is, however, considerable room for improvement, and this applies to other parts of the world as well. In addition, delays to treatment were far greater in Indian patients.

This study also illustrates, and quite dramatically, the impact of socioeconomic status upon outcomes. The gradients of socioeconomic risk or the concept of "health and wealth" is widely documented in North America and Western Europe. It is disconcerting to note that the mortality difference among socioeconomic groups in this registry was almost entirely eliminated after statistical adjustment for differences in treatment received. This study certainly identifies the targets for improvement, including reducing delays to treatment and expanding access to evidence-based therapy. Implementation, however, will be challenging.

B. J. Gersh, MB, ChB, DPhil, FRCP

References

1. Lopez AD, Mathers CD, Ezzati M, Jamison DT, Murray CJ. Global and regional burden of disease and risk factors, 2001: systematic analysis of population health data. *Lancet.* 2006;367:1747-1757.
2. Reddy KS. Cardiovascular disease in non-Western countries. *N Engl J Med.* 2004; 350:2438-2440.

Cardiovascular Risk of Celecoxib in 6 Randomized Placebo-Controlled Trials: The Cross Trial Safety Analysis
Solomon SD, for the Cross Trial Safety Assessment Group (Brigham and Women's Hosp, Boston, MA; et al)
Circulation 117:2104-2113, 2008

Background.—Observational studies and randomized trials have reported increased cardiovascular risk associated with cyclooxygenase-2 inhibitors. Prior placebo-controlled randomized studies had limited ability to assess the relationship of either celecoxib dose or pretreatment cardiovascular status to risk associated with celecoxib. Our aim was to assess the cardiovascular risk associated with celecoxib in 3 dose regimens and to assess the relationship between baseline cardiovascular risk and effect of celecoxib on cardiovascular events.

Methods and Results.—We performed a patient-level pooled analysis of adjudicated data from 7950 patients in 6 placebo-controlled trials comparing celecoxib with placebo for conditions other than arthritis with a planned follow-up of at least 3 years. Patients were administered celecoxib in 3 dose regimens: 400 mg QD, 200 mg BID, or 400 mg BID. From the pooled data, we calculated a hazard ratio for all dose regimens combined and individual hazard ratios for each dose regimen and examined whether celecoxib-related risk was associated with baseline cardiovascular risk. The primary end point was the combination of cardiovascular death, myocardial infarction, stroke, heart failure, or thromboembolic event. With 16 070 patient-years of follow-up, the hazard ratio for the composite end point combining the tested doses was 1.6 (95% CI, 1.1 to 2.3). The risk, which increased with dose regimen ($P=0.0005$), was lowest for the 400-mg-QD dose (hazard ratio, 1.1; 95% CI, 0.6 to 2.0), intermediate for the 200-mg-BID dose (hazard ratio, 1.8; 95% CI, 1.1 to 3.1), and highest for the 400-mg-BID dose (hazard ratio, 3.1; 95% CI, 1.5 to 6.1). Patients at highest baseline risk demonstrated disproportionately greater risk of celecoxib-related adverse events (P for interaction$=0.034$).

Conclusions.—We observed evidence of differential cardiovascular risk as a function of celecoxib dose regimen and baseline cardiovascular risk. By further clarifying the extent of celecoxib-related cardiovascular risk, these findings may help guide treatment decisions for patients who derive clinical benefit from selective cyclooxygenase-2 inhibition.

▶ The finding from observational studies in randomized controlled trials that there is an increased cardiovascular risk associated with cyclooxygenase-2 (COX-2) inhibitors (coxibs) has generated understandable concern, as the drugs are widely used.[1] In addition, experimental studies have identified plausible biological mechanisms to explain the increased cardiovascular risk.[2] Proposed mechanisms include a coxib-induced imbalance between prostacyclin and thromboxane production resulting from inhibition of COX-2-generated prostacyclin without an opposing reduction in thromboxane, and in addition, coxibs can increase blood pressure by a variety of mechanisms as is the case with other nonsteroidal anti-inflammatory agents.

Although cardiovascular risk is clearly increased, overall event rates are low, and this has limited the ability to analyze relationships between coxib dose, pretreatment cardiovascular status, and drug-associated cardiovascular risk. This combined analysis was based upon 6 long-term placebo-controlled trials in 7950 patients with a planned follow-up of 3 years or more, and was commissioned by the National Cancer Institute. What is unique about this analysis is the ability to integrate dosing information with a level of baseline cardiovascular risk. There is a clear interaction between higher doses and cardiovascular events, particularly in groups at moderate or high risk. Among low-risk patients, similar hazard ratios with wide confidence intervals were noted for all 3 doses. The data in regard to celecoxib are clinically relevant, as this remains the only coxib used in the United States and the most widely used worldwide. It should be emphasized, however, that the doses in these trials are higher than those recommended for the treatment of osteoarthritis, but consistent with doses used in rheumatoid arthritis and some other nonarthritic conditions.

The study supports a recent American Heart Association physician statement recommending that the lowest dose possible should be used, particularly in subgroups considered at high cardiovascular risk.[3]

A limitation of this study as recognized by the authors is that none of the trials included in this analysis were designed or powered with cardiovascular endpoints in mind. We also need to be careful not to extrapolate the data to doses not tested. Nonetheless, the data should help to guide rational decision making for patients who derive a clinical benefit from the use of coxibs, and certainly point out that patients who are at a priority risk for cardiovascular events appear to be particularly vulnerable to the effect of the coxibs.

B. J. Gersh, MB, ChB, DPhil, FRCP

References

1. Solomon SD, McMurray JJ, Pfeffer MA, et al. For the Adenoma Prevention with Celecoxib (APC) Study Investigators. Cardiovascular risk associated with celecoxib in a clinical trial for colorectal adenoma prevention. *N Engl J Med.* 2005; 352:1071-1080.
2. Grosser T, Fries S, Fitzgerald GA. Biologic basis for the cardiovascular consequences of COX-2 inhibition: therapeutic challenges and opportunities. *J Clin Invest.* 2006;116:4-15.
3. Antman EM, Bennett JS, Daugherty A, Furberg C, Roberts H, Taubert KA. American Heart Association. Use of nonsteroidal anti-inflammatory drugs; an update for clinicians; a scientific statement from the American Heart Association. *Circulation.* 2007;115:1634-1642.

Intensive Lipid-Lowering With Atorvastatin for Secondary Prevention in Patients After Coronary Artery Bypass Surgery
Shah SJ, Waters DD, Barter P, et al (Univ of California, San Francisco; Heart Research Inst, Sydney, Australia; et al)
J Am Coll Cardiol 51:1938-1943, 2008

Objectives.—The aim of this post hoc analysis from the TNT (Treating to New Targets) trial is to determine whether patients with previous coronary artery bypass grafting (CABG) surgery achieved clinical benefit from intensive low-density lipoprotein (LDL)-cholesterol lowering.

Background.—The development and progression of atherosclerosis is accelerated in coronary venous bypass grafts.

Methods.—A total of 10,001 patients with documented coronary disease, including 4,654 with previous CABG, were randomized to atorvastatin 80 or 10 mg/day and were followed for a median of 4.9 years. The primary end point was the occurrence of a first major cardiovascular event (cardiac death, nonfatal myocardial infarction, resuscitated cardiac arrest, or stroke).

Results.—A first major cardiovascular event occurred in 11.4% of the patients with prior CABG and 8.5% of those without prior CABG (p < 0.001). In CABG patients, mean LDL-cholesterol levels at study end were 79 mg/dl in the 80-mg arm and 101 mg/dl in the 10-mg arm, and the primary event rate was 9.7% in the 80-mg arm and 13.0% in the 10-mg arm (hazard ratio 0.73, 95% confidence interval 0.62 to 0.87, p = 0.0004). Repeat revascularization during follow-up, either CABG or percutaneous coronary intervention, was performed in 11.3% of the CABG patients in the 80-mg arm and 15.9% in the 10-mg arm (hazard ratio 0.70, 95% confidence interval 0.60 to 0.82, p < 0.0001).

Conclusions.—Intensive LDL-cholesterol lowering to a mean of 79 mg/dl with atorvastatin 80 mg/day in patients with previous CABG reduces major cardiovascular events by 27% and the need for repeat coronary revascularization by 30%, compared with less intensive cholesterol-lowering to a mean of 101 mg/dl with atorvastatin 10 mg/day. (A Study to Determine the Degree of Additional Reduction in CV Risk in Lowering LDL Below Minimum Target Levels [TNT]; NCT00327691).

▶ The results of this substudy in 4654 patients with previous coronary bypass surgery, from the Treating to New Targets (TNT) trial of high-dose versus low-dose atorvastatin, should not come as a surprise but are nonetheless of importance. Intensive low-density lipoprotein (LDL) cholesterol lowering to a mean of 79 mg/dL in patients with previous CABG reduced major cardiovascular events by 27% and the need for repeat coronary revascularization by 30% in comparison with less intensive cholesterol lowering to a mean of 101 mg/dL.

This is consistent with the fact that after coronary bypass surgery there is progressive disease in both native vessels and saphenous vein grafts and that LDL cholesterol levels are an important risk factor.[1] One previous large randomized trial with lovastatin demonstrated that saphenous vein graft deterioration was less common, and events were lower with aggressive treatment but the levels achieved were substantially higher than in this study.[2] Nonetheless, the results of the 2 trials are complementary and support the findings of recent studies in a wider group of patients that when LDL cholesterol is the target, "lower is better."[3]

There are limitations to this study as recognized by the authors. The analysis of CABG patients was not prespecified, and there is a great deal about these patients that we do not know (eg, the number and type of grafts, the number of diseased vessels, preoperative symptomatology, and left ventricular function). Moreover, there was no placebo group, although given the results of other studies I do not see this as a problem.

B. J. Gersh, MB, ChB, DPhil, FRCP

References

1. Domanski MJ, Borkowf CB, Campeau L, et al. Prognostic factors for atherosclerosis progression in saphenous vein grafts: the postcoronary artery bypass graft (Post-CABG) trial. Post-CABG Trial Investigators. *J Am Coll Cardiol.* 2000;36: 1877-1883.
2. Knatterud GL, Rosenberg Y, Campeau L, et al. Long-term effects on clinical outcomes of aggressive lowering of low-density lipoprotein cholesterol levels and low-dose anticoagulation in the post coronary artery bypass graft trial. Post CABG Investigators. *Circulation.* 2000;102:157-165.
3. LaRosa JC, Grundy SM, Waters DD, et al. Intensive lipid-lowering with atorvastatin in patients with stable coronary disease. *N Engl J Med.* 2005;352:1425-1435.

Intensive oral antiplatelet therapy for reduction of ischemic events including stent thrombosis in patients with acute coronary syndromes treated with percutaneous coronary intervention and stenting in the TRITON-TIMI 38 trial: a subanalysis of a randomised trial

Wiviott SD, for the TRITON-TIMI 38 investigators (Brigham and Women's Hosp and Harvard Med School, Boston, MA; et al)

Lancet 371:1353-1363, 2008

Background.—Intracoronary stenting can improve procedural success and reduce restenosis compared with balloon angioplasty in patients with acute coronary syndromes, but can also increase the rate of thrombotic complications including stent thrombosis. The TRITON–TIMI 38 trial has shown that prasugrel—a novel, potent thienopyridine—can reduce ischaemic events compared with standard clopidogrel therapy. We assessed the rate, outcomes, and prevention of ischaemic events in patients treated with prasugrel or clopidogrel with stents in the TRITON–TIMI 38 study.

Methods.—Patients with moderate-risk to high-risk acute coronary syndromes were included in our analysis if they had received at least one coronary stent at the time of the index procedure following randomisation in TRITON-TIMI 38, and were further subdivided by type of stent received. Patients were randomly assigned in a 1 to 1 fashion to receive a loading dose of study drug (prasugrel 60 mg or clopidogrel 300 mg) as soon as possible after randomisation, followed by daily maintenance therapy (prasugrel 10 mg or clopidogrel 75 mg). All patients were to receive aspirin therapy. Treatment was to be continued for a minimum of 6 months and a maximum of 15 months. Randomisation was not stratified by stents used or stent type. The primary endpoint was the composite of cardiovascular death, non-fatal myocardial infarction, or non-fatal stroke. Stent thrombosis was assessed using Academic Research Consortium definitions, and analysis was by intention to treat. TRITON-TIMI 38 is registered with ClinicalTrials.gov, number NCT00097591.

Findings.—12 844 patients received at least one coronary stent; 5743 received only drug-eluting stents, and 6461 received only bare-metal stents. Prasugrel compared with clopidogrel reduced the primary endpoint (9·7 *vs* 11·9%, HR 0·81, p=0·0001) in the stented cohort, in patients with only drug-eluting stents (9·0 *vs* 11·1%, HR 0·82, p=0·019), and in patients with only bare-metal stents (10·0 *vs* 12·2%, HR 0·80, p=0·003). Stent thrombosis was associated with death or myocardial infarction in 89% (186/210) of patients. Stent thrombosis was reduced with prasugrel overall (1·13 *vs* 2·35%, HR 0·48, p<0·0001), in patients with drug-eluting stents only (0·84 *vs* 2·31%, HR 0·36, p<0·0001), and in those with bare-metal stents only (1·27 *vs* 2·41%, HR 0·52, p=0·0009).

Interpretation.—Intensive antiplatelet therapy with prasugrel resulted in fewer ischaemic outcomes including stent thrombosis than with standard clopidogrel. These findings were statistically robust irrespective of stent type, and the data affirm the importance of intensive platelet inhibition in patients with intracoronary stents.

▶ The introduction of intracoronary stenting has been a major advance in interventional cardiology, resulting in greater procedural success and lower rates of postprocedure restenosis than after "plain old balloon angioplasty." The Achilles heel of stents, however, is the potential for stent thrombosis early, subacute, and late, and this has led to a series of trials aimed at identifying improved antithrombotic therapies. Approximately 10 years ago, dual antiplatelet therapy with thienopyridine and aspirin became the standard approach to prevent recurrent ischemic events after stent placement.[1] The subsequent introduction of drug-eluting stents demonstrated a low but increased incidence of late stent thrombosis and the need for a much longer duration of clopidogrel therapy.[2] Indeed, the optimal duration of clopidogrel therapy is currently undetermined, but most would recommend therapy for at least 1 year. In addition, there remains a concern about the risk of recurrent ischemic events after coronary stenting, particularly in the setting of acute coronary syndromes and with off-label indications for drug-eluting stents. Another potential concern is the entity of clopidogrel resistance, and there is certainly evidence that patients have variable responses to clopidogrel.[3]

For all of these reasons, the search for newer and better antithrombotic agents continues. Prasugrel, a thienopyridine, was shown in the TRITON-TIMI 38 trial to result in more rapid and consistent platelet inhibition than clopidogrel, and this translated into a 19% reduction in the composite endpoint of cardiovascular death, nonfatal infarction, or nonfatal stroke.[4] The problem is that the more effective a therapy is in preventing thrombosis, the greater the risk of bleeding, and this was indeed the case in this large trial. The anti-ischemic benefits of prasugrel came at a price with higher rates of TIMI major bleeding not related to coronary bypass grafting and although uncommon, higher rates of life-threatening and fatal bleeding. Ongoing trials are currently evaluating different doses of prasugrel so as to enhance safety.

This subset analysis of patients receiving different kinds of stents is encouraging in that ischemic outcomes, including stent thrombosis (both early and late), were reduced by prasugrel. This study also reminds us that late stent thrombosis, although uncommon, is a catastrophic complication leading to death or myocardial infarction in 89% of patients. The anti-ischemic benefits of prasugrel will have to be balanced against the risk of bleeding and ongoing trials will be critically important in this regard—the balance between bleeding and reduced ischemic events is delicate to say the least. Ongoing trials are exploring the optimal dose of the drug.

B. J. Gersh, MB, ChB, DPhil, FRCP

References

1. Leon MB, Baim DS, Popma JJ, et al. A clinical trial comparing three antithrombotic-drug regimens after coronary-artery stenting. Stent Anticoagulation Restenosis Study Investigators. *N Engl J Med.* 1998;339:1665-1671.
2. Pfisterer M, Brunner-La Rocca HP, Buser PT, et al. Late clinical events after clopidogrel discontinuation may limit the benefit of drug-eluting stents: an observational study of drug-eluting versus bare-metal stents. *J Am Coll Cardiol.* 2006;48:2584-2591.
3. Gurbel PA, Bliden KP. Durability of platelet inhibition by clopidogrel. *Am J Cardiol.* 2003;91:1123-1125.
4. Wiviott SD, Braunwald E, McCabe CH, et al. Prasugrel versus clopidogrel in patients with acute coronary syndromes. *N Engl J Med.* 2007;357:2001-2015.

Telmisartan, Ramipril, or Both in Patients at High Risk for Vascular Events
ONTARGET Investigators, Yusuf S, Teo KK, Pogue J, et al (McMaster Univ and Hamilton Health Sciences, Ontario, Canada)
N Engl J Med 358:1547-1559, 2008

Background.—In patients who have vascular disease or high-risk diabetes without heart failure, angiotensin-converting–enzyme (ACE) inhibitors reduce mortality and morbidity from cardiovascular causes, but the role of angiotensin-receptor blockers (ARBs) in such patients is unknown. We compared the ACE inhibitor ramipril, the ARB telmisartan, and the combination of the two drugs in patients with vascular disease or high-risk diabetes.

Methods.—After a 3-week, single-blind run-in period, patients underwent double-blind randomization, with 8576 assigned to receive 10 mg of ramipril per day, 8542 assigned to receive 80 mg of telmisartan per day, and 8502 assigned to receive both drugs (combination therapy). The primary composite outcome was death from cardiovascular causes, myocardial infarction, stroke, or hospitalization for heart failure.

Results.—Mean blood pressure was lower in both the telmisartan group (a 0.9/0.6 mm Hg greater reduction) and the combination-therapy group (a 2.4/1.4 mm Hg greater reduction) than in the ramipril group. At a median follow-up of 56 months, the primary outcome had occurred in 1412 patients in the ramipril group (16.5%), as compared with 1423 patients in the telmisartan group (16.7%; relative risk, 1.01; 95% confidence interval [CI], 0.94 to 1.09). As compared with the ramipril group, the telmisartan group had lower rates of cough (1.1% vs. 4.2%,

P<0.001) and angioedema (0.1% vs. 0.3%, P = 0.01) and a higher rate of hypotensive symptoms (2.6% vs. 1.7%, P<0.001); the rate of syncope was the same in the two groups (0.2%). In the combination-therapy group, the primary outcome occurred in 1386 patients (16.3%; relative risk, 0.99; 95% CI, 0.92 to 1.07); as compared with the ramipril group, there was an increased risk of hypotensive symptoms (4.8% vs. 1.7%, P<0.001), syncope (0.3% vs. 0.2%, P = 0.03), and renal dysfunction (13.5% vs. 10.2%, P<0.001).

Conclusions.—Telmisartan was equivalent to ramipril in patients with vascular disease or high-risk diabetes and was associated with less angioedema. The combination of the two drugs was associated with more adverse events without an increase in benefit. (ClinicalTrials.gov number, NCT00153101.)

▶ This well-done, large trial of patients with vascular disease or high-risk diabetes, but without heart failure, demonstrates that the angiotensin-receptor blocker (ARB) telmisartan is not inferior to ramipril in regard to the primary composite outcome of death from cardiovascular causes, myocardial infarction, stroke, or hospitalization for heart failure. Telmisartan was somewhat better tolerated with a lower rate of angioneurotic edema and cough, but more frequent symptoms of hypotension. Perhaps, surprisingly, the combination of the 2 drugs, despite greater blood pressure lowering, was associated with more adverse events and no increase in benefits. From a practical perspective, therefore, the decision to use an angiotensin-converting enzyme inhibitor (ACEI) or ARB should be based on cost and tolerability.

The results are consistent with those reported in the Valsartan in Acute Myocardial Infarction Trial (VALIANT) of valsartan and captopril in postinfarction patients with congestive heart failure.[1] In contrast, 2 other trials, both carried out in patients with congestive heart failure, demonstrated a reduction in hospital admissions for heart failure and cardiovascular mortality. Of note, the ACEI regimen in these trials was left to the discretion of the physician, whereas evidence-based doses (evidence-based doses of ACEI) were used in The Ongoing Telmisartan Alone and in Combination with Ramipril Global Endpoint Trial (ONTARGET) and VALIANT trial.

The ACEI story is a long and fascinating one. Initially ACEIs were as drugs to control blood pressure; this was followed by trials in patients with and without symptomatic heart failure and, subsequently, the drugs became firmly established in the management of postinfarction patients. Initially, their use was shown to benefit patients with left ventricular function or congestive heart failure, but the indications were subsequently expanded to their use as secondary prevention agents in a wide spectrum in postinfarction patients and in patients with severe vascular disease or diabetes, irrespective of ejection fraction. ACEIs should be considered in all patients with coronary artery disease, but to my mind their use is not mandatory, although this remains an area of controversy. ARBs are an alternative, but the combination adds nothing but side effects with the possible exception of benefit in patients with congestive heart failure. In summary, the ACE inhibitors are like warfarin—these drugs have their problems but they work, and to date they have maintained their place in the therapeutic armamentarium despite competition.

B. J. Gersh, MB, ChB, DPhil, FRCP

References

1. Pfeffer MA, McMurray JJ, Velazquez EJ, et al. Valsartan, captopril, or both in myocardial infarction complicated by heart failure, left ventricular dysfunction, or both. *N Engl J Med.* 2003;349:1893-1906.
2. McMurray JJV. ACE inhibitors in cardiovascular disease – unbeatable? *N Engl J Med.* 2008;385:1615-1616 [editorial].

Vitamins E and C in the Prevention of Cardiovascular Disease in Men: The Physicians' Health Study II Randomized Controlled Trial
Sesso HD, Buring JE, Christen WG, et al (Brigham and Women's Hosp, MA)
JAMA 300:2123-2133, 2008

Context.—Basic research and observational studies suggest vitamin E or vitamin C may reduce the risk of cardiovascular disease. However, few long-term trials have evaluated men at initially low risk of cardiovascular disease, and no previous trial in men has examined vitamin C alone in the prevention of cardiovascular disease.

Objective.—To evaluate whether long-term vitamin E or vitamin C supplementation decreases the risk of major cardiovascular events among men.

Design, Setting, and Participants.—The Physicians' Health Study II was a randomized, double-blind, placebo-controlled factorial trial of vitamin E and vitamin C that began in 1997 and continued until its scheduled completion on August 31, 2007. There were 14,641 US male physicians enrolled, who were initially aged 50 years or older, including 754 men (5.1%) with prevalent cardiovascular disease at randomization.

Intervention.—Individual supplements of 400 IU of vitamin E every other day and 500 mg of vitamin C daily.

Main Outcome Measures.—A composite end point of major cardiovascular events (nonfatal myocardial infarction, nonfatal stroke, and cardiovascular disease death).

Results.—During a mean follow-up of 8 years, there were 1245 confirmed major cardiovascular events. Compared with placebo, vitamin E had no effect on the incidence of major cardiovascular events (both active and placebo vitamin E groups, 10.9 events per 1000 person-years; hazard ratio [HR], 1.01 [95% confidence interval {CI}, 0.90-1.13]; $P = .86$), as well as total myocardial infarction (HR, 0.90 [95% CI, 0.75-1.07]; $P = .22$), total stroke (HR, 1.07 [95% CI, 0.89-1.29]; $P = .45$), and cardiovascular mortality (HR, 1.07 [95% CI, 0.90-1.28]; $P = .43$). There also was no significant effect of vitamin C on major cardiovascular events (active and placebo vitamin E groups, 10.8 and 10.9 events per 1000 person-years, respectively; HR, 0.99 [95% CI, 0.89-1.11];

$P = .91$), as well as total myocardial infarction (HR, 1.04 [95% CI, 0.87-1.24]; $P = .65$), total stroke (HR, 0.89 [95% CI, 0.74-1.07]; $P = .21$), and cardiovascular mortality (HR, 1.02 [95% CI, 0.85-1.21]; $P = .86$). Neither vitamin E (HR, 1.07 [95% CI, 0.97-1.18]; $P = .15$) nor vitamin C (HR, 1.07 [95% CI, 0.97-1.18]; $P = .16$) had a significant effect on total mortality but vitamin E was associated with an increased risk of hemorrhagic stroke (HR, 1.74 [95% CI, 1.04-2.91]; $P = .04$).

Conclusions.—In this large, long-term trial of male physicians, neither vitamin E nor vitamin C supplementation reduced the risk of major cardiovascular events. These data provide no support for the use of these supplements for the prevention of cardiovascular disease in middle-aged and older men.

Trial Registration.—clinicaltrials.gov Identifier: NCT00270647.

▶ The results of this completely neutral trial are not at all unexpected, given the largely neutral previous trials of vitamin E among patients with risk factors or pre-existing cardiovascular disease.[1,2] Nonetheless, there were some positive signals in other earlier trials. In regard to vitamin C, this has either been incorporated into other antioxidant combinations or multivitamin supplements in trials that showed no benefit and in 1 trial of vitamin C alone in women at high risk for cardiovascular disease, the results were entirely neutral.[3]

Nonetheless, a recent survey demonstrated that 12.7% and 12.4% of the United States adults took vitamin E and C supplements, respectively.[4] The herbal drug market and sales of vitamin supplements accounts for millions of dollars in the United States annually, despite the lack of concrete evidence of any benefit—a somewhat paradoxical but, nonetheless, persisting public health phenomenon.

This large, randomized, double-blind, placebo-controlled, factorial trial of vitamin E and vitamin C on United States physicians demonstrates no benefit whatsoever on major cardiovascular events, including myocardial infarction, stroke, cardiovascular death, heart failure, angina, revascularization, and total mortality. Interestingly and of uncertain significance, there did appear to be a slight increase in hemorrhagic stroke with vitamin E use.

As the authors point out, perhaps an even longer period of vitamin administration may be required to show benefit and a randomized multivitamin component of the Physician's Health Study is continuing. Nonetheless, I would certainly be surprised if any of these trials were positive, given the complete absence of any encouraging signals in this and in other trials. It will be interesting to see whether dissemination of the trials into the public domain changes the behaviors or whether money will continue to be wasted on vitamin supplements in people who do not need them.

B. J. Gersh, MB, ChB, DPhil, FRCP

References

1. Dietary supplementation with n-3 polyunsaturated fatty acids and vitamin E after myocardial infarction: results of the GISSI-Prevenzione trial. Gruppo Italiano per

lo Studio della Sopravvive-nza nell'Infarto Miocardico. *Lancet.* 1999;354: 447-455.

2. Yusuf S, Dagenais G, Pogue J, Bosch J, Sleight P. Vitamin E supplementation and cardiovascular events in high-risk patients. Heart Outcomes Prevention Evaluation Study Investigators. *N Engl J Med.* 2000;342:154-160.

3. Cook NR, Albert CM, Gaziano JM, et al. A randomized factorial trial of vitamins C and E and beta carotene in the secondary prevention of cardiovascular events in women: results from the Women's Antioxidant Cardiovascular Study. *Arch Intern Med.* 2007;167:1610-1618.

4. Radimer K, Bindewald B, Hughes J, Ervin B, Swanson C, Picciano MF. Dietary supplement use by US adults: data from the National Health and Nutrition Examination Survey, 1999-2000. *Am J Epidemiol.* 2004;160:339-349.

Optimal Medical Therapy With or Without Percutaneous Coronary Intervention to Reduce Ischemic Burden: Results from the Clinical Outcomes Utilizing Revascularization and Aggressive Drug Evaluation (COURAGE) Trial Nuclear Substudy

Shaw LJ, for the COURAGE Investigators (Univ School of Medicine, Atlanta, GA)
Circulation 117:1283-1291, 2008

Background.—Extent and severity of myocardial ischemia are determinants of risk for patients with coronary artery disease, and ischemia reduction is an important therapeutic goal. The Clinical Outcomes Utilizing Revascularization and Aggressive Drug Evaluation (COURAGE) nuclear substudy compared the effectiveness of percutaneous coronary intervention (PCI) for ischemia reduction added to optimal medical therapy (OMT) with the use of myocardial perfusion single photon emission computed tomography (MPS).

Methods and Results.—Of the 2287 COURAGE patients, 314 were enrolled in this substudy of serial rest/stress MPS performed before treatment and 6 to 18 months (mean = 374 ± 50 days) after randomization using paired exercise (n = 84) or vasodilator stress (n = 230). A blinded core laboratory analyzed quantitative MPS measures of percent ischemic myocardium. Moderate to severe ischemia encumbered $\geq 10\%$ myocardium. The primary end point was $\geq 5\%$ reduction in ischemic myocardium at follow-up. Treatment groups had similar baseline characteristics. At follow-up, the reduction in ischemic myocardium was greater with PCI + OMT (-2.7%; 95% confidence interval, -1.7%, -3.8%) than with OMT (-0.5%; 95% confidence interval, -1.6%, 0.6%; $P<0.0001$). More PCI + OMT patients exhibited significant ischemia reduction (33% versus 19%; $P = 0.0004$), especially patients with moderate to severe pretreatment ischemia (78% versus 52%; $P = 0.007$). Patients with ischemia reduction had lower unadjusted risk for death or myocardial infarction ($P = 0.037$ [risk-adjusted $P = 0.26$]), particularly if baseline ischemia was moderate to severe ($P = 0.001$ [risk-adjusted $P = 0.08$]). Death or myocardial infarction rates ranged from 0% to 39% for patients with no residual ischemia to $\geq 10\%$ residual ischemia on follow-up MPS ($P = 0.002$ [risk-adjusted $P = 0.09$]).

Conclusions.—In COURAGE patients who underwent serial MPS, adding PCI to OMT resulted in greater reduction in ischemia compared with OMT alone. Our findings suggest a treatment target of ≥5% ischemia reduction with OMT with or without coronary revascularization.

▶ This substudy from the Clinical Outcomes Utilizing Revascularization and Aggressive Drug Evaluation (COURAGE) trial adds to our knowledge of the effects of optimal medical therapy (OMT) with or without percutaneous coronary intervention (PCI) on reducing the extent and severity of inducible ischemia in patients with stable coronary artery disease.

The COURAGE trial of 2287 patients with chronic stable angina compared 2 strategies, namely, optimal medical therapy with or without PCI.[1] The trial was basically neutral and demonstrated no difference in the primary endpoint of death or acute myocardial infarction over a median of 4.6 years of follow-up. The results ignited a firestorm of controversy among interventional and noninterventional cardiologists, the media, organizations, and societies in addition to industry. To my mind, the impact of the trial went beyond the implications of the results, which confirm almost 30 years of previous studies of coronary revascularization in low to perhaps moderate risk patients with chronic stable angina, preserved left ventricular function, and preserved left ventricular function in the majority.[2] In any event, the guidelines are highly inclusive and recommend revascularization in any subgroups of patients at high risk with "compelling anatomy."

This substudy does demonstrate the superior efficacy of PCI versus optimal medical therapy (OMT) alone, in regard to the extent of the reduction in inducible ischemia at 18 months. In addition, but not surprisingly, the reduction in ischemic burden translated into a lower unadjusted (but not adjusted) risk of death or myocardial infarction, particularly if the baseline extent of ischemia was moderate to severe. These findings are logical but should not be construed as a negation of the results of the main trial. The substudy involved only 14% of the participants of the main trial, of whom approximately one-third in the PCI group have 5% or greater reduction in ischemic burden versus 18.9% in the OMT alone group. The mean reduction was 2.7% versus 0.5%, and there was no statistically significant difference in the outcomes between the 2 groups, although repeat revascularization was more frequent in the OMT alone group.

Nonetheless, these data do strengthen the argument that significant ischemia in addition to symptoms are valid therapeutic goals in the current era.[3] A critical determinant, however, is the extent of ischemia, and in this study, moderate to severe ischemia was defined as 10% or greater of the myocardium. These results should not be extrapolated to patients with milder degrees of ischemia.

B. J. Gersh, MD, ChB, DPhil, FRCP

References

1. Boden WE, O'Rourke RA, Teo KK, et al. Optimal medical therapy with or without PCI for stable coronary disease. *N Engl J Med.* 2007;356:1503-1516.
2. Holmes DR Jr, Gersh BJ, Whitlow P, et al. Percutaneous coronary intervention for chronic stable angina: a reassessment. *J Am Coll Cardiol Intv.* 2008;1:34-43.

3. Parisi AF, Hartigan PM, Folland ED. Evaluation of exercise thallium scintigraphy versus exercise electrocardiography in predicting survival outcomes and morbid cardiac events in patients with single- and double-vessel disease: findings from the Angioplasty Compared to Medicine Study. *J Am Coll Cardiol.* 1997;30: 1256-1263.

Effect of the Italian Smoking Ban on Population rates of Acute Coronary Events

Cesaroni G, Forastiere F, Agabiti N, et al (Local Health Unit ASL RME, Rome, Italy)
Circulation 117:1183-1188, 2008

Background.—Several countries in the world have not yet prohibited smoking in public places. Few studies have been conducted on the effects of smoking bans on cardiac health. We evaluated changes in the frequency of acute coronary events in Rome, Italy, after the introduction of legislation that banned smoking in all indoor public places in January 2005.

Methods and Results.—We analyzed acute coronary events (out-of-hospital deaths and hospital admissions) between 2000 and 2005 in city residents 35 to 84 years of age. We computed annual standardized rates and estimated rate ratios by comparing the data from prelegislation (2000–2004) and postlegislation (2005) periods. We took into account several time-related potential confounders, including particulate matter (PM_{10}) air pollution, temperature, influenza epidemics, time trends, and total hospitalization rates. The reduction in acute coronary events was statistically significant in 35- to 64-year-olds (11.2%, 95% CI 6.9% to 15.3%) and in 65- to 74-year-olds (7.9%, 95% CI 3.4% to 12.2%) after the smoking ban. No evidence was found of an effect among the very elderly. The reduction tended to be greater in men and among lower socioeconomic groups.

Conclusions.—We found a statistically significant reduction in acute coronary events in the adult population after the smoking ban. The size of the effect was consistent with the pollution reduction observed in indoor public places and with the known health effects of passive smoking. The results affirm that public interventions that prohibit smoking can have enormous public health implications.

▶ The adverse effects of exposure to second-hand smoke are well documented, and 2 previous studies from the United States and Italy found marked reductions in the incidence of myocardial infarction after the introduction of legislation banning smoking in public places.[1,2] The United States study from a small community in Montana counted only a low number of hospital admissions (24 in total), and the previous Italian study was carried out over a short period of time and did not adjust for multiple potential confounding variables.

This much larger study reflects the impact of a comprehensive smoking ban introduced throughout Italy in 2005 and used 2 population registries of hospitalizations and diagnoses in all public and private hospitals in Rome. A strength of this study is the attempt to account for all time-related potential confounders, including particulate matter (PM10), air pollution, temperature, influenza epidemics, time trends, and total hospitalization rates.

This study provides further evidence that public interventions that prohibit smoking are beneficial, and the public health implications are potentially enormous and certainly gratifying. Although smoking bans lead to a reduction in active smoking, the beneficial effects attributable to the population at large are mediated primarily by the significant reduction in exposure to passive smoke among never-smokers and ex-smokers.[3] In this study, there was an approximately 10% reduction in coronary events in individuals aged 35 to 74 years, but there was no effect among the very elderly. Although the reductions are relatively small, the fact that coronary heart diseases are the leading causes of death in Italy and elsewhere would imply that the small reduction has much larger public health implications.

B. J. Gersh, MB, ChB, DPhil, FRCP

References

1. Sargent RP, Shepard RM, Glantz SA. Reduced incidence of admissions for myocardial infarction associated with public smoking ban: before and after study. *BMJ.* 2004;328:977-980.
2. Bartecchi C, Alsever RN, Nevin-Woods C, et al. Reduction in the incidence of acute myocardial infarction associated with a citywide smoking ordinance. *Circulation.* 2006;114:1490-1496.
3. Haw SJ, Gruer L. Changes in exposure of adult non-smokers to secondhand smoke after implementation of smoke-free legislation in Scotland: national cross sectional survey. *BMJ.* 2007;335:549-552.

Spectrum of heart disease and risk factors in a black urban population in South Africa (the Heart of Soweto Study): a cohort study

Sliwa K, Wilkinson D, Hansen C, et al (Univ of the Witwatersrand, Johannesburg; Univ of Queensland, Brisbane; et al)
Lancet 371:915-922, 2008

Background.—The Heart of Soweto Study aims to increase our understanding of the characteristics and burden imposed by heart disease in an urban African community in probable epidemiological transition. We aimed to investigate the clinical range of disorders related to cardiovascular disease in patients presenting for the first time to a tertiary-care centre.

Methods.—From Jan 1 to Dec 31, 2006, we recorded data for 4162 patients with confirmed cases of cardiovascular disease (1593 newly diagnosed and 2569 previously diagnosed and under treatment) who attended the cardiology unit at the Chris Hani Baragwanath Hospital in Soweto, South Africa. We developed a prospectively designed registry and gathered detailed clinical data relating to the presentation, investigations, and treatment of all 1593 patients with newly diagnosed cardiovascular disease.

Findings.—Most patients were black Africans (n=1359 [85%]), and the study population contained more women (n=939 [59%]) than men. Women were slightly younger than were men (mean 53 [SD 16] years vs 55 [15] years; p=0·031), with 399 (25%) patients younger than 40 years. Heart failure was the most common primary diagnosis (704 cases, 44% of total). Moderate to severe systolic dysfunction was evident in 415 (53%) of 844 identified cases of heart failure, 577 (68%) of which were attributable to dilated cardiomyopathy or hypertensive heart disease, or both. Black Africans were more likely to be diagnosed with heart failure than were the rest of the cohort (739 [54%] *vs* 105 [45%]; odds ratio [OR] 1·46, 95% CI 1·11–1·94; p=0·009) but were less likely to be diagnosed with coronary artery disease (77 [6%] *vs* 88 [38%]; OR 0·10, 0·07–0·14; p<0·0001). Prevalence of cardiovascular risk factors was very high, with 897 (56%) patients diagnosed with hypertension (190 [44%] of whom were also obese). Only 209 (13%) patients had no identifiable risk factors, whereas 933 (59%) had several risk factors.

Interpretation.—We noted many threats to the present and future cardiac health of Soweto, including a high prevalence of modifiable risk factors for atherosclerotic disease and a combination of infectious and non-communicable forms of heart disease, with late clinical presentations. Overall, our findings provide strong evidence that epidemiological transition in Soweto, South Africa has broadened the complexity and spectrum of heart disease in this community. This registry will enable continued monitoring of the range of heart disease (Fig 2).

▶ The epidemic of cardiovascular disease in low- and middle-income developing countries has major implications for the rest of the world and argues for a more concerted focus upon cardiovascular disease in addition to communicable diseases, as part of the global health agenda.[1] That cardiovascular disease, including ischemic heart disease has reached epidemic proportions in the Middle East, India, Latin America, and China is not in dispute.[2] The major issues now are the implementation of national policies of primary and secondary prevention.

One of the major problems in the developing world and particularly sub-Saharan Africa is the lack of data and much of what is available is of poor quality. It is crucial for such countries to have a clear picture of the magnitude of the epidemic and its tempo, because these regions face a dual burden of both communicable and noncommunicable disease and a relative lack of resources. It also appears evident that the scope of the epidemic is not the same in all countries in the developing world. This is probably a reflection of differences in the underlying socioeconomic climate and the specific stage in the "epidemiologic transition" to which certain countries and regions within countries belong.

This important study from Soweto, South Africa, comprises a perspective registry of patients with newly diagnosed cardiovascular disease. Eighty-five percent of the population are urban, black African, 59% were women (unlike most epidemiologic studies of cardiovascular disease), and the prevalence of

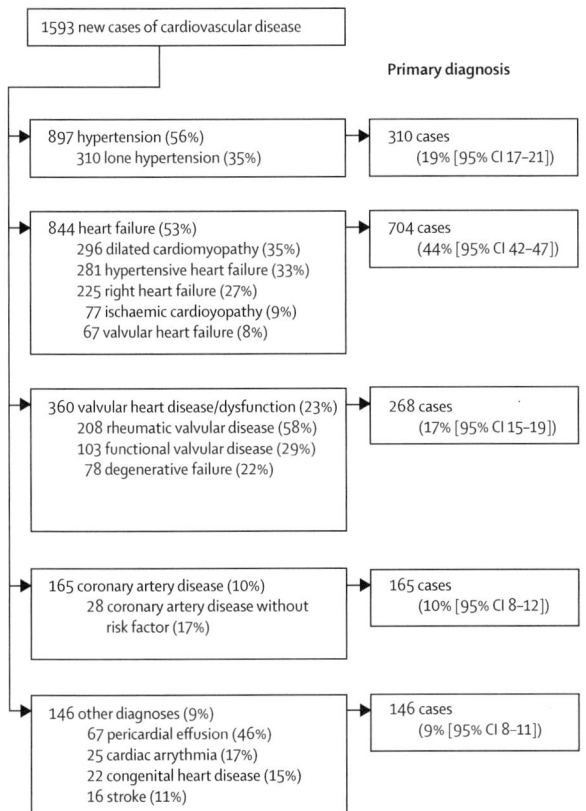

FIGURE 2.—Clinical spectrum of disease. (Reprinted from Sliwa K, Wilkinson D, Hansen C, et al. Spectrum of heart disease and risk factors in a black urban population in South Africa (the Heart of Soweto Study): a cohort study. *Lancet.* 2008;371:915-922, reprinted with permission from Elsevier.)

cardiovascular risk factors was very high. What is extremely interesting is that the dominant disease syndrome was congestive heart failure, secondary to idiopathic dilated cardiomyopathy, hypertensive heart disease, rheumatic fever, valvular disease, and probably HIV cardiomyopathy. Coronary artery disease comprised only 10% of new cases, and among black Africans the incidence was only 6%; 9% had other diagnoses with pericardial effusion due to tuberculosis, HIV infection, or both being the dominant etiologic factor.

It would appear, therefore, that the epidemic of coronary artery disease has not yet affected urban black Africans in South Africa and presumably other regions of sub-Saharan Africa. Nonetheless, the prevalence of risk factors is increasing rapidly, and the likelihood is that the "epidemiologic transition" will result in an epidemic of cardiovascular disease in the future. It is, however, conceivable that there may be a level of genetic protection as has been postulated in the face of the relative lack of coronary heart disease in Japan—the Japanese paradox. The major priority is to establish perspective databases, and South Africa offers a great opportunity to study a potential epidemic of cardiovascular disease, as it probably will evolve. This study from Soweto is a very promising step in that direction.

B. J. Gersh, MB, ChB, DPhil, FRCP

References

1. Fuster V, Voute J, Hunn M, Smith SC Jr. Low priority of cardiovascular and chronic diseases on the global health agenda; a cause for concern. *Circulation.* 2007;116:1966-1970.
2. Murray CJL, Lopez AD. *The Global Burden of Disease; a Comparative Assessment of Mortality and Disability from Diseases, Injuries, and Risk Factors in 1990 and Projected to 2020.* Cambridge, MA: Harvard University Press; 1996.

Day–Night Variation of Acute Myocardial Infarction in Obstructive Sleep Apnea

Kuniyoshi FH, Garcia-Touchard A, Gami AS, et al (Mayo Clinic and Foundation, Rochester, MN; et al)
J Am Coll Cardiol 52:343-346, 2008

Objectives.—This study sought to evaluate the day–night variation of acute myocardial infarction (MI) in patients with obstructive sleep apnea (OSA).

Background.—Obstructive sleep apnea has a high prevalence and is characterized by acute nocturnal hemodynamic and neurohormonal abnormalities that may increase the risk of MI during the night.

Methods.—We prospectively studied 92 patients with MI for which the time of onset of chest pain was clearly identified. The presence of OSA was determined by overnight polysomnography.

Results.—For patients with and without OSA, we compared the frequency of MI during different intervals of the day based on the onset time of chest pain. The groups had similar prevalence of comorbidities. Myocardial infarction occurred between 12 am and 6 am in 32% of OSA patients and 7% of non-OSA patients (p = 0.01). The odds of having OSA in those patients whose MI occurred between 12 am and 6 am was 6-fold higher than in the remaining 18 h of the day (95% confidence interval: 1.3 to 27.3, p = 0.01). Of all patients having an MI between 12 am and 6 am, 91% had OSA.

Conclusions.—The diurnal variation in the onset of MI in OSA patients is strikingly different from the diurnal variation in non-OSA patients. Patients with nocturnal onset of MI have a high likelihood of having OSA. These findings suggest that OSA may be a trigger for MI. Patients having nocturnal onset of MI should be evaluated for OSA, and future research should address the effects of OSA therapy for prevention of nocturnal cardiac events (Fig 1).

▶ Obstructive sleep apnea is an increasingly prevalent condition that remains underdiagnosed and undertreated, although clinical awareness has heightened in recent years.[1] Obstructive sleep apnea is accompanied by a number of potentially deleterious pathophysiologic consequences, including hypoxia and hypercapnia, sympathetic overactivity, hemodynamic stressors, and a prothrombotic and inflammatory state.[2] From a clinical perspective, strong associations with a number of cardiovascular conditions have been documented, including hypertension, myocardial infarction, sudden cardiac death, stroke, atrial fibrillation, and congestive heart failure.

It has been postulated that those nocturnal pathophysiologic responses to obstructive sleep apnea could predispose to plaque rupture, coronary thrombosis, myocardial infarction, and sudden cardiac death. A previous landmark study from the Mayo Clinic demonstrated a striking difference in the diurnal variation in sudden cardiac death in patients with and without obstructive sleep apnea.[3] In patients with obstructive sleep apnea, the peak incidence of sudden cardiac death occurs at night and particularly between midnight and 6 AM as opposed to a peak between 6 AM and mid-day in patients without obstructive sleep apnea.

This study provides additional evidence that obstructive sleep apnea may be causally related to and a trigger of myocardial infarction and demonstrates similar differences in the diurnal variation. An obvious conclusion is that patients with a nocturnal onset of myocardial infarction should be evaluated for underlying obstructive sleep apnea.

A key question for further research is to elucidate the independent effects of obstructive sleep apnea per se as opposed to the associated comorbidities (ie, hypertension, obesity, and diabetes, etc). The second issue is whether treatment of obstructive sleep apnea will reduce the frequency of cardiovascular events, and an accumulating number of studies suggest that this indeed may be the

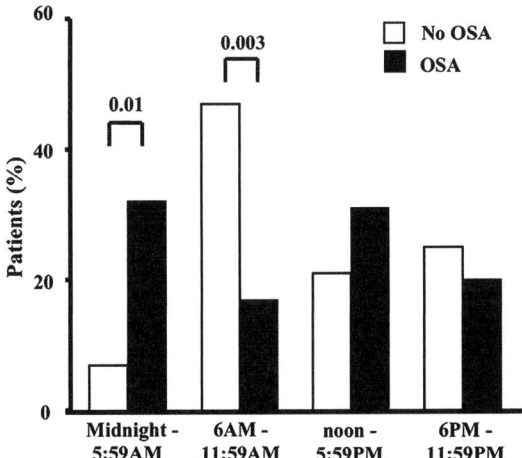

FIGURE 1.—6-h Epochs of MI Occurrence. Day–night pattern of myocardial infarction based on 4 6-h time intervals in OSA (n = 64) and non-OSA (n = 28) patients. (Reprinted from Kuniyoshi FH, Garcia-Touchard A, Gami AS, et al. Day–night variation of acute myocardial infarction in obstructive sleep apnea. *J Am Coll Cardiol*. 2008;52:343-346, with permission from the American College of Cardiology.)

case. Clinicians need to maintain a high index of suspicion because diagnosing and treating obstructive sleep apnea may play an important role in the care of our patients.

B. J. Gersh, MB, ChB, DPhil, FRCP

References

1. Young T, Peppard PE, Gottlieb DJ. Epidemiology of obstructive sleep apnea: a population health perspective. *Am J Respir Crit Care Med.* 2002;165: 1217-1239.
2. Shamsuzzaman AS, Gersh BJ, Somers VK. Obstructive sleep apnea; implications for cardiac and vascular disease. *JAMA.* 2003;290:1906-1914.
3. Gami AS, Howard DE, Olson EJ, Somers VK. Day-night pattern of sudden death in obstructive sleep apnea. *N Engl J Med.* 2005;352:1206-1214.

44 Hypertension

Deteriorating Dietary Habits Among Adults With Hypertension: DASH Dietary Accordance, NHANES 1988-1994 and 1999-2004

Mellen PB, Gao SK, Vitolins MZ, et al (Hattiesburg Clinic, Hattiesburg, MS; Amgen Inc, Thousand Oaks, CA; Wake Forest Univ, Winston-Salem, NC)

Arch Intern Med 168:308-314, 2008

Background.—Although the DASH (Dietary Approaches to Stop Hypertension trial) diet is among the therapeutic lifestyle changes recommended for individuals with hypertension (HTN), accordance with the DASH diet is not known.

Methods.—Using data from the National Health and Nutrition Examination Survey (NHANES) from the 1988-1994 and 1999-2004 periods, DASH accordance among individuals with self-reported HTN was estimated based on 9 nutrient targets (fat, saturated fat, protein, cholesterol, fiber, magnesium, calcium, sodium, and potassium) (score range, 0-9). Using data from 1999-2004, we compared the DASH score among demographic groups in age- and energy-adjusted models and modeled the odds of a DASH-accordant dietary pattern (≥ 4.5) using multivariable logistic regression. The DASH score, DASH accordance, and percentage of participants achieving individual targets were compared with estimates from NHANES 1988-1994 data.

Results.—Based on 4386 participants with known HTN in the recent survey period (1999-2004), the mean (SE) DASH score, after adjustment for age and energy intake, was 2.92 (0.05), with 19.4% (1.2%) classified as DASH accordant. In multivariable logistic regression models, DASH accordance was associated with older age, nonblack ethnicity, higher education, and known diabetes mellitus. Accordance with DASH was 7.3% lower in the recent survey period compared with NHANES 1988-1994 (26.7% [1.1%]) ($P < .001$), reflecting fewer patients with HTN meeting nutrient targets for total fat, fiber, and magnesium.

Conclusion.—The dietary profile of adults with HTN in the United States has a low accordance with the DASH dietary pattern, and the dietary quality of adults with HTN has deteriorated since the introduction of the DASH diet, suggesting that secular trends have minimized the impact of the DASH message.

▶ Although the DASH diet was first shown to lower blood pressure in 1997,[1] and the low-sodium version of the DASH diet was even better in 2001,[2] the authors of this study surveyed the reported dietary habits of adults in large

419

national surveys before and after 1999, to see how many people reported eating what is now considered a "blood-pressure healthy diet." Perhaps, not surprisingly, given the large increase in obesity in both adult and adolescent Americans over the last 20 years,[3,4] they found that few adults were eating a diet that was similar to the DASH diet, and, even more worrisome, that recently, that proportion is decreasing. This is surprising, given the large amount of medical and lay literature introduced since the DASH diet's inception extolling its virtues.[5-8]

When one delves into the details of this article, the results are perhaps even more alarming. The scoring system used to assess accord with the DASH diet provided a maximum of 9 points—presumed complete accordance with the main precepts of 8 target nutrients (total fat, saturated fat, protein, fiber, cholesterol, calcium, magnesium and potassium), as well as sodium. These were indexed to the total energy intake. Interestingly, a participant in the NHANES was considered in accordance with the DASH diet in this study if he/she achieved a score of ≥ 4.5 (ie, half of the point score possible). As 1.2% of the NHANES population was considered in accord with the DASH Diet (ie, with a score of ≥ 4.5), it is likely that few, if any Americans, ingested quantities of all 9 major target nutrients as recommended by the DASH diet.

It is likely that more effort will be needed, on the part of health policymakers and others in the private sector, to make programs such as the Food Guide Pyramid, the 5 A Day program (eat 5 or more servings of fruits and vegetables every day), and some of the recent programs spearheaded by the Whole Grains Council, more well-known, and perhaps, even more acceptable to the contemporary American palate.

W. J. Elliott, MD, PhD

References

1. Appel L, Moore T, Obarzanek E, et al. A clinical trial of the effects of dietary patterns on blood pressure. *N Engl J Med*. 1997;336:1117-1124.
2. Sacks FM, Svetkey LP, Vollmer WM, et al. Effects on blood pressure of reduced dietary sodium and the Dietary Approaches to Stop Hypertension (DASH) diet. *N Engl J Med*. 2001;344:3-9.
3. Hedley AA, Ogden CL, Johnson CL, Carroll MD, Curtin LR, Flegal KM. Prevalence of overweight and obesity among U.S. children, adolescents, and adults, 1999-2002. *JAMA*. 2004;291:2847-2850.
4. Your guide to lowering high blood pressure: healthy eating, http://www.nhlbi.nih.gov/hbp/prevent/h_eating/h_eating.htm. Accessed Oct 3, 08.
5. Moore T, Svetkey L, Lin P-H, Keranja N, Jenkins M. *The DASH* Diet for Hypertension: Lower Your Blood Pressure in 14 Days—Without Drugs*. New York, NY: Simon & Schuster; 2003. 368.
6. Heller M. *The DASH Diet Action Plan Book*. Northbrook, IL: Amidon Press; 2008.
7. Appel LJ, Brands MW, Daniels SR, et al. Dietary approaches to prevent and treat hypertension: a scientific statement from the American Heart Association. *Hypertension*. 2006;47:296-308.
8. Fung TT, Chiuve SE, McCullough ML, Rexrode KM, Logroscino L, Hu FB. Adherence to a DASH-style diet and risk of coronary heart disease and stroke in women. *Arch Intern Med*. 2008;168:713-720.

Case Detection, Diagnosis, and Treatment of Patients with Primary Aldosteronism: An Endocrine Society Clinical Practice Guideline

Funder JW, Carey RM, Fardella C, et al (Prince Henry's Inst of Med Res, Clayton, VIC, Australia; Univ of Virginia Health System, Charlottesville; Universidad Católica de Chile, Santiago; et al)
J Clin Endocrinol Metab 93:3266-3281, 2008

Objective.—Our objective was to develop clinical practice guidelines for the diagnosis and treatment of patients with primary aldosteronism.

Participants.—The Task Force comprised a chair, selected by the Clinical Guidelines Subcommittee (CGS) of The Endocrine Society, six additional experts, one methodologist, and a medical writer. The Task Force received no corporate funding or remuneration.

Evidence.—Systematic reviews of available evidence were used to formulate the key treatment and prevention recommendations. We used the Grading of Recommendations, Assessment, Development, and Evaluation (GRADE) group criteria to describe both the quality of evidence and the strength of recommendations. We used "recommend" for strong recommendations and "suggest" for weak recommendations.

Consensus Process.—Consensus was guided by systematic reviews of evidence and discussions during one group meeting, several conference calls, and multiple e-mail communications. The drafts prepared by the task force with the help of a medical writer were reviewed successively by The Endocrine Society's CGS, Clinical Affairs Core Committee (CACC), and Council. The version approved by the CGS and CACC was placed on The Endocrine Society's Web site for comments by members. At each stage of review, the Task Force received written comments and incorporated needed changes.

Conclusions.—We recommend case detection of primary aldosteronism be sought in higher risk groups of hypertensive patients and those with hypokalemia by determining the aldosterone-renin ratio under standard conditions and that the condition be confirmed/excluded by one of four commonly used confirmatory tests. We recommend that all patients with primary aldosteronism undergo adrenal computed tomography as the initial study in subtype testing and to exclude adrenocortical carcinoma. We recommend the presence of a unilateral form of primary aldosteronism should be established/excluded by bilateral adrenal venous sampling by an experienced radiologist and, where present, optimally treated by laparoscopic adrenalectomy. We recommend that patients with bilateral adrenal hyperplasia, or those unsuitable for surgery, optimally be treated medically by mineralocorticoid receptor antagonists.

▶ This nice review summarizes the current diagnosis and treatment of primary hyperaldosteronism, which is said to be experiencing an epidemic recently.[1,2] For many years, most endocrinologists (and expert panels on which they served) routinely recommended a series of hormonal tests for patients suspected of harboring an adrenal adenoma that autonomously excreted aldosterone, including infusion of 2 liters of saline, measurements of serum levels of several steroids in the supine and standing position in the early morning, and several other maneuvers, in an attempt to distinguish between those individuals with idiopathic hyperaldosteronism and those who had a tumor.[3-5] It is interesting to note that this expert panel now recommends a high-resolution computed tomographic scan of the adrenals as the first step in evaluating a person with a suspected tumor.

The recommendations of this panel were made before the recent articles demonstrating the higher risk of cardiovascular disease often present in these patients at presentation,[6] the recent nice series from France showing a nice and expected blood pressure reduction in patients with a Conn's adenoma that undergo successful surgery,[7] and the single-center study showing the expected prevalence of hyperaldosteronism in resistant hypertension.[8]

It is reassuring to know that after treatment, individuals with hyperaldosteronism do as well as treated essential hypertensive patients, but one wonders if the greater prevalence of cardiovascular disease at diagnosis might be responsible for some of the risk seen after successful treatment.

W. J. Elliott, MD, PhD

References

1. Mulatero P, Stowasser M, Loh K-C, et al. Increased diagnosis of primary aldosteronism, including surgical correctable forms, in centers from five continents. *J Clin Endocrinol Metab.* 2004;89:1045-1050.
2. Kaplan NM. The current epidemic of primary aldosteronism: causes and consequences. *J Hypertens.* 2004;22:863-869.
3. Stewart PM. Mineralocorticoid hypertension. *Lancet.* 1999;353:1341-1347.
4. Young WF Jr. Minireview: primary hyperaldosteronism—changing concepts in diagnosis and treatment. *Endocrinology.* 2003;144:2208-2213.
5. Ganguly A. Primary aldosteronism. *N Engl J Med.* 1998;339:1828-1834.
6. Catena C, Colussi GL, Nadalini E, et al. Cardiovascular outcomes in patients with primary aldosteronism after treatment. *Arch Intern Med.* 2008;168:80-85.
7. Letavernier E, Peyrard S, Amar L, Zinzindohoué F, Fiquet B, Plouin P-F. Blood pressure outcome of adrenalectomy in patients with primary hyperaldosteronemia with or without unilateral adenoma. *J Hypertens.* 2008;26:1816-1823.
8. Douma S, Petidis K, Doumas M, et al. Prevalence of primary hyperaldosteronism in resistant hypertension: a retrospective observational study. *Lancet.* 2008;371:1921-1926.

45 Non-Coronary Heart Disease in Adults

Optimization of the use of B-type natriuretic peptide levels for risk stratification at discharge in elderly patients with decompensated heart failure

Cournot M, Mourre F, Castel F, et al (Centre Hospitalier du Val d'Ariège, Foix, France; et al)

Am Heart J 155:986-991, 2008

Background.—In elderly patients hospitalized for decompensated heart failure, B-type natriuretic peptide (BNP) levels at discharge and the change in BNP during hospitalization may provide different information and may need to be taken into account simultaneously to best reflect the response to therapy. The aim of this study was to determine whether the most accurate risk stratification is obtained using BNP level after stabilization on treatment, the change in BNP under optimal treatment, or a combination of both markers.

Methods.—This prospective cohort study included 157 consecutive patients aged ≥70 (mean, 83 years), hospitalized for decompensated heart failure. Clinical, radiologic, biologic, and ultrasonography data were collected on admission and at discharge.

Results.—The median BNP level on admission was 1,057 pg/mL, and the mean change during hospitalization was −42%. Cardiac death or readmission were independently predicted by both predischarge BNP (best threshold: >360 pg/mL, HR 3.35 [1.94–5.75]) and the change in BNP levels (best threshold: −50%, HR 2.52 [1.59-4.01]). The highest event rate was observed in patients with both a predischarge BNP ≥360 pg/mL and a decrease <50% during hospitalization (HR 5.97 [2.98-11.94] compared with patients with a predischarge BNP <360 pg/mL and a decrease ≥50%, after adjustment for potential confounders). The remaining patients constituted an intermediate risk group (HR 3.13 [1.44-6.77]).

Conclusion.—Predischarge BNP and inhospital BNP change should not be interpreted independently from each other. The highest risk group includes patients with a high predischarge BNP level corresponding to

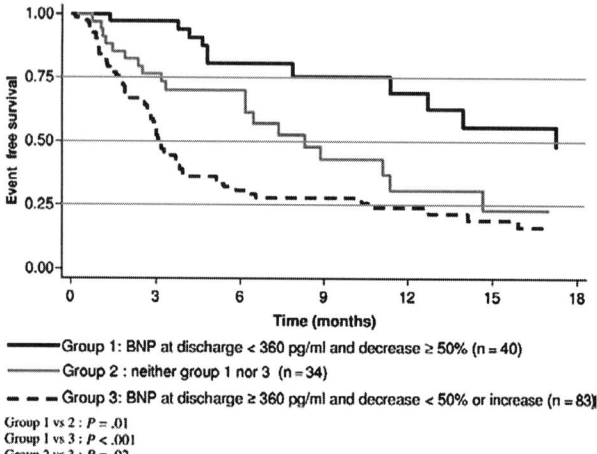

Group 1 vs 2 : $P = .01$
Group 1 vs 3 : $P < .001$
Group 2 vs 3 : $P = .02$

FIGURE 2.—Event free survival curves according to BNP at discharge and change in BNP. (Reprinted from Cournot M, Mourre F, Castel F, et al. Optimization of the use of B-type natriuretic peptide levels for risk stratification at discharge in elderly patients with decompensated heart failure. *Am Heart J.* 2008;155:986-991, with permission from Elsevier.)

more than the half of the BNP on admission. These patients would benefit from close monitoring for signs of decompensation (Fig 2).

▶ B-type naturetic peptide (BNP) has had prognostic value in patients with cardiac dyspnea[1] and chronic heart failure.[2] There are several observational studies that measured BNP during hospitalization for decompensated heart failure (DHF), mostly conducted in younger patients, aged 50 to 65 years, than in this study.[3-6] In these studies, the prognostic usefulness of BNP was investigated either at discharge from the hospital[3,4] or as a change in BNP during the hospitalization.[5,6] Because more than two-thirds of the patients with DHF are ≥70 years of age,[7] account for most of the deaths,[8] and may have different predictive values and prognostic discriminative thresholds, this study has added valuable information to the literature. These authors indicate that the most predictive uses of BNP are the level at admission together with the change in BNP level at discharge (Fig 2). The study is retrospective and the therapy of the patients was clinician-dependent. However, the prognostic value of a high BNP on admission and a failure to drop the BNP value by ≥50% identified a group of elderly patients at high risk of cardiac death or rehospitalization for DHF within a short time after discharge. The use of the combination of admission BNP and the change of BNP at discharge isolates a group with a prognosis 6 times higher than the low-risk group, survival at 3 months of 50% compared with 97%. The value of the prognosis using BNP on admission and at discharge was independent of the altered/preserved left ventricular ejection fraction (LVEF) status because there was no significant statistical interaction between the 3-group variable and the LVEF.

M. D. Cheitlin, MD

References

1. Koglin J, Pehlivanli S, Schwaiblmair M, Vogeser M, Cremer P, vonScheidt W. Role of brain natriuretic peptide in risk stratification of patients with congestive heart failure. *J Am Coll Cardiol.* 2001;38:1934-1941.
2. Doust JA, Pietrzak E, Dobson A, Glasziou P. How well does B-type natriuretic peptide predict death and cardiac events in patients with heart failure: systematic review. *BMJ.* 2005;330:625.
3. Valle R, Prevaldi C, D'Eri A, et al. B-type natriuretic peptide predicts post-discharge prognosis in elderly patients admitted due to cardiogenic pulmonary edema. *Am J Geriatr Cardiol.* 2006;15:202-207.
4. Logeart D, Thabut G, Jourdain P, et al. Peptide assay for identifying patients at high risk of re-admission after decompensated heart failure. *J Am Coll Cardiol.* 2004;43:635-641.
5. Bettencourt P, Azevedo A, Pimenta J, Friões F, Ferreira S, Ferreira A. N-terminal-pro-brain natriuretic peptide predicts outcome after hospital discharge in heart failure patients. *Circulation.* 2004;110:2168-2174.
6. Cournot M, Leprince P, Destrac S, Ferrières J. Usefulness of in-hospital change in B-type natriuretic peptide levels in predicting long-term outcome in elderly patients admitted for decompensated heart failure. *Am J Geriatr Cardiol.* 2007; 16:8-14.
7. Cohen-Solal A, Desnos M, Delahaye F, Emeriau JP, Hanania G. A national survey of heart failure in French hospitals. The Myocardiopathy and Heart Failure Working Group of the French Society of Cardiology, the National College of General Hospital Cardiologists and the French Geriatrics Society. *Eur Heart J.* 2000;21:763-769.
8. Hülsmann M, Berger R, Mörtl D, Pacher R. Influence of age and in-patient care on prescription rate and long-term outcome in chronic heart failure: a data-based sub-study of the EuroHeart Failure Survey. *Eur J Heart Fail.* 2005;7:657-661.

The evolution of diastolic dysfunction in the hypertensive disease

Pavlopoulos H, Grapsa J, Stefanadi E, et al (Hammersmith Hosp, London, UK)
Eur J Echocardiogr 9:772-778, 2008

Aims.—To investigate the effects of cardiac remodelling on left ventricular (LV) diastolic function, as evaluated by tissue Doppler and blood-pool indices, with respect to loading as expressed by wall stress. Cardiac remodelling is the major pathophysiological result of increased blood pressure and manifests as changes in the size, shape, and function of the heart.

Methods and Results.—We evaluated 90 hypertensive patients and 30 healthy volunteers. The hypertensive patients were divided into three groups: (i) HTN-N: normal remodelling ($n = 30$), (ii) HTN-CR: concentric remodelling ($n = 30$), and (iii) HTN-CH: concentric hypertrophy ($n = 30$). Mitral annular early diastolic (Ea) velocities were recorded. Filling pressures (E/Ea), relative wall thickness, LV mass index, DT, isovolumic relaxation time (IVRT), E/A ratio, and longitudinal wall stress (LWS) were also measured. Diastolic dysfunction (DD) was diagnosed based on published criteria. Progressive and increased incidence of DD with advancement of LV remodelling and an increase in LV mass was noted. Wall stress-loading was higher in the HTN-N group and lower in the HTN-CR and HTN-CH groups, despite the more deteriorated diastolic function in the latter groups. DD appeared early, even in the HTN-N group, which had a 36.6% incidence of DD compared to a 13% age-related incidence in the control group ($P < 0.05$). When the control group was used to define the reference values for septal Ea with the cut-off set as 2SD below the mean, the HTN-N, HTN-CR, and HTN-CH groups had abnormal diastolic function at 16.6, 26.6, and 56.6% incidence rates, respectively. Septal (Ea) was correlated with LVMI ($r = -0.55$), RWT ($r = -0.56$), Age ($r = -0.52$), BMI ($r = -0.31$), SBP ($r = -0.54$), PP ($r = -0.55$), and MAP ($r = -0.39$), all at $P < 0.05$. The correlations of blood-pool indices (DT, IVRT, and E/A) with the above parameters were less than that of tissue Doppler imaging (Septal and mean Ea). In a multivariate model, LVMI ($\beta = -0.25$), SBP ($\beta = -0.26$), and age ($\beta = -0.24$) $R^2 = 0.49$ were found to be independent predictors of DD.

Conclusions.—DD appears early in hypertensive disease, before the onset of abnormal remodelling or LV hypertrophy. With progression of the remodelling process and the advance of LVH, diastolic function progressively deteriorates. Tissue Doppler indices are better correlated with clinical and echocardiographic parameters of LV remodelling compared to blood-pool indices.

▶ Diastolic dysfunction (DD) is a cause of heart failure (HF) in ~50% of hypertensive patients admitted with HF.[1] This article investigates the relationship of cardiac remodeling, diastolic function, and ventricular loading expressed as left ventricular wall stress, using tissue Doppler (septal and mean mitral annular early diastolic (Ea) velocities) and blood pool indices (deceleration time, isovolumic relaxation time, and E/A). The authors grouped 90 hypertensive patients according to left ventricular (LV) geometry using the LV mass index (LVMI) and relative wall thickness (RWT), into normal LV geometry, concentric remodeling, and concentric hypertrophy, and compared them with 30 healthy volunteers. They found that LVMI is a continuum from normal to concentric LVH, and that DD starts with hypertensive patients with normal LV geometry. Because wall stress is highest with elevated blood pressure before LV remodeling occurs, this suggests that ventricular loading may be responsible for DD at that stage. As LV remodeling and concentric hypertrophy develop, LV wall stress decreases as the prevalence of DD increases. At these stages, LV wall component changes such as fibrosis,[2,3] myocyte dysfunction,[4] and microvascular ischemia[5] are more important in the development of DD. The tissue Doppler indices of septal and mean Ea correlated better with clinical and echocardiographic parameters of diastolic function than blood pool indices, and LV remodeling based on RWT and LVMI correlated best with tissue Doppler indices of DD.

M. D. Cheitlin, MD

References

1. Levy D, Larson MG, Vasan RS, et al. The progression from hypertension to congestive heart failure. *JAMA.* 1996;275:1557-1562.

2. Conrad CH, Brooks WW, Hayes JA, et al. Myocardial fibrosis and stiffness with hypertrophy and heart failure in the spontaneously hypertensive rat. *Circulation.* 1995;91:161-170.
3. Seccia TM, Belloni AS, Kreutz R, et al. Cardiac fibrosis occurs early and involves endothelin and AT-1 receptors in hypertension due to endogenous angiotensin II. *J Am Coll Cardiol.* 2003;41:666-673.
4. Yelamarty RV, Moore RL, Yu FT, et al. Relaxation abnormalities in single cardiac myocytes from renovascular hypertensive rats. *Am J Physiol.* 1992;262: 980-990.
5. Sasaki O, Hamada M, Hiwada K. Effects of coronary blood flow on left ventricular function in essential hypertensive patients. *Hypertens Res.* 2000;23:239-245.

Outcomes in Adults With Bicuspid Aortic Valves

Tzemos N, Therrien J, Yip J, et al (Univ of Toronto, Ontario, Canada; Natl Univ Hosp, Singapore; McGill Univ, Montreal, Quebec, Canada; et al)
JAMA 300:1317-1325, 2008

Context.—Bicuspid aortic valve is the most common congenital cardiac anomaly in the adult population. Cardiac outcomes in a contemporary population of adults with bicuspid aortic valve have not been systematically determined.

Objective.—To determine the frequency and predictors of cardiac outcomes in a large consecutive series of adults with bicuspid aortic valve.

Design, Setting, and Participants.—Cohort study examining cardiac outcomes in 642 consecutive ambulatory adults (mean [SD] age, 35 [16] years; 68% male) with bicuspid aortic valve presenting to a Canadian congenital cardiac center from 1994 through 2001 and followed up for a mean (SD) period of 9 (5) years. Frequency and predictors of major cardiac events were determined by multivariate analysis. Mortality rate in the study group was compared with age- and sex-matched population estimates.

Main Outcome Measures.—Mortality and cause of death were determined. Primary cardiac events were defined as the occurrence of any of the following complications: cardiac death, intervention on the aortic valve or ascending aorta, aortic dissection or aneurysm, or congestive heart failure requiring hospital admission during the follow-up period.

Results.—During the follow-up period, there were 28 deaths (mean [SD], 4% [1%]). One or more primary cardiac events occurred in 161 patients (mean [SD], 25% [2%]), which included cardiac death in 17 patients (mean [SD], 3% [1%]), intervention on aortic valve or ascending aorta in 142 patients (mean [SD], 22% [2%]), aortic dissection or aneurysm in 11 patients (mean [SD], 2% [1%]), or congestive heart failure requiring hospital admission in 16 patients (mean [SD], 2% [1%]). Independent predictors of primary cardiac events were age older than 30 years (hazard ratio [HR], 3.01; 95% confidence interval [CI], 2.15-4.19; $P<.001$), moderate or severe aortic stenosis (HR, 5.67; 95% CI, 4.16-7.80; $P<.001$), and moderate or severe aortic regurgitation (HR, 2.68; 95% CI, 1.93-3.76; $P<.001$). The 10-year survival rate of the study group (mean [SD], 96% [1%]) was not significantly different from population estimates (mean [SD], 97% [1%]; $P=.71$). At last follow-up, 280 patients (mean [SD], 45% [2%]) had dilated aortic sinus and/or ascending aorta.

Conclusions.—In this study population of young adults with bicuspid aortic valve, age, severity of aortic stenosis, and severity of aortic regurgitation were independently associated with primary cardiac events. Over the mean follow-up duration of 9 years, survival rates were not lower than for the general population.

▶ The bicuspid aortic valve (BAV) is the commonest congenital heart lesion in the population, seen in ~1% of adults.[1] The natural history of the patient with an isolated BAV is difficult to determine because a population echocardiographic survey would have to be done to identify all the patients with BAV and followed their whole life to determine the true incidence of complications. The natural history studies we have of the patients with isolated BAV in the literature are from autopsy or echocardiographic databases. These reports are all selection biased in favor of those patients with BAV who have developed complications and miss many asymptomatic patients with isolated BAV who never had a problem that brought them to medical attention. Michelena and colleagues[2] reported a series of 212 patients with normally functioning isolated BAV from the Olmsted County study found by echocardiography. Twenty years after diagnosis, survival was a mean ± SD of 90% ± 3%, similar to the survival of the general population of the same age and gender. However, there was a significant incidence of cardiovascular events, principally aortic stenosis and regurgitation and ascending aortic aneurysm and dissection. This study is much larger, 642 patients from Canadian databases of congenital heart disease and echocardiography. The findings are similar to those of the Olsted County study: excellent long-term survival similar to the general population of the same age and gender, but with a significant increased incidence of cardiovascular events, mostly aortic stenosis and regurgitation and ascending aortic disease. There are surprisingly few patients who developed infective endocarditis or aortic dissection in this series. The problems are similar to those of other isolated BAV series, that is, selection bias favoring patients who develop complications. Also, the period during which this series was collected was short, a mean ± SD of 9 ± 5 years. On multivariate analysis, independent predictors of cardiovascular events were a mean age older than 30 years and moderate aortic stenosis or regurgitation. The 10-year rate for freedom from a primary cardiac event in patients with no predictors was a mean ± SD of 94% ± 2%, with 1 predictor, 82% ± 3%, and with more than 1 predictor, 35% ± 5%. Although these natural histories do not include all patients with isolated BAV, their high survival rate suggests that even though a large number of patients develop cardiovascular complications in time, with proper therapy, survival is excellent.

M. D. Cheitlin, MD

References

1. Ward C. Clinical significance of the bicuspid aortic valve. *Heart.* 2000;83:81-85.
2. Michelena HI, Desjardins VA, Avierinos JF, et al. Natural history of asymptomatic patients with normally functioning or minimally dysfunctional bicuspid aortic valve in the community. *Circulation.* 2008;117:2776-2784.

Contemporary Epidemiology and Prognosis of Health Care–Associated Infective Endocarditis

Fernández-Hidalgo N, Almirante B, Tornos P, et al (Universitat Autònoma de Barcelona, Spain)
Clin Infect Dis 47:1287-1297, 2008

Background.—The aim of this study was to describe the characteristics of health care–associated infective endocarditis (HAIE) and to establish the risk factors for mortality.

Methods.—We conducted a prospective, observational cohort study. HAIE was defined according to the following conditions: (1) symptom onset >48 h after hospitalization or within 6 months after hospital discharge; or (2) ambulatory manipulations causing endocarditis.

Results.—Eighty-three episodes of HAIE (accounting for 28.4% of all cases of endocarditis) were diagnosed. Compared with patients with community-acquired endocarditis, patients with HAIE were older (median age ± standard deviation, years 65.3 ± 16.4 vs. 57.8 ± 17.0 years; $P = .001$), were in poorer health before disease onset (Charlson index, 2.5 ± 2.3 vs. 1.7 ± 2.1; $P = .006$), had more staphylococcal (55.4% vs. 28.3% of cases) and enterococcal infections (22.9% vs. 7.7% of cases; $P < .005$), underwent fewer surgeries (22.9% vs. 45.9% of cases; $P < .005$), and experienced a higher rate of in-hospital (45.8% vs. 22.0%) and 1-year mortality (59.5% vs. 29.6%; $P < .005$). In the HAIE cohort, independent predictors of in-hospital death were stroke (odds ratio [OR], 8.95; 95% confidence interval [CI], 2.04–39.31; $P = .004$), congestive heart failure (OR, 5.48; 95% CI, 1.77–17.03; $P = .003$), surgery indicated but not performed (OR, 3.74; 95% CI, 1.22–11.45; $P = .021$), and enterococcal infection (OR, 0.18; 95% CI, 0.04–0.78; $P = .022$). Independent predictors of 1-year mortality were surgery indicated but not performed (OR, 7.81; 95% CI, 2.06–29.67; $P = .003$), acute renal failure (OR, 7.18; 95% CI, 1.32–39.18; $P = .023$), and enterococcal infection (OR, 0.18; 95% CI, 0.04–0.81; $P = .026$). For the series overall (292 episodes), HAIE was an independent predictor of in-hospital (OR, 2.83; 95% CI, 1.34–5.98; $P = .007$) and 1-year mortality (OR, 2.59; 95% CI, 1.25–5.39; $P = .011$).

Conclusions.—HAIE is an important health problem associated with considerable mortality. New strategies to prevent HAIE should be assessed.

▶ The problem of nosocomial infective endocarditis (IE) (acquired in hospital) and nosohusial IE (acquired by interventions in the outpatient setting) is increasing in frequency as invasive procedures, including indwelling catheters for chronic intravenous therapy, A-V fistulae for hemodialysis, etc, are used. Existing reports of nosocomial IE place the prevalence at 7.7% to 21.5% for all cases of IE.[1,2] This study reports a prevalence of health care–associated IE (HAIE) of 28.4% of 292 cases of IE. Because HAIE affects mainly elderly men and women with comorbidities and general poor physical condition, the mortality is high, and the complications of IE, such as systemic and cerebral embolism, heart failure, and renal failure, are very high, 85.5% with almost half having more than 1 complication. These patients are likely to be poor surgical risks, and in this study, of the 48 patients with HAIE who had an indication for surgery, 29 (60.4%) did not undergo valve replacement during hospitalization because of high surgical risk. The failure to do indicated surgery was an independent risk factor for in-hospital and 1-year mortality. Because antibiotic prophylaxis is not recommended for these nosocomial and nosohusial procedures,[3] the only hope of preventing these infections is in maximizing the prophylactic measures taken during the placement and manipulation of indwelling catheters and maintaining aseptic measures before and during any invasive procedure.

M. D. Cheitlin, MD

References

1. Martín-Dávila P, Fortućn J, Navas E, et al. Nosocomial endocarditis in a tertiary hospital: an increasing trend in native valve cases. Chest. Am J Infect Control. 2005;128:772-779.
2. Fernández-Guerrero ML, Herrero L, Bellver M, et al. Nosocomial enterococcal endocarditis: a serious hazard for hospitalized patients with enterococcal bacteraemia. J Intern Med. 2002;252:510-515.
3. McDonald JR, Olaison L, Anderson DS, et al. Enterococcal endocarditis: 107 cases from the international collaboration on endocarditis merged database. Am J Med. 2005;118:759-766.

United States Feasibility Study of Transcatheter Insertion of a Stented Aortic Valve by the Left Ventricular Apex
Svensson LG, Dewey T, Kapadia S, et al (Cleveland Clinic, OH; et al)
Ann Thorac Surg 86:46-55, 2008

Background.—Recent US and European registries have indicated 30% to 60% of patients with critical valvular aortic stenosis (AS) are not treated surgically, usually due to advanced age and comorbidities. We report on a Food and Drug Administration approved feasibility study of a less invasive transcatheter approach to potentially treat these high-risk patients.

Methods.—Between December 2006 and February 18, 2008, 40 patients underwent transcatheter insertion of a balloon expandable stainless-steel stent with an internally mounted three-leaflet equine pericardial valve (Edwards Sapien Transcatheter Heart Valve; Edwards Lifesciences, Irvine, CA) into the aortic annulus using a transapical left ventricular insertion (TA-AVI). Patients were inoperable by conventional surgery, or extremely high risk based on Society of Thoracic Surgeons score greater than 15% or other documented risk factors.

Results.—All 40 valves were successfully delivered and 35 were successfully seated. Two valves embolized and required open aortic valve replacement (AVR), and one case of severe regurgitation later required AVR. In a further two patients placed on cardiopulmonary support, one valve later embolized and one migrated. There were 7 (17.5%) deaths within 30 days, and a further 2 (5%) deaths before discharge at 42 and 72 days. There were no immediate postoperative strokes after successful deployment. Valve area improved from 0.62 cm^2 (SD of 0.13) to 1.61 cm^2 (SD 0.37) at 30 days ($p = <0.0001$), with mean perivalvular regurgitation of 1.19 (SD 0.80). Mean follow-up was 143 days (SD 166 days) with 6 further deaths from comorbid disease, none valve or cardiac related. The Kaplan-Meier survival was 81.8% ± 6.2% at 1 month and 71.7% ± 7.7% at 3 months.

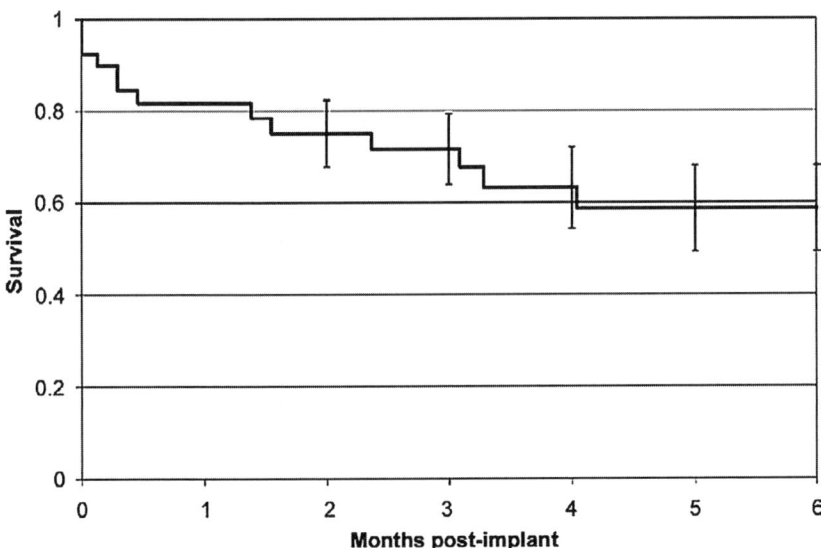

FIGURE 1.—Kaplan-Meier survival for all trans-left ventricular apex aortic valve insertion patients. Error bars at ± 1 standard error. (Reprinted from Svensson LG, Dewey T, Kapadia S, et al. United States feasibility study of transcatheter insertion of a stented aortic valve by the left ventricular apex. *Ann Thorac Surg.* 2008;86:46-55, with permission from The Society of Thoracic Surgeons.)

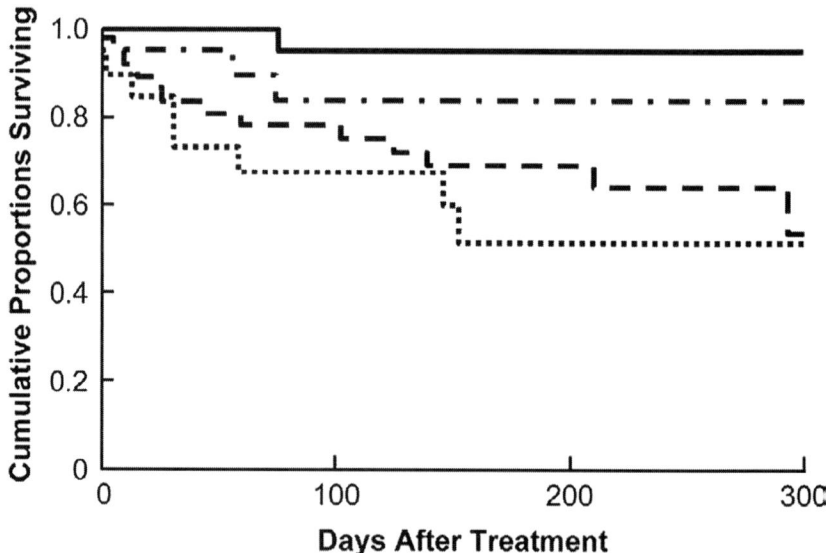

FIGURE 2.—Kaplan-Meier survival for patients referred to Cleveland Clinic for possible percutaneous trans-left ventricular apex aortic valve insertion or transfemoral aortic valve insertion. (AVR = conventional open aortic valve replacement; — = surgical AVR; - · - = percutaneous AVR; - - - = no intervention; · · · = aortic valvuloplasty.) (Reprinted from Svensson LG, Dewey T, Kapadia S, et al. United States feasibility study of transcatheter insertion of a stented aortic valve by the left ventricular apex. *Ann Thorac Surg.* 2008;86:46-55, with permission from The Society of Thoracic Surgeons.)

Conclusions.—Transapical insertion of a balloon expandable stented valve is feasible but carries considerable risk and will be further evaluated in the PARTNER (Placement of AoRTic traNscathetER valve) randomized trial (Figs 1 and 2).

▶ Aortic valve replacement (AVR) for critical aortic stenosis (AS) is one of the most successful surgical procedures for alleviating symptoms and extending life. In the United States, there are 125 000 patients with critical AS, most of them elderly, and only about 40% undergo AVR.[1] The common reason for deciding against surgery is that the patient is considered to be an unacceptable surgical risk, usually because of age and serious comorbidities. Because only about one-third of symptomatic patients with AS will be alive by 1 year,[2] alternative methods for treating such patients such as balloon angioplasty have been tried, but the most intriguing intervention is that of percutaneous catheter-based AV insertion, either through the femoral venous route, first reported by Cribier and colleagues[3] in 2002, or more recently transapical insertion through a localized thoracic incision.[4] The problems with percutaneous AV insertion by the femoral route, either venous or retrograde arterial, concern the many patients with extensive iliofemoral atherosclerosis, resulting in inability to pass the catheter, stroke, embolization of the valve, and difficulty in properly seating the valve. The transapical approach was developed to overcome some of these problems.[5] This article reports a feasibility study in the United States of the transapical approach attempted in 40 patients with critical AS. Unfortunately, the patients in this study were chosen for the transapical approach because of lack of access transfemorally due to severe atherosclerosis. They also had a higher Society of Thoracic Surgeons (STS) score then patients sent for the transfemoral route, (> 15% vs > 10%), so the 2 different approaches cannot be compared. As stated, the usual reason for not sending patients for AVR is the assumption that the patient is high-risk perioperatively. With this transapical route, in this study and the European transapical series, the 1-year survival of 60%[4] is better than the dismal survival with medical management alone. With recent advances in balloon valvuloplasty, in patients thought to be too high a risk for AVR, the effective aortic orifice achieved is comparable with that of the inserted percutaneous biologic valve, and the 1-year survival is 70%.[6] So, there are other interventional options in these sick patients. In the Euro-Heart survey, 33% of extremely symptomatic patients with critical AS were not referred for surgery based on estimation of surgical risk.[7] However, the estimation of risk by models such as the Euro-Score and the STS score are not specifically designed for AS surgery and tend to overestimate the risk.[8] Surgical AVR remains preferable to these still experimental interventions in patients with critical AS, if deemed possible by experienced surgeons.

M. D. Cheitlin, MD

References

1. Stuge O, Liddicoat J. Emerging opportunities for cardiac surgeons within structural heart disease. *J Thorac Cardiovasc Surg.* 2006;132:1258-1261.
2. Lindroos M, Kupari M, Heikkilä J, Tilvis R. Prevalence of aortic valve abnormalities in the elderly: an echocardiographic study of a random population sample. *J Am Coll Cardiol.* 1993;21:1220-1225.
3. Cribier A, Eltchaninoff H, Bash A, et al. Percutaneous transcatheter implantation of an aortic valve prosthesis for calcific aortic stenosis: first human case description. *Circulation.* 2002;106:3006-3008.
4. Walther T, Simon P, Dewey T, et al. Transapical minimally invasive aortic valve implantation: multicenter experience. *Circulation.* 2007;116:I240-I245.
5. Walther T, Simon P, Dewey T, Wimmer-Greinecker G, et al. Transapical minimally invasive aortic valve implantation: multicenter experience. *Circulation.* 2007;116:240-245.
6. Sack S, Kahlert P, Khandanpour S, et al. Revival of an old method with new techniques: balloon aortic valvuloplasty of the calcified aortic stenosis in the elderly. *Clin Res Cardiol.* 2008;97:288-297.
7. Iung B, Baron G, Butchart EG, et al. A prospective survey of patients with valvular heart disease in Europe: The Euro Heart Survey on valvular disease. *Eur Heart J.* 2003;24:1231-1243.
8. Dewey TM, Brown D, Ryan WH, Herbert MA, Prince SL, Mack MJ. Reliability of risk algorithms in predicting early and late operative outcomes in high-risk patients undergoing aortic valve replacement. *J Thorac Cardiovasc Surg.* 2008; 135:180-187.

46 Pediatric Cardiovascular Disease

Cardiac Resynchronization Therapy (and Multisite Pacing) in Pediatrics and Congenital Heart Disease: Five Years Experience in a Single Institution
Cecchin F, Frangini PA, Brown DW, et al (Harvard Med School, Boston, MA)
J Cardiovasc Electrophysiol 20:58-65, 2009

Introduction.—Clinical evidence supports the use of cardiac resynchronization therapy (CRT) in adults with heart failure, but experience in pediatrics and congenital heart disease (CHD) is limited in terms of patient numbers and follow-up. We sought to determine the functional assessment and clinical outcomes in pediatric and CHD CRT patients followed uniformly at one institution.

Methods.—Retrospective review of 60 consecutive patients who underwent CRT between 2002 and 2007.

Results.—At implantation, median age was 15.0 years (5 months to 47 years). Overall, 46 patients had CHD (77%) and 14 had dilated cardiomyopathy. Prior to CRT, 92% were on heart failure treatment drugs and 55% had pacemakers. Median follow-up time was 0.7 years (1 day–5.3 years). Median QRS width decreased from 149 to 120 ms (P < 0.001). Median ejection fraction (EF) increased from 36% to 42% (P < 0.001) and improvement was particularly evident in the group with CHD. Of note, 8 of 13 patients with single ventricle morphology had a "strong CRT response," defined as either an improvement of 2–3 ordinal points in NYHA classification and/or increased ventricular function by ≥ 10 EF units. Overall, an improvement in functional status was observed in 39 of 45 patients (87%) with sufficient follow-up data.

Conclusions.—Children and CHD patients treated with CRT have acute improvement in ventricular function, but implantation may require individualized planning and unconventional approaches. Future important goals include preimplant determination of CRT responders in pediatric and CHD patients, optimizing lead placement and programing, as well as long-term CRT device management issues.

▶ These are encouraging results for this therapy in patients who were mildly to severely symptomatic by NYHA class in 73%. Improvement in functional class and ejection fraction (EF) was remarkable and better in most cases than has been reported with medications. There is still work to be done with more follow-up and improved methods of lead placement, but these data do hold out another form of treatment for these patients who frequently are near the end of their treatment options.

T. P. Graham, MD

Natural history of ventricular premature contractions in children with a structurally normal heart: does origin matter?
Beaufort-Krol GCM, Dijkstra SSP, Bink-Boelkens MTE (Univ of Groningen, The Netherlands)
Europace 10:998-1003, 2008

Aims.—Premature ventricular contractions (PVCs) are thought to be innocent in children with normal hearts, especially if they disappear during exercise. The aim of our study was to study the natural history of PVCs in childhood and whether there is a difference between PVCs originating from the right [premature ventricular contraction with left bundle branch block (PVC-LBBB)] or the left ventricle [premature ventricular contraction with right bundle branch block (PVC-RBBB)].

Methods and Results.—We evaluated children with frequent PVCs and anatomically normal hearts ($n = 59$; 35M/24F) by 12-lead ECG, echocardiography, Holter recording, and an exercise test. Age at the first visit was 7.1 ± 4.3 years (mean $\pm$ SD), and follow-up was 3.1 ± 3.1 years. We could evaluate each child for 2.5 ± 1.5 times. Premature ventricular contraction with left bundle branch block was seen in 41% of the children; PVC-RBBB in 36%; and undetermined in 23%. Mean percentage PVCs in the Holter recording decreased ($14.3 \pm 13.7\%$ in the age group 1–3 years to $4.8 \pm 7.2\%$ in the age group ≥ 16 years; $P = 0.08$). Mean percentage PVC-LBBB did not change (12.3 ± 21.4 vs. $11.7 \pm 5.5\%$), whereas PVC-RBBB decreased (16.3 ± 4.2 to $0.6 \pm 1.4\%$; $P < 0.02$).

Conclusion.—We conclude that there is a difference in the natural history between PVC-LBBB and PVC-RBBB in children with an anatomically normal heart. Premature ventricular contraction with right bundle branch block disappears during childhood. Follow-up of these children seems not necessary. Premature ventricular contraction with left bundle branch block does not disappear and, therefore, it may be necessary to follow these children even during adulthood.

▶ The current dogma has been that premature ventricular contractions (PVCs) in children with a normal heart are benign. This study generally supports that hypothesis with the caveat that those PVCs with a left bundle branch block (LBBB) pattern (right ventricular in origin) should be followed re the question of late onset of RV arrhythmogenic dysplasia. This may represent somewhat of an overkill, but hopefully data can be collected to determine if this approach is necessary.

T. P. Graham, MD

Functional Status After Operation for Ebstein Anomaly: The Mayo Clinic Experience

Brown ML, Dearani JA, Danielson GK, et al (Mayo Clinic and Found, Rochester, MN)
J Am Coll Cardiol 52:460-466, 2008

Objectives.—The objective of this study was to review the long-term functional outcome of patients with Ebstein anomaly who had cardiac operation at our institution.

Background.—Ebstein anomaly is a spectrum of tricuspid valvular and right ventricular dysplasia. Many patients will require operation in an attempt to improve quality of life.

Methods.—From April 1, 1972, to January 1, 2006, 539 patients with Ebstein anomaly underwent 604 cardiac operations at the Mayo Clinic in Rochester, Minnesota. Patient records were reviewed, and all patients known to still be alive were mailed a medical questionnaire or contacted by telephone.

Results.—At the initial operation at our institution, the mean age of the patients was 24 years (range 8 days to 79 years) and 53% were female patients. Survival at 5, 10, 15, and 20 years was 94%, 90%, 86%, and 76%, respectively. Survival free of late reoperation was 86%, 74%, 62%, and 46% at 5, 10, 15, and 20 years, respectively. Surveys were returned by 285 of 448 (64%) patients known to be alive at the time of this study. Two hundred thirty-seven (83%) patients were in New York Heart Association functional class I or II, and 34% were taking no cardiac medication. One hundred three patients (36%) reported an incident of atrial fibrillation or flutter, 5 patients (2%) reported having had endocarditis, and 1 patient (<1%) reported having a stroke. There were 275 pregnancies among 82 women. The recurrence of congenital heart disease was reported in 9 of 232 (3.9%) liveborn children.

Conclusions.—Patients have good long-term survival and functional outcomes after undergoing surgery for Ebstein anomaly. Atrial arrhythmias are common both before and after surgery. Many patients have had one or more successful pregnancies with a low-recurrence risk of congenital heart disease.

▶ The Mayo Clinic group has a very large and successful experience with Ebstein anomaly, particularly in those patients who are not severely symptomatic as neonates or young infants. Despite an overall excellent success story, issues remain with arrhythmias, right ventricular dysfunction, and repeat operations for those with a valve replacement.

T. P. Graham, MD

Remote ischemic preconditioning elaborates a transferable blood-borne effector that protects mitochondrial structure and function and preserves myocardial performance after neonatal cardioplegic arrest

Wang L, Oka N, Tropak M, et al (Hosp for Sick Children, Toronto, Ontario, Canada)

J Thorac Cardiovasc Surg 136:335-342, 2008

Objective.—Remote ischemic preconditioning is known to elicit production of a blood-borne cardioprotective factor that is infarct sparing in models of ischemia–reperfusion injury and myocardial damage reducing after cardiopulmonary bypass in human subjects. The mechanism of protection remains incompletely understood. In this study, we examined effects on mitochondrial structure and function in a noninfarct model of cardioplegic arrest.

Methods.—Explanted neonatal rabbit hearts were mounted in a Langendorff preparation and perfused with dialysate of blood taken from sham-treated or remotely preconditioned rabbits. Each heart was subsequently subjected to 1-hour cardioplegic arrest and 30-minute reperfusion periods, during which hemodynamic responses were measured. Mitochondria were isolated for structural and functional measurements.

Results.—Relative to hearts with sham-treated dialysate, myocardial performance (systolic pressure, maximum positive and negative first derivatives of left ventricular pressure, and left ventricular end-diastolic pressure) was better preserved with dialysate from preconditioned rabbits. Similarly, mitochondria isolated from hearts with dialysate from preconditioned rabbits showed preserved respiration at complex I and IV in the electron transport chain ($P < .01$ and $P < .05$, respectively). Mitochondrial outer membrane integrity was also preserved, with diminished sensitivity of mitochondrial respiration to exogenous cytochrome c ($P < .01$) and less cytosolic diffusion of cytochrome c ($P < .01$). Mitochondrial resistance to calcium-mediated mitochondrial permeability transition pore opening was not affected.

Conclusion.—The cardioprotective factor in plasma dialysate after remote preconditioning preserves mitochondrial structure and function in a noninfarct cardioplegic arrest model. This protection is associated with preservation of global myocardial performance.

▶ Usually I do not choose animal studies for review in this medium, but the extraordinary results of this whole story of remote ischemic preconditioning by the Toronto group is too good to pass up. I urge readers to become familiar with this series of articles and to participate in clinical trials as they become available.

T. P. Graham, MD

Implantable Cardioverter-Defibrillators in Tetralogy of Fallot
Khairy P, Harris L, Landzberg MJ, et al (Canadian Adult Congenital Heart (CACH) Network, Canada; Children's Hosp, Boston, MA; et al)
Circulation 117:363-370, 2008

Background.—Tetralogy of Fallot is the most common form of congenital heart disease in implantable cardioverter-defibrillator (ICD) recipients, yet little is known about the value of ICDs in this patient population.

Methods and Results.—We conducted a multicenter cohort study in high-risk patients with Tetralogy of Fallot to determine actuarial rates of ICD discharges, identify risk factors, and characterize ICD-related complications. A total of 121 patients (median age 33.3 years; 59.5% male) were enrolled from 11 sites and followed up for a median of 3.7 years. ICDs were implanted for primary prevention in 68 patients (56.2%) and for secondary prevention in 53 (43.8%), defined by clinical sustained ventricular tachyarrhythmia or resuscitated sudden death. Overall, 37 patients (30.6%) received at least 1 appropriate and effective ICD discharge, with a median ventricular tachyarrhythmia rate of 213 bpm. Annual actuarial rates of appropriate ICD shocks were 7.7% and 9.8% in primary and secondary prevention, respectively ($P=0.11$). A higher left ventricular end-diastolic pressure (hazard ratio 1.3 per mm Hg, $P=0.004$) and nonsustained ventricular tachycardia (hazard ratio 3.7, $P=0.023$) independently predicted appropriate ICD shocks in primary prevention. Inappropriate shocks occurred in 5.8% of patients yearly. Additionally, 36 patients (29.8%) experienced complications, of which 6 (5.0%) were acute, 25 (20.7%) were late lead-related, and 7 (5.8%) were late generator-related complications. Nine patients died during follow-up, which corresponds to an actuarial annual mortality rate of 2.2%, which did not differ between the primary and secondary prevention groups.

Conclusions.—Patients with tetralogy of Fallot and ICDs for primary and secondary prevention experience high rates of appropriate and effective shocks; however, inappropriate shocks and late lead-related complications are common.

▶ This relatively large retrospective study indicates that this therapy, probably, is useful to prevent sudden death in high-risk postoperative tetralogy patients. It is a mixed bag, however, in that complications are frequent and inappropriate discharges remain a problem. Identifying the high-risk patients who are unlikely to have serious complications is a difficult endeavor and appropriate patient counseling before embarking on this therapy will be mandatory.

T. P. Graham, MD

PART SEVEN

THE DIGESTIVE SYSTEM

NICHOLAS J. TALLEY, MD, PHD

47 Colon

Effect of Aspirin or Resistant Starch on Colorectal Neoplasia in the Lynch Syndrome

Burn J, for the CAPP2 Investigators (Newcastle Univ, UK; et al)
N Engl J Med 359:2567-2578, 2008

Background.—Observational and epidemiologic data indicate that the use of aspirin reduces the risk of colorectal neoplasia; however, the effects of aspirin in the Lynch syndrome (hereditary nonpolyposis colon cancer) are not known. Resistant starch has been associated with an antineoplastic effect on the colon.

Methods.—In a randomized, placebo-controlled trial, we used a two-by-two design to investigate the effects of aspirin, at a dose of 600 mg per day, and resistant starch (Novelose), at a dose of 30 g per day, in reducing the risk of adenoma and carcinoma among persons with the Lynch syndrome.

Results.—Among 1071 persons in 43 centers, 62 were ineligible to participate in the study, 72 did not enter the study, and 191 withdrew from the study. These three categories were equally distributed across the study groups. Over a mean period of 29 months (range, 7 to 74), colonic adenoma or carcinoma developed in 141 participants. Of 693 participants randomly assigned to receive aspirin or placebo, neoplasia developed in 66 participants receiving aspirin (18.9%), as compared with 65 receiving placebo (19.0%) (relative risk, 1.0; 95% confidence interval [CI], 0.7 to 1.4). There were no significant differences between the two groups with respect to the development of advanced neoplasia (7.4% and 9.9%, respectively; P = 0.33). Among the 727 participants receiving resistant starch or placebo, neoplasia developed in 67 participants receiving starch (18.7%), as compared with 68 receiving placebo (18.4%) (relative risk, 1.0; 95% CI, 0.7 to 1.4). Advanced adenomas and colorectal cancers were evenly distributed in the two groups. The prevalence of serious adverse events was low, and the events were evenly distributed.

Conclusions.—The use of aspirin, resistant starch, or both for up to 4 years has no effect on the incidence of colorectal adenoma or carcinoma among carriers of the Lynch syndrome (Table 3). (Current Controlled Trials number, ISRCTN59521990.)

▶ Lynch syndrome (hereditary non-polyposis colon cancer [HNPCC]) is an autosomal dominant disorder with defective mismatch repair (MMR) that

TABLE 3.—Outcomes According to Study Group

Variable	All Participants No. (%)	Participants Assigned to Both Interventions				Participants Assigned to a Single Intervention			
		Aspirin Plus Resistant Starch	Aspirin Plus Placebo	Resistant Starch Plus Placebo	Placebo Plus Placebo	Aspirin Only	Placebo Only	Resistant Starch Only	Placebo Only
No neoplasia — no./total no. (%)	605/746 (81.1)	142	137	127	143	5	8	22	21
Neoplasia — no./total no. (%)	141/746 (18.9)	33	29	30	33	4	2	4	6
Adenoma only	118/746 (15.8)	29	24	24	29	3	2	4	3
Colorectal cancer only	13/746 (1.7)	2	2	4	3	1	0	0	1
Adenoma and colorectal cancer	10/746 (1.3)	2	3	2	1	0	0	0	2
Advanced adenoma or colorectal cancer	68/746 (9.1)	10	15	18	15	1	1	3	5
Largest dimension of neoplasm — mm									
Mean	137	8.0	10.3	10.8	8.3	2.9	8	11.5	13.0
Range		1–68	2–39	1–70	1–40	1–5	8–8	3–23	2–55
No. of adenomas — no./total no. (%)									
1	97/128 (75.8)	24	21	19	23	3	1	3	3
2	20/128 (15.6)	5	4	3	5	0	1	0	2
3	6/128 (4.7)	1	1	3	1	0	0	0	0
4	2/128 (1.6)	1	0	0	1	0	0	0	0
5	3/128 (2.3)	0	1	1	0	0	0	1	0
Total	128/128 (100)	31	27	26	30	3	2	4	5

(Reprinted from Burn J, for the CAPP2 Investigators. Effect of aspirin or resistant starch on colorectal neoplasia in the Lynch syndrome. N Engl J Med. 2008;359:2567-2578.)

predisposes to colon, endometrial, uroepithelial, and small intestinal cancer. The risk of colon cancer in mutation carriers is approximately 10%/decade and it occurs at a mean age of 45 years with a cumulative risk of colonic neoplasia approaching 70% by age 60.

This burden of colon cancer would make Lynch syndrome an ideal condition for chemoprevention. The regular use of aspirin (ASA) and other inhibitors of cyclo-oxygenase has been shown to reduce the risk of adenomas and colorectal cancer in multiple epidemiological and randomized clinical trials in average risk and familial adenomatous polyposis populations. Fermentation of "resistant starch" (RS, carbohydrate that escapes digestion in the small intestine) leads to the production of short-chain fatty acids in the colon, which have antineoplastic properties and an attractive chemopreventive strategy.

This multicenter, randomized, placebo-controlled trial investigated the potential for aspirin (600 mg/d) and resistant starch (30 g/d) or the combination as chemopreventive agents in HNPCC using a two-by-two design. Subjects ($n = 1071$) were either proven carriers of a known mutation in MMR by genetic testing or had a clinical diagnosis based on Amsterdam criteria and a personal history of an HNPCC-related cancer. A polyp-clearing colonoscopy was required within 3 months of enrollment; subjects were randomized and then followed up to 4 years with endoscopic surveillance with the rate of recurrent colon neoplasia the primary endpoint.

Table 3 summarizes the primary outcomes in the study. Powered to detect a 40% reduction in neoplasms, ASA, RS, or both had no effect on the rate of adenoma, advanced adenoma, or colorectal cancer development over 4 years. Indeed, the rates were remarkably similar between the groups, making it unlikely that a larger study would detect a clinically significant chemopreventive effect.

Therefore, in spite of considerable evidence in other populations, ASA or related NSAIDs (such as celecoxib or sulindac) cannot be recommended for use as chemoprevention in Lynch syndrome based on this large, well-designed clinical trial. The development of advanced adenoma and invasive cancer in 10% of these subjects over 4 years highlights the need for aggressive colonoscopic surveillance in this high-risk population.

R. K. Pearson, MD

Adalimumab for the treatment of fistulas in patients with Crohn's disease
Colombel J-F, Schwartz DA, Sandborn WJ, et al (Centre Hospitalier Universitaire de Lille, France; Vanderbilt Univ Med Ctr, Nashville, TN; Mayo Clinic, Rochester, MN; et al)
Gut 58:940-948, 2009

Objective.—To evaluate the efficacy of adalimumab in the healing of draining fistulas in patients with active Crohn's disease (CD).

Design.—A phase III, multicentre, randomised, double-blind, placebo controlled study with an open-label extension was conducted in 92 sites.

Patients.—A subgroup of adults with moderate to severely active CD (CD activity index 220–450) for ≥4 months who had draining fistulas at baseline.

Interventions.—All patients received initial open-label adalimumab induction therapy (80 mg/40 mg at weeks 0/2). At week 4, all patients were randomly assigned to receive double-blind placebo or adalimumab 40 mg every other week or weekly to week 56 (irrespective of fistula status). Patients completing week 56 of therapy were then eligible to enroll in an open-label extension.

Main Outcome Measures.—Complete fistula healing/closure (assessed at every visit) was defined as no drainage, either spontaneous or with gentle compression.

Results.—Of 854 patients enrolled, 117 had draining fistulas at both screening and baseline (70 randomly assigned to adalimumab and 47 to placebo). The mean number of draining fistulas per day was significantly decreased in adalimumab-treated patients compared with placebo-treated patients during the double-blind treatment period. Of all patients with healed fistulas at week 56 (both adalimumab and placebo groups), 90% (28/31) maintained healing following 1 year of open-label adalimumab therapy (observed analysis).

Conclusions.—In patients with active CD, adalimumab therapy was more effective than placebo for inducing fistula healing. Complete fistula healing was sustained for up to 2 years by most patients in an open-label extension trial.

▶ This study reports the efficacy of adalimumab in penetrating (fistulizing) Crohn's disease (CD). Patients who completed the previously published 56-week, Crohn's Trial of the Fully Human Antibody Adalimumab for Remission Maintenance (CHARM) and were entered in the Additional Long-Term Dosing with HUMIRA to Evaluate Sustained Remission on Efficacy in Crohn's Disease (ADHERE) study were the basis for the analysis. It is important to note that the primary intent (although it was a secondary endpoint) of these studies was not to measure fistula closure rates. Patients who met study criteria for active CD based on CD activity index (CDAI) score who also happened to have fistulas were the basis for the analysis. Adalimumab was effective at closing fistulas although differences compared with placebo took 16 weeks to appreciate. While previous immunosuppressant and antibiotic use did not influence findings, numbers were small. Because treatment decisions were not based on fistula closure but on CDAI, the authors present 2 analyses. The first was based on 2-year data of only those who received adalimumab at randomization in CHARM and entered ADHERE. The second analysis assumed that all patients who left the trial or had incomplete data were therapeutic failures. This resulted in best- and worst-case fistula closure rates that ranged from 46% to 55% at 6 months in CHARM to 31% to 59% closure rates at 60 weeks in ADHERE (2-year follow-up). A remarkable finding was that among patients whose fistulas had closed after CHARM, 75% (worst case)—90% (best case) maintained closure in ADHERE. The results of this study are quite encouraging. Previously, there was very little information on tumour necrosis factor (TNF) antagonists other then infliximab for fistulizing CD. This study demonstrated similar efficacy as infliximab despite that most of these fistula patients (62%) had previous TNF antagonist exposure, which has been associated with lower response rates in CD. While infliximab continues to have the best evidence, this study suggests that adalimumab may be an acceptable alternative for patients with penetrating CD.

M. F. Picco, MD, PhD

Budesonide Is Effective in Treating Lymphocytic Colitis: A Randomized Double-Blind Placebo-Controlled Study

Miehlke S, Madisch A, Karimi D, et al (Technical Univ Hosp, Dresden, Germany; Inst for Pathology, Klinikum Bayreuth, Germany; et al)
Gastroenterology 136:2092-2100, 2009

Background & Aims.—Budesonide is effective in treating collagenous colitis, but no treatment is established for lymphocytic colitis. We performed a randomized, double-blind, placebo-controlled study to evaluate the effects of budesonide in patients with lymphocytic colitis.

Methods.—Forty-two patients (median age, 61 years) with lymphocytic colitis and chronic diarrhea were randomly assigned to groups that were given oral doses of budesonide (9 mg/d) or placebo for 6 weeks. Non-responders at week 6 were given open-label budesonide (9 mg/d) for 6 additional weeks. A complete colonoscopy and histologic and quality-of-life analyses were performed at baseline and at week 6. The primary end point was clinical remission at 6 weeks, with last observation carried forward (LOCF). All patients who left the study in clinical remission were followed for relapse.

Results.—At week 6, 86% of patients given budesonide were in clinical remission (with LOCF) compared with 48% of patients given placebo (*P* = .010). Furthermore, open-label budesonide therapy induced clinical remission in 7 of 8 patients given placebo. Histologic remission was observed in 73% of patients given budesonide compared with 31% given placebo (*P* = .030). Only 1 patient discontinued budesonide therapy prematurely. During a mean follow-up period of 14 months, 15 patients (44.1%) experienced a clinical relapse (after a mean of 2 months); 8 of the relapsing patients were retreated with and responded again to budesonide.

Conclusions.—Budesonide effectively induces clinical remission in patients with lymphocytic colitis and significantly improves histology results after 6 weeks. Clinical relapses occur but can be treated again with budesonide.

▶ Budesonide is commonly used in the treatment of both collagenous and lymphocytic colitis. The evidence for its use in lymphocytic colitis has been lacking until now. In this study, oral enteric-coated, pH-dependent release budesonide was found to have efficacy in lymphocytic colitis similar to collagenous colitis. The majority of patients also had biopsy data available confirming high histologic remission rates. The authors point out that histologic data were only available on 28 of 42 patients, so that any conclusions regarding histology were "observational." While they may be observational, they are quite compelling. Quality-of-life data was a little more difficult to interpret, which may be more a result of how quality of life was measured. As with data in collagenous colitis, 6-week treatment at 9 mg daily results in the highest efficacy. The drug was very well tolerated. As with other studies on microscopic colitis, relapse rates after cessation of treatment were high. Other studies have supported efficacy and safety of low-dose budesonide over 6 months, but longer follow-up studies are needed. As with collagenous colitis, the clinical presentation of lymphocytic colitis can vary from mild irritable bowel–like symptoms that may respond to conservative measures (antidiarrheal therapies) to severe diarrhea. The selection of budesonide should be patient specific, but it is safe and effective for the induction of remission for this disorder.

M. F. Picco, MD, PhD

Long-term budesonide treatment of collagenous colitis: a randomised, double-blind, placebo-controlled trial
Bonderup OK, Hansen JB, Teglbjærg PS, et al (Randers Regional Hosp, Denmark; Aalborg Hosp, Denmark; et al)
Gut 58:68-72, 2009

Objective.—To evaluate the efficacy and safety of long-term budesonide therapy for the maintenance of clinical remission in patients with collagenous colitis.

Design.—Randomised, placebo-controlled study with a 24-week, blinded follow-up period without any treatment.

Setting.—Three gastroenterology clinics in Denmark.

Patients.—Forty-two patients with histologically confirmed collagenous colitis and diarrhoea (more than three stools/day).

Interventions.—Patients in clinical remission after 6 weeks' open-label therapy with oral budesonide (Entocort CIR capsules, 9 mg/day) received 24 weeks' double-blind maintenance therapy with budesonide 6 mg/day or placebo. Thereafter, patients entered the 24-week, blinded follow-up period.

Main Outcome Measure.—The proportion of patients in clinical remission (three or fewer stools/day) at the end of maintenance therapy.

Findings.—A total of 34 patients in remission at week 6 were randomly assigned to budesonide 6 mg/day (n = 17) or placebo (n = 17). After 24 weeks' maintenance treatment, the proportions of patients in clinical remission were 76.5% (13 of 17) with budesonide and 12% (2 of 17) with placebo (p<0.001). At 48 weeks (the end of the follow-up period, without any treatment) these values were 23.5% (4 of 17) and 12% (2 of 17), respectively (p = 0.6). The median times to relapse after stopping active treatment (6 plus 24 weeks in the budesonide group; 6 weeks in the placebo group) were 39 and 38 days, respectively. Long-term treatment with budesonide was well tolerated.

Conclusions.—Long-term maintenance therapy with oral budesonide is efficacious and well tolerated for preventing relapse in patients with collagenous colitis. The risk of relapse after 24 weeks' maintenance treatment is similar to that observed after 6 weeks' induction therapy.

▶ This trial adds to the growing body of literature of the effectiveness of oral budesonide (Entocort CIR) in the treatment of collagenous colitis. The trial carries treatment beyond induction of remission into maintenance therapy, showing that this agent is superior to placebo at 24 weeks with very high relapse rates with treatment discontinuation. The results, while impressive, do not necessarily translate into using oral budesonide as an induction and/or maintenance agent for all patients with collagenous colitis. One could argue that many patients meeting minimum study entry criteria would clinically have mild disease and might not need oral budesonide therapy. Collagenous colitis has a wide spectrum of presentations ranging from mild symptoms reminiscent of irritable bowel syndrome to severe diarrhea and dehydration. Patients with mild symptoms are often adequately treated with dietary modification or antidiarrheal therapy. While these approaches may lack clinical studies proving efficacy, they have minimal toxicity. Budesonide is often reserved for those with more severe symptoms, because of concerns regarding its long-term safety. While this and other studies including trials using this agent for Crohn's disease have shown significantly fewer adverse events than traditional corticosteroids, these events do occur and long-term follow-up is limited. More time may be needed document adverse events such as osteoporosis. Budesonide is an excellent choice for patients with debilitating disease. Many of these patients will have flare-ups with tapering of this agent despite use of other less toxic agents. These are the patients where the benefit of long-term budesonide therapy may outweigh the potential long-term risk of this agent.[1]

M. F. Picco, MD, PhD

Reference

1. Chande N, McDonald J. Interventions for treating collagenous colitis. *Cochrane Database Syst Rev.* 2008;16:CD006096.

Long-term outcome of treatment with infliximab in 614 patients with Crohn's disease: results from a single-centre cohort
Schnitzler F, Fidder H, Ferrante M, et al (Univ Hosp Gasthuisberg, Leuven, Belgium; et al)
Gut 58:492-500, 2009

Background and Aims.—This observational study assessed the long-term clinical benefit of infliximab (IFX) in 614 consecutive patients with Crohn's disease (CD) from a single centre during a median follow-up of 55 months (interquartile range (IQR) 27–83).

Methods.—The primary analysis looked at the proportion of patients with initial response to IFX who had sustained clinical benefit at the end of follow-up. The long-term effects of IFX on the course of CD as reflected by the rate of surgery and hospitalisations and need for corticosteroids were also analysed.

Results.—10.9% of patients were primary non-responders to IFX. Sustained benefit was observed in 347 of the 547 patients (63.4%) receiving long-term treatment. In 68.3% of these, treatment with IFX was ongoing and in 31.7% IFX was stopped, with the patient being in remission. Seventy patients (12.8%) had to stop IFX due to side effects and 118 (21.6%) due to loss of response. Although the yearly drop-out rates of IFX in patients with episodic (10.7%) and scheduled treatment (7.1%) were similar, the need for hospitalisations and surgery decreased less in the episodic than in the scheduled group. Steroid discontinuation also occurred in a higher proportion of patients in the scheduled group than in the episodic group.

Conclusions.—In this large real-life cohort of patients with CD, long-term treatment with IFX was very efficacious to maintain improvement during a median follow-up of almost 5 years and changed disease outcome by decreasing the rate of hospitalisations and surgery.

▶ Current practice for patients treated with inhibitors of tumor necrosis factor (TNF) alpha is induction therapy and, among responders, indefinite commitment to long-term therapy. This has raised questions about long-term efficacy and safety since after one year only about 40% of responders will remain in remission. We have very little data on outcomes after 1 year. This study followed patients receiving either episodic or scheduled infliximab for 5 years, one of the longest follow-up periods to date. These data do suggest that long-term treatment remains effective in the majority of patients, especially those on scheduled rather than episodic therapy. While the results are encouraging, the study does have some limitations. It is a longitudinal follow-up study so that treatment assignments were known. The initial response rates to infliximab were very high compared with what has been published in randomized controlled studies. The definition of "sustained clinical benefit" was "lasting control of the disease activity during follow-up with persistent improvement of symptoms," which is quite nonspecific. That being said, the data do support the common practice of continued use of infliximab, but more studies are needed. The long-term outcomes are very favorable with sustained responses and lower hospitalization rates in the infliximab group. The article also presents an interesting finding among the episodic treatment group. After receiving infliximab for a median of 6 months, over 2/3 of these patients stayed in remission for a median of 47.3 months with no further infliximab. While this may have been the result of a selection bias, no specific features identified patients who were more likely to remain in remission. However, the majority of these patients remained on immunomodulator therapy after their last dose of infliximab. The questions of when to start and when to stop (if ever) anti-TNF agents remain, but this study does suggest that the current practice of indefinite therapy does lead to better patient outcomes.

M. F. Picco, MD, PhD

48 Pancreas

Are there roles for intraductal US and saline solution irrigation in ensuring complete clearance of common bile duct stones?
Ang TL, Teo EK, Fock KM, et al (Changi General Hosp, Singapore)
Gastrointest Endosc 69:1276-1281, 2009

Background.—Persistent small common bile duct (CBD) stones after endoscopic sphincterotomy (EST) and stone extraction may be a nidus for stone growth and could be detected by intraductal US (IDUS). CBD saline solution irrigation may flush out residual stones.

Objectives.—Our purpose was to determine the frequency of residual CBD stones after EST and basket/balloon extraction by using IDUS and to assess the effectiveness of saline solution irrigation in clearing remnant CBD stones.

Design.—Prospective study.

Setting.—General Hospital Singapore.

Patients.—Seventy patients (mean age 62 years, 51% male) were recruited.

Interventions.—In the presence of CBD stones, EST and stone extraction were performed, followed by IDUS. If residual stones were detected, a catheter was inserted into the proximal CBD, saline solution irrigation performed, and IDUS repeated.

Main Outcome Measurements.—(1) The frequency of residual stones detected by IDUS after EST and basket/balloon extraction and (2) the effect of saline solution irrigation in clearing residual CBD stones.

Results.—Cholangiogram showed CBD stones in 38 of 70 patients (median 1 [range 1-5], mean size 7.6 mm [range 3.0-12.0 mm]). IDUS showed CBD stones in 32 of 32 with normal cholangiogram (median 2 [range 1-8], mean size 2.6 mm [range 0.9-7.2 mm]). After EST and stone extraction, IDUS showed persistent stones in 28 of 70 (median: 2 [range 1-5], mean size 2.2 mm [range 1.1-4.6 mm]). The CBD was irrigated with a mean of 48 mL of saline solution. Repeat IDUS showed persistent CBD stones in 2 of 70, and these were flushed out by further saline solution irrigation.

Limitations.—Single-center study.

Conclusion.—IDUS detected small residual CBD stones that persisted after EST and basket/balloon extraction. Saline solution irrigation appeared useful in clearing residual small stones.

▶ It has long been suspected and now well documented with use of intraductal ultrasound (IDUS) and cholangioscopy that residual gravel or stones are frequently missed after endoscopic sphincterotomy (EST) and stone extraction from the common bile duct (CBD). Risk factors appear to include common duct diameter > 1 cm, multiple stones at start, pneumobilia which limits cholangiogram accuracy, and fragmentation of stones during extraction. Although it is assumed residual gravel or small stones will pass spontaneously through an adequate sphincterotomy, these stones likely play a significant role in recurrent biliary tract disease in these patients, reported to occur in up to 25% of cases over time.

In this prospective single-center study, 70 patients with CBD stones subjected to EST and stone extraction, IDUS documented a median of 2 residual stones (range 1-5) in 40% (28/40) of patients with a mean diameter of 2.2 mm. With a catheter placed to the level of the hilum, the CBD was irrigated with 20 to 80 cc of normal saline (mean volume 48 cc). Adequacy of irrigation was assessed by complete clearance of biliary dye. Direct inspection of the ampulla often confirmed clearance of residual stones. After one irrigation repeat, IDUS confirmed clearance of residual stones in (97%) 38/40. Clearance of the other 2 residual stones was documented by IDUS after a second irrigation. There was no evidence for complications (worsening cholangitis, increased pancreatitis) resulting from irrigation.

This study confirms residual stones after EST and standard stone extraction are common. Because IDUS is not widely available, this study would suggest CBD irrigation is safe and effective in clearing residual CBD debris but probably should be reserved for patients at higher risk.

S. M. Lange, MD

Branch duct intraductal papillary mucinous neoplasms in a retrospective series of 190 patients
Woo SM, Ryu JK, Lee SH, et al (Seoul Natl Univ College of Medicine, Yeongeon-dong, Jongno-gu, Korea)
Br J Surg 96:405-411, 2009

Background.—A consensus conference has recommended close observation of branch duct intraductal papillary mucinous neoplasms (BD-IPMNs) smaller than 30 mm, without symptoms or mural nodules. This study investigated whether these recommendations could be validated in a single-centre experience of BD-IPMNs.

Methods.—Some 190 patients with radiological imaging or histological findings consistent with BD-IPMN were enrolled between 1998 and 2005. Those with less than 6 months' follow-up and no histological confirmation were excluded.

Results.—BD-IPMN was diagnosed by computed tomography and pancreatography in 105 patients and pathologically in 85. Eighteen patients had adenoma, 53 borderline malignancy, five carcinoma *in situ* and nine invasive carcinoma. Findings associated with malignancy were the presence of radiologically suspicious features ($P < 0·001$) and a cyst size of at least 30 mm ($P = 0·001$). Had consensus guidelines been applied,

54 patients would have undergone pancreatic resection, whereas only 28 of these patients actually had a resection; 12 of the latter patients had a malignancy compared with none of the 26 patients who were treated conservatively.

Conclusion.—A simple increase in cyst size is not a reliable predictor of malignancy. Observation is recommended for patients with a BD-IPMN smaller than 30 mm showing no suspicious features on imaging.

▶ Intraductal papillary mucinous neoplasms (IPMNs) of the pancreas are sub-divided into main duct and branch duct groups based on well-defined imaging criteria due to differences in prognosis. Prevalence of cancer ranges from 52% to 92% in main duct IPMNs and 6% to 46% in branch duct IPMNs. Consensus management is to resect main duct IPMNs if operative risk is acceptable. Branch duct IPMNs may be observed if they are less than 30 mm and have no suspicious clinical or imaging criteria (symptoms, elevated CA19-9, mural nodules, thick walls, suspicious cytology).

This single-center retrospective analysis of 190 patients with branch duct IPMNs assessed the validity of published consensus guidelines for resection and significance of change in cyst characteristics during follow-up. For cysts > 30 mm or with mural nodules at presentation, 33% (12/36) contained invasive malignancy, but 100% (4/4) of cysts > 30 mm with mural nodules contained malignancy at resection. Although only 15% of cysts with at least one criterion for resection had invasive malignancy, when borderline malig-nancy and carcinoma in situ are included, 61% of cysts had significant pathology. Only 2/14 patients with malignancy had lesions less than 30 mm and no suspicious imaging features. These 2 cases represented only 1% of patients not meeting criteria for resection. Of interest, as with adenocarcinoma of the pancreas, diabetes was associated with underlying malignancy. During a mean follow-up of 24 months, 10.5% of cysts (11) enlarged by > 20% from baseline. None contained mural nodules or other suspicious imaging criteria. Six underwent resection and 1(16%) contained malignancy.

Overall, these results reaffirm current management guidelines for branch duct IPMNs. When operative risk is acceptable and life expectancy > 3 to 5 years, resection of lesions with associated symptoms or elevated CA19-9, cysts > 30 mm, and/or those containing suspicious imaging criteria (mural nodules, thick wall) is justified based on risk for advanced histology. Likewise, when cysts enlarge > 20% during observation, resection should be considered. The development of diabetes may be an additional risk factor to consider. Iden-tification of additional criteria to refine selection of patients for resection is required to reduce unnecessary surgery.

S. M. Lange, MD

Comparison of carcinoembryonic antigen and molecular analysis in pancreatic cyst fluid

Sawhney MS, Devarajan S, O'Farrel P, et al (Beth Israel Deaconess Med Ctr and Harvard Med School, Boston, MA)
Gastrointest Endosc 69:1106-1110, 2009

Background.—Pancreatic-cyst fluid carcinoembryonic antigen (CEA) levels and molecular analysis are useful diagnostic tests in differentiating mucinous from nonmucinous cysts.

Objective.—To assess agreement between CEA and molecular analysis for differentiating mucinous from nonmucinous cysts.

Design.—Retrospective analysis.

Setting.—Academic medical center.

Methods.—Patients who underwent EUS-guided FNA for evaluation of pancreatic cysts were identified. The following information was used to designate a cyst mucinous: the CEA criterion was CEA level $\geq$192 ng/mL and the molecular analysis criteria were DNA quantity $\geq$40 ng/μL and/or k-ras 2-point mutation and/or $\geq$2 allelic imbalance mutations. Pathologic analysis of cysts served as the criterion standard.

Results.—From 2006 to 2007, 100 patients met the study criteria. The average age of the patients was 63 years, 65% were women, and 30% were symptomatic. The mean diameter of pancreatic cysts was 2.5 cm. The median CEA value was 83 ng/mL (range 1-50,000 ng/mL), the mean DNA content was 16 ng/μL (range 1-212 ng/μL), 11% had K-*ras* mutations, and 43% had $\geq$2 allelic imbalance mutations. When using pre-specified criteria, there was poor agreement between CEA and molecular analysis for the classification of mucinous cysts (kappa = 0.2). Poor agreement existed between CEA and DNA quantity (Spearman correlation = 0.2; P = .1), K-*ras* mutation (kappa = 0.3), and $\geq$2 allelic imbalance mutations (kappa = 0.1). Of the 19 patients for whom a final pathologic diagnosis was available, CEA had a sensitivity of 82% compared with 77% for molecular analysis. When CEA and molecular analysis were combined, 100% sensitivity was achieved.

Limitations.—Retrospective analysis and small sample size.

Conclusion.—There was poor agreement between CEA levels and molecular analysis for diagnosis of mucinous cysts. Diagnostic sensitivity was improved when results of CEA levels and molecular analysis were combined.

▶ In clinical practice, pancreatic cysts that can't be classified as inflammatory (pseudocysts) or serous cystadenomas by clinical and imaging criteria must be assumed to be mucin-producing cysts, which carry the potential for malignant degeneration. Imaging (MRI or endoscopic ultrasound [EUS]) can often identify characteristics compatible with main duct or side branch intraductal papillary mucinous neoplasms and appropriate intervention or surveillance undertaken. The remaining pancreatic cysts are indeterminate. Additional testing to define their nature and associated risk for malignant degeneration would contribute to more cost-effective surveillance programs. Fine needle aspiration (FNA) of these cysts for cytology and cyst-fluid analysis is feasible and safe. To date, cyst-fluid carcinoembryonic antigen (CEA) level > 190 ng/mL is the only widely accepted candidate to help differentiate mucinous from nonmucinous cysts and therefore malignant potential of indeterminate cysts.

In this retrospective single-center study of 100 patients with pancreatic cysts subjected to FNA, cyst-fluid CEA and molecular analysis to include DNA quantity, K-*ras* mutation, and/or allelic imbalance mutations were assessed alone and in combination to differentiate mucinous from nonmucinous cysts. When using prespecified criteria based on the literature for each metric, there was poor agreement between CEA level and all 3 components of molecular analysis for classification of mucinous cysts. When 19 patients for whom a final pathologic diagnosis was available were analyzed, CEA > 192 ng/mL had a sensitivity of 82% compared with 77% for molecular analysis. When CEA and molecular analysis were combined, sensitivity was 100%.

The small sample size and availability of molecule analysis limit conclusions and widespread application to daily practice, but these results clearly suggest focusing on cyst-fluid analysis represents the best candidate to further refine management algorithms for indeterminate pancreatic cysts.

S. M. Lange, MD

Incidental Cystic Neoplasms of Pancreas: What Is the Optimal Interval of Imaging Surveillance?

Das A, Wells CD, Nguyen CC (Mayo Clinic Arizona, Scottsdale)
Am J Gastroenterol 103:1657-1662, 2008

Background.—The optimal interval of imaging studies for surveillance of incidental pancreatic cystic neoplasms is not known.

Objective.—A retrospective analysis of longitudinal medical records of patients with pancreatic cystic neoplasms was performed to examine the natural history of incidentally detected cystic pancreatic neoplasms with respect to the development of significant growth and to identify predictors of such growth.

Results.—After excluding patients with small (<10 mm) cysts (N = 144) and inadequate clinical follow-up of less than 6 months (N = 79) and those with a clinical diagnosis of pancreatic pseudocysts, serous cystadenoma, main duct intraductal papillary mucinous neoplasm (N = 29), and neuroendocrine tumor (N = 3), in total, 166 cysts in 150 patients were available for analysis. The working diagnoses on these cysts (based on clinical, radiological features, aspiration cytology, cyst fluid analysis, and surgical pathology data when available) were mucinous cystic neoplasm in 117 and branch-type intraductal papillary mucinous neoplasm in 49. The mean standard error (SE) initial size of these cysts was 2 (0.1) cm. Over a median period of follow-up of 32 (IQR [inter-quartile range] 19–48) months, 89% of all the cysts did not show significant growth during the follow-up. In a multivariate Cox proportional hazards model, the initial size of the cystic lesion was an independent predictor of significant growth during follow-up (relative risk 1.28, 95% confidence interval [CI] 1.08–1.61, $P = 0.01$); the only other significant variable was the presence of intracystic or mural nodule (relative risk 38.6, 95% CI 2.3–654, $P = 0.01$).

Conclusion.—Most incidentally detected cystic neoplasms of the pancreas did not have significant growth during follow-up. Such growth is unlikely to occur before 2 yr of the baseline evaluation, and we suggest that the optimal imaging interval during follow-up of these patients should be at 2 yr from the baseline evaluation, particularly in cystic lesions 3.0 cm or less in size and without intracystic or mural nodules.

▶ Cystic neoplasms of the pancreas primarily refer to serous cystadenomas, mucinous cystadenomas, and intraductal papillary mucinous neoplasms (IPMN). Serous cystadenomas have little to no risk for malignant degeneration, and most can be differentiated from other pancreatic cysts on cross-sectional imaging by distinct imaging features. Surveillance after diagnosis for malignant degeneration is not required.

In contrast, mucin-producing neoplasms of the pancreas carry a small but significant risk for malignant degeneration. Criteria used to stratify risk among indeterminate cysts or those felt to be mucinous include: associated symptoms, age, male gender, internal septations or calcification, mural nodules or associated mass, association to the main pancreatic duct, presence of mucin, and carcinoembryonic antigen (CEA) level determined by fine needle aspiration. Size, presence of mural nodules, and cyst characteristics compatible with IPMN are clinically most useful. Cysts less than 3 cm and lack of mural nodules and side branch IPMNs identify cysts with significantly less risk over time for malignant degeneration. Current recommendations for surveillance with CT, MRI, or endoscopic ultrasound (EUS) are yearly for cysts < 1 cm, every 6 months for cysts measuring 1 to 2 cm, and every 3 to 6 months for cysts > 3 cm if resection is not undertaken. However, these recommendations are not based on strong clinical evidence.

In this retrospective analysis of 150 patients (166 cysts) with cysts > 1 cm felt to be mucin-producing lesions (117 mucinous cystic neoplasms, 49 branch duct IPMNs) with median cross-sectional imaging follow-up greater of 32 months, 89% of all cysts did not show significant growth, defined as an increase in diameter by > 10 mm. Of the 18 cysts that demonstrated significant growth, none changed within 12 months and only 3 showed significant growth within 24 months of the initial imaging study. Initial size > 3 cm was an independent predictor for growth versus smaller lesions (44% vs 5.6%). The only other independent predictor for growth was intracystic or mural nodules. The authors conclude optimal imaging interval during follow-up should be at 2 yr from the baseline evaluation, particularly in cystic lesions 3.0 cm or less in size and without intracystic or mural nodules.

These data clearly suggest reevaluation of current recommendations for initial follow-up surveillance of small indeterminate or mucin-producing cysts is justified. However, longer-term studies are required to determine the best approach over the subsequent lifetime of an individual patient.

S. M. Lange, MD

49 Liver

Meta-analysis: Combination Endoscopic and Drug Therapy to Prevent Variceal Rebleeding in Cirrhosis

Gonzalez R, Zamora J, Gomez-Camarero J, et al (Hosp Universitario Ramón y Cajal, Madrid, Spain; Hosp General Universitario Gregorio Marañón, Madrid, Spain; et al)

Ann Intern Med 149:109-122, 2008

Background.—Combining endoscopic therapy and β-blockers may improve outcomes in patients with cirrhosis and bleeding esophageal varices.

Purpose.—To assess whether a combination of endoscopic and drug therapy prevents overall and variceal rebleeding and improves survival better than either therapy alone.

Data Sources.—MEDLINE, EMBASE, the Cochrane Central Register of Controlled Trials, the Cochrane Database of Systematic Reviews, and conference proceedings through 30 December 2007.

Study Selection.—Randomized trials comparing endoscopic plus β-blocker therapy with either therapy alone, without language restrictions.

Data Extraction.—Two reviewers independently extracted data on interventions and the primary study outcomes of overall rebleeding and mortality. Metaregression and stratified analysis were used to explore heterogeneity.

Data Synthesis.—23 trials (1860 patients) met inclusion criteria. Combination therapy reduced overall rebleeding more than endoscopic therapy alone (pooled relative risk, 0.68 [95% CI, 0.52 to 0.89]; $I^2 = 61\%$) or β-blocker therapy alone (pooled relative risk, 0.71 [CI, 0.59 to 0.86]; $I^2 = 0\%$). Combination therapy also reduced variceal rebleeding and variceal recurrence. Reduction in mortality from combination therapy did not statistically significantly differ from that from endoscopic (Peto odds ratio, 0.78 [CI, 0.58 to 1.07) or drug therapy (Peto odds ratio, 0.70 [CI, 0.46 to 1.06]). Effects were independent of the endoscopic procedure (injection sclerotherapy or banding). No trial-level variable associated with the effect was identified through metaregression or stratified analysis.

Limitation.—Statistically significant heterogeneity in trial quality and evidence for selective reporting and publication bias were found.

Conclusion.—A combination of endoscopic and drug therapy reduces overall and variceal rebleeding in cirrhosis more than either therapy alone.

▶ Patients with cirrhosis who survive an episode of variceal bleeding have a greater than 60% risk of rebleeding at 1 year. The mortality from rebleeding is 20%. The 2 primary interventions used to prevent esophageal variceal rebleeding include endoscopic banding or sclerotherapy and drug therapy. Endoscopic therapy induces fibrosis and thrombosis in the varix but does not alter the portal hypertension. The drug therapy is targeted at reducing portal pressures and splanchnic blood flow. Although studies have shown each therapy to be efficacious, the combination therapy could be more effective than either therapy alone. Several studies have shown that combination therapy works better than endoscopic therapy alone; however, the impact on survival is unclear.

This study by Gonzales et al is an analysis of randomized trials comparing endoscopic therapy plus β-blocker therapy with either therapy alone. A total of 23 trials or 1860 patients met inclusion criteria, and their data were extracted and reviewed. The study demonstrated that combination therapy was more effective in preventing rebleeding than either therapy alone, but mortality rates were not changed by the combination therapy.

This study strengthens the recommendation that patients who develop bleeding from varices should be considered for treatment with endoscopic therapy and β blocker to prevent rebleeding complications. There is still no documented survival benefit from combination therapy.

D. M. Harnois, DO

Causes, Clinical Features, and Outcomes From a Prospective Study of Drug-Induced Liver Injury in the United States

Chalasani N, Fontana RJ, Bonkovsky HL, et al (Indiana Univ School of Medicine, Indianapolis; Univ of Michigan Med School, Ann Arbor; Carolinas Med Ctr, Charlotte, NC; et al)
Gastroenterology 135:1924-1934, 2008

Background & Aims.—Idiosyncratic drug-induced liver injury (DILI) is among the most common causes of acute liver failure in the United States, accounting for approximately 13% of cases. A prospective study was begun in 2003 to recruit patients with suspected DILI and create a repository of biological samples for analysis. This report summarizes the causes, clinical features, and outcomes from the first 300 patients enrolled.

Methods.—Patients with suspected DILI were enrolled based on pre-defined criteria and followed up for at least 6 months. Patients with acetaminophen liver injury were excluded.

Results.—DILI was caused by a single prescription medication in 73% of the cases, by dietary supplements in 9%, and by multiple agents in 18%. More than 100 different agents were associated with DILI; antimicrobials

(45.5%) and central nervous system agents (15%) were the most common. Causality was considered to be definite in 32%, highly likely in 41%, probable in 14%, possible in 10%, and unlikely in 3%. Acute hepatitis C virus (HCV) infection was the final diagnosis in 4 of 9 unlikely cases. Six months after enrollment, 14% of patients had persistent laboratory abnormalities and 8% had died; the cause of death was liver related in 44%.

Conclusions.—DILI is caused by a wide array of medications, herbal supplements, and dietary supplements. Antibiotics are the single largest class of agents that cause DILI. Acute HCV infection should be excluded in patients with suspected DILI by HCV RNA testing. The overall 6-month mortality was 8%, but the majority of deaths were not liver related.

▶ Drug-induced liver injury is a leading cause of acute liver injury and failure in the United States. The Drug Induced Liver Injury Network is a NIH/NIDDK sponsored network formed in 2003 and investigates in retrospective and prospective fashion cases of liver toxicity. This report summarizes the cause, clinical features, and outcomes of the first 300 patients enrolled.

A detailed medical and laboratory history was obtained on all cases with follow-up at 6, 12, and up to 24 months. Based on the dominant type of injury pattern the cases were divided into hepatocellular, cholestatic, or mixed type of injury. The severity of injury was also recorded.

The drug-induced liver injury was caused by a single prescription medication in most cases (73%), a dietary agent in 9%, and a combination of agents in 18% of patients. The median duration between first exposure and liver injury was 42 days.

The drug-induced liver injury was hepatocellular in 57%, cholestatic in 23%, and mixed in 20%. In a multivariate analysis, the presence of diabetes and alcohol consumption were independent predictors of severe injury.

The mortality was higher in patients with hepatocellular liver injury with peak serum total bilirubin level of > 2.5 mg/dL. At 6 months of follow-up 13.6% of patients had evidence of chronic liver disease, 2.1% had a liver transplant, and 8% had died.

This study is the first to provide prospective analysis of patients developing drug-induced liver injury.

D. M. Harnois, DO

Sorafenib in Advanced Hepatocellular Carcinoma
Llovet JM, for the SHARP Investigators Study Group (Centro de Investigaciones en Red de Enfermedades Hepáticas y Digestivas Hospital Clínic Barcelona, et al)
N Engl J Med 359:378-390, 2008

Background.—No effective systemic therapy exists for patients with advanced hepatocellular carcinoma. A preliminary study suggested that sorafenib, an oral multikinase inhibitor of the vascular endothelial growth factor receptor, the platelet-derived growth factor receptor, and Raf may be effective in hepatocellular carcinoma.

Methods.—In this multicenter, phase 3, double-blind, placebo-controlled trial, we randomly assigned 602 patients with advanced hepatocellular carcinoma who had not received previous systemic treatment to receive either sorafenib (at a dose of 400 mg twice daily) or placebo. Primary outcomes were overall survival and the time to symptomatic progression. Secondary outcomes included the time to radiologic progression and safety.

Results.—At the second planned interim analysis, 321 deaths had occurred, and the study was stopped. Median overall survival was 10.7 months in the sorafenib group and 7.9 months in the placebo group (hazard ratio in the sorafenib group, 0.69; 95% confidence interval, 0.55 to 0.87; P<0.001). There was no significant difference between the two groups in the median time to symptomatic progression (4.1 months vs. 4.9 months, respectively, P = 0.77). The median time to radiologic progression was 5.5 months in the sorafenib group and 2.8 months in the placebo group (P<0.001). Seven patients in the sorafenib group (2%) and two patients in the placebo group (1%) had a partial response; no patients had a complete response. Diarrhea, weight loss, hand–foot skin reaction, and hypophosphatemia were more frequent in the sorafenib group.

Conclusions.—In patients with advanced hepatocellular carcinoma, median survival and the time to radiologic progression were nearly 3 months longer for patients treated with sorafenib than for those given placebo. (ClinicalTrials.gov number, NCT00105443.)

▶ Hepatocellular cancer (HCC) is the fifth most common cancer worldwide and the third leading cause of death from cancer. The major risk factors for the development of HCC include chronic viral hepatitis B and C infection, alcoholic cirrhosis, nonalcoholic steatohepatitis, and most particularly the development of cirrhosis. The treatment of liver cancer is complicated by the coexistence of hepatic dysfunction from liver disease in most patients requiring treatment for HCC.

This study by Llovet et al describes the positive results of a phase 3 study assessing the use of sorafenib in patients with unresectable HCC. Sorafenib is a potent inhibitor of Raf-1 and both variants of B-Raf. In addition, it has activity against multiple receptor tyrosine kinases involved in tumor growth and angiogenesis including endothelial growth factor receptors (VEGFR) and platelet-derived growth factors.

Investigators in this trial observe that in the population of patients with preserved liver function (Child-Pugh class A cirrhosis), the use of sorafenib resulted in a modest gain in survival of 3 months. Survival was improved because the drug slowed tumor progression. Because of this evidence, the drug sorafenib was approved by the Food and Drug Administration for the treatment of HCC.

This is an important first step toward the development of targeted therapies in the treatment of HCC and now serves as the benchmark for future studies. In particular, there is a need to understand the application of this and other treatments in patients with more advanced liver disease (Child-Pugh class B cirrhosis).

D. M. Harnois, DO

Hyponatremia and Mortality among Patients on the Liver-Transplant Waiting List
Kim WR, Biggins SW, Kremers WK, et al (Mayo Clinic College of Medicine, Rochester, MN; Univ of California at San Francisco; et al)
N Engl J Med 359:1018-1026, 2008

Background.—Under the current liver-transplantation policy, donor organs are offered to patients with the highest risk of death.

Methods.—Using data derived from all adult candidates for primary liver transplantation who were registered with the Organ Procurement and Transplantation Network in 2005 and 2006, we developed and validated a multivariable survival model to predict mortality at 90 days after registration. The predictor variable was the Model for End-Stage Liver Disease (MELD) score with and without the addition of the serum sodium concentration. The MELD score (on a scale of 6 to 40, with higher values indicating more severe disease) is calculated on the basis of the serum bilirubin and creatinine concentrations and the international normalized ratio for the prothrombin time.

Results.—In 2005, there were 6769 registrants, including 1781 who underwent liver transplantation and 422 who died within 90 days after registration on the waiting list. Both the MELD score and the serum sodium concentration were significantly associated with mortality (hazard ratio for death, 1.21 per MELD point and 1.05 per 1-unit decrease in the serum sodium concentration for values between 125 and 140 mmol per liter; P<0.001 for both variables). Furthermore, a significant interaction was found between the MELD score and the serum sodium concentration, indicating that the effect of the serum sodium concentration was greater in patients with a low MELD score. When applied to the data from 2006, when 477 patients died within 3 months after registration on the waiting list, the combination of the MELD score and the serum sodium concentration was considerably higher than the MELD score alone in 32 patients who died (7%). Thus, assignment of priority according to the MELD score combined with the serum sodium concentration might have resulted in transplantation and prevented death.

Conclusions.—This population-wide study shows that the MELD score and the serum sodium concentration are important predictors of survival among candidates for liver transplantation.

▶ The allocation of grafts for liver transplantation from deceased donors in the United States is based on medical urgency as estimates according to the Model of End-Stage Liver Disease (MELD) score. This score is based on total serum bilirubin, the international normalized ratio (INR) for prothrombin time, and the serum creatinine concentration. In the United States, the MELD score has been the system of allocation of liver graft organs since 2002.

Serum sodium concentration has also been recognized as an important prognostic factor for patients with liver cirrhosis. This study, published by Kim et al in the *New England Journal of Medicine* using data derived from all adult candidates registered for primary liver transplant with the Organ Procurement and Transplantation Network in 2005 and 2006, showed that MELD score and serum sodium concentration are important predictors of survival among candidates for liver transplantation.

D. M. Harnois, DO

Predicting survival after liver transplantation in patients with hepatocellular carcinoma beyond the Milan criteria: a retrospective, exploratory analysis

Mazzaferro V, on behalf of the Metroticket Investigator Study Group (Natl Cancer Inst, Milan, Italy; et al)
Lancet Oncol 10:35-43, 2009

Background.—Patients undergoing liver transplantation for hepatocellular carcinoma within the Milan criteria (single tumour ≤5 cm in size or ≤3 tumours each ≤3 cm in size, and no macrovascular invasion) have an excellent outcome. However, survival for patients with cancers that exceed these criteria remains unpredictable and access to transplantation is a balance of maximising patients' chances of cure and organ availability. The aim of this study was to explore the survival of patients with tumours that exceed the Milan criteria, to assess whether the criteria could be less restrictive, enabling more patients to qualify as transplant candidates, and to derive a prognostic model based on objective tumour characteristics, to see whether the Milan criteria could be expanded.

Methods.—Data on patients who underwent transplantation for hepatocellular carcinoma despite exceeding Milan criteria at different centres were recorded via a web-based survey completed by specialists from each centre. The survival of these patients was correlated retrospectively with the size of the largest tumour nodule, number of nodules, and presence or absence of microvascular invasion detected at pathology. Contoured multivariable regression Cox models produced survival estimates by means of different combinations of the covariates. The primary aim of this study was to derive a prognostic model of overall survival based on tumour characteristics, according to the main parameters used in the Tumour Node Metastasis classification. The secondary aim was the identification of a subgroup of patients with hepatocellular carcinoma exceeding the Milan criteria, who achieved a 5-year overall survival of at least 70%—ie, similar to the outcome expected for patients who meet the Milan criteria.

Findings.—Over a 10-month period, between June 25, 2006, and April 3, 2007, data for 1556 patients who underwent transplantation for hepatocellular carcinoma were entered on the database by 36 centres. 1112 patients had hepatocellular carcinoma exceeding Milan criteria and 444 patients had hepatocellular carcinoma shown not to exceed Milan criteria at post-transplant pathology review. In the group of patients with hepatocellular carcinomas exceeding the criteria, the median size of the largest nodule was 40 mm (range 4–200) and the median number of nodules was four (1–20). 454 of 1112 patients (41%) had microvascular invasion and, for those transplanted outside the Milan criteria, 5-year overall survival was $53 \cdot 6\%$ (95% CI $50 \cdot 1$–$57 \cdot 0$), compared with $73 \cdot 3\%$ ($68 \cdot 2$–$77 \cdot 7$) for those that met the criteria. Hazard ratios (HR) associated with increasing values of size and number were $1 \cdot 34$ ($1 \cdot 25$–$1 \cdot 44$) and $1 \cdot 51$ ($1 \cdot 21$–$1 \cdot 88$), respectively. The effect was linear for size, whereas for number of tumours, the effect tended to plateau above three tumours. The effect of tumour size and number on survival was mediated by recurrence (b=$0 \cdot 08$, SE=$0 \cdot 12$, p=$0 \cdot 476$). The presence of microvascular invasion doubled HRs in all scenarios. The 283 patients without microvascular invasion, but who fell within the Up-to-seven criteria (hepatocellular carcinomas with seven as the sum of the size of the largest tumour [in cm] and the number of tumours) achieved a 5-year overall survival of $71 \cdot 2\%$ ($64 \cdot 3$–$77 \cdot 0$).

Interpretation.—More patients with hepatocellular carcinoma could be candidates for transplantation if the current dual (yes/no) approach to candidacy, based on the strict Milan criteria, were replaced with a more precise estimation of survival contouring individual tumour characteristics and use of the up-to-seven criteria.

▶ In 1996, Mazzaferro et al published their results of liver transplantation for small hepatocellular cancers (HCC) in the *New England Journal of Medicine*. This and subsequent studies demonstrated that liver transplant could be successfully performed with reasonable survival in patients transplanted within criteria eventually termed the Milan criteria (a single tumor < 5 cm in size or < 3 tumors < 3 cm in size).

It has been shown more recently that patients exceeding these criteria can have a favorable outcome in liver transplant, but extended criteria have not been clearly agreed upon. The data presented in this study by Mazzafero et al in the *Lancet Oncology* demonstrate that tumor size and number continue to have an impact on survival and recurrence. In addition, the presence of microvascular invasion on explant also increased recurrence risk. This study proposes that a new expanded criterion for liver transplant be defined by the "up to

7 criteria." According to this study, patients transplanted with tumors meeting the "up to 7 criteria" (7 as the total sum of the size of the largest tumor [in cm] and the number of tumors) achieved a reasonable overall 5-year survival of 71.2%.

This article adds to the discussion to attempt to find the appropriate extension of the initial Milan criteria for liver transplant in HCC without compromising results.

D. M. Harnois, DO

Reassessing Selection Criteria Prior to Liver Transplantation for Hepatocellular Carcinoma Utilizing the Scientific Registry of Transplant Recipients Database

Toso C, Asthana S, Bigam DL, et al (Univ of Alberta, Edmonton, Canada)
Hepatology 49:832-838, 2009

The current model of liver graft allocation in place in the United States favors transplantation of patients with small hepatocellular carcinomas (HCCs) within the Milan criteria (a single tumor up to 5 cm in diameter or up to three lesions, none larger than 3 cm). Although several reports have suggested that these criteria could be extended, there is currently no agreement on new selection tools. In this study, we performed an overview of 6478 adult recipients of an isolated first liver transplant registered in the Scientific Registry of Transplant Recipients (SRTR) database. From March 2002 to January 2008, increasing numbers of patients outside Milan criteria ($P \leq 0.001$) have been registered for a transplant, but they still represent less than 5% of the transplants performed for HCC. Of all the tested variables (tumor number, largest tumor size, and Milan and University of California San Francisco criteria), only total tumor volume (TTV; $P \leq 0.05$) and alpha fetoprotein (AFP; $P \leq 0.001$) could predict patient survival. While these two parameters demonstrated independent behaviors (no patient demonstrated an increase in both values), a composite score was defined, with patients with a TTV > 115 cm^3 or an AFP > 400 ng/mL being outside criteria. The combined TTV/AFP score efficiently predicted posttransplant survival (hazard ratio = 2, 95% confidence interval = 1.7-2.4, $P \leq 0.001$); patients not meeting these criteria had a survival below 50% at 3 years.

Conclusion.—According to the present SRTR data, Milan criteria are too restrictive, and patients with larger TTV can enjoy satisfactory posttransplant survivals. A composite patient selection score combining TTV and AFP was the most effective of all tested staging criteria for the prediction of posttransplant patient survival for candidates with HCC.

▶ Hepatocellular carcinoma (HCC) is a frequent complication of patients with cirrhosis and is commonly the cause of death in these patients. Among carefully selected individuals, liver transplant (LT) has an excellent 5-year survival for patients transplanted with HCC. The current United Network of Organ Sharing

(UNOS) approved criteria for transplant in HCC are defined by the Milan criteria (a single lesion less than or equal to 5 cm or no more than 3 lesions with none larger than 3 cm). For some time liver transplant centers have argued that there are individuals with HCC who benefit from transplant with tumors beyond the Milan criteria. Attempts to define these "expanded criteria" have been proposed by several centers.

The first well-documented evidence was reported by Yao et al from the University of California San Francisco (UCSF), who demonstrated maintenance of good outcomes with the transplantation of patients with a single HCC up to 6.5 cm in diameter or with up to 3 HCCs, none larger than 4.5 cm, with a cumulative diameter up to 8 cm. Although their first study was based on retrospective review of explant tumor characteristics, the same group demonstrated more recently that similar excellent outcomes (93.6% of patients free of recurrence at 5 years) can be achieved on the basis of prospective radiological data. Despite good outcomes, the expansion of liver transplant criteria to the UCSF, criteria has neither been uniformly accepted nor adopted.

The authors of the this article in *Hepatology* 2009 have previously demonstrated in a 3-center study, including 288 patients, that the total tumor volume (TTV) was the most accurate morphological criterion for selecting HCC patients before transplantation. Those with a TTV up to 115 cm^3 demonstrated 79% 5-year survival, without tumor number restriction.

This study by Toso et al used data from the Scientific Registry of Transplant Recipients (SRTR) to confirm their previous results in a larger cohort of patients. The SRTR data system includes data on all donors, wait-listed candidates, and transplant recipients in the United States submitted by the members of the Organ Procurement and Transplantation Network (OPTN). The Health Resources and Services Administration (United States Department of Health and Human Services) provides oversight of the activities of the OPTN and SRTR contractors. The study population included all adult (18 years) patients who received a first isolated liver transplant from March 2002 to January 2008 for a diagnosis of HCC.

This study looked at a number of predictive variables for HCC. Of all the tested variables (tumor number, largest tumor size, and Milan and University of California San Francisco criteria), only total tumor volume (TTV; $P \leq .05$) and alpha fetoprotein (AFP; $P \leq .001$) could predict patient survival. While these 2 parameters demonstrated independent behaviors (no patient demonstrated an increase in both values), a composite score was defined, with patients with a TTV > 115 cm^3 or an AFP > 400 ng/mL being outside criteria. The combined TTV/AFP score efficiently predicted post-transplant survival (hazard ratio = 2, 95% confidence interval = 1.7-2.4, $P \leq .001$).

As discussed in an editorial by William Sanchez in the same journal, many of the limitations of the current study are inherent to its retrospective nature, and include the lack of standardization of imaging modalities used and the variable use of pretransplant loco-regional therapy. In addition, as the editorial points out, several important questions remain unanswered. The primary endpoint of this study was all-cause mortality. The study did not assess the other important outcome of interest, namely recurrence-free survival after transplant.

Furthermore, the median duration of follow-up after LT was relatively short at 13.4 months.

Clearly, biological parameters rather than morphologic parameters need to be established to define those who would benefit most from the resource of LT. At this time, however, we are left with only morphologic criteria. There is a great debate developing in the transplant community over the definition of the limits of acceptable "expanded criteria" for HCC in LT. Despite the limitations of this study, the information provided by this analysis of a large number of patients will help shape what will be the final new model of criteria for HCC in LT.

D. M. Harnois, DO

2-Year GLOBE Trial Results: Telbivudine Is Superior to Lamivudine in Patients With Chronic Hepatitis B

Liaw Y-F, The GLOBE Study Group (Chang Gung Univ College of Medicine, Taipei, Taiwan; et al)
Gastroenterology 136:486-495, 2009

Background & Aims.—The GLOBE trial has compared the efficacy and safety of telbivudine versus lamivudine treatment over 2 years in patients with chronic hepatitis B.

Methods.—Hepatitis B e antigen (HBeAg)-positive (n = 921) and HBeAg-negative (n = 446) patients received telbivudine or lamivudine once daily for 104 weeks. The primary outcome, assessed in the intent-to-treat population, was therapeutic response (hepatitis B virus DNA <5 $\log_{10}$ copies/mL and either HBeAg loss or normalization of alanine amino-transferase [ALT] level).

Results.—The therapeutic response to telbivudine was superior to that of lamivudine in HBeAg-positive (63% vs 48%; $P < .001$) and HBeAg-negative (78% vs 66%; $P = .007$) patients. HBeAg-positive patients given telbivudine also had better outcomes compared with lamivudine in terms of nondetectable viremia (<300 copies/mL) at 55.6% versus 38.5% ($P < .001$), HBeAg loss at 35.2% versus 29.2% ($P = .056$), and viral resistance at 25.1% versus 39.5% ($P < .001$). Hepatitis B e antigen seroconversion was 29.6% versus 24.7% ($P = .095$) in all patients and 36% versus 27% ($P = .022$) in patients with baseline ALT level ≥2 times normal. Telbivudine-treated HBeAg-negative patients showed higher rates of nondetectable viremia compared with lamivudine at 82.0% versus 56.7% ($P < .001$) and less resistance at 10.8% versus 25.9% ($P < .001$). Adverse events occurred with similar frequency, whereas grade 3/4 increases in creatine kinase levels were more common in patients given telbivudine (12.9% vs 4.1%, $P < .001$). Multivariate logistic regression analyses identified telbivudine treatment, among other variables, as an independent predictor of better week 104 outcomes.

Conclusions.—Telbivudine is superior to lamivudine in treating patients with chronic hepatitis B over a 2-year period.

▶ The incidence of acute hepatitis B (HBV) in the United States is declining according to most recent statistics from the Centers for Disease Control, noting an 80% decline from 1987 to 2004. This is largely related to the program of vaccination for HBV. Yet, estimates are that between 1.1 and 2.0 million individuals are chronically infected with HBV in the United States.

There are now 7 drugs available to treat HBV infection. This study, together with other studies, demonstrates that antiviral agents can reduce the morbidity and improve clinical outcomes in selected individuals with HBV infection as summarized at the recent National Institutes of Health (NIH) consensus conference on HBV.

This study reports the results of the 2-year GLOBE trial, demonstrating a significantly better response of telbivudine compared with lamivudine in 921 HBeAg-positive (63% vs 48%; $P < 0.001$) and 446 HBeAg-negative patients (78% vs 66%; $P = 0.007$). However, the frequency of telbivudine resistance in HBeAg positive patients also increased from 5% at 1 year to 25.1% at 2 years. There was also an associated increase in lamivudine resistance of 11% at 1 year and 39.5% at 2 years.

The GLOBE trial demonstrates the importance of ongoing measurement of HBV DNA to ensure drug resistance has not occurred. The trial clearly demonstrated the superiority of telbivudine over lamivudine in treating patients with HBV infection; however, the high resistance rate will likely limit its utility in the management of chronic HBV infection as other agents have been shown to have equal efficacy and less development of resistance.

D. M. Harnois, DO

National Institutes of Health Consensus Development Conference Statement: Management of Hepatitis B
Sorrell MF, Belongia EA, Costa J, et al (Univ of Nebraska Med Ctr, Omaha, NE; Marshfield Clinic Research Found, WI; Yale Univ School of Medicine, New Haven, CT; et al)
Ann Intern Med 150:104-110, 2009

Hepatitis B is a major cause of liver disease worldwide, ranking as a substantial cause of cirrhosis and hepatocellular carcinoma. The development and use of a vaccine for hepatitis B virus (HBV) has resulted in a substantial decline in the number of new cases of acute hepatitis B among children, adolescents, and adults in the United States. However, this success has not yet been duplicated worldwide, and both acute and chronic HBV infection continue to represent important global health problems.

Seven treatments are currently approved for adult patients with chronic HBV infection in the United States: interferon-α, pegylated interferon-α, lamivudine, adefovir dipivoxil, entecavir, telbivudine, and tenofovir disoproxil fumarate. Interferon-α and lamivudine have been approved for children with HBV infection. Although available randomized, controlled trials (RCTs) show encouraging short-term results—demonstrating the favorable effect of these agents on such intermediate markers of disease as HBV DNA level, liver enzyme tests, and liver histology—limited rigorous evidence exists demonstrating the effect of these therapies on important long-term clinical outcomes, such as the development of hepatocellular carcinoma or a reduction in deaths. Questions therefore remain about which groups of patients benefit from therapy and at which point in the course of disease this therapy should be initiated.

▶ The incidence of acute hepatitis B (HBV) in the United States is declining according to most recent statistics from the Center for Disease Control (an 80% decline from 1987 to 2004). This is largely related to the program of vaccination for HBV. Yet, estimates are that between 1.1 and 2.0 million individuals are chronically infected with HBV in the United States.

In October 2008, the National Institutes of Health (NIH) brought together the world's leading researchers and clinicians in the area of hepatitis B and developed a consensus statement on the current understanding of the hepatitis B virus and recommended guidelines for treatment and follow-up. These results were published in a supplement to *Hepatology* in May 2009. This article is the introduction and summary statement of the guidelines, though I strongly recommend readers review the entire supplement for a greater understanding of the current knowledge of HBV.

D. M. Harnois, DO

Nonhospital Health Care–Associated Hepatitis B and C Virus Transmission: United States, 1998–2008

Thompson ND, Perz JF, Moorman AC, et al (Ctrs for Disease Control and Prevention, Atlanta, GA)
Ann Intern Med 150:33-39, 2009

In the United States, transmission of hepatitis B virus (HBV) and hepatitis C virus (HCV) from health care exposures has been considered uncommon. However, a review of outbreak information revealed 33 outbreaks in nonhospital health care settings in the past decade: 12 in outpatient clinics, 6 in hemodialysis centers, and 15 in long-term care facilities, resulting in 448 persons acquiring HBV or HCV infection. In each setting, the putative mechanism of infection was patient-to-patient transmission through failure of health care personnel to adhere to fundamental principles of infection control and aseptic technique (for example, reuse of syringes or lancing devices).

Difficult to detect and investigate, these recognized outbreaks indicate a wider and growing problem as health care is increasingly provided in outpatient settings in which infection control training and oversight may be inadequate. A comprehensive approach involving better viral hepatitis surveillance and case investigation, health care provider education and training, professional oversight, licensing, and public awareness is needed to ensure that patients are always afforded basic levels of protection against viral hepatitis transmission.

▶ In the United States, transmission of viral hepatitis through health care exposure is considered rare. A majority of reported cases occur in acute care hospitals. Previously, the documentation of outbreaks in outpatient practices has not been well described. One recent example of an outpatient-related transmission of viral infection at a Nevada endoscopy unit resulted in the mandatory screening of 40 000 persons for possible exposure.

In this article from the *Annals of Internal Medicine*, Thompson and colleagues review 33 outbreaks of viral hepatitis B (HBV) and C (HCV) in nonhospital health care settings, which were documented by the Centers for Disease Control (CDC) between 1998 and 2008. A total of 448 persons were infected over this 10-year period through exposures in outpatient medical systems that included outpatient practices, hemodialysis units, and long-term care facilities. These numbers likely underestimate the actual number of patient exposures.

Patient-to-patient transmission in these cases was linked primarily to syringe reuse, lapses in contamination of injectable medications, or flush solutions. In several outbreaks, contamination from inappropriate use of single-use medication vials, eg, propofol, was the source of exposure. Anesthesia delivery was a common factor in 6 outbreaks. In the long-term care facilities, most of the 15 outbreaks involved patient-to-patient transmission of HBV infection through reuse of fingerstick devices (10 outbreaks) or blood glucose monitors (3 outbreaks).

These outbreaks emphasize the importance of developing and monitoring adherence to safety precautions intended to minimize the potential transmission of viral hepatitis.

D. M. Harnois, DO

Prolonged Therapy of Advanced Chronic Hepatitis C with Low-Dose Peginterferon

Di Bisceglie AM, HALT-C Trial Investigators (Saint Louis Univ School of Medicine; et al)
N Engl J Med 359:2429-2441, 2008

Background.—In patients with chronic hepatitis C who do not have a response to antiviral treatment, the disease may progress to cirrhosis, liver failure, hepatocellular carcinoma, and death. Whether long-term antiviral therapy can prevent progressive liver disease in such patients remains uncertain.

Methods.—We conducted a randomized, controlled trial of peginterferon alfa-2a at a dosage of 90 μg per week for 3.5 years, as compared with no treatment, in 1050 patients with chronic hepatitis C and advanced fibrosis who had not had a response to previous therapy with peginterferon and ribavirin. The patients, who were stratified according to stage of fibrosis (622 with noncirrhotic fibrosis and 428 with cirrhosis), were seen at 3-month intervals and underwent liver biopsy at 1.5 and 3.5 years after randomization. The primary end point was progression of liver disease, as indicated by death, hepatocellular carcinoma, hepatic decompensation, or, for those with bridging fibrosis at baseline, an increase in the Ishak fibrosis score of 2 or more points.

Results.—We randomly assigned the patients to receive peginterferon (517 patients) or no therapy (533 patients) for 3.5 years. The level of serum aminotransferases, the level of serum hepatitis C virus RNA, and histologic necroinflammatory scores all decreased significantly (P<0.001) with treatment, but there was no significant difference between the groups in the rate of any primary outcome (34.1% in the treatment group and 33.8% in the control group; hazard ratio, 1.01; 95% confidence interval, 0.81 to 1.27; P=0.90). The percentage of patients with at least one serious adverse event was 38.6% in the treatment group and 31.8% in the control group (P=0.07).

Conclusions.—Long-term therapy with peginterferon did not reduce the rate of disease progression in patients with chronic hepatitis C and advanced fibrosis, with or without cirrhosis, who had not had a response to initial treatment with peginterferon and ribavirin.

▶ The Hepatitis C Antiviral Long Term Treatment against Cirrhosis (HALT-C) study is a prospective, randomized study to determine whether maintenance therapy with low-dose pegylated interferon alpha in patients with chronic hepatitis C (HCV) who had failed to clear virus following a standard course of treatment would slow progression of disease. The primary end point of the study was progression of disease as determined by the development of complications of end-stage liver disease including hepatocellular cancer (HCC), liver failure, and the need for liver transplant or an increase in fibrosis score (Ishak fibrosis score increase of 2 or more points).

Patients were randomly selected to receive therapy with peginterferon alfa 2a for 3.5 years versus no treatment. The treatment group had improvement in serum aminotransferases, level of serum HCV RNA, and histology. However, there was no statistical difference in primary end points in the treated and untreated group. And so the conclusions of the trial are that long-term therapy with peginterferon did not reduce the rate of disease progression in patients with chronic HCV and advanced fibrosis in individuals who had not had an initial response to treatment with peginterferon and ribavirin.

The publication of the results of the HALT-C trial is the final chapter in the use of maintenance therapy as an effective approach in nonresponders with chronic HCV infection. The trial has left us a great deal of knowledge on HCV-related liver disease as yet to be fully understood and has led to the publication of a large number of articles in top-ranking medical journals.

D. M. Harnois, DO

Telaprevir and Peginterferon with or without Ribavirin for Chronic HCV Infection

Hézode C, for the PROVE2 Study Team (Univ of Paris, Créteil, France; et al)
N Engl J Med 360:1839-1850, 2009

Background.—In patients with chronic infection with hepatitis C virus (HCV) genotype 1, treatment with peginterferon alfa and ribavirin for 48 weeks results in rates of sustained virologic response of 40 to 50%. Telaprevir is a specific inhibitor of the HCV serine protease and could be of value in HCV treatment.

Methods.—A total of 334 patients who had chronic infection with HCV genotype 1 and had not been treated previously were randomly assigned to receive one of four treatments involving various combinations of telaprevir (1250 mg on day 1, then 750 mg every 8 hours), peginterferon alfa-2a (180 µg weekly), and ribavirin (dose according to body weight). The T12PR24 group (81 patients) received telaprevir, peginterferon alfa-2a, and ribavirin for 12 weeks, followed by peginterferon alfa-2a and ribavirin for 12 more weeks. The T12PR12 group (82 patients) received telaprevir, peginterferon alfa-2a, and ribavirin for 12 weeks. The T12P12 group (78 patients) received telaprevir and peginterferon alfa-2a without ribavirin for 12 weeks. The PR48 (control) group (82 patients) received peginterferon alfa-2a and ribavirin for 48 weeks. The primary end point, a sustained virologic response (an undetectable HCV RNA level 24 weeks after the end of therapy), was compared between the control group and the combined T12P12 and T12PR12 groups.

Results.—The rate of sustained virologic response for the T12PR12 and T12P12 groups combined was 48% (77 of 160 patients), as compared with 46% (38 of 82) in the PR48 (control) group (P = 0.89). The rate was 60% (49 of 82 patients) in the T12PR12 group (P = 0.12 for the comparison with the PR48 group), as compared with 36% (28 of 78 patients) in the T12P12 group (P = 0.003; P = 0.20 for the comparison with the PR48 group). The rate was significantly higher in the T12PR24 group (69% [56 of 81 patients]) than in the PR48 group (P = 0.004). The adverse events with increased frequency in the telaprevir-based groups were pruritus, rash, and anemia.

Conclusions.—In this phase 2 study of patients infected with HCV genotype 1 who had not been treated previously, one of the three telaprevir groups had a significantly higher rate of sustained virologic response than that with standard therapy. Response rates were lowest with the regimen that did not include ribavirin. (ClinicalTrials.gov number, NCT00372385.)

▶ Current standard treatment for chronic hepatic C virus (HCV) infection is pegylated interferon and ribavirin. The response rate varies according to HCV genotype. Among patients with genotype 2 or 3 the rates of sustained virologic response (SVR) were 70% to 80% and were achieved with a 24-week course of treatment (even with lower doses of ribavirin). In contrast, the response rate for patients infected with the genotype 1 virus was substantially lower (ranging from 40%-50%) and required longer duration of therapy (48 weeks) and higher doses of ribavirin.

In 10 years, the treatment of hepatitis C has changed very little. A greater understanding of the viral structure of HCV has now led to the development of targeted HCV therapy. One of these new drugs is telaprevir, a specific inhibitor of the HCV protease.

Telaprevir has profound effects in HCV replication in cell culture and animal models. If used alone, viral levels rebounded after the drug was discontinued and telaprevir resistance appeared. The combination of telaprevir and peginterferon provided greater viral suppression and less viral resistance.

D. M. Harnois, DO

Telaprevir with Peginterferon and Ribavirin for Chronic HCV Genotype 1 Infection

McHutchison JG, for the PROVE1 Study Team (Duke Clinical Res Inst and Duke Univ, Durham, NC; et al)
N Engl J Med 360:1827-1838, 2009

Background.—Current therapy for chronic hepatitis C virus (HCV) infection is effective in less than 50% of patients infected with HCV genotype 1. Telaprevir, a protease inhibitor specific to the HCV nonstructural 3/4A serine protease, rapidly reduced HCV RNA levels in early studies.

Methods.—We randomly assigned patients infected with HCV genotype 1 to one of three telaprevir groups or to the control group. The control group (called the PR48 group) received peginterferon alfa-2a (180 μg per week) and ribavirin (1000 or 1200 mg per day, according to body weight) for 48 weeks, plus telaprevir-matched placebo for the first 12 weeks (75 patients). The telaprevir groups received telaprevir (1250 mg on day 1 and 750 mg every 8 hours thereafter) for 12 weeks, as well as peginterferon alfa-2a and ribavirin (at the same doses as in the PR48 group) for the same 12 weeks (the T12PR12 group, 17 patients) or for a total of 24 weeks (the T12PR24 group, 79 patients) or 48 weeks (the T12PR48 group, 79 patients). The primary outcome was a sustained virologic response (an undetectable HCV RNA level 24 weeks after the end of therapy).

Results.—The rate of sustained virologic response was 41% (31 of 75 patients) in the PR48 group, as compared with 61% (48 of 79 patients) in the T12PR24 group (P = 0.02), 67% (53 of 79 patients) in the T12PR48 group (P = 0.002), and 35% (6 of 17 patients) in the T12PR12 group (this group was exploratory and not compared with the control group). Viral breakthrough occurred in 7% of patients receiving telaprevir. The rate of discontinuation because of adverse events was higher in the three telaprevir-based groups (21%, vs. 11% in the PR48 group), with rash the most common reason for discontinuation.

Conclusions.—Treatment with a telaprevir-based regimen significantly improved sustained virologic response rates in patients with genotype

1 HCV, albeit with higher rates of discontinuation because of adverse events. (ClinicalTrials.gov number, NCT00336479.)

▶ Current standard treatment for chronic hepatic C virus (HCV) infection is pegylated interferon and ribavirin. The response rate varies according to HCV genotype. Among patients with genotype 2 or 3 the rates of sustained virologic response (SVR) were 70% to 80% and were achieved with a 24-week course of treatment (even with lower doses of ribavirin). In contrast, the response rate for patients infected with the genotype 1 virus was substantially lower (ranging from 40%-50%) and required longer duration of therapy (48 weeks) and higher doses of ribavirin.

In 10 years, the treatment of hepatitis C has changed very little. A greater understanding of the viral structure of HCV has now led to the development of targeted HCV therapy. One of these new drugs is telaprevir, a specific inhibitor of the HCV protease.

Telaprevir has profound effects in HCV replication in cell culture and animal models. If used alone, viral levels rebounded after the drug was discontinued and telaprevir resistance appeared. The combination of telaprevir and peginterferon provided greater viral suppression and less viral resistance.

In the study by McHutchinson et al, patients infected with HCV genotype 1 were randomly assigned to 1 of 3 groups. The control group PR 48 received peginterferon alfa-2a and weight-based ribavirin for 48 weeks and a telaprevir placebo for the first 12 weeks. The telaprevir groups received telaprevir for 12 weeks as well as peginterferon alfa-2a, and ribavirin for 12 weeks (T12PR12), 24 weeks (T12PR24), and 48 weeks (T12PR48). The primary outcome was SVR (undetectable HCV RNA at 24 weeks after end of therapy).

The rate of SVR was 41% in the PR 48 control group, as compared with 61% in the T12PR24 (telaprevir for 12 weeks as well as peginterferon alfa-2a, and ribavirin for 24 weeks), and 67% in the T12PR48 group (telaprevir for 12 weeks as well as peginterferon alfa-2a, and ribavirin for 48 weeks). Viral breakthrough occurred in 7% of patients receiving telaprevir.

The adverse events were increased in the telaprevir group and included anemia, gastrointestinal side effects, pruritus, and a rash. The rash tended to be severe, to arise 8 weeks into treatment, and resulted in discontinuation of therapy in a number of patients.

These results suggest that the addition of telaprevir to peginterferon alfa-2a and ribavirin may improve the SVR in patients with chronic HCV genotype 1 infection. However, larger and longer studies are needed to look at both issues of safety and efficacy.

D. M. Harnois, DO

50 Miscellaneous

Community Subgroups in Dyspepsia and Their Association With Weight Loss

Jones MP, Talley NJ, Eslick GD, et al (Macquarie Univ, North Ryde, Australia; Mayo Clinic Jacksonville, FL; Univ of Sydney at Nepean Hosp, Penrith, Australia; et al)

Am J Gastroenterol 103:2051-2060, 2008

Objective.—A link between dyspepsia symptoms and weight loss is controversial. We aimed to determine whether or not weight loss is a marker of dyspepsia.

Methods.—Independent community-based cross-sectional studies. Subjects were randomly selected from the general population in Sydney, Australia. All subjects completed validated community health surveys. Two distinct data collections were used; the first as a training sample (N = 888) and the second as a validation sample to confirm the findings of the first (N = 2,907). The study was focused on weight loss, which was categorized as (a) any weight loss, (b) substantive weight loss (≥3 kg), and (c) weight loss expressed as percentage of body weight.

Results.—All dyspepsia symptoms studied were positively associated with weight loss although the strength of association did vary. Nausea and vomiting were most strongly associated with weight loss as were meal-related complaints such as postprandial fullness. Similarly, clusters formed based on symptoms were strongly differentiated in terms of weight loss with clusters characterized by nausea, vomiting, and early satiety/ postprandial fullness reporting 25–30% weight loss prevalence over the previous 3 months compared with around 10% prevalence in clusters characterized by low dyspepsia symptom burden. Weight loss ≥3 kg followed a similar pattern but with a prevalence approximately half that of any weight loss, while weight loss expressed as percentage of body weight followed the same pattern.

Conclusions.—Dyspepsia symptoms are clearly and, in some cases, strongly associated with weight loss, both any loss of weight and substantive weight loss. Weight loss should be considered a warning symptom of dyspepsia.

▶ The cardinal symptoms of dyspepsia include epigastric pain, epigastric discomfort, postprandial fullness, and early satiation (inability to finish a normal size meal). This study suggests that weight loss is an additional cardinal dyspeptic symptom. Weight loss has been observed to occur in patients with functional dyspepsia seen in tertiary referral patients, but this community study indicates that the association is not just due to referral bias. Weight loss may occur in dyspepsia because patients are unable to eat as much because eating induces major symptoms. In turn, their inability to finish a normal size meal may reflect the fact that their gastric fundus cannot appropriately relax (fundic disaccommodation). Dyspeptic patients with meal-related symptoms may be less likely to be obese based on these data.

N. J. Talley, MD, PhD

Components of placebo effect: randomised controlled trial in patients with irritable bowel syndrome
Kaptchuk TJ, Kelley JM, Conboy LA, et al (Harvard Med School, Boston, MA; Endicott College, Beverly, MA; et al)
BMJ 336:999-1003, 2008

Objective.—To investigate whether placebo effects can experimentally be separated into the response to three components—assessment and observation, a therapeutic ritual (placebo treatment), and a supportive patient-practitioner relationship—and then progressively combined to produce incremental clinical improvement in patients with irritable bowel syndrome. To assess the relative magnitude of these components.

Design.—A six week single blind three arm randomised controlled trial.

Setting.—Academic medical centre.

Participants.—262 adults (76% women), mean (SD) age 39 (14), diagnosed by Rome II criteria for and with a score of ≥150 on the symptom severity scale.

Interventions.—For three weeks either waiting list (observation), placebo acupuncture alone ("limited"), or placebo acupuncture with a patient-practitioner relationship augmented by warmth, attention, and confidence ("augmented"). At three weeks, half of the patients were randomly assigned to continue in their originally assigned group for an additional three weeks.

Main Outcome Measures.—Global improvement scale (range 1-7), adequate relief of symptoms, symptom severity score, and quality of life.

Results.—At three weeks, scores on the global improvement scale were 3.8 (SD 1.0) v 4.3 (SD 1.4) v 5.0 (SD 1.3) for waiting list versus "limited" versus "augmented," respectively (P<0.001 for trend). The proportion of patients reporting adequate relief showed a similar pattern: 28% on waiting list, 44% in limited group, and 62% in augmented group (P<0.001 for trend). The same trend in response existed in symptom severity score (30 (63) v 42 (67) v 82 (89), P<0.001) and quality of life (3.6 (8.1) v 4.1 (9.4) v 93 (14.0), P<0.001). All pairwise comparisons between augmented and limited patient-practitioner relationship were significant: global improvement scale (P<0.001), adequate relief of symptoms (P<0.001), symptom severity score (P=0.007), quality of life (P=0.01). Results were similar at six week follow-up.

Conclusion.—Factors contributing to the placebo effect can be progressively combined in a manner resembling a graded dose escalation of component parts. Non-specific effects can produce statistically and clinically significant outcomes and the patient-practitioner relationship is the most robust component.

Trial Registration.—Clinical Trials NCT00065403.

▶ Maximizing the therapeutic encounter in patients with irritable bowel syndrome (IBS) and other chronic gastrointestinal illnesses is relevant for the clinical practitioner, as this may help to obtain the best outcomes. The data from this novel, randomized controlled trial suggest that the placebo response can be augmented by very simple office techniques. The augmented interaction tested comprised asking questions about symptom relationships and lifestyle, assessing nongastrointestinal complaints, probing how the patient understood the causes and meaning of their condition, being warm and friendly in manner, listening actively, being empathetic, and communicating a positive expectation and confidence in the outcome. Exactly which of these components has the most effect remains unclear, but presumably a combination of them is required to obtain the best outcome. The patient-physician relationship has been known for a long time to be the centerpiece of the clinical encounter. This randomized trial confirms this belief in a scientific and robust fashion.

N. J. Talley, MD, PhD

Development of Functional Diarrhea, Constipation, Irritable Bowel Syndrome, and Dyspepsia During and After Traveling Outside the USA
Tuteja AK, Talley NJ, Gelman SS, et al (George E. Wahen V.A. Med Ctr, Salt Lake City, UT; Univ of Utah, Salt Lake City; Mayo Clinic College of Medicine, Rochester, MN)
Dig Dis Sci 53:271-276, 2008

Background.—Persistent gastrointestinal (GI) symptoms after travel abroad may be common. It remains unclear how often subjects who developed new GI symptoms while abroad have persistent symptoms on return. The objective of this retrospective study was to evaluate the prevalence of persistent GI symptoms in a healthy cohort of travelers.

Methods.—One hundred and eight consecutive patients, mostly returned missionaries, attending the University of Utah International Travel Clinic for any reason (but mostly GI symptoms) had data recorded about their bowel habits before, during, and after travel abroad. All subjects had standard hematological, biochemical, and microbiological tests to exclude known causes of their symptoms. Endoscopic procedures were performed when considered necessary by the treating physician. Diarrhea, constipation, irritable bowel syndrome (IBS), bloating, and dyspepsia were defined according to the Rome II Criteria.

Results.—Eighty three (82% men and 18% women, median age 21 years) completed the survey with 68 subjects completing the questionnaire about bowel habits before and during travel. Among the respondents, 55 (82.1%) did not have any symptoms before travel. During travel, 41 (63%) developed new onset diarrhea; 6 (9%) developed constipation; 16 (24%) IBS, 29 (45%) bloating; and 11 (16%) dyspepsia. Of those who developed symptoms during travel, 27 (68%) had persistent diarrhea, 3 (50%) had persistent constipation, 10 (63%) had persistent IBS, 12 (43%) had persistent bloating and 8 (73%) had persistent dyspepsia. The presence of bowel symptoms during and after travel was not associated with age, gender, travel destination, or duration of travel.

Conclusions.—This study suggests that new onset of diarrhea, IBS, constipation, and dyspepsia are common among subjects traveling abroad. Gastrointestinal symptoms that develop during travel abroad usually persist on return.

▶ Over 50 million people travel from the industrialized world to the developing world each year, and traveler's diarrhea is a known risk factor for the irritable bowel syndrome (IBS). The prevalence of transient or persistent other gastrointestinal problems after travel is less well documented. The study identified travel as a risk factor for the development of symptoms that were not limited to diarrhea. Bloating, dyspepsia, as well as IBS can be persistent and develop after travel abroad. The exact mechanisms that account for these associations, however, remain to be clarified. Colonic infection, low-grade inflammation, and the increased stress of travel may all be relevant. The retrospective nature of this study, the relatively small sample size, and the high proportion of men reduce the generalizability of the data.

N. J. Talley, MD, PhD

Effect and cost-effectiveness of step-up versus step-down treatment with antacids, H$_2$-receptor antagonists, and proton pump inhibitors in patients with new onset dyspepsia (DIAMOND study): a primary-care-based randomised controlled trial

van Marrewijk CJ, Mujakovic S, Fransen GAJ, et al (Radboud Univ Nijmegen Med Centre, Netherlands; Utrecht Univ Med Centre, Netherlands; Care and Public Health Res Inst (Caphri) Maastricht Univ, Netherlands)
Lancet 373:215-225, 2009

Background.—Substantial physician workload and high costs are associated with the treatment of dyspepsia in primary health care. Despite the availability of consensus statements and guidelines, the most cost-effective empirical strategy for initial management of the condition remains to be determined. We compared step-up and step-down treatment strategies for initial management of patients with new onset dyspepsia in primary care.

Methods.—Patients aged 18 years and older who consulted with their family doctor for new onset dyspepsia in the Netherlands were eligible for enrolment in this double-blind, randomised controlled trial. Between October, 2003, and January, 2006, 664 patients were randomly assigned to receive stepwise treatment with antacid, H₂-receptor antagonist, and proton pump inhibitor (step-up; n=341), or these drugs in the reverse order (step-down; n=323), by use of a computer-generated sequence with blocks of six. Each step lasted 4 weeks and treatment only continued with the next step if symptoms persisted or relapsed within 4 weeks. Primary outcomes were symptom relief and cost-effectiveness of initial management at 6 months. Analysis was by intention to treat (ITT); the ITT population consisted of all patients with data for the primary outcome at 6 months. This trial is registered with ClinicalTrials.gov, number NCT00247715.

Findings.—332 patients in the step-up, and 313 in the step-down group reached an endpoint with sufficient data for evaluation; the main reason for dropout was loss to follow-up. Treatment success after 6 months was achieved in 238 (72%) patients in the step-up group and 219 (70%) patients in the step-down group (odds ratio 0·92, 95% CI 0·7–1·3). The average medical costs were lower for patients in the step-up group than for those in the step-down group (€228 *vs* €245; p=0·0008), which was mainly because of costs of medication. One or more adverse drug events were reported by 94 (28%) patients in the step-up and 93 (29%) patients in the step-down group. All were minor events, including (other) dyspeptic symptoms, diarrhoea, constipation, and bad/dry taste.

Interpretation.—Although treatment success with either step-up or step-down treatment is similar, the step-up strategy is more cost effective at 6 months for initial treatment of patients with new onset dyspeptic symptoms in primary care.

▶ Guidelines around the world have varied in their recommendations for initial therapy in patients with new onset dyspepsia (defined as epigastric pain or discomfort). In the United States, empiric treatment with acid suppression typically with a proton pump inhibitor (PPI), or testing and treating for *Helicobacter pylori* are the currently recommended alternatives. In Europe, however, empiric treatment with antacids or H₂-receptor antagonists is still recommended for new onset dyspepsia in some places, reserving PPI therapy for those who continue to be symptomatic. There have been no previous trials of step-up versus step-down therapy in dyspepsia (step-up referring to treatment steps of 4 weeks duration, beginning with an antacid and then stepping up to H₂-receptor antagonist twice daily and finally a PPI once daily, versus starting with a PPI and then stepping down). This excellent randomized control trial did allow patients with heartburn into the study, and over two-thirds had reflux symptoms. Only about one-third were *H pylori* infected. There was a similar treatment success in each arm, with about 70% benefiting in the step-up and step-down groups. However, the step-up strategy was slightly more cost-effective, although this result is driven by the price of medication. This is the first study to focus on dyspepsia rather than reflux disease when comparing step-up with step-down therapy. Unfortunately, reflux disease confounded the results. Nevertheless, the data suggest that for the management of dyspepsia in primary care, starting with simple empiric therapy, including an over-the-counter medicine, is a reasonable option.

N. J Talley, MD, PhD

Helicobacter pylori test and treat versus proton pump inhibitor in initial management of dyspepsia in primary care: multicentre randomised controlled trial (MRC-CUBE trial)
Delaney BC, Qume M, Moayyedi P, et al (Univ of Birmingham; McMaster Univ, Hamilton, Ontario, Canada; et al)
BMJ 336:651-654, 2008

Objective.—To determine the cost effectiveness of *Helicobacter pylori* "test and treat" compared with empirical acid suppression in the initial management of patients with dyspepsia in primary care.

Design.—Randomised controlled trial.

Setting.—80 general practices in the United Kingdom.

Participants.—699 patients aged 18-65 who presented to their general practitioner with epigastric pain, heartburn, or both without "alarm symptoms" for malignancy.

Intervention.—*H pylori* [13]C urea breath test plus one week of eradication treatment if positive or proton pump inhibitor alone; subsequent management at general practitioner's discretion.

Main Outcome Measures.—Cost effectiveness in cost per quality adjusted life year (QALY) (EQ-5D) and effect on dyspeptic symptoms at one year measured with short form Leeds dyspepsia questionnaire.

Results.—343 patients were randomised to testing for *H pylori*, and 100 were positive. The successful eradication rate was 78%. 356 patients received proton pump inhibitor for 28 days. At 12 months no significant differences existed between the two groups in QALYs, costs, or dyspeptic symptoms. Minor reductions in costly resource use over the year in the test and treat group "paid back" the initial cost of the intervention.

Conclusions.—Test and treat and acid suppression are equally cost effective in the initial management of dyspepsia. Empirical acid suppression is an appropriate initial strategy. As costs are similar overall, general practitioners should discuss with patients at which point to consider *H pylori* testing.

Trial Registration.—Current Controlled Trials ISRCTN87644265.

▶ United States guidelines currently recommend either empiric proton pump inhibitor [PPI] therapy or *Helicobacter pylori* testing and treatment as the initial management of dyspepsia when there are no alarm features. Canadian data have suggested that *H pylori* test and treatment may be cost saving. This pragmatic, multicenter, primary care-based, randomized controlled trial assessed the cost-effectiveness of *H pylori* test and treatment versus empiric acid suppression. The study was particularly of high quality, and showed that testing and treating *H pylori* at the initial consultation provided similar outcomes to acid suppression therapy alone. Indeed, the costs were similar at 1 year for both strategies. Notably, those who were randomized to the *H pylori* test and treatment arm but were *H pylori* negative received the same treatment as those randomized to the empiric acid suppression treatment arm (omeprazole 20 mg once daily for 1 month). As only 29% of patients randomized to the test and treat arm were infected with *H pylori*, the results of this trial may not apply to regions where the prevalence of *H pylori* is higher. However, in relatively low *H pylori* prevalence regions, either strategy provides similar outcomes, and the choice depends on the clinician's judgment. This reviewer believes that *H pylori* test and treat makes the most sense, as those in the *H pylori*-positive arm who have successful eradication will also have the additional benefit of unrecognized peptic ulcer disease being eliminated.

N. J. Talley, MD, PhD

Heme Oxygenase-1 Protects Interstitial Cells of Cajal From Oxidative Stress and Reverses Diabetic Gastroparesis

Choi KM, Gibbons SJ, Nguyen TV, et al (Mayo Clinic, Rochester, MN)
Gastroenterology 135:2055-2064, 2008

Background & Aims.—Diabetic gastroparesis (delayed gastric emptying) is a well-recognized complication of diabetes that causes considerable morbidity and makes glucose control difficult. Interstitial cells of Cajal, which express the receptor tyrosine kinase Kit, are required for normal gastric emptying. We proposed that Kit expression is lost during diabetic gastroparesis due to increased levels of oxidative stress caused by low levels of heme oxygenase-1 (HO-1), an important cytoprotective molecule against oxidative injury.

Methods.—Gastric emptying was measured in nonobese diabetic mice and correlated with levels of HO-1 expression and activity. Endogenous HO-1 activity was increased by administration of hemin and inhibited by chromium mesoporphyrin.

Results.—In early stages of diabetes, HO-1 was up-regulated in gastric macrophages and remained up-regulated in all mice that were resistant to development of delayed gastric emptying. In contrast, HO-1 did not remain up-regulated in all the mice that developed delayed gastric emptying; expression of Kit and neuronal nitric oxide synthase decreased markedly in these mice. Loss of HO-1 up-regulation increased levels of reactive oxygen species. Induction of HO-1 by hemin decreased reactive oxygen species, rapidly restored Kit and neuronal nitric oxide synthase expression, and completely normalized gastric emptying in all mice. Inhibition of HO-1 activity in mice with normal gastric emptying caused a loss of Kit expression and development of diabetic gastroparesis.

Conclusions.—Induction of the HO-1 pathway prevents and reverses cellular changes that lead to development of gastrointestinal complications of diabetes. Reagents that induce this pathway might therefore be developed as therapeutics.

▶ New treatments for diabetic gastroparesis and other forms of gastroparesis are desperately needed, as current management options are remarkably limited. Indeed, prokinetics and antiemetics only treat the symptoms, not the pathogenesis. It is known that the enzyme heme oxygenase-1 provides a defense against oxidative stress. Using an animal model of type I diabetes (nonobese diabetic mice), the investigators assessed whether the development of delayed gastric emptying in diabetes mellitus could be reversed by giving hemin, which induces the enzyme heme oxygenase. They found that inhibition of heme oxygenase activity leads to the development of slow gastric emptying and loss of the gut pacemaker cells, the interstitial cells of Cajal. Introduction of heme oxygenase reversed gastroparesis, a remarkable observation. This is really important new data because if confirmed in humans, the results suggest that the drugs that induce the heme oxygenase pathway may reverse the loss of cells that cause slow gastric emptying and may even be able to normalize gastric emptying. Watch out for more on this topic in the future.

N. J. Talley, MD, PhD

High- *Versus* Low-Dose Proton Pump Inhibitors After Endoscopic Hemostasis in Patients With Peptic Ulcer Bleeding: A Multicentre, Randomized Study

Andriulli A, Loperfido S, Focareta R, et al (IRCCS, Rotondo, Italy; Regional Hosp, Treviso, Italy; " S. Sebastiano" Hosp, Caserta, Italy; et al)
Am J Gastroenterol 103:3011-3018, 2008

Background.—The most effective schedule of proton pump inhibitor (PPI) administration following endoscopic hemostasis of bleeding ulcers remains uncertain.

Methods.—Patients with actively bleeding ulcers and those with non-bleeding visible vessel or adherent clot were treated with epinephrine injection and/or thermal coagulation, and randomized to receive intravenous PPIs according to an intensive regimen (80 mg bolus followed by 8 mg/h as continuous infusion for 72 h) or a standard regimen (40 mg bolus daily followed by saline infusion for 72 h). After the infusion, all patients were given 20 mg PPI twice daily orally. The primary end point was the in-hospital rebleeding rate, as ascertained at the repeat endoscopy.

Results.—Bleeding recurred in 28 of 238 patients (11.8%) receiving the intensive regimen, and in 19 of 236 (8.1%) patients receiving the standard regimen ($P = 0.18$). Most rebleeding episodes occurred during the initial 72-h infusion: 18 (7.6%) and 19 events (8.1%) in the intensive and standard groups, respectively ($P = 0.32$). Mean units of blood transfused were

1.7 ± 2.1 in the intensive and 1.5 ± 2.1 in the standard regimen group ($P = 0.34$). The duration of hospital stay was <5 days for 88 (37.0%) and 111 patients (47.0%) in the intensive and standard groups ($P = 0.03$). There were fewer surgical interventions in the standard versus intensive regimen (1 vs 3). Five patients in each treatment group died.

Conclusions.—Following endoscopic hemostasis of bleeding ulcers, standard-dose PPIs infusion was as effective as a high-dose regimen in reducing the risk of recurrent bleeding.

▶ This is an important article that I would suggest all read. In those patients treated during endoscopy, the authors found no evidence that high-dose proton pump inhibitor (PPI) treatment reduced rebleeding, transfusion requirements, or need for surgery. The proposed mechanism of benefit of a high-dose regimen is to promote clot stability by sustaining the intragastic pH above 6. Clinical trials show that a high-dose PPI infusion is superior to placebo; however, this study and others now report no difference in risk reduction of high- versus low-dose PPI therapy. The strength of this study is that it was a multicenter, randomized, controlled trial of a large number of patients. Four previous studies have reported similar results. This study also has important cost-saving advantages that should be highlighted. This study also gives emphasis to the role of adequate endoscopic hemostasis, which may perhaps be more important than the PPI dose.

J. S. Scolapio, MD

Increased faecal serine protease activity in diarrhoeic IBS patients: a colonic lumenal factor impairing colonic permeability and sensitivity

Gecse K, Róka R, Ferrier L, et al (Neuro-Gastroenterology and Nutrition Unit, Toulouse, France; Univ of Szeged, Hungary)
Gut 57:591-598, 2008

Objectives.—Diarrhoea-predominant irritable bowel syndrome (IBS-D) is characterised by elevated colonic lumenal serine protease activity. The aims of this study were (1) to investigate the origin of this elevated serine protease activity, (2) to evaluate if it may be sufficient to trigger alterations in colonic paracellular permeability (CPP) and sensitivity, and (3) to examine the role of the proteinase-activated receptor-2 (PAR-2) activation and signalling cascade in this process.

Patients and Methods.—Faecal enzymatic activities were assayed in healthy subjects and patients with IBS, ulcerative colitis and acute infectious diarrhoea. Following mucosal exposure to supernatants from control subjects and IBS-D patients, electromyographic response to colorectal balloon distension was recorded in wild-type and PAR-2$^{-/-}$ mice, and CPP was evaluated on colonic strips in Ussing chambers. Zonula occludens-1 (ZO-1) and phosphorylated myosin light chain were detected by immunohistochemistry.

Results.—The threefold increase in faecal serine protease activity seen in IBS-D patients compared with constipation-predominant IBS (IBS-C) or infectious diarrhoea is of neither epithelial nor inflammatory cell origin, nor is it coupled with antiprotease activity of endogenous origin. Mucosal application of faecal supernatants from IBS-D patients in mice evoked allodynia and increased CPP by 92%, both of which effects were prevented by serine protease inhibitors and dependent on PAR-2 expression. In mice, colonic exposure to supernatants from IBS-D patients resulted in a rapid increase in the phosphorylation of myosin light chain and delayed redistribution of ZO-1 in colonocytes.

Conclusions.—Elevated colonic lumenal serine protease activity of IBS-D patients evokes a PAR-2-mediated colonic epithelial barrier dysfunction and subsequent allodynia in mice, suggesting a novel organic background in the pathogenesis of IBS.

▶ The search for biomarkers in IBS continues with great enthusiasm. In this landmark study, serine protease activity was identified to be significantly greater in the stool of patients with IBS and diarrhea by Rome II criteria, but was not increased in IBS with constipation or mixed IBS. Furthermore, the fecal supernatants of patients with IBS and diarrhea have levels of serine protease activity comparable with patients with ulcerative colitis. These serine proteases are signaling molecules that activate protease-activated receptors (PARs); PAR-2 is known to be expressed in intestinal epithelial cells and modulates motility and sensation. A further interesting twist here was that the fecal supernatants from IBS diarrhea patients changed visceral hypersensitivity in mice when the supernates were applied intra-colonically; these effects were blocked by using serine protease inhibitors dependent on PAR-2 expression. Other experiments have suggested that infusing the supernatants from IBS diarrhea patients can disrupt the epithelial type junctions and hence alter permeability. Where these serine proteases arise from is unclear, but colonic microbes may be to blame. This study is important because it provides evidence for a pathobiology in IBS with diarrhea. The observations also suggest that new approaches to therapy, including alterations of colonic microbia and direct inhibitors of fecal serine protease, may yield a benefit for diarrhea-type IBS in the future. IBS with diarrhea likely is an organic gut disease!

N. J. Talley, MD, PhD

Increased Prevalence and Mortality in Undiagnosed Celiac Disease
Rubio-Tapia A, Kyle RA, Kaplan EL, et al (Mayo Clinic, Rochester, MN; Univ of Minnesota Med School, Minneapolis; et al)
Gastroenterology 137:88-93, 2009

Background & Aims.—The historical prevalence and long-term outcome of undiagnosed celiac disease (CD) are unknown. We investigated the long-term outcome of undiagnosed CD and whether the prevalence of undiagnosed CD has changed during the past 50 years.

Methods.—This study included 9133 healthy young adults at Warren Air Force Base (sera were collected between 1948 and 1954) and 12,768 gender-matched subjects from 2 recent cohorts from Olmsted County, Minnesota, with either similar years of birth ($n = 5558$) or age at sampling ($n = 7210$) to that of the Air Force cohort. Sera were tested for tissue transglutaminase and, if abnormal, for endomysial antibodies. Survival was measured during a follow-up period of 45 years in the Air Force cohort. The prevalence of undiagnosed CD between the Air Force cohort and recent cohorts was compared.

Results.—Of 9133 persons from the Air Force cohort, 14 (0.2%) had undiagnosed CD. In this cohort, during 45 years of follow-up, all-cause mortality was greater in persons with undiagnosed CD than among those who were seronegative (hazard ratio = 3.9; 95% confidence interval, 2.0–7.5; $P < .001$). Undiagnosed CD was found in 68 (0.9%) persons with similar age at sampling and 46 (0.8%) persons with similar years of birth. The rate of undiagnosed CD was 4.5-fold and 4-fold greater in the recent cohorts, respectively, than in the Air Force cohort (both $P \leq .0001$).

Conclusions.—During 45 years of follow-up, undiagnosed CD was associated with a nearly 4-fold increased risk of death. The prevalence of undiagnosed CD seems to have increased dramatically in the United States during the past 50 years.

▶ This is an excellent article on celiac disease (CD) and one of the few that has this length of follow-up (ie, 45 years). The 2 most important messages from this article are that the prevalence of CD has increased significantly over the past 50 years and that undiagnosed CD is associated with increased mortality. The most likely reason for the increased prevalence of CD is environmental changes (ie, change in the quantity, quality, and processing of cereals). The potential role of highly processed nutrients as modifiers of gene expression may alter the risk for development of CD in genetically susceptible individuals. Limitations of this study include the lack of diagnostic confirmation of CD by intestinal biopsy. I would also caution the readers regarding the conclusion that mortality is 4 times higher in untreated CD. These conclusions are based on limited number of cases, and smoking habits are not known and therefore not reported.

J. S. Scolapio, MD

Intravenous Esomeprazole for Prevention of Recurrent Peptic Ulcer Bleeding

Sung JJY, for the Peptic Ulcer Bleed Study Group (Chinese Univ of Hong Kong, China; et al)
Ann Intern Med 150:455-464, 2009

Background.—Use of proton-pump inhibitors in the management of peptic ulcer bleeding is controversial because discrepant results have been reported in different ethnic groups.

Objective.—To determine whether intravenous esomeprazole prevents recurrent peptic ulcer bleeding better than placebo in a multiethnic patient sample.

Design.—Randomized trial conducted between October 2005 and December 2007; patients, providers, and researchers were blinded to group assignment.

Setting.—91 hospital emergency departments in 16 countries.

Patients.—Patients 18 years or older with peptic ulcer bleeding from a single gastric or duodenal ulcer showing high-risk stigmata.

Intervention.—Intravenous esomeprazole bolus, 80 mg, followed by 8-mg/h infusion, over 72 hours or matching placebo, each given after successful endoscopic hemostasis. Intervention was allocated by computer-generated randomization. After infusion, both groups received oral esomeprazole, 40 mg/d, for 27 days.

Measurements.—The primary end point was rate of clinically significant recurrent bleeding within 72 hours. Recurrent bleeding within 7 and 30 days, death, surgery, endoscopic re-treatment, blood transfusions, hospitalization, and safety were also assessed.

Results.—Of 767 patients randomly assigned, 764 provided data for an intention-to-treat analysis (375 esomeprazole recipients and 389 placebo recipients). Fewer patients receiving intravenous esomeprazole (22 of 375) had recurrent bleeding within 72 hours than those receiving placebo (40 of 389) (5.9% vs. 10.3%; difference, 4.4 percentage points [95% CI, 0.6% to 8.3%]; $P = 0.026$). The difference in bleeding recurrence remained significant at 7 days and 30 days ($P = 0.010$). Esomeprazole also reduced endoscopic retreatment (6.4% vs. 11.6%; difference, 5.2 percentage points [95% CI of difference, 1.1 percentage points to 9.2 percentage points]; $P = 0.012$), surgery (2.7% vs. 5.4%), and all-cause mortality rates (0.8% vs. 2.1%) more than placebo, although differences for the latter 2 comparisons were not significant. About 10% and 40% of patients in both groups reported serious and nonserious adverse events, respectively.

Limitation.—Endoscopic therapy was not completely standardized; some patients received epinephrine injection, thermal coagulation, or hemoclips alone, whereas others received combination therapy, but there were similar proportions with single therapy in each group.

Conclusion.—High-dose intravenous esomeprazole given after successful endoscopic therapy to patients with high-risk peptic ulcer bleeding reduced recurrent bleeding at 72 hours and had sustained clinical benefits for up to 30 days.

▶ This is a must read article that has very important clinical application. This is the first international trial to provide strong evidence supporting the use of high-dose IV esomeprazole as adjuvant therapy to endoscopic therapy for patients with high-risk GI bleeding. The strength of this article, besides its clinical importance, is its robust experimental design. These authors also do a very good job of describing the shortcomings of previous studies. It is important to note that despite a consistent reduction in recurrent bleeding and improvement in many secondary outcomes with intravenous esomeprazole, the study did not demonstrate statistically significant differences in deaths or requirements for surgery (just short of statistical difference). This may be because the study was not powered to detect differences in mortality rates. Infusion site reactions (phlebitis) were the only reported complication of the esomeprazole infusion.

J. S. Scolapio, MD

Irritable Bowel Syndrome: A 10-Yr Natural History of Symptoms and Factors That Influence Consultation Behavior

Ford AC, Forman D, Bailey AG, et al (Leeds General Infirmary, UK; Leeds Univ, UK; et al)
Am J Gastroenterol 103:1229-1239, 2008

Objective.—Irritable bowel syndrome (IBS) is a chronic functional gastrointestinal disorder. The natural history of the condition has been studied extensively, but few studies have examined factors that predict its new onset or health care-seeking behavior.

Methods.—Individuals, now aged 50–59 yr, originally enrolled in a population-screening program for *Helicobacter pylori* (*H. pylori*) were contacted via postal questionnaire, utilizing the Manning criteria for IBS diagnosis. Baseline demographic data, quality of life, and IBS and dyspepsia symptom data were already on file. Consent to examine primary care records was sought, and data regarding IBS- and dyspepsia-related consultations were extracted.

Results.—Of 8,407 individuals originally involved, 3,873 (46%) provided symptom data at baseline and 10-yr follow-up. Of 3,659 individuals without IBS at baseline, 542 (15%) developed new-onset IBS at 10-yr follow-up. After multivariate logistic regression, lower quality of life at baseline (odds ratio [OR] 4.41, 99% confidence interval [CI] 2.92–6.65), dyspepsia at baseline (OR 1.77, 99% CI 1.28–2.46), and female gender (OR 2.14, 99% CI 1.56–2.94) were significant risk factors for new-onset IBS. Of 651 individuals with IBS at either baseline or 10-yr follow-up, 113 (17%) consulted a primary care physician with symptoms. *H. pylori* infection (OR 1.93, 99% CI 1.03–3.62) and any dyspepsia-related consultation (OR 2.14, 99% CI 1.15–4.00) significantly increased the likelihood of consultation.

Conclusions.—Poor quality of life at baseline was a strong predictor of new-onset IBS, but not of IBS-related consultation behavior, which was associated with consultation for dyspepsia during the study period.

▶ It is well known that IBS relapses and remits, but many do not seek medical care. Therefore, understanding the natural history of IBS requires population-based studies. Remarkably, little is known about risk factors for the onset of new IBS. In this 10-year follow-up study of a large British population, the authors observed that a lower quality of life at study entry and the presence of dyspepsia were both significant risk factors for the new onset of IBS symptoms (two-thirds of those with IBS had persistent symptoms at the 10-year follow-up).

An association between impaired quality of life and IBS has been well described in cross-sectional studies, and it has been assumed that IBS causes impaired quality of life. This study suggests that to the contrary, a low quality of life for whatever reason may lead to the development of IBS. Whether the application of interventions to improve quality of life will reduce the incidence of IBS is unknown.

N. J. Talley, MD, PhD

Long-term budesonide treatment of collagenous colitis: a randomised, double-blind, placebo-controlled trial

Bonderup OK, Hansen JB, Teglbjærg PS, et al (Randers Regional Hosp, Denmark; Aalborg Hosp, Denmark; et al)
Gut 58:68-72, 2009

Objective.—To evaluate the efficacy and safety of longterm budesonide therapy for the maintenance of clinical remission in patients with collagenous colitis.

Design.—Randomised, placebo-controlled study with a 24-week, blinded follow-up period without any treatment.

Setting.—Three gastroenterology clinics in Denmark.

Patients.—Forty-two patients with histologically confirmed collagenous colitis and diarrhoea (more than three stools/day).

Interventions.—Patients in clinical remission after 6 weeks' open-label therapy with oral budesonide (Entocort CIR capsules, 9 mg/day) received 24 weeks' double-blind maintenance therapy with budesonide 6 mg/day or placebo. Thereafter, patients entered the 24-week, blinded follow-up period.

Main Outcome Measure.—The proportion of patients in clinical remission (three or fewer stools/day) at the end of maintenance therapy.

Findings.—A total of 34 patients in remission at week 6 were randomly assigned to budesonide 6 mg/day (n = 17) or placebo (n = 17). After 24

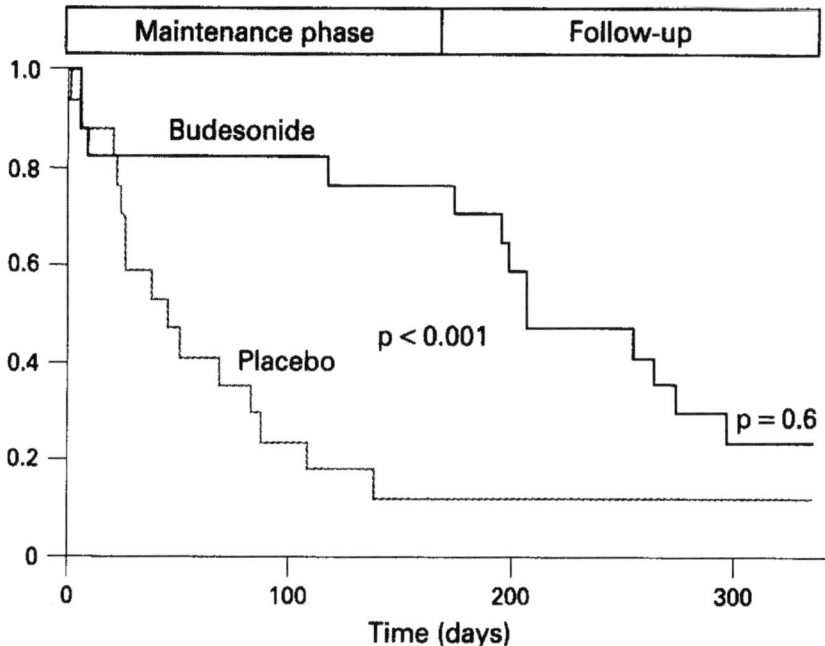

FIGURE 3.—Kaplan–Meier curves of relapse-free survival during maintenance and follow-up (untreated); p value correspond to the between-group difference at the end of maintenance and follow-up, respectively. (Courtesy of Bonderup OK, Hansen JB, Teglbjærg PS, et al. Long-term budesonide treatment of collagenous colitis: a randomised, double-blind, placebo-controlled trial. *Gut.* 2009;58:68-72.)

weeks' maintenance treatment, the proportions of patients in clinical remission were 76.5% (13 of 17) with budesonide and 12% (2 of 17) with placebo (p<0.001). At 48 weeks (the end of the follow-up period, without any treatment) these values were 23.5% (4 of 17) and 12% (2 of 17), respectively (p = 0.6). The median times to relapse after stopping active treatment (6 plus 24 weeks in the budesonide group; 6 weeks in the placebo group) were 39 and 38 days, respectively. Long-term treatment with budesonide was well tolerated.

Conclusions.—Long-term maintenance therapy with oral budesonide is efficacious and well tolerated for preventing relapse in patients with collagenous colitis. The risk of relapse after 24 weeks' maintenance treatment is similar to that observed after 6 weeks' induction therapy.

▶ This is an excellent article from Denmark that reports the results of budesonide treatment for collagenous colitis. There remains a high risk of clinical relapse after stopping maintenance therapy with budesonide. This study would support that the risk of relapse after 24 weeks of treatment is much improved compared with placebo (Fig 3). What I would like to highlight from this study is that budesonide was well tolerated and that most side effects were tolerated and transient. There were no serious side effects reported. Leg cramps were the most common reported side effect (4 reports) of the medication. There were 2 reports of worsening diabetes in the budesonide group as well. This study, however, fails to state if patients were also taking an antidiarrheal agent during the maintenance phase of the study.

J. S. Scolapio, MD

Methylnaltrexone for Opioid-Induced Constipation in Advanced Illness
Thomas J, Karver S, Cooney GA, et al (San Diego Hospice and the Inst for Palliative Medicine, CA; Gulfside Regional Hospice, New Port Richey, FL; Hospice of Palm Beach County, West Palm Beach, FL; et al)
N Engl J Med 358:2332-2343, 2008

Background.—Constipation is a distressing side effect of opioid treatment. As a quaternary amine, methylnaltrexone, a μ-opioid–receptor antagonist, has restricted ability to cross the blood–brain barrier. We investigated the safety and efficacy of subcutaneous methylnaltrexone for treating opioid-induced constipation in patients with advanced illness.

Methods.—A total of 133 patients who had received opioids for 2 or more weeks and who had received stable doses of opioids and laxatives for 3 or more days without relief of opioid-induced constipation were randomly assigned to receive subcutaneous methylnaltrexone (at a dose of 0.15 mg per kilogram of body weight) or placebo every other day for 2 weeks. Coprimary outcomes were laxation (defecation) within 4 hours after the first dose of the study drug and laxation within 4 hours after two or more of the first four doses. Patients who completed this phase were eligible to enter a 3-month, open-label extension trial.

Results.—In the methylnaltrexone group, 48% of patients had laxation within 4 hours after the first study dose, as compared with 15% in the placebo group, and 52% had laxation without the use of a rescue laxative within 4 hours after two or more of the first four doses, as compared with 8% in the placebo group (P<0.001 for both comparisons). The response rate remained consistent throughout the extension trial. The median time to laxation was significantly shorter in the methylnaltrexone group than in the placebo group. Evidence of withdrawal mediated by central nervous system opioid receptors or changes in pain scores was not observed. Abdominal pain and flatulence were the most common adverse events.

Conclusions.—Subcutaneous methylnaltrexone rapidly induced laxation in patients with advanced illness and opioid-induced constipation. Treatment did not appear to affect central analgesia or precipitate opioid withdrawal. (Clinical Trials.gov number, NCT00402038.)

▶ Treatment of severe constipation in hospital or in advanced illness can be challenging. In patients with cancer who need opiates, blockade of only peripheral opioid receptors theoretically should relieve constipation without loss of analgesia. Methylnaltrexone crosses the blood-brain barrier in a restricted amount and therefore was tested in opioid-induced constipation. In this well-conducted, randomized, placebo-controlled trial, those who failed standard laxative therapy did benefit from methylnaltrexone given subcutaneously at a dose of 0.15 mg per kg on alternate days for 2 weeks. The patients enrolled in the study were receiving a median opioid dose of about 100 mg of oral morphine equivalent. In the patients who received methylnaltrexone, the response was rapid although about half of the patients did not respond to the first dose. Notably, opioid withdrawal was not an issue. Based on these data, the management of opioid-induced constipation can be considered in a stepwise fashion. It is still reasonable to try and prevent the onset of constipation with the use of simple stimulant laxatives in patients newly receiving opiates. In those who develop constipation, after obstruction and impaction has been ruled out, use of an osmotic laxative, such as polyethylene glycol, is a reasonable first-line step. Patients who are refractory may next be offered methylnaltrexone.

N. J. Talley, MD, PhD

Multicenter, 4-Week, Double-Blind, Randomized, Placebo-Controlled Trial of Lubiprostone, a Locally-Acting Type-2 Chloride Channel Activator, in Patients With Chronic Constipation

Johanson JF, Morton D, Geenen J, et al (Univ of Illinois College of Medicine, Rockford; GANT Res, Ft Worth, TX; Gastroenterology Consultants, Ltd, Milwaukee, WI; et al)
Am J Gastroenterol 103:170-177, 2008

Objectives.—To assess the efficacy and safety of lubiprostone in adults with chronic constipation.

Methods.—This multicenter, parallel-group, double-blind controlled trial enrolled 242 patients with constipation and randomized them to receive oral lubiprostone 24 mcg or placebo twice daily for 4 wk. The primary efficacy end point was the number of spontaneous bowel movements (SBMs; those occurring without use of constipation relieving medications) after 1 wk of double-blind treatment. Other evaluations included SBMs at weeks 2, 3, and 4; bowel movement (BM) characteristics (*i.e.*, consistency and straining); constipation severity; abdominal bloating/discomfort; global treatment effectiveness ratings; and safety assessments.

Results.—The 120 lubiprostone-treated patients reported a greater mean number of SBMs at week 1 compared with the 122 placebo-treated patients (5.69 *vs* 3.46, $P = 0.0001$), with a greater frequency of SBMs also reported at weeks 2, 3, and 4 ($P \leq 0.002$). Within 24 h of the first dose of study drug, 56.7% of those given lubiprostone reported a SBM compared with 36.9% of those given placebo ($P = 0.0024$); within 48 h, 80% and 60.7% of these patients reported a SBM ($P = 0.0013$), respectively. Stool consistency, straining, and constipation severity, as well as patient-reported assessments of treatment effectiveness, were significantly improved with lubiprostone compared with placebo at all weeks

($P \leq 0.0003$). The two most common treatment-related adverse events were nausea (31.7%) and headache (11.7%).

Conclusions.—In patients with chronic constipation, treatment with lubiprostone produces a BM in the majority of individuals within 24–48 h of initial dosing and improves the frequency as well as other characteristics associated with BMs with short-term (*i.e.*, 4 wk) treatment. The most commonly reported adverse event was mild to moderate nausea, which resulted in treatment discontinuation in 5% of treated patients.

▶ Lubiprostone is a new type of drug for the treatment of chronic constipation. It acts locally in the small intestine opening the chloride channels and leading to fluid secretion. Data from this randomized controlled trial indicate that lubiprostone is efficacious in chronic constipation. Just over half the patients who received lubiprostone had a spontaneous bowel movement within 1 day. Nausea was a significant side effect in about 30% of those receiving lubiprostone, although this may be somewhat ameliorated by giving the drug with meals. The pathogenesis of the nausea is unknown, although it may reflect an interaction with taste receptors. The fact that lubiprostone acts locally rather than systemically suggests that the drug otherwise is likely to be safe.

N. J. Talley, MD, PhD

Randomized clinical trial of botulinum toxin injection for pain relief in patients with thrombosed external haemorrhoids

Patti R, Arcara M, Bonventre S, et al (Univ of Palermo, Italy)
Br J Surg 95:1339-1343, 2008

Background.—Thrombosed external haemorrhoids are one of the most frequent anorectal emergencies. They are associated with swelling and intense pain. Internal sphincter hypertonicity plays a role in the aetiology of the pain. This study evaluated the efficacy and safety of an intrasphincteric injection of botulinum toxin for pain relief in patients with thrombosed external haemorrhoids.

Methods.—Thirty patients with thrombosed external haemorrhoids who refused surgical operation were randomized into two groups. Patients received an intrasphincteric injection of either $0 \cdot 6$ ml saline or $0 \cdot 6$ ml of a solution containing 30 units botulinum toxin. Anorectal manometry was performed before treatment and 5 days afterwards.

Results.—After 5 days of treatment, the maximum resting pressure fell in both groups, but was significantly lower in the botulinum toxin group ($P = 0 \cdot 004$). Pain intensity was significantly reduced within 24 h of botulinum toxin treatment ($P < 0 \cdot 001$), but only after 1 week in the placebo group ($P = 0 \cdot 019$).

Conclusion.—A single injection of botulinum toxin into the anal sphincter seems to be effective in rapidly controlling the pain associated with thrombosed external haemorrhoids, and could represent an effective conservative treatment for this condition. Registration number: NCT00717782 (http://www.clinicaltrials.gov).

▶ Thrombosed external hemorrhoids are a common cause of severe perianal pain. The intensity of the pain is often determined by the size and extent of the thrombosis and the time from the inciting event. A constant finding is the marked severity of pain at the outset. Treatment for the condition varies from ice packs to emergent excision in either an emergency department or an operating room.

Patti and colleagues from the University of Palermo performed a randomized trial to examine the effect of intrasphincteric botulinum toxin injection in patients with thrombosed external hemorrhoids. They noted rapid control of pain when the toxin was injected when compared with saline controls.

Strengths of this study include its prospective design and inclusion of appropriate controls (saline injected). Additionally, pain control was carefully monitored. An important finding was a significant reduction in the time to return to work in the botulinum toxin group. Surprisingly, anal manometry was tolerated before treatment. In my experience, many of these patients would refuse this evaluation due to the severity of pain.

Study weaknesses include the lack of information concerning the time from onset of symptoms until injection treatment. Additionally, direct injection into the internal sphincter can be somewhat challenging in the office, and it is occasionally difficult to be certain if the toxin is inserted directly into the sphincter rather than extrasphincteric tissue. Finally, there was no significant difference in clot resorption between the 2 groups.

In summary, the injection of botulinum toxin appears to be effective in reducing pain in patients with thrombosed external hemorrhoids. Other institutions are encouraged to perform similar trials in larger numbers of patients with the hope of replicating these excellent results.

J. L. Rombeau, MD

The effect of a low-fat, high-protein or high-carbohydrate *ad libitum* diet on weight loss maintenance and metabolic risk factors

Claessens M, Van Baak MA, Monsheimer S, et al (Maastricht Univ, The Netherlands)
Int J Obes 33:296-304, 2009

Background.—High-protein (HP) diets are often advocated for weight reduction and weight loss maintenance.

Objective.—The aim was to compare the effect of low-fat, high-carbohydrate (HC) and low-fat, HP *ad libitum* diets on weight maintenance after weight loss induced by a very low-calorie diet, and on metabolic and cardiovascular risk factors in healthy obese subjects.

Design.—Forty-eight subjects completed the study that consisted of an energy restriction period of 5–6 weeks followed by a weight maintenance period of 12 weeks. During weight maintenance subjects received malto-dextrin (HC group) or protein (HP group) (casein (HPC subgroup) or whey (HPW subgroup)) supplements (2×25 g per day), respectively and consumed a low-fat diet.

Results.—Subjects in the HP diet group showed significantly better weight maintenance after weight loss (2.3 kg difference, $P = 0.04$) and fat mass reduction (2.2 kg difference, $P = 0.02$) than subjects in the HC group. Triglyceride (0.6 mM difference, $P = 0.01$) and glucagon (9.6 pg ml^{-1} difference, $P = 0.02$) concentrations increased more in the HC diet group, while glucose (0.3 mM difference, $P = 0.02$) concentration increased more in the HP diet group. Changes in total cholesterol, low-density lipoprotein-cholesterol, high-density lipoprotein-cholesterol, insulin, HOMAir index, HbA1c, leptin and adiponectin concentrations did not differ between the diets. No differences were found between the casein- or whey-supplemented HP groups.

Conclusions.—These results show that low-fat, high-casein or whey protein weight maintenance diets are more effective for weight control than low-fat, HC diets and do not adversely affect metabolic and cardio-vascular risk factors in weight-reduced moderately obese subjects without metabolic or cardiovascular complications.

▶ Many "fad" diets have been suggested for weight loss over the years. Despite initial weight loss, many patients eventually fail these diets at the 1-year mark usually as a result of noncompliance with the diet. Only surgical treatment (lap banding or gastric bypass) has shown sustained weight loss beyond a year. In the current articles the authors compare a low-fat, high-carbohydrate diet to a low-fat, high-protein *ad libitum* diet on "weight maintenance" after weight loss induced by a very low calorie diet. The results of this study, like most other diet studies, is flawed by the number of patients studied (too few) and length of time to follow-up (not long enough). This study is limited by its short follow-up period of only 12 weeks. I do not believe this study offers much practical application to the care of our obese patients. Behavior modification, ie, total caloric intake reduction coupled with increased physical activity, will ultimately determine weight loss and weight maintenance. In select patients with BMI's greater than 40, lap banding or gastric bypass appear to have results superior to diet alone. As gastroenterologists, we will be caring for more individuals that have had these surgical procedures and should be knowledgeable of the complications associated with each.

J. S. Scolapio, MD

The effect of metabolic risk factors on the natural course of gastro-oesophageal reflux disease
Lee Y-C, Yen AM-F, Tai JJ, et al (Natl Taiwan Univ, Taipei; et al)
Gut 58:174-181, 2009

Background and Aims.—The effect of metabolic risk factors on the natural course of gastro-oesophageal reflux disease (GORD), which remains elusive, was quantified.

Methods.—The population included 3669 subjects undergoing repeated upper endoscopy. Data were analysed using a three-state Markov model to estimate transition rates (according to the Los Angeles classification) regarding the natural course of the disease. Individual risk score together with the kinetic curve was derived by identifying significant factors responsible for the net force between progression and regression.

Results.—During three consecutive study periods, 12.2, 14.9 and 17.9% of subjects, respectively, progressed from non-erosive to erosive disease, whereas 42.5, 37.3 and 34.6%, respectively, regressed to the non-erosive stage. The annual transition rate from non-erosive to class A–B disease was 0.151 per person year (95% CI 0.136 to 0.165) and from class A–B to C–D was 0.079 per person year (95% CI 0.063 to 0.094). The regression rate from class A–B to non-erosive disease was 0.481 per person year (95% CI 0.425 to 0.536). Class C–D, however, appeared to be an absorbing state when not properly treated. Being male (relative risk (RR) 4.31; 95% CI 3.22 to 5.75), smoking (RR 1.20; 95% CI 1.03 to 1.39) or having metabolic syndrome (RR 1.75; 95% CI 1.29 to 2.38) independently increased the likelihood of progressing from a non-erosive to an erosive stage of disease and/or lowered the likelihood of disease regression. The short-term use of acid suppressants (RR 0.54; 95% CI 0.39 to 0.75) raised the likelihood of regression from erosive to non-erosive disease.

Conclusions.—Intraoesophageal damage is a dynamic and migratory process in which the metabolic syndrome is associated with accelerated progression to or attenuated regression from erosive states. These findings have important implications for the design of effective prevention and screening strategies.

▶ Nonerosive reflux disease is considered by some authorities to be a distinct disease entity from reflux oesophagitis. Little is known about the rate of progression from nonerosive disease to reflux oesophagitis, and the risk factors for such progression are not well documented. This important study from Taiwan evaluated 3669 patients who had 2 upper endoscopy examinations as part of health screening in otherwise healthy people. Over the study period, the observed rate of transition from nonerosive reflux disease to reflux oesophagitis ranged from 12% to 18%. Male sex, smoking, and the metabolic syndrome were independent risk factors for progression of reflux disease. These data suggest that nonerosive reflux disease and reflux oesophagitis are part of the same continuum, and there may be reversible risk factors for progression. The link of gastro-esophageal reflux disease (GERD) progression to metabolic syndrome is particularly interesting, and may not all be explained by obesity. The role of genetics and environment, and the inter-relationships with metabolic syndrome in GERD deserves serious attention.

N. J. Talley, MD, PhD

Yield of Diagnostic Tests for Celiac Disease in Individuals With Symptoms Suggestive of Irritable Bowel Syndrome: Systematic Review and Meta-analysis

Ford AC, Chey WD, Talley NJ, et al (McMaster Univ, Ontario, Canada; Univ of Michigan Med Ctr, Ann Arbor; Mayo Clinic Florida, Jacksonville; et al)
Arch Intern Med 169:651-658, 2009

Background.—Individuals with irritable bowel syndrome (IBS) report abdominal pain, bloating, and diarrhea, symptoms similar to those in celiac disease. Studies suggest that the prevalence of celiac disease is increased in individuals with IBS; however, evidence is conflicting, and current guidelines do not always recommend screening for celiac disease in these individuals.

Methods.—We conducted a systematic review and meta-analysis to estimate prevalence of celiac disease in unselected adults who met diagnostic criteria for IBS. MEDLINE (1950 to May 31, 2008) and EMBASE (1980 to May 31, 2008) were searched. Case series and case-control studies that used serologic tests for celiac disease were eligible for inclusion. Prevalence of positive serologic indications of celiac disease and biopsy-proved celiac disease were extracted and pooled for all studies and were compared between cases and controls using an odds ratio and 95% confidence interval.

Results.—Fourteen studies were identified comprising 4204 individuals, of whom 2278 (54%) met diagnostic criteria for IBS. Pooled prevalence of positive IgA-class antigliadin antibodies, either positive endomysial antibodies or tissue transglutaminase, and biopsy-proved celiac disease were 4.0% (95% confidence interval, 1.7-7.2), 1.63% (0.7-3.0), and 4.1% (1.9-7.0), respectively. Pooled odds ratios (95% confidence intervals) for positive IgA-class antigliadin antibodies, either positive endomysial antibodies or tissue transglutaminase, and biopsy-proved celiac disease in cases meeting diagnostic criteria for IBS compared with controls without IBS were 3.40 (1.62-7.13), 2.94 (1.36-6.35), and 4.34 (1.78-10.6).

Conclusion.—Prevalence of biopsy-proved celiac disease in cases meeting diagnostic criteria for IBS was more than 4-fold that in controls without IBS.

▶ This is an excellent systematic review that all GI physicians should read. We all have seen patients in our GI clinics complaining of abdominal pain, bloating, and diarrhea. I think we are often quick to label these patients as having irritable bowel syndrome (IBS) without further evaluation. Celiac disease as well as lactose intolerance should be considered. This article would suggest that the prevalence of biopsy-proven celiac disease with IBS symptoms is 4-fold that of controls. I would suggest, based on the results of this article, that screening for celiac disease should be undertaken in those patients who have IBS symptoms. If screening is to be done, the endomysial antibody (EMA) and tissue transglutaminase antibody (tTGA) testing is preferred.

J. S. Scolapio, MD

Radiofrequency Ablation in Barrett's Esophagus with Dysplasia
Shaheen NJ, Sharma P, Overholt BF, et al (The Univ of North Carolina at Chapel Hill; Univ of Kansas School of Medicine; Gastrointestinal Associates, Knoxville, TN; et al)
N Engl J Med 360:2277-2288, 2009

Background.—Barrett's esophagus, a condition of intestinal metaplasia of the esophagus, is associated with an increased risk of esophageal adenocarcinoma. We assessed whether endoscopic radiofrequency ablation could eradicate dysplastic Barrett's esophagus and decrease the rate of neoplastic progression.

Methods.—In a multicenter, sham-controlled trial, we randomly assigned 127 patients with dysplastic Barrett's esophagus in a 2:1 ratio to receive either radiofrequency ablation (ablation group) or a sham procedure (control group). Randomization was stratified according to the grade of dysplasia and the length of Barrett's esophagus. Primary outcomes at 12 months included the complete eradication of dysplasia and intestinal metaplasia.

Results.—In the intention-to-treat analyses, among patients with low-grade dysplasia, complete eradication of dysplasia occurred in 90.5% of those in the ablation group, as compared with 22.7% of those in the control group (P<0.001). Among patients with high-grade dysplasia, complete eradication occurred in 81.0% of those in the ablation group, as compared with 19.0% of those in the control group (P<0.001). Overall, 77.4% of patients in the ablation group had complete eradication of intestinal metaplasia, as compared with 2.3% of those in the control group (P<0.001). Patients in the ablation group had less disease progression (3.6% vs. 16.3%, P = 0.03) and fewer cancers (1.2% vs. 9.3%, P = 0.045). Patients reported having more chest pain after the ablation procedure than after the sham procedure. In the ablation group, one patient had upper gastrointestinal hemorrhage, and five patients (6.0%) had esophageal stricture.

Conclusions.—In patients with dysplastic Barrett's esophagus, radiofrequency ablation was associated with a high rate of complete eradication

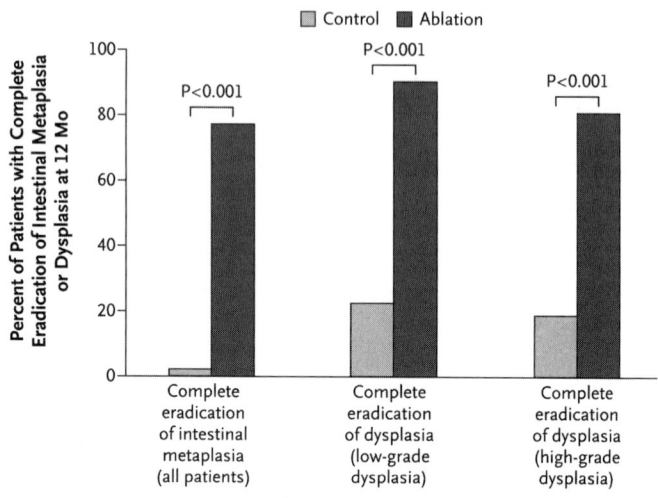

of both dysplasia and intestinal metaplasia and a reduced risk of disease progression. (ClinicalTrials.gov number, NCT00282672.).

▶ Barrett's esophagus with dysplasia has a risk of progression to invasive cancer reported at 1%/year for low-grade and up to 10%/year for high-grade dysplasia. Despite this clinical challenge, optimal management of dysplastic Barrett's has not been established. For high-grade dysplasia, guidelines have been published endorsing a variety of strategies ranging from surgical esophagectomy to endoscopic ablation to conservative management directed by intensive endoscopic surveillance (invasive intervention only when cancer is identified). Endoscopic therapy hinges on the idea that destruction of the Barrett's will revert to healthy squamous epithelium.

This multicenter, randomized, and sham-controlled trial of endoscopic radiofrequency ablation (RFA) with a commercially available catheter (HALO BarrX Medical) used circumferential contact tissue ablation coupled with intensive acid suppression to assess the rate of eradication of dysplasia and intestinal metaplasia. Stratified on the basis of degree of dysplasia (high vs low grade), 127 patients were randomized 2:1 to ablation vs sham and followed with a rigorous endoscopic biopsy surveillance, including the use of jumbo forceps (4 quadrant biopsies every 1 cm of Barrett's) for up to 1 year.

Fig 3 shows that the ablation arms met all 3 primary outcomes with statistically and clinically significant rates of complete eradication of intestinal metaplasia and dysplasia in both high-grade and low-grade cohorts compared with sham controls. An important secondary outcome was also met; in the high-grade dysplasia group, ablation lowered the risk of cancer (1.2% vs 9.3%). While this is the penultimate outcome sought in Barrett's management trials, the authors caution that the result in this trial represents an absolute difference of 4 versus 1 cancer development because of the relatively small size of the control group with high-grade dysplasia ($n = 21$). A concern with any ablative technique is persistence of dysplastic epithelium beneath the neo-squamous mucosa; this was uncommon at 1 year in this trial (5% vs 40% in the control group).

Finally, RFA competes with endoscopic photodynamic therapy (PDT), previously shown to be effective in Barrett's ablation.[1] Complications in this study were uncommon; chest pain with the initial ablation was frequent but self-limited (median 8 days); serious adverse events occurred in only 3 patients. A predicted adverse outcome from thermal injury to the mucosa includes the development of esophageal strictures; this developed in only 6% in the RFA trial vs 39% with PDT.[1]

It is important to acknowledge that this study uses eradication of metaplasia/dysplasia as a surrogate for cancer prevention and the durability of squamous reversion after any endoscopic ablation remains to be proven. In addition, any endoscopic therapy is costly. However, this study shows that RFA is safe and effective for eradication of dysplastic Barrett's. Given the ominous risk associated with Barrett's with high-grade dysplasia and the morbidity associated with surgical esophagectomy, the risks and cost of RFA appear justifiable. The role of endoscopic therapy in the more common Barrett's with low-grade dysplasia remains to be elucidated.

R. K. Pearson, MD

Reference

1. Overholt BF, Lightdale CJ, Wang KK, et al. Photodynamic therapy with porfimer sodium for ablation of high-grade dysplasia in Barrett's esophagus: international, partially blinded, randomized phase III trial. *Gastrointest Endosc.* 2005;62:488-498.

PART EIGHT

ENDOCRINOLOGY, DIABETES, AND METABOLISM

DEREK LEROITH, MD, PHD

51 Adrenal Cortex

Adrenocortical carcinoma survival rates correlated to genomic copy number variants
Stephan EA, Chung T-H, Grant CS, et al (Translational Genomics Res Inst, Phoenix, AZ; Mayo Clinic, Rochester, MN; et al)
Mol Cancer Ther 7:425-431, 2008

Adrenocortical carcinoma (ACC) is a rare endocrine malignancy accounting for between 0.02% and 0.2% of all cancer deaths. Surgical removal offers the only current potential for cure. Unfortunately, ACC has undergone metastatic spread in 40% to 70% of patients at the time of diagnosis. Standard chemotherapy with mitotane is often ineffective with intolerable side effects. The modern molecular technology of comparative genomic hybridization allows the examination of DNA for chromosomal alterations, which can lend biological insight into cancer processes. Genomes of 25 ACC clinical samples were queried on the Agilent 44K Human Genome comparative genomic hybridization array detecting regions of chromosomal gain and loss within the tumor population. Commonly shared amplifications appearing in $\geq 50\%$ of tumors at $P \leq 10^{-4}$ include regions within chromosomes 5, 7, 12, 16q, and 20. Deleted genomic regions within ACC include portions of chromosomes 1, 3p, 10q, 11, 14q, 15q, 17, and 22q. Genomic aberrations in regions associated with differential survival ($P \leq 0.05$) and presence in $\geq 20\%$ of tumors include amplifications of 6q, 7q, 12q, and 19p. Deletions within stratified survival groups include localized regions within 3, 8, 10p, 16q, 17q, and 19q. Statistical analysis of this genetic landscape reveals a set of chromosomal aberrations strongly associated with survival in an accumulation-dependent fashion. These regions may hold prognostic indicators and offer therapeutic targets that can be used to develop novel treatments for aggressive tumors.

▶ The identification of sensitive biomarkers in cancer is an important step in determining malignancy grade and ultimately prognosis and stratification of therapy. The chromosomal aberrations in adrenal cortical carcinoma have been well described with observed chromosomal gains and deletions. This study is descriptive, but helps establish a correlation between alterations in specific regions and survival. In the future, the clustering of chromosomal and specific gene overexpression or underexpression may help map the potential biological behavior of these tumors.

D. E. Schteingart, MD

Waiting for change: Symptom resolution after adrenalectomy for Cushing's syndrome

Sippel RS, Elaraj DM, Kebebew E, et al (Univ of Wisconsin Madison; Univ of California San Francisco)

Surgery 144:1054-1061, 2008

Background.—The debilitating symptoms and physical changes from Cushing's syndrome may resolve after treatment, but the time course to resolution is not well established.

Methods.—Between February 1995 and May 2007, 60 patients underwent adrenalectomy for Cushing's syndrome. Pre-operative and operative variables were collected from a prospective database. Long-term follow-up was obtained via patient survey.

Results.—Unilateral adrenalectomy was performed in 53% and a bilateral adrenalectomy in 47% of patients. Median time to diagnosis was 24 months (range, 1–384). Three percent had intra-operative complications, and 28% developed post-operative complications. Steroids were required post-operatively for a median of 30 months after unilateral adrenalectomy (range, 0–96). At a median follow-up of 3.7 years (range, 0–13.3), 85% of patients are still alive. The majority of the physical changes resolved after adrenalectomy. The time to symptom resolution varied from a few weeks to up to 4 years. Most of the physical changes resolved by a mean of 7–9 months after surgery. Quality of life improved in 78% of patients, with 68% improving dramatically ($P < .001$).

Conclusion.—Adrenalectomy can provide excellent palliation of the symptoms of cortisol excess and can dramatically improve patient quality of life, but both patients and physicians must know that these changes may take years.

▶ The recovery from the devastating consequence of hypercortisolism in patients with Cushing's disease successfully treated with transsphenoidal surgery is often long, and patients complain of a variety of symptoms. We normally advise patients it may take 6 to 12 months for the clinical manifestations of Cushing's to resolve. This study provides objective chronology of what patients can expect following normalization of cortisol levels. Many of the complaints during the first few months are related to withdrawal from high levels of cortisol and consist of arthralgia, myalgia, fatigue, nausea, and variable mood. Symptoms occasionally improve by increasing the replacement dose of glucocorticoids, but this strategy delays recovery of the HPA axis. Patients need to be encouraged to continue their steroid taper, in spite of these symptoms. The chronology described in this article could be useful in reassuring patients about their eventual improvement.

D. E. Schteingart, MD

52 Calcium and Bone Metabolism

Serum 25-Hydroxyvitamin D Concentrations and Risk for Hip Fractures
Cauley JA, LaCroix AZ, Wu L, et al (Univ of Pittsburgh; Fred Hutchinson Cancer Res Ctr, Seattle, WA; et al)
Ann Intern Med 149:242-250, 2008

Background.—The relationship between serum 25-hydroxyvitamin D [25(OH) vitamin D] concentration and hip fractures is unclear.

Objective.—To see whether low serum 25(OH) vitamin D concentrations are associated with hip fractures in community-dwelling women.

Design.—Nested case–control study.

Setting.—40 clinical centers in the United States.

Participants.—400 case-patients with incident hip fracture and 400 control participants matched on the basis of age, race or ethnicity, and date of blood draw. Both groups were selected from 39 795 postmenopausal women who were not using estrogens or other bone-active therapies and who had not had a previous hip fracture.

Measurements.—Serum 25(OH) vitamin D was measured and patients were followed for a median of 7.1 years (range, 0.7 to 9.3 years) to assess fractures.

Results.—Mean serum 25(OH) vitamin D concentrations were lower in case-patients than in control participants (55.95 nmol/L [SD, 20.28] vs. 59.60 nmol/L [SD, 18.05]; $P = 0.007$), and lower serum 25(OH) vitamin D concentrations increased hip fracture risk (adjusted odds ratio for each 25-nmol/L decrease, 1.33 [95% CI, 1.06 to 1.68]). Women with the lowest 25(OH) vitamin D concentrations ($\leq$47.5 nmol/L) had a higher fracture risk than did those with the highest concentrations ($\geq$70.7 nmol/L) (adjusted odds ratio, 1.71 [CI, 1.05 to 2.79]), and the risk increased statistically significantly across quartiles of serum 25(OH) vitamin D concentration (P for trend = 0.016). This association was independent of number of falls, physical function, frailty, renal function, and sex-steroid hormone levels and seemed to be partially mediated by bone resorption.

Limitations.—Few case-patients were nonwhite women. Bone mineral density and parathyroid hormone levels were not accounted for in the analysis.

Conclusion.—Low serum 25(OH) vitamin D concentrations are associated with a higher risk for hip fracture.

▶ Vitamin D deficiency is commonly associated with fractures,[1,2] but whether vitamin D deficiency independently increases fracture risk has not been clear in all studies. A recent evidence-based study of serum 25-hydroxyvitamin D level and fracture risk concluded that the available evidence did not support an association.[3] Another recent nested case-control study reported no association between serum 25-hydroxyvitamin D and fracture risk,[4] and a third study using NHANES III data showed that hip fracture risk was reduced with serum 25-hydroxyvitamin D level of > 60 nmol/L.[5]

The authors performed a nested case-control study of 400 postmenopausal women with incident hip fracture who were enrolled in the Women's Health Initiative Observational Study to see whether baseline serum 25-hydroxyvitamin D level correlated with hip fracture risk over a median of 7.1 years. Neither the cases nor the controls were treated with hormone or estrogen therapy, and none of the subjects had a history of previous hip fracture. Subjects with incident hip fractures had a median baseline serum 25-hydroxyvitamin D level of 55.95 ± 20.28 nmol/L, whereas control subjects had a median baseline level of 59.6 ± 18.05 nmol/L ($P = 0.007$). Lower serum 25-hydroxyvitamin D level increased the relative risk of hip fracture risk by 1.33 for each 25 nmol/L decrease. Women within the lowest quartile of baseline serum 25-hydroxyvitamin D had higher fracture risk than women within the highest baseline quartile, and hip fracture risk increased significantly across quartiles of serum 25-hydroxyvitamin D. The association between serum 25-hydroxyvitamin D and hip fracture was independent of number of falls, physical function, frailty, renal function, and sex steroid hormone levels, and was partially mediated by bone resorption.

These findings from a very large study of community-dwelling postmenopausal women suggest that vitamin D deficiency is associated with hip fracture risk. The association between baseline serum 25-hydroxyvitamin D and hip fracture risk in this study was linear and did not seem to differ by age. The reason for the association is not clear, but it may be due in part to increased bone resorption reflected by increased serum CTx-telopeptide in subjects in the lowest quartile of serum 25-hydroxyvitamin D, presumably driven by higher parathyroid hormone levels in this group. Another explanation could be impaired muscle strength, balance, and/or poor physical function, all of which could increase the risk of falls. The optimal serum 25-hydroxyvitamin D level to maintain bone health has not yet been established, but the level at which serum parathyroid hormone plateaus in the normal range is around 78 nmol/L,[6] similar to the optimal serum 25-hydroxyvitamin D threshold level of at least 78 nmol/L based on bone mineral density.[7] Further studies will help clarify these issues.

B. L. Clarke, MD

References

1. Thomas MK, Lloyd-Jones DM, Thadhani RI, et al. Hypovitaminosis D in medical inpatients. *N Engl J Med.* 1998;338:777-783.
2. Leboff MS, Kohlmeier L, Hurwitz S, et al. Occult vitamin D deficiency in postmenopausal US women with acute hip fracture. *JAMA.* 1999;281:1505-1511.
3. Cranney A, Horsley T, O'Donnell S, et al. *Effectiveness and safety of vitamin D in relation to bone health.* Rockville, MD: Agency for Healthcare Research and Quality; 2007. Available at: www.ahrq.gov/clinic/tp/vitadtp.htm; 2007. Accessed May 3, 2009.
4. Roddam AW, Neale R, Appleby P, et al. Association between plasma 25-hydroxyvitamin D levels and fracture risk: the EPIC-Oxford study. *Am J Epidemiol.* 2007; 166:1327-1336.
5. Looker AC, Mussolino ME. Serum 25-hydroxyvitamin D and hip fracture risk in older U.S. white adults. *J Bone Miner Res.* 2008;23:143-150.
6. Bischoff-Ferrari HA. The 25-hydroxyvitamin D threshold for better health. *J Steroid Biochem Mol Biol.* 2007;103:614-619.
7. Bischoff-Ferrari HA, Dietrich T, Orav EJ, Dawson-Hughes B. Positive association between 25-hydroxy vitamin D levels and bone mineral density: a population-based study of younger and older adults. *Am J Med.* 2004;116:634-639.

Benefit of Adherence With Bisphosphonates Depends on Age and Fracture Type: Results From an Analysis of 101,038 New Bisphosphonate Users

Curtis JR, Westfall AO, Cheng H, et al (Univ of Alabama at Birmingham; et al)
J Bone Miner Res 23:1435-1441, 2008

The relationship between high adherence to oral bisphosphonates and the risk of different types of fractures has not been well studied among adults of different ages. Using claims data from a large U.S. health care organization, we quantified adherence after initiating bisphosphonate therapy using the medication possession ratio (MPR) and identified fractures. Cox proportional hazards models were used to evaluate the rate of fracture among nonadherent persons (MPR < 50%) compared with highly adherent persons (MPR ≥ 80%) across several age strata and a variety of types of clinical fractures. In conjunction with fracture incidence rates among the nonadherent, these estimates were used to compute the number needed to treat with high adherence to prevent one fracture, by age and fracture type. Among 101,038 new bisphosphonate users, the proportion of persons with high adherence at 1, 2, and 3 yr was 44%, 39%, and 35%, respectively. Among 65- to 78-yr-old persons with a physician diagnosis of osteoporosis, the crude and adjusted rate of hip fracture among the nonadherent was 1.96 (95% CI, 1.48–2.60) and 1.74 (95% CI, 1.30–2.31), respectively, resulting in a number needed to treat with high adherence to prevent one hip fracture of 107. The impact of high adherence was substantially less for other types of fractures and for younger persons. Analysis of adherence in a non–time-dependent fashion artifactually magnified differences in fracture rates between adherent and nonadherent persons. The antifracture effectiveness associated with high adherence to oral bisphosphonates varied substantially by age and fracture type. These results provide estimates of absolute fracture effectiveness across age subgroups and fracture types that have been minimally evaluated in clinical trials and may be useful for future cost-effectiveness studies.

▶ As for most diseases, success of treatment of osteoporosis with bisphosphonates depends on the effectiveness of the medication and patient adherence to treatment. Previously published studies have shown that long-term adherence to oral bisphosphonates is relatively poor,[1-4] in that roughly 50% of patients discontinue taking oral bisphosphonates after 1 to 2 years. These observations have led to the formulation of longer-acting bisphosphonates taken less frequently, and the development of intravenous bisphosphonates that can be given once every 3 months or once a year.

This study evaluated adherence to oral bisphosphonates and the risk of fracture in a very large claims database from a large United States health care organization covering about 17 million persons. Nonadherent subjects were defined as those with a medication possession ratio of less than 50% of the time, and highly adherent subjects as those with a medication possession ratio of more than 80% of the time. Among over 100 000 new users of bisphosphonates, high adherence at 1, 2, and 3 years was only 44%, 39%, and 35%, respectively. Among 65- to 78-year-old subjects diagnosed with osteoporosis, nonadherence led to crude and adjusted rates of hip fracture that were 96% and 74%, respectively, higher than in adherent subjects. The number of adherent older subjects needed to treat to prevent a hip fracture was 107, but antifracture efficacy associated with high adherence to oral bisphosphonates varied widely by age and fracture type. The authors concluded that analysis of adherence in a non-time-dependent fashion artifactually magnifies differences in fracture rates between adherent and nonadherent persons, and that high adherence has less impact on fractures other than hip fractures and in younger individuals.

The findings in this article are important because they highlight the importance of adherence to oral bisphosphonate medication to achieve fracture reduction. Analysis of time-dependent medication possession ratio showed a strong linear relationship between increasing adherence and decreasing fracture rate without a threshold effect. High adherence was less effective in reducing wrist and nonvertebral fractures, particularly in younger subjects. These findings indicate that adherence to oral bisphosphonate therapy has the greatest benefit for fracture reduction in older subjects diagnosed with osteoporosis.

For further reading on this subject I suggest an article by Caro et al.[5]

B. L. Clarke, MD

References

1. Recker RR, Gallagher R, MacCosbe PE. Effect of dosing frequency on bisphosphonate medication adherence in a large longitudinal cohort of women. *Mayo Clin Proc.* 2005;80:856-861.
2. Curtis JR, Westfall AO, Allison JJ, et al. Channeling and adherence with alendronate and risedronate among chronic glucocorticoid users. *Osteoporosis Int.* 2006; 17:1268-1274.

3. Gold DT, Safi W, Trinh H. Patient preference and adherence: comparative US studies between two bisphosphonates, weekly risedronate and monthly ibandronate. *Curr Med Res Opin.* 2006;22:2383-2391.
4. Siris ES, Harris ST, Rosen CT, et al. Adherence to bisphosphonate therapy and fracture rates in osteoporotic women: relationship to vertebral and nonvertebral fractures from two US claims databases. *Mayo Clin Proc.* 2006;81:1013-1022.
5. Caro JJ, Ishak KJ, Huybrechts KF, et al. The impact of compliance with osteoporosis therapy on fracture rates in actual practice. *Osteoporosis Int.* 2004;15: 1003-1008.

The Natural History of Primary Hyperparathyroidism with or without Parathyroid Surgery after 15 Years

Rubin MR, Bilezikian JP, McMahon DJ, et al (Columbia Univ, NY)
J Clin Endocrinol Metab 93:3462-3470, 2008

Context.—Primary hyperparathyroidism (PHPT) often presents without classical symptoms such as overt skeletal disease or nephrolithiasis. We previously reported that calciotropic indices and bone mineral density (BMD) are stable in untreated patients for up to a decade, whereas after parathyroidectomy, normalization of biochemistries and increases in BMD ensue.

Objective.—The objective of the study was to provide additional insights in patients with and without surgery for up to 15 yr.

Design.—The study had an observational design.

Setting.—The setting was a referral center.

Patients.—Patients included 116 patients (25 men, 91 women); 99 (85%) were asymptomatic.

Intervention.—Fifty-nine patients (51%) underwent parathyroidectomy and 57 patients were followed up without surgery.

Main Outcome Measure.—BMD was measured.

Results.—Lumbar spine BMD remained stable for 15 yr. However, BMD started to fall at cortical sites even before 10 yr, ultimately decreasing by $10 \pm 3\%$ (mean $\pm$ SEM; $P < 0.05$) at the femoral neck, and $35 \pm 5\%$; $P < 0.05$ at the distal radius, in the few patients observed for 15 yr. Thirty-seven percent of asymptomatic patients showed disease progression (one or more new guidelines for surgery) at any time point over the 15 yr. Meeting surgical criteria at baseline did not predict who would have progressive disease. BMD increases in patients who underwent surgery were sustained for the entire 15 yr.

Conclusions.—Parathyroidectomy led to normalization of biochemical indices and sustained increases in BMD. Without surgery, PHPT progressed in one third of individuals over 15 yr; meeting surgical criteria at the outset did not predict this progression. Cortical bone density decreased in the majority of subjects with additional observation time points and long-term follow-up. These results raise questions regarding how long patients with PHPT should be followed up without intervention.

▶ The authors previously reported that patients with asymptomatic primary hyperparathyroidism who were not sent to parathyroid surgery generally maintained their calciotropic indices and bone mineral density stability over the next 10 years.[1] This landmark article demonstrated the generally benign clinical course of primary hyperparathyroidism in patients who did not present initially with classical features such as overt skeletal disease or calcium nephrolithiasis. About 27% of the patients not sent to surgery at baseline eventually developed a reason(s) for surgery later. Surgical cure of those patients electing to have surgery at baseline, or surgery later for complications that eventually developed, led to normalization of biochemistries and improvement in bone mineral density.

This study reports the 15-year follow-up of the initial cohort of patients with asymptomatic primary hyperparathyroidism. The initial cohort included 116 patients, 99 (85%) of whom were asymptomatic. Of the original 116 patients, 59 (51%) chose to undergo surgery at baseline, and 57 were followed without surgery. Lumbar spine bone density remained stable over the 15 years of follow-up, but cortical bone density started to decrease even before 10 years of follow-up, and eventually decreased by 10% ± 3% at the femoral neck, and by 35% ± 5% at the distal radius, in the few patients followed out to 15 years.

In the 57 patients with asymptomatic primary hyperparathyroidism at baseline, 37% eventually developed disease progression such that they met surgical criteria. Patients who met surgical criteria at baseline did not necessarily develop progressive disease. Patients who underwent parathyroidectomy at baseline had improved bone mineral density that was sustained over the entire follow-up period.

This study is important because it clarifies the natural history of asymptomatic primary hyperparathyroidism. It is clear that patients with symptomatic primary hyperparathyroidism should generally be referred for surgery to treat complications they already have, and to minimize the likelihood of development of future complications. Patients with asymptomatic primary hyperparathyroidism are typically counseled to not have surgery based on the original 10-year study.[1,2] This longer-term follow-up study indicates that a third of the patients eventually develop indications for surgery over 15 years, with the implication being that longer follow-up would likely lead to an even higher percentage for whom surgery would eventually be recommended. It is not possible to predict which asymptomatic patients will not develop complications leading to eventual recommendation for surgery, and it is clear that patients meeting criteria for parathyroidectomy at baseline do not predictably worsen over time if they choose to avoid surgery. The study suggests that patients with asymptomatic primary hyperparathyroidism would probably benefit from surgery at some point, primarily to prevent distal radial bone loss. Some of these asymptomatic patients may also benefit from surgery because of improved quality of life.[3]

B. L. Clarke, MD

References

1. Silverberg SJ, Shane E, Jacobs TP, et al. A 10-year prospective study of primary hyperparathyroidism with or without parathyroid surgery. *N Engl J Med.* 1999; 341:1249-1255.
2. Bilezikian JP, Khan AA, Potts JT Jr. Third International Workshop on the Management of Asymptomatic Primary Hyperparathyroidism. Guidelines for the management of asymptomatic primary hyperparathyroidism: summary statement from the third international workshop. *J Clin Endocrinol Metab.* 2009;94:335-339.
3. Ambrogini E, Cetani F, Cianferotti L, et al. Surgery or surveillance for mild asymptomatic primary hyperparathyroidism: a prospective randomized clinical trial. *J Clin Endocrinol Metab.* 2007;92:3114-3121.

Early Responsiveness of Women with Osteoporosis to Teriparatide After Therapy with Alendronate or Risedronate

Miller PD, Delmas PD, Lindsay R, et al (Colorado Ctr for Bone Res, Lakewood; Claude Bernard Univ Lyon 1, France; Helen Hayes Hosp, West Haverstraw, NY; et al)
J Clin Endocrinol Metab 93:3785-3793, 2008

Background.—Anabolic responsiveness to teriparatide can be blunted or delayed in patients previously treated with alendronate. The extent of this effect is different for other antiresorptives. This study evaluated the early anabolic effects of teriparatide in postmenopausal women with osteoporosis previously treated with alendronate or risedronate.

Methods.—Patients treated for at least 24 months with alendronate or risedronate discontinued their bisphosphonate and received teriparatide for 12 months. The primary endpoint was a comparison of changes from baseline in N-terminal propeptide of type 1 collagen after 3 months between prior bisphosphonate groups. We also examined changes in other bone turnover markers, bone mineral density (BMD), and relationships between early changes in bone turnover markers and 12-month areal and volumetric BMD.

Results.—In the prior risedronate group, the N-terminal propeptide of type 1 collagen increase was significantly greater after 3 months of teriparatide than in the prior alendronate group (mean ± SE, 86.0 ± 5.6 *vs.* 61.2 ± 5.3 ng/ml, respectively; $P < 0.001$). Findings were similar for the other bone turnover markers. The changes in areal BMD and trabecular spine volumetric BMD were also greater in the prior risedronate group ($P < 0.05$). Early changes in bone turnover markers correlated with changes in trabecular spine volumetric BMD at 12 months (Spearman $r = 0.45$). Teriparatide was well tolerated.

Conclusion.—This nonrandomized but prospective study suggests that there may be differences in anabolic responsiveness to teriparatide as a function of the type of prior bisphosphonate exposure.

▶ Simultaneous administration of teriparatide (recombinant human parathyroid hormone 1-34) or parathyroid hormone (PTH) 1-84 and alendronate blunts the bone density response to teriparatide or PTH 1-84 alone.[1-3] Correspondingly, administration of alendronate prior to teriparatide may delay or blunt the anabolic responsiveness to teriparatide. Other antiresorptive agents may also limit the responsiveness to teriparatide when given prior to or simultaneously with teriparatide,[4-7] but perhaps less effectively than the more potent bisphosphonates.

This open-label study evaluated the early anabolic responsiveness of postmenopausal women previously treated with alendronate or risedronate for at least 24 months. Patients discontinued their alendronate or risedronate and substituted teriparatide 20 μg each day by subcutaneous injection for 12 months. Second morning void urinary NTx-telopeptide, and other serum and urinary markers of bone turnover, and bone mineral density were followed over the 12 months during treatment with teriparatide. The authors report that urinary NTx-telopeptide and other markers of bone turnover increased more over the first 3 months of teriparatide treatment in subjects previously treated with risedronate, and that increases in areal and volumetric bone mineral density over 12 months were greater in subjects previously treated with risedronate. The early changes in markers of bone turnover correlated with changes in lumbar spine trabecular volumetric bone mineral density at 12 months.

This study demonstrates that the response to anabolic agents after previous treatment with antiresorptive drugs may be greater in those treated with less potent anticatabolic agents. This distinction is clinically important because most patients considering treatment with an anabolic agent have previously been treated with an antiresorptive drug, in many cases with potent bisphosphonates. Further studies will be required to show that this phenomenon is true for all antiresorptive drugs.

B. L. Clarke, MD

References

1. Black DM, Greenspan SL, Ensrud KE, et al. The effects of parathyroid hormone and alendronate alone or in combination in postmenopausal osteoporosis. *N Engl J Med.* 2003;349:1207-1215.
2. Neer R, Hayes A, Rao A, Finkelstein J. Effects of parathyroid hormone, alendronate, or both on bone density in osteoporotic postmenopausal women [abstract 1039]. *J Bone Miner Res.* 2002;17:S135.
3. Finkelstein JS, Leder BZ, Burnett SM, et al. Effects of teriparatide, alendronate, or both on bone turnover in men. *J Clin Endocrinol Metab.* 2006;91:2882-2887.
4. Deal C, Omizo M, Schwartz EN, et al. Combination teriparatide and raloxifene therapy for postmenopausal osteoporosis: results from a 6-month double-blind placebo-controlled trial. *J Bone Miner Res.* 2005;20:1905-1911.
5. Lindsay R, Nieves J, Formica C, et al. Randomized controlled study of effect of parathyroid hormone on vertebral bone mass and fracture incidence among postmenopausal women on oestrogen with osteoporosis. *Lancet.* 1997;350:550-555.
6. Cosman F, Nieves JW, Zion M, Barbuto N, Lindsay R. Effect of prior and ongoing raloxifene therapy on response to PTH and maintenance of BMD after PTH therapy. *Osteoporos Int.* 2008;19:529-535.
7. Ettinger B, San Martin JA, Crans G, Pavo I. Differential effects of teriparatide on BMD after treatment with raloxifene or alendronate. *J Bone Miner Res.* 2004;19:745-751.

Efficacy of Bazedoxifene in Reducing New Vertebral Fracture Risk in Postmenopausal Women With Osteoporosis: Results From a 3-Year, Randomized, Placebo-, and Active-Controlled Clinical Trial

Silverman SL, Christiansen C, Genant HK, et al (Cedars-Sinai Med Ctr, Los Angeles, CA; Ctr for Clinical and Basic Research, Ballerup, Denmark; Univ of California, San Francisco; et al)
J Bone Miner Res 23:1923-1934, 2008

In this 3-yr, randomized, double-blind, placebo- and active-controlled study, healthy postmenopausal women with osteoporosis (55–85 yr of age) were treated with bazedoxifene 20 or 40 mg/d, raloxifene 60 mg/d, or placebo. The primary endpoint was incidence of new vertebral fractures after 36 mo; secondary endpoints included nonvertebral fractures, BMD, and bone turnover markers. Among 6847 subjects in the intent-to-treat population, the incidence of new vertebral fractures was significantly lower ($p < 0.05$) with bazedoxifene 20 mg (2.3%), bazedoxifene 40 mg (2.5%), and raloxifene 60 mg (2.3%) compared with placebo (4.1%), with relative risk reductions of 42%, 37%, and 42%, respectively. The treatment effect was similar among subjects with or without prevalent vertebral fracture ($p = 0.89$ for treatment by baseline fracture status interaction). The incidence of nonvertebral fractures with bazedoxifene or raloxifene was not significantly different from placebo. In a posthoc analysis of a subgroup of women at higher fracture risk (femoral neck T-score ≤ -3.0 and/or ≥ 1 moderate or severe vertebral fracture or multiple mild vertebral fractures; $n = 1772$), bazedoxifene 20 mg showed a 50% and 44% reduction in nonvertebral fracture risk relative to placebo ($p = 0.02$) and raloxifene 60 mg ($p = 0.05$), respectively. Bazedoxifene significantly improved BMD and reduced bone marker levels ($p < 0.001$ versus placebo). The incidence of vasodilatation, leg cramps, and venous thromboembolic events was higher with bazedoxifene and raloxifene compared with placebo. In conclusion, bazedoxifene significantly reduced the risk of new vertebral fracture in postmenopausal women with osteoporosis and decreased the risk of nonvertebral fracture in subjects at higher fracture risk.

▶ The selective estrogen receptor modulator (SERM) raloxifene was previously approved for prevention and treatment of postmenopausal osteoporosis on the basis of a large phase III, prospective, randomized, controlled clinical trial.[1,2] This drug interacts with estrogen receptor (ER)-alpha and ER-beta in bone to improve bone density and reduce vertebral fractures, but not hip or nonvertebral fractures. Given the central role that estrogen deficiency plays in the pathogenesis of postmenopausal osteoporosis, other agents that more potently modulate the estrogen receptor have been investigated to determine whether their effects might be more favorable.

Bazedoxifene is a novel SERM that has been shown to have improved tissue-selective activities on bone and lipid metabolism, without adverse effects on uterine or breast tissue.[3,4] Bazedoxifene was shown to prevent bone loss and decrease bone turnover without stimulating the uterus in a 2-year randomized controlled trial in healthy postmenopausal women with normal or low bone density.[5] The current 3-year randomized, double-blind, placebo- and active-controlled study demonstrates that bazedoxifene also reduced vertebral fracture risk in 6847 healthy postmenopausal women randomized to receive bazedoxifene 20 or 40 mg/day, raloxifene 60 mg/day, or placebo. Vertebral fractures were reduced by 42% in the bazedoxifene 20 mg/day group, compared with 37% in the bazedoxifene 40 mg/day group, and 42% in the raloxifene group, compared with placebo. Vertebral fractures were reduced similarly, regardless of baseline vertebral fracture status. Hip and nonvertebral fractures were not reduced, except in a high-risk subset of women with baseline femoral neck T-score < −3.0 and/or at least one moderate or severe vertebral fracture or multiple mild vertebral fractures. In the high-risk subjects, bazedoxifene 20 mg/day reduced nonvertebral fractures by 50% compared with placebo, and by 44% compared with raloxifene. The authors concluded that bazedoxifene reduced the risk of new vertebral fractures in postmenopausal women, and decreased the risk of nonvertebral fractures in women at higher fracture risk.

These findings suggest that the novel SERM bazedoxifene appears to reduce vertebral fracture risk in postmenopausal women similarly to raloxifene, and that, like raloxifene, it does not reduce nonvertebral fracture risk except in high-risk patients. It is not yet clear why drugs in the SERM category are not able to reduce hip or nonvertebral fractures except in more severely affected patients, but this will continue to limit their use in treating patients with post-menopausal osteoporosis. Drugs in the SERM category may ultimately find their broadest application in treatment of patients with postmenopausal osteoporosis who have a higher risk of breast cancer or other diseases that respond favorably to estrogen receptor modulation.

B. L. Clarke, MD

References

1. Ettinger B, Black DM, Mitlak BH, et al. Reduction of vertebral fracture risk in postmenopausal women with osteoporosis treated with raloxifene: results from a 3-year randomized clinical trial. Multiple Outcomes of Raloxifene Evaluation (MORE) Investigators. *JAMA.* 1999;282:637-645.
2. Ensrud KE, Stock JL, Barrett-Connor E, et al. Effects of raloxifene on fracture risk in postmenopausal women: the Raloxifene Use for the Heart Trial. *J Bone Miner Res.* 2008;23:112-120.
3. Komm BS, Kharode YP, Bodine PV, et al. Bazedoxifene acetate: a selective estrogen receptor modulator with improved selectivity. *Endocrinology.* 2005;146: 3999-4008.
4. Ronkin S, Northington R, Baracat E, et al. Endometrial effects of bazedoxifene acetate, a novel selective estrogen receptor modulator, in postmenopausal women. *Obstet Gynecol.* 2005;105:1397-1404.
5. Miller PD, Chines AA, Christiansen C, et al. Effects of bazedoxifene on BMD and bone turnover in postmenopausal women: 2-year results of a randomized, double-blind, placebo- and active-controlled study. *J Bone Miner Res.* 2008;23:525-535.

The Antiresorptive Effects of a Single Dose of Zoledronate Persist for Two Years: A Randomized, Placebo-Controlled Trial in Osteopenic Postmenopausal Women

Grey A, Bolland MJ, Wattie D, et al (Univ of Auckland, New Zealand)
J Clin Endocrinol Metab 94:538-544, 2009

Context.—Annual iv administration of 5 mg zoledronate decreases fracture risk. The optimal dosing interval of 5 mg zoledronate is not known.

Objective.—Our objective was to determine the duration of antiresorptive action of a single 5-mg dose of iv zoledronate.

Design, Setting, and Participants.—We conducted a double-blind, randomized, placebo-controlled trial over 2 yr at an academic research center, in a volunteer sample of 50 postmenopausal women with osteopenia.

Intervention.—Intervention included 5 mg zoledronate.

Main Outcome Measures.—Biochemical markers of bone turnover and bone mineral density of the lumbar spine, proximal femur, and total body.

Results.—Compared with placebo, zoledronate treatment decreased mean levels of each of four markers of bone turnover by at least 38% (range 38–45%) for the duration of the study ($P < 0.0001$ for each marker). After 2 yr, bone mineral density was higher in the zoledronate group than the placebo group by an average of 5.7% (95% confidence interval = 4.0–7.4) at the lumbar spine, 3.9% (2.2–5.7) at the proximal femur, and 1.7% (0.8–2.5) at the total body ($P < 0.0001$ for each skeletal site). Between-groups differences in markers of bone turnover and bone mineral density were similar at 12 and 24 months. Mild secondary hyperparathyroidism was present throughout the study in the zoledronate group.

Conclusion.—The antiresorptive effects of a single 5-mg dose of zoledronate are sustained for at least 2 yr. The magnitudes of the effects on markers of bone turnover and bone mineral density are comparable at 12 and 24 months. Administration of zoledronate at intervals of up to 2 yr may be associated with antifracture efficacy; clinical trials to investigate this possibility are justified.

▶ The optimal dosing interval for many bisphosphonates used for treatment of osteoporosis has not been investigated thoroughly. Because the introduction of bisphosphonates as therapeutic agents for prevention and treatment of osteoporosis, more potent and longer acting bisphosphonates have been approved, and several earlier approved bisphosphonates have been reformulated to allow weekly or monthly dosing. Zoledronic acid is currently the most potent and long-acting bisphosphonate available.[1-5] This compound is approved for once-yearly intravenous treatment of postmenopausal osteoporosis, male osteoporosis, glucocorticoid-induced osteoporosis, and Paget's disease, in addition to more frequent treatment of multiple myeloma and metastatic breast and prostate cancer. The optimal dosing interval of zoledronic acid for osteoporosis is not yet known.

The authors of this study evaluated the effects of a single 5 mg intravenous dose of zoledronic acid compared with placebo over 2 years on bone mineral density and biochemical markers of bone turnover in 50 volunteer postmenopausal women with osteopenia. It was shown that 2 markers of bone resorption, serum β-C-terminal telopeptide of type I collagen (CTX), and urine N-telopeptide of type 1 collagen (NTx), and 2 markers of bone formation, serum osteocalcin, and procollagen type-I N-terminal propeptide (P1NP) had sustained decreases of 38% to 45% from baseline over 2 years, with all markers equally suppressed at 12 and 24 months. After 2 years, bone mineral density increased in the patients treated with zoledronic acid by a mean of 5.7% at the lumbar spine, and 3.9% at the proximal femur, compared with placebo. The zoledronic acid group had sustained mild physiological hyperparathyroidism for the duration of the study.

This study demonstrates that a single infusion of zoledronic acid 5 mg causes suppression of bone turnover for up to 2 years, with bone resorption equally suppressed at 12 and 24 months. Because the study was not powered to show fracture reduction efficacy, it is not yet clear whether fractures may also be reduced at this dosing interval. Clinical trials to demonstrate fracture efficacy with less than once-yearly zoledronic acid would help clarify this issue.

B. L. Clarke, MD

References

1. Black DM, Delmas PD, Eastell R, et al. Once-yearly zoledronic acid for treatment of postmenopausal osteoporosis. *N Engl J Med.* 2007;356:1809-1822.
2. Lyles KW, Colon-Emeric CS, Magaziner JS, et al. Zoledronic acid and clinical fractures and mortality after hip fracture. *N Engl J Med.* 2007;357:1799-1809.
3. Reid IR, Brown JP, Burckhardt P, et al. Intravenous zoledronic acid in postmenopausal women with low bone mineral density. *N Engl J Med.* 2002;346:653-661.
4. Devogelaer JP, Brown JP, Burckhardt P, et al. Zoledronic acid efficacy and safety over five years in postmenopausal women. *Osteoporosis Int.* 2007;18:1211-1218.
5. Bolland M, Grey A, Horne A, et al. Effects of intravenous zoledronate on bone turnover and BMD persist for at least 24 months. *J Bone Miner Res.* 2008;23:1304-1308.

Zoledronic acid and risedronate in the prevention and treatment of glucocorticoid-induced osteoporosis (HORIZON): a multicentre, double-blind, double-dummy, randomised controlled trial

Reid DM, Devogelaer J-P, Saag K, et al (Univ of Aberdeen, UK; Université Catholique de Louvain, Brussels, Belgium; Univ of Alabama at Birmingham; et al)

Lancet 373:1253-1263, 2009

Background.—Persistent use of glucocorticoid drugs is associated with bone loss and increased fracture risk. Concurrent oral bisphosphonates increase bone mineral density and reduce frequency of vertebral fractures, but are associated with poor compliance and adherence. We aimed to assess whether one intravenous infusion of zoledronic acid was non-inferior to daily oral risedronate for prevention and treatment of glucocorticoid-induced osteoporosis.

Methods.—This 1-year randomised, double-blind, double-dummy, non-inferiority study of 54 centres in 12 European countries, Australia, Hong Kong, Israel, and the USA, tested the effectiveness of 5 mg intravenous infusion of zoledronic acid versus 5 mg oral risedronate for prevention and treatment of glucocorticoid-induced osteoporosis. 833 patients were randomised 1:1 to receive zoledronic acid (n=416) or risedronate (n=417). Patients were stratified by sex, and allocated to prevention or treatment subgroups dependent on duration of glucocorticoid use immediately preceding the study. The treatment subgroup consisted of those treated for more than 3 months (272 patients on zoledronic acid and 273 on risedronate), and the prevention subgroup of those treated for less than 3 months (144 patients on each drug). 62 patients did not complete the study because of adverse events, withdrawal of consent, loss to follow-up, death, misrandomisation, or protocol deviation. The primary endpoint was percentage change from baseline in lumbar spine

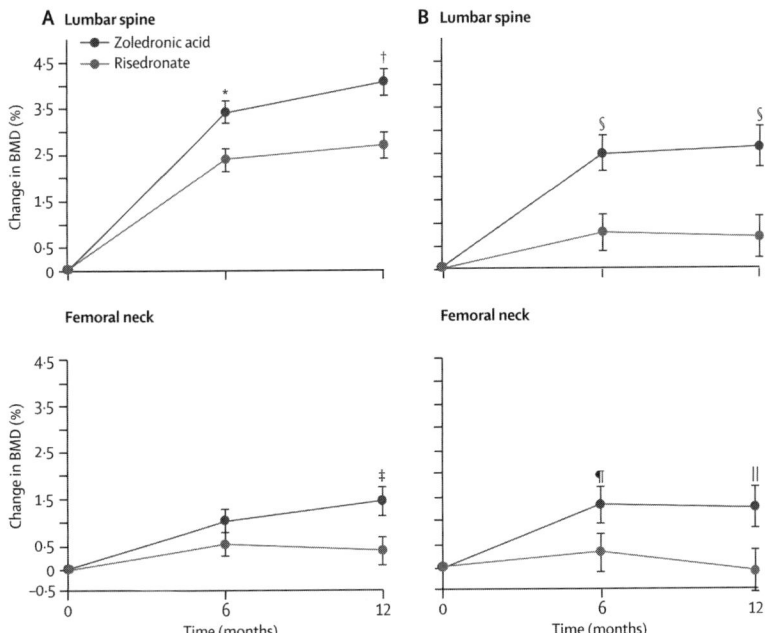

FIGURE 2.—Change in mean bone mineral density of lumbar spine and femoral neck for (A) treatment and (B) prevention subgroups (modified intention-to-treat group) Data are least-squares mean. Error bars=95% CI. BMD=bone mineral density. p values compare change in bone mineral density relative to baseline between drug groups, calculated from a three-way analysis of variance with adjustment for drug group, study region, and sex. *p=0·0005. †p=0·0001. ‡p=0·0050. §p<0·0001. ¶p=0·0156. ||p=0·0049. (Reprinted from Reid DM, Devogelaer J-P, Saag K, et al. Zoledronic acid and risedronate in the prevention and treatment of glucocorticoid-induced osteoporosis (HORIZON): a multicentre, double-blind, double-dummy, randomised controlled trial. *Lancet.* 2009;373:1253-1263, with permission from Elsevier Ltd.)

bone mineral density. Drug efficacy was assessed on a modified intention-to-treat basis and safety was assessed on an intention-to-treat basis. This trial is registered with ClinicalTrials.gov, number NCT00100620.

Findings.—Zoledronic acid was non-inferior and superior to risedronate for increase of lumbar spine bone mineral density in both the treatment (least-squares mean 4·06% [SE 0·28] *vs* 2·71% [SE 0·28], mean difference 1·36% [95% CI 0·67–2·05], p=0·0001) and prevention (2·60% [0·45] *vs* 0·64% [0·46], 1·96% [1·04–2·88], p<0·0001) subgroups at 12 months. Adverse events were more frequent in patients given zoledronic acid than in those on risedronate, largely as a result of transient symptoms during the first 3 days after infusion. Serious adverse events were worsening rheumatoid arthritis for the treatment subgroup and pyrexia for the prevention subgroup.

Interpretation.—A single 5 mg intravenous infusion of zoledronic acid is non-inferior, possibly more effective, and more acceptable to patients than is 5 mg of oral risedronate daily for prevention and treatment of bone loss that is associated with glucocorticoid use (Fig 2).

▶ Few head-to-head comparison studies are available for current drugs used to prevent or treat osteoporosis, and no studies are available that compare fracture reduction efficacy of any of the agents, due to the very large, long-term, and expensive studies that would be needed to demonstrate differences in fracture reduction.[1] A variety of agents have been approved to prevent or treat glucocorticoid-induced osteoporosis based on comparison with placebo.[2-4] For patients with glucocorticoid-induced osteoporosis, the only comparison study published to date showed that teriparatide was more effective than alendronate in preventing bone loss,[5] but this study was not powered to show fracture reduction. No studies have been available that compare the bone density or other effects of oral versus intravenous bisphosphonates in patients with glucocorticoid-induced osteoporosis.

This randomized, double-blind, double-dummy, non-inferiority study was conducted to determine whether zoledronic acid 5 mg intravenously over 15 minutes once a year was as effective as risedronate 5 mg orally once daily at preventing bone loss in patients treated with glucocorticoids. Over 800 patients taking glucocorticoids in 16 countries were randomized 1:1 to receive zoledronic acid or risedronate for 1 year. Zoledronic acid was shown to be non-inferior and superior to risedronate due to the increase in lumbar spine, femoral neck, total hip, and distal radius bone mineral density in both the treatment and prevention subgroups at 12 months (Fig 2). Adverse events were more frequent for the zoledronic acid group due to acute phase reactions during the first three days after infusions. The authors concluded that zoledronic acid was non-inferior, possibly more effective, and more acceptable to patients than risedronate for prevention and treatment of glucocorticoid-induced bone loss.

This study shows that intravenous and oral bisphosphonates may cause different magnitudes of beneficial effect on bone density at different skeletal sites in patients being treated for glucocorticoid-induced bone loss. While the study was not powered to show differences in fracture reduction, the greater improvement in bone density at all skeletal sites measured with zoledronic acid implies that fewer vertebral fractures might occur with zoledronic acid treatment. Future trials powered to show fracture reduction will be required to prove that zoledronic acid is more effective than risedronate in reducing fractures.

B. L. Clarke, MD

References

1. MacLean C, Newberry S, Maglione M, et al. Systematic review: comparative effectiveness of treatments to prevent fractures in men and women with low bone density or osteoporosis. *Ann Intern Med.* 2008;148:197-213.
2. Saag KG, Emkey R, Schnitzer TJ, et al. Alendronate for the prevention and treatment of glucocorticoid-induced osteoporosis. Glucocorticoid-Induced Osteoporosis Intervention Study Group. *N Engl J Med.* 1998;339:292-299.
3. Cohen S, Levy RM, Keller M, et al. Risedronate therapy prevents corticosteroid-induced bone loss: a twelve-month, multicenter, randomized, double-blind, placebo-controlled, parallel-group study. *Arthritis Rheum.* 1999;42:2309-2318.
4. Reid DM, Hughes RA, Laan RF, et al. Efficacy and safety of daily risedronate in the treatment of corticosteroid-induced osteoporosis in men and women: a randomized trial. European Corticosteroid-Induced Osteoporosis Treatment Study. *J Bone Miner Res.* 2000;15:1006-1013.
5. Saag KG, Shane E, Boonen S, et al. Teriparatide or alendronate in glucocorticoid-induced osteoporosis. *N Engl J Med.* 2007;357:2028-2039.

53 Diabetes

Effect of a Multifactorial Intervention on Mortality in Type 2 Diabetes
Gæde P, Lund-Andersen H, Parving H-H, et al (Steno Diabetes Ctr,
Copenhagen, Denmark; Copenhagen Univ Hosp, Denmark; et al)
N Engl J Med 358:580-591, 2008

Background.—Intensified multifactorial intervention — with tight glucose regulation and the use of renin–angiotensin system blockers, aspirin, and lipid-lowering agents — has been shown to reduce the risk of nonfatal cardiovascular disease among patients with type 2 diabetes mellitus and microalbuminuria. We evaluated whether this approach would have an effect on the rates of death from any cause and from cardiovascular causes.

Methods.—In the Steno-2 Study, we randomly assigned 160 patients with type 2 diabetes and persistent microalbuminuria to receive either intensive therapy or conventional therapy; the mean treatment period was 7.8 years. Patients were subsequently followed observationally for a mean of 5.5 years, until December 31, 2006. The primary end point at 13.3 years of follow-up was the time to death from any cause.

Results.—Twenty-four patients in the intensive-therapy group died, as compared with 40 in the conventional-therapy group (hazard ratio, 0.54; 95% confidence interval [CI], 0.32 to 0.89; $P = 0.02$). Intensive therapy was associated with a lower risk of death from cardiovascular causes (hazard ratio, 0.43; 95% CI, 0.19 to 0.94; $P = 0.04$) and of cardiovascular events (hazard ratio, 0.41; 95% CI, 0.25 to 0.67; $P<0.001$). One patient in the intensive-therapy group had progression to end-stage renal disease, as compared with six patients in the conventional-therapy group ($P = 0.04$). Fewer patients in the intensive-therapy group required retinal photocoagulation (relative risk, 0.45; 95% CI, 0.23 to 0.86; $P = 0.02$). Few major side effects were reported.

Conclusions.—In at-risk patients with type 2 diabetes, intensive intervention with multiple drug combinations and behavior modification had sustained beneficial effects with respect to vascular complications and on rates of death from any cause and from cardiovascular causes. (ClinicalTrials.gov number, NCT00320008.)

▶ This study is an observational follow-up study of the participants of the Steno-2 study, a randomized, controlled trial.

The Steno-2 study randomly assigned 160 subjects with type 2 diabetes and microalbuminuria to an intensive therapy or a conventional arm for a total of almost 8 years. In this observational follow-up study, subjects were followed for over 5 years after finishing the active treatment period.

After the end of the active study period, all patients and their primary care physicians were informed of the study finding. Their treatment then becomes much similar, and both groups were then managed with the same degree of intensity. Although the groups' glucose, blood pressure, and lipid control were similar during the follow-up period, their cardiovascular outcomes and mortality were very different, almost half in the previously intensively treated group.

These findings are consistent with those of the Diabetes Control and Complications Trial (DCCT), Epidemiology of Diabetes Interventions and Complications (EDIC), and UK Prospective Diabetes Study (UKPDS) follow-up studies underscoring the need and significant benefit of early aggressive treatment in diabetes. The reason for the continued and progressively larger difference in cardiovascular and mortality outcomes is not well understood, but has been ascribed to a so-called "metabolic memory" or "legacy effect."

F. Ovalle, MD

Effect of a Low–Glycemic Index or a High–Cereal Fiber Diet on Type 2 Diabetes: A Randomized Trial

Jenkins DJA, Kendall CWC, McKeown-Eyssen G, et al (Clinical Nutrition and Risk Factor Modification Ctr, Toronto, Ontario, Canada; Dalla Lana School of Public Health, Toronto, Ontario, Canada; et al)
JAMA 300:2742-2753, 2008

Context.—Clinical trials using antihyperglycemic medications to improve glycemic control have not demonstrated the anticipated cardiovascular benefits. Low–glycemic index diets may improve both glycemic control and cardiovascular risk factors for patients with type 2 diabetes but debate over their effectiveness continues due to trial limitations.

Objective.—To test the effects of low–glycemic index diets on glycemic control and cardiovascular risk factors in patients with type 2 diabetes.

Design, Setting, and Participants.—A randomized, parallel study design at a Canadian university hospital research center of 210 participants with type 2 diabetes treated with antihyperglycemic medications who were recruited by newspaper advertisement and randomly assigned to receive 1 of 2 diet treatments each for 6 months between September 16, 2004, and May 22, 2007.

Intervention.—High–cereal fiber or low–glycemic index dietary advice.

Main Outcome Measures.—Absolute change in glycated hemoglobin A_{1c} (HbA_{1c}), with fasting blood glucose and cardiovascular disease risk factors as secondary measures.

Results.—In the intention-to-treat analysis, HbA_{1c} decreased by -0.18% absolute HbA_{1c} units (95% confidence interval [CI], -0.29% to -0.07%) in the high–cereal fiber diet compared with -0.50% absolute HbA_{1c} units (95% CI, -0.61% to -0.39%) in the low–glycemic index diet ($P < .001$). There was also an increase of high-density lipoprotein cholesterol in the low–glycemic index diet by 1.7 mg/dL (95% CI, 0.8-2.6 mg/dL) compared with a decrease of high-density lipoprotein cholesterol by −0.2 mg/dL (95% CI, −0.9 to 0.5 mg/dL) in the high–cereal fiber diet ($P = .005$). The reduction in dietary glycemic index related positively to the reduction in HbA$_{1c}$ concentration ($r = 0.35$, $P < .001$) and negatively to the increase in high-density lipoprotein cholesterol ($r = −0.19$, $P = .009$).

Conclusion.—In patients with type 2 diabetes, 6-month treatment with a low–glycemic index diet resulted in moderately lower HbA$_{1c}$ levels compared with a high–cereal fiber diet.

Trial Registration.—clinicaltrials.gov identifier: NCT00438698.

▶ What is the best diet for subjects with diabetes? That is a question that remains unanswered.

Measuring the effect of diets on surrogate markers for cardiovascular disease is standard in clinical trials. However, the only way we will ever answer the question of which is the best diet will be by performing a prospective, randomized clinical trial comparing the effects of diets on patient-important outcomes, ie, cardiovascular events, sensation of well being, and mortality. After all, we need to remember that what patients want is for us (the physicians) to make them feel better, live happier, and live longer.

In the meantime, studies like this need to be viewed with some skepticism as long as the differences between treatment arms are small, which was the case in this study. The study was otherwise well conducted in a randomized, controlled fashion. The groups were well matched at baseline and the caloric content and overall macronutrient distribution for their diets was rather similar. The only major difference was that created by the intervention: low-glycemic index diet versus high-cereal fiber diet. The investigators concluded that a low-glycemic index diet results in a slightly better A$_{1c}$ and high-density lipoprotein (HDL) level than a high-cereal fiber diet.

F. Ovalle, MD

Effect of a Multifactorial Intervention on Mortality in Type 2 Diabetes

Gæde P, Lund-Andersen H, Parving H-H, et al (Steno Diabetes Ctr, Copenhagen; Glostrup Univ Hosp, Glostrup; et al)
N Engl J Med 358:580-591, 2008

Background.—Intensified multifactorial intervention — with tight glucose regulation and the use of renin–angiotensin system blockers, aspirin, and lipid-lowering agents — has been shown to reduce the risk of nonfatal cardiovascular disease among patients with type 2 diabetes mellitus and microalbuminuria. We evaluated whether this approach would have an effect on the rates of death from any cause and from cardio-vascular causes.

Methods.—In the Steno-2 Study, we randomly assigned 160 patients with type 2 diabetes and persistent microalbuminuria to receive either intensive therapy or conventional therapy; the mean treatment period was 7.8 years. Patients were subsequently followed observationally for a mean of 5.5 years, until December 31, 2006. The primary end point at 13.3 years of follow-up was the time to death from any cause.

Results.—Twenty-four patients in the intensive-therapy group died, as compared with 40 in the conventional-therapy group (hazard ratio, 0.54; 95% confidence interval [CI], 0.32 to 0.89; P = 0.02). Intensive therapy was associated with a lower risk of death from cardiovascular causes (hazard ratio, 0.43; 95% CI, 0.19 to 0.94; P = 0.04) and of cardiovascular events (hazard ratio, 0.41; 95% CI, 0.25 to 0.67; P < 0.001). One patient in the intensive-therapy group had progression to end-stage renal disease, as compared with six patients in the conventional-therapy group (P = 0.04). Fewer patients in the intensive-therapy group required retinal photocoagulation (relative risk, 0.45; 95% CI, 0.23 to 0.86; P = 0.02). Few major side effects were reported.

Conclusions.—In at-risk patients with type 2 diabetes, intensive intervention with multiple drug combinations and behavior modification had sustained beneficial effects with respect to vascular complications and on rates of death from any cause and from cardiovascular causes. (ClinicalTrials.gov number, NCT00320008.)

▶ Gæde et al report the follow-up data from the Steno-2 study. This is a multifactorial intervention study including glucose control, inhibition of the renin-angiotensin system, aspirin, and lipid lowering in patients with type 2 diabetes mellitus and microalbuminuria. The treatment goals were similar to those recommended by the American Diabetes Association (ADA). This included an HbA1c < 6.5%, fasting serum cholesterol < 175 mg/dl, fasting serum triglycerides < 150 mg/dl, and blood pressure < 130/80 mm Hg.

The initial trial ended after 7.8 years and showed risk reductions for vascular endpoints.

This recent follow-up study investigated the mortality after 13.3 years; the primary endpoint was death from any cause and from cardiovascular causes. 160 patients were included in the follow-up. As the initial results were positive, intensive therapy was recommended for all patients included in the study at the end of the original trial. As a result, HbA1c, blood pressure and lipids were comparable between the 2 groups at the end of the follow-up (13.3 years).

At the end of the follow-up, the intensive therapy led to a significant reduction in overall mortality by 20%, as well as to significant reductions in cardiovascular events and progression to end-stage renal disease.

Although the number of patients included was relatively small, the Steno-2 study is an important example to support the value of multifactorial interventions. This appears especially true in patients shortly after type 2 diabetes mellitus has been diagnosed. Of note, 50% of the patients in the conventional group died during the follow-up period. This underlines the importance of adequate and stringent therapy for those patients.

For further reading on this subject I suggest an article by Gaede et al.[1]

S. Schinner, MD

Reference

1. Gaede P, Vedel P, Larsen N, Jensen GV, Parving HH, Pedersen O. Multifactorial intervention and cardiovascular disease in patients with type 2 diabetes. *N Engl J Med.* 2003;348:383-393.

Intensive Blood Glucose Control and Vascular Outcomes in Patients with Type 2 Diabetes
The ADVANCE Collaborative Group (George Inst for International Health, Sydney, NSW, Australia; et al)
N Engl J Med 358:2560-2572, 2008

Background.—In patients with type 2 diabetes, the effects of intensive glucose control on vascular outcomes remain uncertain.

Methods.—We randomly assigned 11,140 patients with type 2 diabetes to undergo either standard glucose control or intensive glucose control, defined as the use of gliclazide (modified release) plus other drugs as required to achieve a glycated hemoglobin value of 6.5% or less. Primary end points were composites of major macrovascular events (death from cardiovascular causes, nonfatal myocardial infarction, or nonfatal stroke) and major microvascular events (new or worsening nephropathy or retinopathy), assessed both jointly and separately.

Results.—After a median of 5 years of follow-up, the mean glycated hemoglobin level was lower in the intensive-control group (6.5%) than in the standard-control group (7.3%). Intensive control reduced the incidence of combined major macrovascular and microvascular events (18.1%, vs. 20.0% with standard control; hazard ratio, 0.90; 95% confidence interval [CI], 0.82 to 0.98; P = 0.01), as well as that of major microvascular events (9.4% vs. 10.9%; hazard ratio, 0.86; 95% CI, 0.77 to 0.97; P = 0.01), primarily because of a reduction in the incidence of nephropathy (4.1% vs. 5.2%; hazard ratio, 0.79; 95% CI, 0.66 to 0.93; P = 0.006), with no significant effect on retinopathy (P = 0.50). There were no significant effects of the type of glucose control on major macrovascular events (hazard ratio with intensive control, 0.94; 95% CI, 0.84 to 1.06; P = 0.32), death from cardiovascular causes (hazard ratio with intensive control, 0.88; 95% CI, 0.74 to 1.04; P = 0.12), or death from any cause (hazard ratio with intensive control, 0.93; 95% CI, 0.83 to 1.06; P = 0.28). Severe hypoglycemia, although uncommon, was more common in the intensive-control group (2.7%, vs. 1.5% in the standard-control group; hazard ratio, 1.86; 95% CI, 1.42 to 2.40; P < 0.001).

Conclusions.—A strategy of intensive glucose control, involving gliclazide (modified release) and other drugs as required, that lowered the glycated hemoglobin value to 6.5% yielded a 10% relative reduction in the combined outcome of major macrovascular and microvascular events, primarily as a consequence of a 21% relative reduction in nephropathy. (ClinicalTrials.gov number, NCT00145925.)

▶ The Action in Diabetes and Vascular Disease: Preterax and Diamicron Modified Release Controlled Evaluation (ADVANCE) study investigated the effect of glucose lowering to an HbA1c target of < 6.5% on micro and macrovascular endpoints, and on mortality in patients with type 2 diabetes mellitus. The international multicenter study included 11 000 patients with a mean age of 66 years. The mean duration of diabetes was 7 years.

Glucose lowering to an HbA1c target in the intervention group was achieved primarily by the sulfonylurea gliclazide in addition to pre-existing medication. The control group was treated according to "standard treatment" to reach an HbA1c of 7.5%.

The intervention group received additional medication (oral antidiabetic drugs or insulin if needed) in addition to pre-existing drugs and gliclazide. Furthermore, these patients were encouraged for lifestyle modifications.

The primary endpoint was a composite of microvascular (nephropathy, retinopathy) and macrovascular (nonfatal myocardial infarction, nonfatal stroke, death from cardiovascular causes) events. After a median follow-up of 5 years, the HbA1c in the control group was 7.3% and 6.5% in the study group.

The primary endpoint (HR 0.90 [95% CI, 0.82-0.98]) as well as the incidence of microvascular events (HR 0.86 [95% CI, 0.77-0.97]) were significantly reduced in the intervention group ($P = 0.01$). However, the effect on microvascular events was significant only for nephropathy, not for retinopathy. In addition, the intervention group showed a 6% reduction in macrovascular events and a decrease in mortality (HR 0.93 [95% CI, 0.83-1.06] $P = 0.28$) (However, neither effect reached statistical significance.) This important multicenter study confirms the benefits of glucose lowering strategies for nephropathy. This is in line with data from the original U.K. Prospective Diabetes Study (UKPDS) that demonstrated a significant benefit for microvascular endpoints with an HbA1c target of 7% while macrovascular benefits did not reach statistical significance.[1,2] The data from the ADVANCE study is seemingly in contrast to the Action to Control Cardiovascular Risk in Diabetes (ACCORD) study[3] that demonstrated an increase in mortality with an HbA1c target < 6%. Notably, the patients in the ADVANCE study were younger and had less of a cardiovascular burden than those in the ACCORD study. In addition, the approach to glucose lowering was less aggressive in the ADVANCE study.

It is also interesting to compare ADVANCE with the 10 year follow-up data of the UKPDS study,[4] which indicated that macrovascular effects of glucose-lowering therapies need more time to become evident than microvascular effects.

The ADVANCE study confirms the importance of early treatment of patients with type 2 diabetes mellitus to avoid diabetes-related long-term complications.

S. Schinner, MD

References

1. UK Prospective Diabetes Study (UKPDS) Group. Intensive blood-glucose control with sulphonylureas or insulin compared with conventional treatment and risk of complications in patients with type 2 diabetes (UKPDS 33). *Lancet.* 1998; 352:837-853 [Erratum, Lancet 1999;354:602.].
2. UK Prospective Diabetes Study (UKPDS) Group. Effect of intensive blood-glucose control with metformin on complications in overweight patients with type 2 diabetes (UKPDS 34). *Lancet.* 1998;352:854-865 [Erratum, Lancet 1998;352:1558.].
3. The Action to Control Cardiovascular Risk in Diabetes (ACCORD) Study Group. Effects of intensive glucose lowering in type 2 diabetes. *N Engl J Med.* 2008;358: 2545-2559.
4. Holman RR, et al. 10 year follow-up of intensive glucose control in type 2 diabetes mellitus. *N Engl J Med.* 2008;359:15.

10-Year Follow-up of Intensive Glucose Control in Type 2 Diabetes

Holman RR, Paul SK, Bethel MA, et al (Diabetes Trials Unit, Oxford, UK; et al)
N Engl J Med 359:1577-1589, 2008

Background.—During the United Kingdom Prospective Diabetes Study (UKPDS), patients with type 2 diabetes mellitus who received intensive glucose therapy had a lower risk of microvascular complications than did those receiving conventional dietary therapy. We conducted post-trial monitoring to determine whether this improved glucose control persisted and whether such therapy had a long-term effect on macrovascular outcomes.

Methods.—Of 5102 patients with newly diagnosed type 2 diabetes, 4209 were randomly assigned to receive either conventional therapy (dietary restriction) or intensive therapy (either sulfonylurea or insulin or, in overweight patients, metformin) for glucose control. In post-trial monitoring, 3277 patients were asked to attend annual UKPDS clinics for 5 years, but no attempts were made to maintain their previously assigned therapies. Annual questionnaires were used to follow patients who were unable to attend the clinics, and all patients in years 6 to 10 were assessed through questionnaires. We examined seven prespecified aggregate clinical outcomes from the UKPDS on an intention-to-treat basis, according to previous randomization categories.

Results.—Between-group differences in glycated hemoglobin levels were lost after the first year. In the sulfonylurea–insulin group, relative reductions in risk persisted at 10 years for any diabetes-related end point (9%, P = 0.04) and microvascular disease (24%, P = 0.001), and risk reductions for myocardial infarction (15%, P = 0.01) and death from any cause (13%, P = 0.007) emerged over time, as more events occurred. In the metformin group, significant risk reductions persisted for any diabetes-related end point (21%, P = 0.01), myocardial infarction (33%, P = 0.005), and death from any cause (27%, P = 0.002).

Conclusions.—Despite an early loss of glycemic differences, a continued reduction in microvascular risk and emergent risk reductions for myocardial infarction and death from any cause were observed during 10 years of post-trial follow-up. A continued benefit after metformin therapy was evident among overweight patients. (UKPDS 80; Current Controlled Trials number, ISRCTN75451837.)

▶ Holman and colleagues report the 10-year follow-up of the United Kingdom Prospective Diabetes Study (UKPDS). In this initial study, 5000 patients newly diagnosed with type 2 diabetes mellitus were treated either with conventional therapy (ie, diet) or with intensive therapy (ie, sulfonylurea/insulin or metformin [when overweight]). The target fasting blood glucose level in the intensively treated group was <110 mg/dl (6.0 mmol/l). The HbA1c reached was 7.0 in the sulfonylurea/insulin group, 7.4 in the metformin group, and 8.0 in the conventional group. Importantly, the patients were relatively young (53 years) and healthy (virtually no cardiovascular disease) when they entered the study. The mean duration of treatment was 10.7 years, but patients could have been in the trial for 6 to 20 years. Thereafter, the intervention study was stopped and patients were treated in community hospitals according to "normal standards."

This recent study by Holman et al investigated the follow-up results as a post-interventional study. Patients had yearly clinical and biochemical examinations for 5 years, and yearly questionnaires for another 5 years.

As expected, the HbA1c control was lost postinterventionally after 1 year (ie, 1 year after the intervention stopped); there was no statistical difference in the HbA1c levels in initially intensively versus conventionally treated patients. There were no differences in lipid profiles or blood pressure between the groups at any time.

However, after 10 years, the intensively treated patients had a significant reduction in the prevalence for any diabetes-related end point (ie, sudden death, death from hyperglycemia or hypoglycemia, fatal or nonfatal myocardial infarction, angina, heart failure, fatal or nonfatal stroke, renal failure, amputation, vitreous hemorrhage, retinal photocoagulation, blindness, cataract extraction). In addition, they had significantly less diabetes-related causes of death, death from any cause, myocardial infarction, and microvascular disease (only significant in the sulfonylurea-insulin group).

This is an extremely important study as it demonstrates the benefits of early treatment of type 2 diabetes mellitus. A number of studies had previously shown that glycemic control improves microvascular complications while failing statistical significance for macrovascular end points. However, in this study macrovascular complications were significantly reduced by targeting glycemic control. This suggests that it takes years until the benefits of glucose control become evident for macrovascular end points. At the same time, it is interesting that the patients in this study took advantage of diabetes control 10 years after the intervention trial was stopped. This implies a "glucose memory" (so-called legacy effect) over years, or even decades, and poses a very strong argument for early treatment of type 2 diabetes mellitus.[1-3]

S. Schinner, MD

References

1. UK Prospective Diabetes Study (UKPDS) Group. Intensive blood-glucose control with sulphonylureas or insulin compared with conventional treatment and risk of complications in patients with type 2 diabetes (UKPDS 33). *Lancet.* 1998; 352:837-853 [Erratum, Lancet 1999;354:602].
2. Gaede P, Lund-Andersen H, Parving HH, Pedersen O. Effect of a multifactorial intervention on mortality in type 2 diabetes. *N Engl J Med.* 2008;358:580-591.
3. The Diabetes Control and Complications Trial Research Group. The effect of intensive treatment of diabetes on the development and progression of long-term complications of insulin-dependent diabetes mellitus. *N Engl J Med.* 1993;329: 977-986.

Can metabolic syndrome usefully predict cardiovascular disease and diabetes? Outcome data from two prospective studies
Sattar N, McConnachie A, Shaper AG, et al (Univ of Glasgow, UK; Royal Free and Univ College Med School, London, UK; et al)
Lancet 371:1927-1935, 2008

Background.—Clinical use of criteria for metabolic syndrome to simultaneously predict risk of cardiovascular disease and diabetes remains uncertain. We investigated to what extent metabolic syndrome and its individual components were related to risk for these two diseases in elderly populations.

Methods.—We related metabolic syndrome (defined on the basis of criteria from the Third Report of the National Cholesterol Education Program) and its five individual components to the risk of events of incident cardiovascular disease and type 2 diabetes in 4812 non-diabetic individuals aged 70–82 years from the Prospective Study of Pravastatin in the Elderly at Risk (PROSPER). We corroborated these data in a second prospective study (the British Regional Heart Study [BRHS]) of 2737 non-diabetic men aged 60–79 years.

Findings.—In PROSPER, 772 cases of incident cardiovascular disease and 287 of diabetes occurred over 3·2 years. Metabolic syndrome was not associated with increased risk of cardiovascular disease in those without baseline disease (hazard ratio 1·07 [95% CI 0·86–1·32]) but was associated with increased risk of diabetes (4·41 [3·33-5·84]) as was each of its components, particularly fasting glucose (18·4 [13·9–24·5]). Results were similar in participants with existing cardiovascular disease. In BRHS, 440 cases of incident cardiovascular disease and 105 of diabetes occurred over 7 years. Metabolic syndrome was modestly associated with incident cardiovascular disease (relative risk 1·27 [1·04–1·56]) despite strong association with diabetes (7·47 [4·90–11·46]). In both studies, body-mass index or waist circumference, triglyceride, and glucose cutoff points were not associated with risk of cardiovascular disease, but all five components were associated with risk of new-onset diabetes.

Interpretation.—Metabolic syndrome and its components are associated with type 2 diabetes but have weak or no association with vascular risk in elderly populations, suggesting that attempts to define criteria that simultaneously predict risk for both cardiovascular disease and diabetes are unhelpful. Clinical focus should remain on establishing optimum risk algorithms for each disease.

▶ The concept of the "metabolic syndrome" (ie, the cluster of xxx) has received substantial attention over the past decades. In particular, this concept has improved our understanding of the interplay of obesity and insulin resistance with comorbidities like diabetes mellitus, arterial hypertension, and dyslipidemia. However, it is not clear whether the definition of the metabolic syndrome allows a prediction of clinical outcome parameters like cardiovascular disease or the manifestation of diabetes mellitus.

In the present report by Sattar et al, a total number of approximately 7500 patients were included consisting of 2 separate prospective studies (PROSPER and BRHS). Notably, the mean age of the patients at entry in the study was 75 years and 68 years respectively. The patients were screened for components of the metabolic syndrome at the beginning of the study. The diagnosis of diabetes mellitus at the beginning of the study was an exclusion criterion. After follow-up of 3.2 years the authors found a strong correlation of the metabolic syndrome and its individual components (BMI, waist circumference, triglyceride levels, fasting glucose) with the onset of diabetes mellitus. However, the association with cardiovascular disease was only weak. The metabolic syndrome was not a better predictor of cardiovascular disease than the individual components, but predicted future diabetes better than the single components (besides the fasting blood glucose level) in elderly people. Similarly, previous studies showed inferiority of the metabolic to conventional risk scores like the Framingham risk score in predicting cardiovascular disease in middle-aged men. This might be explained by the inclusion of smoking as a major risk factor in conventional cardiovascular risk scores, but not in the metabolic syndrome.

Therefore, the sum of the components defining the metabolic syndrome appears not to be a stronger predictor of cardiovascular events or the manifestation of diabetes mellitus than the individual components.

However, the major limitation of the study is the relatively short follow-up (3.2 years). Other studies with vascular endpoints pointed out that cardiovascular benefits might take time to develop (see UKPDS 10 year follow-up).

For further reading on this subject I suggest articles by Wannamethee et al,[1] Gami et al,[2] and Stern et al.[3]

S. Schinner, MD

References

1. Wannamethee SG, Shaper AG, Lennon L, Morris RW. Metabolic syndrome vs Framingham Risk Score for prediction of coronary heart disease, stroke, and type 2 diabetes mellitus. *Arch Intern Med.* 2005;165:2644-2650.
2. Gami AS, Witt BJ, Howard DE, et al. Metabolic syndrome and risk of incident cardiovascular events and death: a systematic review and meta-analysis of longitudinal studies. *J Am Coll Cardiol.* 2007;49:403-414.
3. Stern MP, Williams K, Gonzalez-Villalpando C, Hunt KJ, Haffner SM. Does the metabolic syndrome improve identification of individuals at risk of type 2 diabetes and/or cardiovascular disease? *Diabetes Care.* 2004;27:2676-2681.

54 Lipoproteins and Atherosclerosis

Adherence to the Mediterranean Diet Is Inversely Associated With Circulating Interleukin-6 Among Middle-Aged Men: A Twin Study
Dai J, Miller AH, Bremner JD, et al (Emory Univ, Atlanta, GA; Emory Univ School of Medicine, Atlanta, GA; et al)
Circulation 117:169-175, 2008

Background.—The Mediterranean diet is protective against cardiovascular disease; a proposed mechanism is through a reduction in systemic inflammation. It is unknown to what extent the association between the Mediterranean diet and inflammation is due to genetic or other familial factors.

Methods and Results.—We administered the Willett food frequency questionnaire to 345 middle-aged male twins and assessed adherence to the Mediterranean diet using a published adherence score. Fasting plasma levels of interleukin-6, C-reactive protein, and known cardiovascular risk factors were measured. Mixed-effect regression analyses were used to examine the relationship between diet score and inflammatory biomarkers after accounting for known cardiovascular risk factors. Adherence to the Mediterranean diet was associated with reduced levels of interleukin-6 ($P<0.001$) but not C-reactive protein ($P = 0.10$) after adjustment for total energy intake, other nutritional factors, known cardiovascular risk factors, and use of supplements and medications. When the overall association of adherence to the diet with interleukin-6 levels was partitioned into between- and within-pair effects, the between-pair effect was not significant ($P = 0.9$) and the within-pair effect was highly significant ($P<0.0001$). A 1-unit within-pair absolute difference in the diet score was associated with a 9% (95% CI, 4.5 to 13.6) lower interleukin-6 level.

Conclusions.—Shared environmental and genetic factors are unlikely to play a major role in the association between adherence to the Mediterranean diet and systemic inflammation. These results support the hypothesis that reduced inflammation is an important mechanism linking Mediterranean diet to reduced cardiovascular risk.

▶ The Mediterranean diet has beneficial effects on cardiovascular disease. Metabolic diseases like obesity with insulin resistance and type 2 diabetes mellitus predisposing to coronary heart disease are associated with chronic, subclinical inflammation.

These metabolic disorders are characterized by elevated serum levels of the proinflammatory cytokines. Consistently, the proinflammatory cytokine IL-6 is elevated in obesity, impaired glucose tolerance (IGT), and type 2 diabetes mellitus. However, the relative contributions of genetic and environmental factors to systemic inflammation are not known. Therefore, this article investigated diet-mediated effects on proinflammatory serum markers in twins. Three hundred and forty-five male twins were included and followed by a food questionnaire. Adherence to Mediterranean diet was significantly inversely associated with the IL-6 levels, but not with C-reactive protein. This effect persisted within pairs, but was not significant between pairs.

The latter might be due to the common family environment.

The subject of the study is of great public interest, as Mediterranean diet habits have become more popular in western societies. At the same time, feasible primary prevention strategies for cardiovascular disease have become more important. However, one must add that this study included only middle-aged men, and can therefore only be translated to women with caution.

The strength of the study is clearly the inclusion of twins, thereby having a better estimate of environmental factors contributing to proinflammation and cardiovascular risk.

To date there is increasing evidence from a number of in vitro, ex vivo, and clinical studies for the association of subclinical inflammation with obesity and type 2 diabetes mellitus. It has been shown that circulating leukocytes from patients with type 2 diabetes mellitus are activated. In line with this, the levels of cytokines and chemokines are elevated in serum and plasma of (pre) diabetic subjects. Consistently, subclinical inflammation has been shown to induce insulin resistance. Adipose tissue seems to play an important role in this process: On one hand, the adipose tissue is characterized by macrophage accumulation and local inflammation in obesity; on the other hand adipocytes can secrete proinflammatory cytokines on their own. These factors can thereafter contribute to local inflammation within the walls of blood vessels. In line with this, an accumulation of macrophages is a typical feature of atherosclerotic lesions.

Therefore, antiinflammatory strategies, either pharmacological or diet based, are important tools for the prevention of atherosclerosis.[1-4]

S. Schinner, MD

M. Schott, MD, PhD

References

1. Forst T, Hohberg C, Pfützner A. Cardiovascular effects of disturbed insulin activity in metabolic syndrome and in type 2 diabetic patients. *Horm Metab Res.* 2009;41: 123-131.
2. Averill MM, Bornfeldt KE. Lipids versus glucose in inflammation and the pathogenesis of macrovascular disease in diabetes. *Curr Diab Rep.* 2009;9:18-25. Review.

3. Trichopoulou A, Costacou T, Bamia C, Trichopoulos D. Adherence to a Mediterranean diet and survival in a Greek population. *N Engl J Med.* 2003;348: 2599-2608.
4. Serra-Majem L, Roman B, Estruch R. Scientific evidence of interventions using the Mediterranean diet: a systematic review. *Nutr Rev.* 2006;64:S27-S47.

Alcohol consumption and blood lipids in elderly coronary patients

de Jong HJI, de Goede J, Oude Griep LM, et al (Wageningen Univ, The Netherlands)
Metabolism 57:1286-1292, 2008

Alcohol may have a beneficial effect on coronary heart disease (CHD) that could be mediated by elevation of high-density lipoprotein cholesterol (HDLC). Data on alcohol consumption and blood lipids in coronary patients are scarce. We studied whether total ethanol intake and consumption of specific types of beverages are associated with blood lipids in older subjects with CHD. Blood lipids were measured in 1052 myocardial infarction patients aged 60 to 80 years (78% male). Intake of alcoholic beverages, total ethanol, and macronutrients was assessed by food frequency questionnaire. Seventy percent of the subjects used lipid-lowering medication. Total cholesterol was on average 5.14 mmol/L, and HDLC was on average 1.28 mmol/L. Among men, total ethanol intake was positively associated with HDLC (difference of 0.094 mmol/L for ≥ 15 g/d vs 0 g/d, $P = .024$), whereas the association with HDLC among women was not significant (difference of 0.060 mmol/L for ≥ 5 g/d vs 0 g/d, $P = .560$) after adjustment for dietary, lifestyle, and CHD risk factors. Liquor consumption was weakly positively associated with HDLC in men $(P = .045)$. Beer consumption in men and wine consumption in women were also positively associated with HDLC, but were not significant in the fully adjusted model. In conclusion, moderate alcohol consumption may elevate HDLC in treated post–myocardial infarction patients. This may be due to ethanol and not to other beneficial substances in alcoholic beverages. Based on this finding, further research needs to be done to examine the effects of the residual substances from different types of alcoholic beverages on HDLC.

▶ Moderate alcohol intake (2 alcoholic drinks per day, corresponding to 20-40 g alcohol) decreases the risk for cardiovascular disease. This has led to the so-called French paradox (ie, the lower risk for cardiovascular disease in France which was initially thought to be mediated by polyphenols like resveratrol that are contained in red wine). Nowadays, there is evidence that white wine might have similar effects. Several mechanisms of action have been proposed to explain the beneficial effects of moderate alcohol consumption:

1. An altered lipoprotein pattern: high-density lipoprotein (HDL) is increased and low-density lipoprotein (LDL) decreased in individuals with moderate alcohol consumption.

2. Moderate alcohol consumption can have favorable effects on platelet coagulation.

The purpose of this study was to evaluate the effect of alcohol consumption on lipid profiles in 4837 elderly patients (68 and 70 years of age in men and women respectively) with coronary heart disease. The results were slightly different between men and women: In men, there was a significant positive correlation between alcohol intake and HDL cholesterol levels; this was not significant in women. Interestingly, this trend was also seen for beer and liquor, although with weak or no statistical significance. This study adds further evidence for beneficial effects of moderate alcohol consumption on cardiovascular risk parameters. It is still a matter of debate how this protective effect can be explained, and whether it is linked to wine consumption. There is a lot of basic science done on molecular effects of polyphenols on cellular aging and stress response in in vitro and animal studies. It will be a future challenge to test whether these cellular effects can be translated into clinical medicine.[1-3]

S. Schinner, MD
M. Schott, MD, PhD

References

1. Opie LH, Lecour S. The red wine hypothesis: from concepts to protective signalling molecules. *Eur Heart J.* 2007;28:1683-1693.
2. Das S, Das DK. Resveratrol: a therapeutic promise for cardiovascular diseases. *Recent Pat Cardiovasc Drug Discov.* 2007;2:133-138.
3. Zhuang H, Kim YS, Koehler RC, Doré S. Potential mechanism by which resveratrol, a red wine constituent, protects neurons. *Ann N Y Acad Sci.* 2003;993:276-286.

Dietary fat and sleep duration in Chinese men and women

Shi Z, McEvoy M, Luu J, et al (Univ of Newcastle, NSW, Australia; John Hunter Hosp, Newcastle, NSW, Australia)
Int J Obes (Lond) 32:1835-1840, 2008

Background.—Many recent studies have highlighted the complex interaction between sleep duration, food intake and metabolic balance. Although a causal link is yet to be established, emerging evidence suggests that short sleep duration may alter the balance between energy intake and energy expenditure. Thus far, most research has focussed on the link between sleep duration and carbohydrate metabolism. The role of sleep duration in fat intake and vice versa remains relatively unknown.

Objective.—The aim of this analysis was to determine whether there exists a significant association between sleep duration and fat intake.

Design.—Data from 2828 adults living in Jiangsu province, China, collected during a national survey of nutrition and health conducted in 2002.

Results.—The analysis showed a statistically significant association between sleep duration and fat and carbohydrate intake but not protein or fasting blood glucose. Those who slept for less than 7 h a day had significantly higher ($P = 0.005$) percentage of energy from fat intake than those who slept for 7–9 h per day. Analysis of the influence of high fat intake upon sleep demonstrated a trend to reduced sleep duration between the highest and lowest quartiles of fat intake ($P = 0.056$).

Conclusions.—To our knowledge, this is the first data from a large cross-sectional study to show an association between decreased sleep duration and increased fat intake in humans. Given the trend towards decreased sleep duration in modern societies and the parallel obesity epidemic, the significance of this association warrants more research.

▶ Western lifestyle promotes the prevalence of obesity. The western food composition and sedentary lifestyle contribute to adiposity. However, more recent data suggest a role for sleep duration in regulating eating habits. Short sleep duration correlates with the body mass index (BMI), and sleep duration is nowadays shorter (7 h) than 50 years ago (9 h).

The study by Shi et al reports on a large-scale epidemiologic survey in China; 2828 adults were included. The data showed increased fat intake when the sleep duration per day was less than 7 h. Surprisingly, the carbohydrate intake was decreased with a sleep duration of less than 7 h. This might be explained by local (ie, Chinese) dietary habits.

This study is one of few large-scale reports on the interaction between sleep duration and food intake in humans. The most important limitation is the fact that sleeping and eating habit data are based on self-report. However, in such large populations it is hard to collect data on eating and sleeping by direct external measurement.

What are the potential mechanisms linking sleep duration with obesity?

(1) Adipokines regulate food intake. Leptin suppresses appetite and ghrelin increases appetite. Shorter sleep duration leads to decreased levels of leptin and increased levels of ghrelin. Interestingly, sleep duration also directs our appetite toward energy-dense food.

(2) The regulation of metabolism is governed by the so-called circadian clock. On the molecular levels, this means a circadian regulation of transcriptional processes, leading to timely regulated hormone secretion. Of note, also adipocytes as endocrine active cells were shown to have circadian regulation.

(3) Altered hypothalamic secretion of hormones regulates food intake (eg, orexin).

Further studies are needed to evaluate epidemiological data in large samples of different ethnic origin. Moreover, future basic science studies will help to understand the underlying mechanisms.

For further reading on this subject I suggest articles by Cizza et al,[1] Taheri,[2] and Spiegal et al.[3]

S. Schinner, MD
M. Schott, MD, PhD

References

1. Cizza G, Skarulis M, Mignot E. A link between short sleep duration and obesity: building the evidence for causation. *Sleep*. 2005;28:1217-1220.
2. Taheri S. The link between short sleep duration and obesity: we should recommend more sleep to prevent obesity. *Arch Dis Child*. 2006;91:881-884.
3. Spiegal K, Leproult R, Van Cauter E. Impact of sleep debt on metabolic and endocrine function. *Lancet*. 1999;354:1435-1439.

55 Neuroendocrinology

High prevalence of biochemical acromegaly in primary care patients with elevated IGF-1 levels

Schneider HJ, Sievers C, Saller B, et al (Ludwig-Maximilian-Univ, Munich, Germany; Max Planck Inst of Psychiatry, Munich, Germany; Pfizer Ltd, EBT Endocrine Care, Walton Oaks, UK; et al)

Clin Endocrinol 69:432-435, 2008

Objective.—The estimated prevalence of acromegaly is 40–125 per million. The diagnosis of acromegaly is often delayed due to deficits in recognizing the signs of the disease. It is not known how many subjects with increased IGF-1 levels have acromegaly. We aimed to assess the prevalence of acromegaly in primary care by screening for elevated IGF-1 levels.

Design.—A cross-sectional, epidemiological study (the DETECT study).

Patients.—A total of 6773 unselected adult primary care patients were included.

Measurements.—We measured IGF-1 in all patients and recommended further endocrine evaluation in all patients with elevated IGF-1 levels (> 2 age-dependent SDS).

Results.—Of 125 patients with elevated IGF-1 levels, 76 patients had indeterminate results and acromegaly could be excluded in 42 patients. One patient had known florid acromegaly. Two patients had newly diagnosed acromegaly and pituitary adenomas. Four patients had biochemical acromegaly but refused further diagnostics. This corresponds to a prevalence of 1034 per million patients.

Conclusions.—Our study shows a high prevalence of undiagnosed acromegaly in primary care. These results imply that acromegaly is underdiagnosed and stress the importance of detecting acromegaly.

▶ The incidence of acromegaly is commonly reported to be about 3.5 cases per million, with the incidence as high as 125 cases per million. However, because of the rarity of the disease and the prolonged clinical onset of symptoms, some investigators question whether the diagnosis is substantially underappreciated. To address this concern, these authors assessed the insulin-like growth factor-I (IGF-1) levels of 6773 patients from multiple centers in a cross-sectional, epidemiological study (the Diabetes Cardiovascular Risk-Evaluation: Targets and Essential Data for Commitment of Treatment [DETECT] study). In this analysis, 125 patients were noted to have elevated IGF-1. After excluding those patients with indeterminate follow-up testing, they determined that 7 of the 6773 patients screened had acromegaly. This corresponds to a prevalence of 1034 cases per million. This data dramatically brings into question the accuracy of previous estimates of the prevalence of acromegaly in the general population. It further supports the impetus to implement broad screening for the disease in the general population because screening in only those patients with marked clinical signs of acromegaly may miss a substantial proportion of patients with active disease.

W. H. Ludlam, MD, PhD

Growth Hormone Treatment on Atherosclerosis: Results of a 5-Year Open, Prospective, Controlled Study in Male Patients with Severe Growth Hormone Deficiency
Colao A, Di Somma C, Spiezia S, et al ("Federico II" Univ of Naples, Italy; "S. Maria degli Incurabili" Hosp of Naples, Italy)
J Clin Endocrinol Metab 93:3416-3424, 2008

Background.—Severe GH deficiency (GHD) is associated with increased cardiovascular risk and intima-media thickness (IMT) at major arteries.

Objective.—The objective of the study was to investigate the 5-yr effects of GH replacement on common carotid IMT and insulin resistance syndrome (IRS) (at least two of the following: triglycerides levels ≥ 1.7 mmol/liter, high-density lipoprotein-cholesterol levels ≤ 1.0 mmol/liter, blood pressure above 130/85 mm Hg, fasting glucose 6.1–7 or 2 hr after glucose 7.7–11.1 mmol/liter).

Design.—This was an interventional, open, prospective, controlled study.

Patients.—Patients included 35 men with severe GHD and 35 age-matched healthy men as controls.

Intervention.—All patients received standard replacement therapy; GH replacement was added in 22 patients (group A) and refused by 13 others (group B).

Measurements.—Five-year changes in IMT and IRS prevalence were measured.

Results.—At baseline, IMT was higher in the patients with ($P < 0.001$) and without IRS ($P = 0.004$) than in controls. Eighteen patients (51.4%) and two controls (5.7%; $P < 0.0001$) had IRS. At study end, use of lipid-lowering drugs (92.3, *vs.* 13.6 and 34.3%, $P < 0.0001$), glucose-lowering drugs (69.2 *vs.* 31.4 and 22.7%; $P = 0.016$), and antihypertensive drugs (61.5 vs. 20.0 and 4.5%; $P < 0.0001$) was higher in group B patients than controls and group A patients. IGF-I levels normalized in all group A patients and remained lower than -1 sd score in 77% of group B patients. IMT significantly decreased only in group A and significantly increased in controls and nonsignificantly in group B patients. IRS prevalence significantly reduced only in group A patients.

Conclusions.—Severely hypopituitary GHD men have more frequently increased IMT at common carotid arteries and IRS than controls. After 5 years, only in GH replaced patients, IMT and prevalence of IRS decreased.

▶ Growth hormone deficiency (GHD) is associated with a variety of cardiovascular risks, including anomalies in lipid metabolism, increased visceral fat distribution, glucose intolerance, insulin resistance, hypertension, and increased intima-media thickness (IMT) of major arteries. Although many of these parameters improve with GH treatment, a previously performed 2-year study failed to show improvement in IMT. To address the question of whether longer GH treatment is necessary to reduce progression of early atherosclerosis, these authors designed a 5-year observational, prospective, controlled study to investigate the effects of long-term GH replacement on common carotid artery IMT and insulin resistance syndrome. These authors noted that IMT and insulin resistance was higher in 35 severe GHD patients than 35 controls at baseline. However, after 5 years of GH treatment in 22 of the 35 GHD patients, both IMT and insulin resistance significantly decreased compared with the 13 GHD that were not treated with GH. These authors also noted that the use of lipid-lowering, glucose-lowering, and antihypertensive medications was higher in the GHD patients not treated with GH. These results further support the positive effects of GH replacement in GHD individuals on cardiovascular risk reduction.

W. H. Ludlam, MD, PhD

Quality of Life in Acromegalic Patients during Long-Term Somatostatin Analog Treatment with and without Pegvisomant

Neggers SJCMM, van Aken MO, de Herder WW, et al (Erasmus Univ Med Ctr Rotterdam, The Netherlands; et al)
J Clin Endocrinol Metab 93:3853-3859, 2008

Objective.—The objective of the study was to assess whether weekly administration of 40 mg pegvisomant (PEG-V) improves quality of life (QoL) and metabolic parameters in acromegalic patients with normal age-adjusted IGF-I concentrations during long-acting somatostatin analog (SSA) treatment.

Design.—This was a prospective, investigator-initiated, double blind, placebo-controlled, crossover study. Twenty acromegalic subjects received either PEG-V or placebo for two consecutive treatment periods of 16 wk, separated by a washout period of 4 wk. Efficacy was assessed as change between baseline and end of each treatment period. QoL was assessed by the Acromegaly Quality of Life Questionnaire (AcroQoL) and the Patient-Assessed Acromegaly Symptom Questionnaire (PASQ).

Results.—The AcroQoL (P = 0.008) and AcroQoL physical (P = 0.002) improved significantly after PEG-V was added. The addition of PEG-V also significantly improved the PASQ (P = 0.038) and the single PASQ questions, perspiration (P = 0.024), soft tissue swelling (P = 0.036), and overall health status (P = 0.035). No significant change in Z-score of IGF-I (P = 0.34) was observed during addition of PEG-V. Transient liver enzyme elevations were observed in five subjects (25%).

Conclusion.—Improvement in quality of life was observed without significant change in IGF-I after the addition of 40 mg pegvisomant weekly to monthly SSA therapy in acromegalic patients who had normalized IGF-I on SSA monotherapy. These data question the current recommendations in how to assess disease activity in acromegaly. Moreover, the findings question the validity of the current approach of medical treatment in which pegvisomant is used only when SSA therapy has failed to normalize IGF-I.

▶ Quality of life is often suboptimal in acromegaly patients effectively treated biochemically. This issue poses a significant challenge for the treating physician. One possible explanation for the discordance between the normalization of growth hormone (GH) levels and persistent symptoms is that achieving traditionally accepted biochemical treatment goals may not truly normalize the effects of GH overproduction. To address this question, these authors performed a double-blinded, placebo-controlled, crossover study in which patients who were already "well controlled" on long-term somatostatin analog (SA) treatment (ie, had normal insulin-like growth factor 1 [IGF-1] levels) were additionally treated with 40 mg pegvisomant per week. They found that quality of life in patients treated with both SA and pegvisomant had significant improvement in quality of life as measured by both the Acromegaly Quality of Life Questionnaire (AcroQoL) and the Patient-Assessed Acromegaly Symptom Questionnaire (PASQ). These authors believe that their data (1) challenge the biochemical parameters that are considered acceptable in assessing effective treatment of acromegaly, and (2) the algorithm that pegvisomant should only be used when SA monotherapy is inadequate to normalize IGF-1.

W. H. Ludlam, MD, PhD

Effects of an Oral Growth Hormone Secretagogue in Older Adults
White HK, Petrie CD, Landschulz W, et al (Durham Veterans Affairs (VA) Med Ctr, Durham, NC; Pfizer Global Res and Development, Groton, CT; Eli Lilly and Co., Indianapolis, IN; et al)
J Clin Endocrinol Metab 94:1198-1206, 2009

Context.—GH secretion declines with age, possibly contributing to reduced muscle mass, strength, and function. GH secretagogues (GHS) may increase muscle mass and physical performance.

Objectives/Design.—We conducted a randomized, double-masked, placebo-controlled, multicenter study to investigate the hormonal, body composition, and physical performance effects and the safety of the orally active GHS capromorelin in older adults with mild functional limitation.

Intervention/Participants.—A total of 395 men and women aged 65–84 yr were randomized for an intended 2 yr of treatment to four dosing groups (10 mg three times/week, 3 mg twice a day, 10 mg each night, and 10 mg twice a day) or placebo. Although the study was terminated early according to predetermined treatment effect criteria, 315 subjects completed 6 months of treatment, and 284 completed 12 months.

Results.—A sustained dose-related rise in IGF-I concentrations occurred in all active treatment groups. Each capromorelin dose prompted a rise in peak nocturnal GH, which was greatest with the least frequent dosing. At 6 months, body weight increased 1.4 kg in subjects receiving capromorelin and decreased 0.2 kg in those receiving placebo ($P = 0.006$). Lean body mass increased 1.4 *vs.* 0.3 kg ($P = 0.001$), and tandem walk improved by 0.9 sec ($P = 0.02$) in the pooled treatment *vs.* placebo groups. By 12 months, stair climb also improved ($P = 0.04$). Adverse events included fatigue, insomnia, and small increases in fasting glucose, glycosylated hemoglobin, and indices of insulin resistance.

Conclusions.—In healthy older adults at risk for functional decline, administration of the oral GHS capromorelin may improve body composition and physical function.

▶ Muscle mass decreases during the aging process, and is associated with a decline in functionality. Aging is also associated with a decline in growth hormone (GH), and GH deficiency is known to lead to a decrease in muscle mass. This study investigates the long-term treatment (4 different dosing patterns) of the oral GH secretagogue, capromorelin, for safety and effect on GH and IGF-1 level, body composition, and physical performance in 395 elderly patients (age 65 to 84 yr) with mild limitation in function. Although the intended 2-year study was terminated early (at 6 months) due to a lack of statistically significant improvement in percent lean body mass (LBM), 315 patients completed 6 months of treatment and 284 patients completed 12 months. These authors found that the oral GH secretagogue increased IGF-1 and nocturnal GH levels, and that there was an associated increase in body weight as well as walking and stair climbing ability. Although the study was ended early, the data suggest an exciting potential role for this agent in improving functionality in the aging.

W. H. Ludlam, MD, PhD

Increased Prevalence of Tricuspid Regurgitation in Patients with Prolactinomas Chronically Treated with Cabergoline

Colao A, Galderisi M, Di Sarno A, et al (Federico II Univ of Napoli, Italy)

J Clin Endocrinol Metab 93:3777-3784, 2008

Background.—Cabergoline, a dopamine receptor-2 agonist used to treat prolactinomas, was associated with increased risk of cardiac valve disease in Parkinson's disease.

Objective.—Our objective was to evaluate prevalence of cardiac valve regurgitation in cabergoline-treated patients with prolactinomas.

Design and Setting.—An observational, case-control study was conducted at a university hospital.

Patients.—Fifty treated patients (44 women and six men) and 50 sex- and age-matched control subjects participated; 20 *de novo* patients were also studied.

Intervention.—In the treated patients, the last cabergoline dose was 1.3 ± 1.3 mg/wk (<1 mg/wk in 44%, 1–3 mg/wk in 46%, and >3 mg/wk in 10%). Treatment duration was 12–60 months in 32% and more than 60 months in 68%. The cumulative (milligrams × months of treatment) dose of cabergoline ranged from 32–1938 mg (median 280 mg).

Measurements.—Valve regurgitation was assessed according to the recommendations of the American Society of Echocardiography.

Results.—In *de novo* patients, treated patients, and controls, the prevalence of mild regurgitation of mitral (35, 22, and 12%, $P = 0.085$), aortic (0, 4, and 2%, $P = 0.59$), tricuspid (55, 30, and 42%, $P = 0.13$) or pulmonic (20, 12, and 6%, $P = 0.22$) valves was similar. Conversely, the prevalence of moderate tricuspid regurgitation was higher in the treated patients (54%) than in *de novo* patients (0%) and controls (18%, $P < 0.0001$). Moderate tricuspid regurgitation was more frequent in patients receiving a cumulative dose above the median (72%) than in those receiving a lower dose (36%, $P = 0.023$). A higher systolic ($P = 0.03$) and diastolic blood pressure ($P < 0.0001$) was found in patients with than in those without moderate tricuspid regurgitation.

Conclusion.—Moderate tricuspid regurgitation is more frequent in patients taking cabergoline (at higher cumulative doses) than in *de novo* patients and control subjects, but the clinical significance of this finding has not been established. A complete echocardiographic assessment is indicated in patients treated long term with cabergoline, particularly in those requiring elevated doses.

▶ Cabergoline treatment has been associated with increased risk of valvular heart disease in patients receiving prolonged exposure with this agent in Parkinson's disease. Although the average dose of cabergoline used to treat Parkinson's disease patients is many fold higher than the dose typically used to treat prolactinomas, endocrinologists have developed increasing concern regarding the prolonged use of this agent. To address this concern, these authors developed an observational, case-control study in which 50 cabergoline-treated patients were compared with 50 age and sex-matched controls, and the incidence of valvular heart disease was assessed. The authors noted an increasingly higher incidence (in a dose-dependent manner) of tricuspid valvular heart disease in patients taking cabergoline than in either *de novo* patients or controls, but these differences did not reach statistical significance. The authors conclude that cabergoline treatment of prolactinomas is associated with increased risk of tricuspid regurgitation, and that a complete echocardiographic exam is warranted in all patients being exposed to long-term cabergoline administration, particularly at higher doses.

W. H. Ludlam, MD, PhD

56 Obesity

Long-Term Effects of Roux-en-Y Gastric Bypass Surgery on Plasma Glucagon-Like Peptide-1 and Islet Function in Morbidly Obese Subjects
Vidal J, Nicolau J, Romero F, et al (Hospital Clínic Universitari, Barcelona, Spain)
J Clin Endocrinol Metab 94:884-891, 2009

Context.—An enlarged incretin response after Roux-en-Y gastric bypass (RYGBP) has been proposed to promote excessive β-cell function and mass.

Objective.—The objective of the study was to determine whether RYGBP is associated with a steadily increased glucagon-like peptide 1 (GLP-1) response and a disruption of the relationship between insulin sensitivity and insulin secretion required to maintain plasma glucose in the normal range.

Design and Patients.—This was a cross-sectional study. Twenty-four women divided into three groups according to time after RYGBP (9–15, 21–30, and more than 36 months). Eight normal-weight and eight morbidly obese women served as controls.

Main Outcome Measures.—GLP-1 was determined after a standardized test meal. Insulin secretion (AIRg) and insulin sensitivity (S_I) were derived from an iv glucose tolerance test. Postprandial glucose profile was recorded with a continuous glucose monitoring system.

Results.—Area under the curve$_{0-120}$ of GLP-1 was larger after RYGBP compared with controls ($P < 0.01$) but was comparable among surgical groups ($P = 0.314$). Time after surgery was not associated with changes in S_I ($P = 0.657$), AIRg ($P = 0.329$), or the disposition index (DI = AIRgS$_I$, $P = 0.915$). After surgery, the GLP-1 response and the DI were not significantly correlated ($P = 0.304$). Glucose less than 50 mg/dl was found in operated subjects, but the proportion did not increase with time after surgery ($P = 0.459$). Neither the GLP-1 response ($P = 0.620$) nor the DI ($P = 0.457$) differed significantly between those with or without hypoglycemic episodes.

Conclusions.—Although the GLP-1 response to meal intake is steadily elevated after RYGBP, this does not result over time in the development of an inappropriate insulin secretion relative to the prevailing insulin sensitivity or the occurrence of hypoglycemic episodes.

▶ The prevalence of obesity has increased dramatically over the past decades. Obesity is a major contributor to the development of type 2 diabetes mellitus, arterial hypertension, and dyslipidemia. Conventional therapy strategies for obesity include nutrition counseling, physical exercise training, and medical treatment. However, the long-term effects of these approaches are often discouraging. Therefore, bariatric surgery is becoming more common to treat morbidly obese patients. Recent trials showed promising results for bariatric surgery with respect to weight loss, remission, or improvement of type 2 diabetes mellitus and mortality.

However, alterations in the incretin response have been reported. An increase in glucagon-like peptide-1 (GLP-1) secretion has been reported after bariatric surgery in response to meal intake. GLP-1 stimulates insulin release and the proliferation of pancreatic beta cells. Therefore, this increase in GLP-1 levels has been associated with episodes of postprandial hypoglycemia as a rare complication.

This study by Vidal et al investigated long-term effects of Roux-en Y gastric bypass surgery on GLP-1 response to a meal in relation to insulin sensitivity and insulin resistance. This approach was chosen in order to determine whether the insulin response was appropriate with respect to the given insulin sensitivity. The authors found the GLP-1 response to a meal to be increased after Roux-en Y gastric bypass surgery. Interestingly, this did not necessarily lead to an inappropriate insulin release over time.

The subject of the study is important as the number of patients undergoing bariatric surgery increases. It is of clinical and scientific relevance to understand the physiological adaptations after this intervention. However, the study has some limitations: (a) the number of patients included is relatively small (24 operated patients and 16 controls); (b) the study claims that the increase in GLP-1 does not necessarily result in inappropriate insulin secretion. On the other hand, the study does not explain the increase in hypoglycemic episodes in operated patients. More mechanistic studies are needed to broaden our understanding of the adaptation processes after bariatric surgery.

For further reading on this subject I suggest articles by Adams et al,[1] Dixon et al,[2] and Service et al.[3]

S. Schinner, MD

References

1. Adams TD, Gress RE, Smith SC, et al. Long-term mortality after gastric bypass surgery. *N Engl J Med.* 2007;357:753-761.
2. Dixon JB, O'Brien PE, Playfair J, et al. Adjustable gastric banding and conventional therapy for type 2 diabetes: a randomized controlled trial. *JAMA.* 2008; 299:316-323.
3. Service GJ, Thompson GB, Service FJ, Andrews JC, Collazo-Clavell ML, Lloyd RV. Hyperinsulinemic hypoglycemia with nesidioblastosis after gastric-bypass surgery. *N Engl J Med.* 2005;353:249-254.

Nonsurgical Management of Obesity in Adults

Eckel RH (Univ of Colorado Denver, Aurora)
N Engl J Med 358:1941-1950, 2008

A 44-year-old woman desires weight reduction. Her history is notable for hypertension, snoring, daytime somnolence, and osteoarthritis. Her father was obese and had type 2 diabetes. On physical examination, her weight is 215 lb (98 kg), her body-mass index (BMI) (the weight in kilograms divided by the square of the height in meters) 32.7, her waist circumference 40 in. (102 cm), and her blood pressure 140/92 mm Hg. The stigmata of Cushing's syndrome are not present. The fasting glucose level is 112 mg per deciliter (6.2 mmol per liter). The fasting cholesterol level is 205 mg per deciliter (5.3 mmol per liter), triglyceride level 224 mg per deciliter (2.5 mmol per liter), high-density lipoprotein (HDL) cholesterol level 40 mg per deciliter (1.0 mmol per liter), and low-density lipoprotein (LDL) cholesterol level 120 mg per deciliter (3.1 mmol per liter). The thyrotropin level is normal. What would you advise?

▶ This review by Eckel summarizes the medical therapy for obesity. The assessment of the obese patient should include the history of weight gain, medical therapy with focus on drugs that may cause weight gain or prevent weight loss, history of comorbidities, and the patient's readiness to enroll in a weight loss program. The cornerstone of medical therapy for obesity is lifestyle changes. There is a brief review of macronutrient composition of diets and its effect on weight loss. Pharmacological therapy for obesity includes the present FDA-approved medications, and by the time the review was written, rimonabant, a cannabinoid receptor antagonist (CB1R antagonist), was approved for the treatment of obesity in Europe and other countries. But, on November 2008 this drug was withdrawn from the market because of increased risk of depressive symptoms and anxiety in patients treated with rimonabant. These side effects were already observed during clinical trials, in spite of the fact that patients who suffered from depression were not included.[1] It is emphasized in the review that present medical therapy for obesity is still inadequate, and more research should be done to improve adherence to lifestyle changes and maintain the weight loss.

R. Ness-Abramof, MD

Reference

1. Pi-Sunyer FX, Aronne LJ, Heshmati HM, Devin J, Rosenstock J. RIO-North America Study Group. Effect of rimonabant, a cannabinoid-1 receptor blocker, on weight and cardiometabolic risk factors in overweight or obese patients: RIO-North America: a randomized controlled trial. *JAMA.* 2006;295:761-775.

Factors Associated With Weight Loss After Gastric Bypass

Campos GM, Rabl C, Mulligan K, et al (Univ of California, San Francisco)
Arch Surg 143:877-884, 2008

Background.—Gastric bypass (GBP) is the most common operation performed in the United States for morbid obesity. However, weight loss is poor in 10% to 15% of patients. We sought to determine the independent factors associated with poor weight loss after GBP.

Design.—Prospective cohort study. We examined demographic, operative, and follow-up data by means of multivariate analysis. Variables investigated were age, sex, race, marital and insurance status, initial weight and body mass index (BMI) (calculated as weight in kilograms divided by height in meters squared), comorbidities (diabetes mellitus, hypertension, joint disease, sleep apnea, hyperlipidemia, and psychiatric disease), laparoscopic vs open surgery, gastric pouch area, gastrojejunostomy technique, and alimentary limb length.

Setting.—University tertiary referral center.

Patients.—All patients at our institution who underwent GBP from January 1, 2003, through July 30, 2006.

Main Outcome Measures.—Weight loss at 12 months defined as poor (≤40% excess weight loss) or good (>40% excess weight loss).

Results.—Follow-up data at 12 months were available for 310 of the 361 patients (85.9%) undergoing GBP during the study period. Mean preoperative BMI was 52 (range, 36-108). Mean BMI and excess weight loss at follow-up were 34 (range, 17-74) and 60% (range, 8%-117%), respectively. Thirty-eight patients (12.3%) had poor weight loss. Of the 4 variables associated with poor weight loss in the univariate analysis (greater initial weight, diabetes, open approach, and larger pouch size), only diabetes (odds ratio, 3.09; 95% confidence interval, 1.35-7.09 [$P = .007$]) and larger pouch size (odds ratio, 2.77; 95% confidence interval, 1.81-4.22 [$P < .001$]) remained after the multivariate analysis.

Conclusions.—Gastric bypass results in substantial weight loss in most patients. Diabetes and larger pouch size are independently associated with poor weight loss after GBP.

▶ The beneficial effects of a substantial weight loss through bariatric surgery includes improved metabolic profile, better quality of life, and an increased life span compared to matched obese individuals.[1] Roux-en-Y gastric bypass (RYBG) is the most common bariatric surgery performed in North America. RYBG combines a restrictive and malabsorptive procedure in which a small pouch is created at the proximal part of the stomach and it is anastomosed to the proximal jejunum, therefore bypassing part of the stomach, duodenum and part of the jejunum. The weight loss achieved with RYBG is greater compared to pure gastric restrictive procedures.[2] In spite of the fact that there is an expected weight loss of more than 40% of excess body weight, some patients will lose substantially less weight. Factors associated with a lower weight loss include older age, male sex, greater initial weight and BMI, and the presence of diabetes among others.

Campos et al designed a prospective study in which they investigated whether age, sex, race, marital and insurance status, initial body weight and BMI, comorbidities, surgical procedure (laparoscopic vs open surgery, pouch area (assessed by swallow studies of the upper gastrointestinal tract on postoperative day 1), gastrojejunostomy technique, and alimentary limb length are related to poor weight loss. The authors defined "poor weight loss" as ≤ 40% excess weight loss within 1 year. From the 361 patients recruited, the data from 310 patients were available for analysis. The mean excess weight loss was 60% (range 8%-117%), while 12.3% of patients had poor weight loss. On univariate analysis, just diabetes and larger pouch size were independently associated with poor weight loss after RYGB.

The relation between pouch size and subsequent weight loss is clear. The problem is standardizing the desired pouch size during surgery, since the pouch size depends on a patient's body habitus and the surgeon's technique. The reason why diabetic patients lose less weight is less clear. Some plausible explanations are the use of medications that promote weight gain (such as insulin, sulfonylureas, and glitazones), hypoglycemia and improved glucose control with less glycosuria.[3] On the other hand, a drastic reduction in the need for diabetes medications is seen immediately after surgery, even before any weight loss is achieved. We need more prospective studies to evaluate whether the connection between poor weight loss and diabetes is related to their specific medical therapy or hormonal/metabolic factors as shown in an article by Somma et al in which the authors find that patients with GH and IGF-1 deficiency lose less fat mass after gastric banding.

R. Ness-Abramof, MD

References

1. Adams TG, Gress RE, Smith SC, et al. Long-term mortality after gastric bypass surgery. *N Engl J Med.* 2007;357:753-761.
2. Mechanick JI, Kushner RF, Sugerman HJ, et al. American Association of Clinical Endocrinologists, The Obesity Society, and American Society for Metabolic & Bariatric Surgery medical guidelines for clinical practice for the perioperative nutritional, metabolic, and nonsurgical support of the bariatric surgery patient. *Obesity (Silver Spring).* 2009;17:S1-70.
3. Ness-Abramof R, Apovian CM. Drug-induced weight gain. *Drugs of today.* 2005; 41:547-555.

Orlistat Inhibition of Intestinal Lipase Acutely Increases Appetite and Attenuates Postprandial Glucagon-Like Peptide-1-(7–36)-Amide-1, Cholecystokinin, and Peptide YY Concentrations
Ellrichmann M, Kapelle M, Ritter PR, et al (Ruhr-Univ Bochum, Germany; et al)
J Clin Endocrinol Metab 93:3995-3998, 2008

Introduction.—Intestinal lipase inhibition using tetrahydrolipstatin (Orlistat) has been widely used in the pharmacotherapy of morbid obesity.

However, the effects of Orlistat on the secretion of appetite regulating gastrointestinal hormones and appetite sensations are still debated. We addressed whether Orlistat alters the secretion of glucagon-like peptide-1-(7–36)-amide (GLP-1), cholecystokinin (CCK), peptide YY (PYY), and ghrelin as well as postprandial appetite sensations.

Methods.—Twenty-five healthy human volunteers were examined with a solid-liquid test meal after the oral administration of Orlistat or placebo. Gastric emptying, gallbladder volume and the plasma levels of CCK, PYY, GLP-1, and ghrelin were determined and appetite sensations were measured using visual analogue scales.

Results.—Gastric emptying was accelerated by Orlistat administration ($P < 0.0001$), whereas gall-bladder emptying was inhibited ($P < 0.0001$). Plasma levels of CCK (by ~53%), PYY (by ~40%), and GLP-1 (by ~20%) were significantly lowered by Orlistat ($P < 0.001$), whereas ghrelin levels were unaffected by Orlistat treatment ($P = 0.18$). Satiety and fullness were lowered by Orlistat ($P < 0.0001$), whereas appetite and prospective food consumption increased ($P < 0.0001$). The changes in CCK and PYY levels and the mean hunger ratings after Orlistat treatment were closely related to the inhibition of gallbladder motility.

Conclusions.—Orlistat alters gastric and gallbladder emptying and reduces the postprandial secretion of GLP-1, PYY and CCK. These changes in gastrointestinal hormone concentrations may raise appetite sensations and increase food consumption and should therefore be considered as potential side effects when applying lipase inhibitors for the treatment of morbid obesity.

▶ It is known that body weight control is very complex, involving neural and hormonal signals from the adipose tissue, brain, and gastrointestinal tract. The role of the gastrointestinal tract in satiety and weight maintenance has been thoroughly studied during the last 2 decades. It is known that cholecystokinin (CCK), glucagon-like peptide 1 (GLP-1), and peptide YY (PYY) increase satiety, while ghrelin is an orexogenic hormone. Orlistat is a reversible pancreatic, gastric, and intestinal lipase inhibitor that reduces the absorption of approximately 30% of alimentary fat.[1] It is an approved medication for weight loss when prescribed in combination with a calorie-restricted diet. Orlistat has been shown to promote weight loss and improve glucose control, but its effect on the postprandial secretion of gastrointestinal hormones CCK, PYY, GLP-1, and ghrelin is not clear, with conflicting results in the literature.

Ellrichmann et al examined 25 healthy volunteers with a solid-liquid test meal after the oral administration of orlistat or placebo. They measured gastric emptying, gallbladder volume, appetite sensations, and the plasma levels of CCK, PYY, GLP-1, and ghrelin. It was found that gastric emptying was accelerated by orlistat, consistent with previous data, while gallbladder emptying was inhibited. Plasma levels of CCK, PYY, and GLP-1 were significantly decreased by orlistat compared with placebo. Ghrelin levels were not affected by orlistat. Satiety and fullness were lowered by orlistat.

These results support previous reports showing that orlistat acutely enhances gastric emptying and decreases the secretion of anorexogenic gut hormones.[2,3] Because orlistat is a weight loss medication, the decreased satiety may diminish its weight loss effectiveness. Furthermore, increased gastric motility coupled with a decrease in GLP-1 may increase postprandial glucose levels, particularly in diabetic patients. Although Sahin et al did not show a greater postprandial glucose excursion with orlistat, their study population included obese nondiabetic subjects. Whether this effect is clinically significant and if it persists with chronic use of orlistat should be evaluated, because orlistat has been shown to be effective in the prevention of diabetes, particularly in patients with impaired glucose tolerance.[4]

R. Ness-Abramof, MD

References

1. McNeely W, Benfield P. Orlistat. *Drugs*. 1998;56:241-249.
2. Pilichiewicz A, O'Donovan C, Feinle C, et al. Effect of lipase inhibition on gastric emptying of, and the glycemic and incretin responses to, an oil/aqueous drink in type 2 diabetes mellitus. *J Clin Endocrinol Metab*. 2003;88:3829-3834.
3. Sahin M, Tanaci N, Yucel M, Tutuncu NB, Guvener N. The effect of single-dose orlistat on postprandial serum glucose, insulin and glucagon-like peptide-1 levels in nondiabetic obese patients. *Clin Endocrinol*. 2007;67:346-350.
4. Torgerson JS, Hauptman J, Boldrin MN, Sjöström L. XENical in the prevention of diabetes in obese subjects (XENDOS) study: a randomized study of orlistat as an adjunct to lifestyle changes for the prevention of type 2 diabetes in obese patients. *Diabetes Care*. 2004;27:155-161. Erratum in: *Diabetes Care*. 2004 Mar;27(3):856.

Association of breakfast energy density with diet quality and body mass index in American adults: National Health and Nutrition Examination Surveys, 1999–2004

Kant AK, Andon MB, Angelopoulos TJ, et al (Queens College of the City Univ of New York, Flushing; Quaker-Tropicana-Gatorade Res and Development Dept, Barrington, IL; Univ of Central Florida, Orlando; et al)
Am J Clin Nutr 88:1396-1404, 2008

Background.—Recent reports suggest that dietary energy density (ED) is associated with diet quality, energy intake, and body weight. Breakfast consumption was also associated with diet quality and body weight; however, little is known about the association of breakfast consumption with dietary ED.

Objectives.—We examined differences in the ED (in energy content/g of food) of diets between breakfast consumers and nonconsumers, and in breakfast reporters we examined the association of ED of breakfast foods with ED of nonbreakfast foods, diet quality, and body mass index (BMI; in kg/m^2).

Design.—We combined dietary data from the 3 continuous National Health and Nutrition Examination Surveys (1999–2004) to determine the ED (in kcal/g) of foods and nutritive beverages and the ED of foods only ($n = 12\,316$; ≥ 20 y). Linear and logistic regression methods were used to examine the independent associations of breakfast reporting or breakfast ED with 24-h ED, nonbreakfast ED, diet quality, and BMI.

Results.—The ED of 24-h dietary intake was lower among breakfast reporters than among nonreporters. Women breakfast reporters (but not men) had lower BMI than did nonreporters (27.9 ± 0.2 compared with 29.4 ± 0.4; $P = 0.001$). With increasing breakfast ED, nonbreakfast ED and fat intake increased, but micronutrient intake and the likelihood of mention of all 5 food groups declined. BMI increased with increasing breakfast ED in men but with increasing nonbreakfast ED in women ($P \leq 0.001$).

Conclusions.—Our results support recommendations to encourage breakfast consumption and suggest that the ED of breakfast was associated with diet quality, overall diet ED, and body weight.

▶ Breakfast consumption has been associated with lower body weight, and therefore in most lifestyle programs, patients are advised to eat breakfast. Kant et al evaluated breakfast energy density and energy intake, and its correlation to body mass index (BMI), in subjects surveyed by the National Health and Nutrition Examination Surveys, 1999-2004. They report that most women (not men) who skipped breakfast had higher BMIs than those who did not skip breakfast. Men with higher BMIs reported more energy-dense breakfasts, but the energy density of nonbreakfast meals did not predict BMI.

The authors conclude that shifting breakfast eating habits in men toward a lower energy-dense breakfast may prevent weight gain. Whether or not advising women who skip breakfast to eat a low-energy-density breakfast will also decrease other caloric intake during the day needs to be further evaluated.

R. Ness-Abramof, MD

57 Pediatric Endocrinology

Consensus Statement on the Use of Gonadotropin-Releasing Hormone Analogs in Children
Carel J-C, Eugster EA, Rogol A, et al (Robert Debré Hosp, Paris, France; Indiana Univ, Indianapolis; et al)
Pediatrics 123:e752-e762, 2009

Objective.—Gonadotropin-releasing hormone analogs revolutionized the treatment of central precocious puberty. However, questions remain regarding their optimal use in central precocious puberty and other conditions. The Lawson Wilkins Pediatric Endocrine Society and the European Society for Pediatric Endocrinology convened a consensus conference to review the clinical use of gonadotropin-releasing hormone analogs in children and adolescents.

Participants.—When selecting the 30 participants, consideration was given to equal representation from North America (United States and Canada) and Europe, an equal male/female ratio, and a balanced spectrum of professional seniority and expertise.

Evidence.—Preference was given to articles written in English with long-term outcome data. The US Public Health grading system was used to grade evidence and rate the strength of conclusions. When evidence was insufficient, conclusions were based on expert opinion.

Consensus Process.—Participants were put into working groups with assigned topics and specific questions. Written materials were prepared and distributed before the conference, revised on the basis of input during the meeting, and presented to the full assembly for final review. If consensus could not be reached, conclusions were based on majority vote. All participants approved the final statement.

Conclusions.—The efficacy of gonadotropin-releasing hormone analogs in increasing adult height is undisputed only in early-onset (girls <6 years old) central precocious puberty. Other key areas, such as the psychosocial effects of central precocious puberty and their alteration by gonadotropin-releasing hormone analogs, need additional study. Few controlled prospective studies have been performed with gonadotropin-releasing hormone analogs in children, and many conclusions rely in part on collective expert opinion. The conference did not endorse commonly voiced concerns regarding the use of gonadotropin-releasing hormone analogs, such as promotion of weight gain or long-term diminution of bone mineral density. Use of gonadotropin-releasing hormone analogs for conditions other than central precocious puberty requires additional investigation and cannot be suggested routinely.

▶ Despite widespread use of GnRH analogs (GnRHa) for the treatment of central precocious puberty (CPP) worldwide for more than 2 decades, significant questions remain about this therapeutic modality. The goals of this consensus conference, which was jointly sponsored by North American and European pediatric endocrine societies, was to review existing literature with the aim of deriving consensus recommendations, and to identify areas in which a particular dearth of information is present. A notable strength of this consensus conference, which has been lacking from previous similar efforts, was the application of a grading system to indicate quality of the evidence and strength of the recommendations made. Several of the group's findings (there were 30 participants) are worth noting. One of those is that a significant and predictable increase in adult height can be guaranteed only in girls with early-onset (less than age 6), rapidly progressing CPP. This is an important caveat for pediatric endocrinologists, since the vast majority of the children that we treat with GnRHa do not fit within this category. Another finding of surprise to many attendees was that, contrary to popular opinion, GnRHa do not cause or aggravate obesity. Beyond the realm of CPP, the consensus group also examined the use of GnRHa for other indications, which have included a broad range of conditions such as children with early normal puberty, idiopathic short stature, congenital adrenal hypoplasia, long-standing primary hypothyroidism, small for gestational age, and growth hormone deficiency. Across the board, scientific support for the routine use of these agents for indications other than CPP was found to be lacking. Similarly, concerns about negative psychological consequences of CPP, which are often used to justify treatment, simply could not be substantiated. While each of these conclusions should give us pause, perhaps the most troubling was a more general yet consistent thread that ran through every aspect of the consensus conference proceedings. This was a glaring lack of controlled and rigorously conducted clinical studies on which to base treatment recommendations. Although hardly unique to pediatric endocrinology, it reminds us of the importance of actively pursuing opportunities to engage in scrupulous scientific investigation, even in areas that fall under the rubric of "common clinical practice." Only then will we truly be assured of benefiting our patients through medical intervention.

E. Eugster, MD, PhD

Consensus Statement on the Diagnosis and Treatment of Children with Idiopathic Short Stature: A Summary of the Growth Hormone Research Society, the Lawson Wilkins Pediatric Endocrine Society and the European Society for Paediatric Endocrinology Workshop
Cohen P, Rogol AD, Deal CL, et al (Mattel Children's Hosp at UCLA, Los Angeles, CA; Univ of Virginia, Charlottesville; Sainte-Justine Hosp, Montreal, Quebec, Canada; et al)
J Clin Endocrinol Metab, 2008 Sep 9, Epub ahead of print

Objective.—To summarize important advances in the management of children with idiopathic-short-stature (ISS).

Participants.—32 invited leaders in the field.

Evidence.—Extensive literature-review and clinical-experience.

Consensus.—Participants reviewed discussion-summaries, voted and reached a majority-decision on each document-section.

Conclusions.—ISS is defined auxologically by a height below -2 SDS without findings of disease as evident by a complete evaluation by a pediatric endocrinologist including stimulated-GH levels. An MRI is not necessary in patients with ISS. ISS may be a risk factor for psychosocial problems, but true psychopathology is rare. In the US and seven other countries, the regulatory authorities approved GH treatment (at doses up to 53 mcg/kg/day) for children shorter than -2.25 SDS while in other countries lower cut-offs are proposed. Aromatase-inhibition increases predicted-adult-height in males with ISS, but adult-height data are not available. Psychological-counseling is worthwhile to consider instead of or as an adjunct to hormone treatment. The predicted-height may be inaccurate and is not an absolute criterion for GH-treatment decisions. The shorter the child, the more consideration should be given to GH. Successful first-year response to GH-treatment includes an increase in height SDS > 0.3 to 0.5. The mean increase in adult-height in children with ISS attributable to GH-therapy (average duration of 4-7 years) is 3.5-7.5 cm. Responses are highly variable. IGF-I levels may be helpful in assessing compliance and GH-sensitivity; levels that are consistently elevated (>2.5 SDS) should prompt consideration of GH-dose-reduction. GH-therapy for children with ISS has a similar safety profile to other GH-indications.

▶ Although consensus conferences have their critics,[1] these exercises nonetheless represent a collaborative and extensive review of existing literature and thoughtful deliberation of the issues impacting clinical care by presumed experts in the field. Therefore, it behooves all pediatric endocrinologists to have some familiarity with the conclusions that are made and the gaps in current knowledge that are identified as a result of this process. As with similar consensus meetings, a notable strength of this one is that it was a joint effort between North American and European societies, allowing a multinational perspective to be brought to the table. Several key findings are worth noting. Although the designation of idiopathic-short-stature (ISS) is an auxological one (height < −2.25 SDS), the use of growth hormone (GH) for this indication in the United States also requires a predicted adult height of < 4'11" in girls and < 5'2" in boys. In contrast, the consensus document definition of ISS includes children with constitutional delay of growth and puberty (most of whom do not end up short) as well as those with genetic short stature, conditions which comprise the bulk of referrals to pediatric endocrinologists and have long been considered normal variants. The categorization of these common entities as "idiopathic" and the implication that all of these children should be considered for growth hormone therapy indeed gives one pause. Despite the consensus definition, the concept of prescribing growth hormone to a child with a normal growth velocity and a predicted height that is normal for the family and the general population, just because he or she is at the first percentile, is highly controversial.[2] The mean increase in height after 4 to 7 years of daily growth hormone injections in children with ISS is 3.5 to 7.5 cm, or 1.4 to 2.9 inches, at a cost of $25 400 to $50 800 per inch. Obviously, growth hormone in this population does not make children tall, or even of average stature. Although the assumption is that a couple of extra inches will improve quality of life, the consensus conference rightly concludes that "It is presently unknown if, and how, a gain in height relates to change in quality of life." Until sufficient data from studies that are rigorously executed and free of bias are available with which to answer these questions, the debate about growth hormone therapy in healthy short children will continue.

E. Eugster, MD, PhD

References

1. Rivkees SA. Why the consensus for consensus? *J Pediatr Endocrinol Metab.* 2008; 21:503-505.
2. Lee MM. Idiopathic short stature. *N Engl J Med.* 2006;354:2576-2582.

58 Reproductive Endocrinology

Oral but not transdermal estrogen replacement therapy changes the composition of plasma lipoproteins

Vrablik M, Fait T, Kovar J, et al (Charles Univ, Prague, Czech Republic; Inst for Clinical and Experimental Medicine, Prague, Czech Republic)
Metab Clin Exp 57:1088-1092, 2008

The role of hormone replacement therapy and estrogen replacement therapy (ERT) in cardiovascular disease prevention has not been unambiguously defined yet. The metabolic effects of estrogens may vary depending upon the route of administration. Therefore, we compared the impact of unopposed oral or transdermal ERT on plasma lipids and lipoproteins in 41 hysterectomized women. This was an open-label, randomized, crossover study (with 2 treatments and 2 periods). The 41 hysterectomized women were randomized to receive oral or transdermal 17β-estradiol in the first or second of two 12-week study periods. Plasma lipid and lipoprotein levels were assayed before and after each treatment using standard automated methods. Lipid content of lipoprotein subclasses was assessed by sequential ultracentrifugation. The atherogenic index of plasma (AIP) was calculated as log(triglyceride [TG]/high-density lipoprotein [HDL] cholesterol). The difference between the 2 forms of administration was tested using a linear mixed model. The change from baseline for each of the forms was tested using paired t test. Oral ERT resulted in a significant increase in HDL cholesterol and apolipoprotein A-I levels, whereas it significantly decreased total and low-density lipoprotein (LDL) cholesterol and increased TG concentrations. Transdermal ERT had no such effect. Oral ERT led to a significant TG enrichment of HDL (0.19 ± 0.06 vs 0.27 ± 0.07 mmol/L, $P < .001$) and LDL particles (0.23 ± 0.08 vs 0.26 ± 0.10 mmol/L, $P < .001$) compared with baseline, whereas transdermal therapy did not have any effect on lipoprotein subclasses composition. The difference between the 2 treatments was statistically significant for HDL-TG and LDL-TG (0.27 ± 0.07 vs 0.19 ± 0.05 mmol/L, $P < .001$ and 0.26 ± 0.10 vs 0.22 ± 0.07 mmol/L, $P < .001$, respectively). The transdermal but not oral ERT significantly reduced the AIP compared with baseline (-0.17 ± 0.26 vs -0.23 ± 0.25, $P = .023$), making the difference between the therapies statistically significant (-0.23 ± 0.25 vs -0.18 ± 0.22, $P = .017$). Oral administration of ERT resulted in TG

TABLE 1.—Lipid, Lipoprotein, and Apolipoprotein Levels at Baseline and After Oral and Transdermal Estradiol

	Baseline	Oral	Transdermal
TC (mmol/L)	5.5 ± 1.1	$5.3 \pm 0.9^*$	5.5 ± 1.2
TG (mmol/L)	1.4 ± 0.8	$1.6 \pm 0.8^*$	$1.3 \pm 0.7\dagger$
HDL-C (mmol/L)	1.9 ± 0.4	$2.1 \pm 0.4^*$	$2.0 \pm 0.4\dagger$
LDL-C (mmol/L)	3.1 ± 1.0	$2.5 \pm 0.7^*$	$3.0 \pm 1.0\dagger$
Apo B (g/L)	1.1 ± 0.4	$1.0 \pm 0.3^*$	1.0 ± 0.4
Apo A-I (g/L)	1.5 ± 0.2	$1.6 \pm 0.2^*$	$1.5 \pm 0.2\dagger$

TC indicates total cholesterol.
*Significantly different from baseline, $P < .01$.
$\dagger$Significantly different between treatments, $P < .01$.
(Reprinted from Vrablik M, Fait T, Kovar J, et al. Oral but not transdermal estrogen replacement therapy changes the composition of plasma lipoproteins. *Metab Clin Exp.* 57:1088-1092, 2008, with permission from Elsevier.)

enrichment of LDL and HDL particles. Transdermal ERT did not change the composition of the lipoproteins and produced a significant improvement of AIP. Compared with transdermal ERT, orally administered ERT changes negatively the composition of plasma lipoproteins (Table 1).

▶ Postmenopausal hormone replacement with estrogen and progestin in clinical trials has been shown to positively affect plasma lipid profiles but have a negative impact on cardiovascular outcomes. Transdermal estrogen therapy compared with oral estrogen combination therapy did not have the same adverse outcome. Low-density lipoprotein (LDL) particle size is variable and small dense LDL particles have proatherogenic actions. The proportion of these harmful particles rises with increasing plasma triglycerides (TG). This study was designed to compare the effect of unopposed oral or transdermal estrogen on plasma lipids and lipoproteins in hysterectomized women. Oral but not transdermal estrogen resulted in TG enrichment of LDL and high-density lipoprotein (HDL) particles, and transdermal estrogen significantly improved the atherogenic index, whereas it was worse with oral estrogen. The route of administration of estrogen must be considered when estrogen replacement therapy is deemed necessary. Further long-term study is needed to validate the findings of the study on cardiovascular outcomes.

A. W. Meikle, MD

Older Men With Low Serum Estradiol and High Serum SHBG Have an Increased Risk of Fractures

Mellström D, Vandenput L, Mallmin H, et al (Univ of Gothenburg, Sweden; Univ of Uppsala, Sweden; et al)
J Bone Miner Res 23:1552-1560, 2008

Osteoporosis-related fractures constitute a major health concern not only in women but also in men. To study the predictive role of serum sex steroids for fracture risk in men, serum sex steroids were analyzed by the specific gas chromatography-mass spectrometry technique at baseline in older men ($n = 2639$; mean, 75 yr of age) of the prospective population-based MrOS Sweden cohort. Fractures occurring after baseline were validated (average follow-up of 3.3 yr). The incidence for having at least one validated fracture after baseline was 20.9/1000 person-years. Estradiol (E2; hazard ratio [HR] per SD decrease, 1.34; 95% CI, 1.22–1.49), free estradiol (fE2; HR per SD decrease, 1.41; 95% CI, 1.28–1.55), testosterone (T; HR per SD decrease, 1.27; 95% CI, 1.16–1.39), and free testosterone (fT; HR per SD decrease, 1.32; 95% CI, 1.21–1.44) were all inversely, whereas sex hormone-binding globulin (SHBG; HR per SD increase, 1.41; 95% CI, 1.22–1.63) was directly related to fracture risk. Multivariable proportional hazards regression

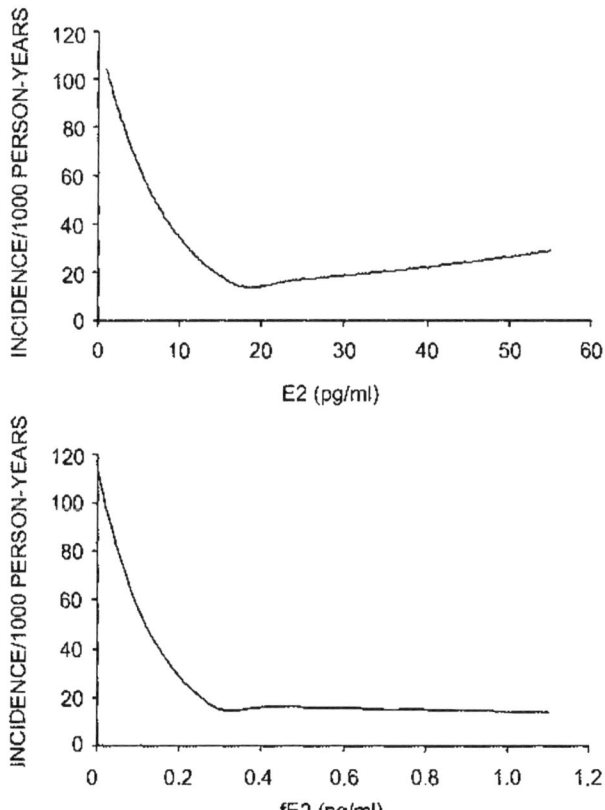

FIGURE 1.—Yearly incidence of fracture in relation to total E2 and fE2. Poisson regression models were used to determine the relation between serum hormone levels and fracture risk (all validated fractures). (Reprinted from Mellström D, Vandenput L, Mallmin H, et al. Older men with low serum estradiol and high serum SHBG have an increased risk of fractures. *J Bone Miner Res.* 2008;23:1552-1560, with permission from the American Society for Bone and Mineral Research.)

models, adjusted for age, suggested that fE2 and SHBG ($p < 0.001$), but not fT, were independently associated with fracture risk. Further subanalyses of fracture type showed that fE2 was inversely associated with clinical vertebral fractures (HR per SD decrease, 1.57; 95% CI, 1.36–1.80), nonvertebral osteoporosis fractures (HR per SD decrease, 1.42; 95% CI, 1.23–1.65), and hip fractures (HR per SD decrease, 1.44; 95% CI, 1.18–1.76). The inverse relation between serum E2 and fracture risk was nonlinear with a strong relation <16 pg/ml for E2 and 0.3 pg/ml for fE2. In conclusion, older Swedish men with low serum E2 and high SHBG levels have an increased risk of fractures (Fig 1).

▶ Osteoporotic fractures in both aging men and women cause substantial morbidity and mortality. Risk factors for osteoporosis have been more extensively studied in women than in men. Sex steroids are important for bone health in both sexes. The relative contribution of androgens and estrogens on bone mass and the development of osteoporosis are less clear in men. This is in part because testosterone is a precursor for estradiol, which is known to have major influence on bone integrity in men. In cross-sectional studies, correlations of hormone concentrations and risk of fractures are used in an attempt to find the main hormone that might influence fracture risk. This study included the measurement of both free and total testosterone and estradiol and sex hormone binding globulin (SHBG) in older Swedish men and related these serum concentrations to fracture risk. They concluded that low serum estradiol and free estradiol concentrations and high SHBG posed the greatest risk for fracture. This conclusion supports the results of other studies that infer that estradiol concentrations are critical in sustaining bone health in aging men.

A. W. Meikle, MD

A comparison between rimonabant and metformin in reducing biochemical hyperandrogenaemia and insulin resistance in patients with polycystic ovary syndrome (PCOS): a randomized open-label parallel study
Sathyapalan T, Cho LW, Kilpatrick ES, et al (Univ of Hull, UK; Hull Royal Infirmary, UK; et al)
Clin Endocrinol 69:931-935, 2008

Context.—Weight loss and metformin therapy are reported to be beneficial in improving the biochemical hyperandrogenaemia and insulin resistance of polycystic ovary syndrome (PCOS). Rimonabant has been found to reduce weight and improve the metabolic profile in patients with obesity, type 2 diabetes and metabolic syndrome.

Objective.—To compare the effects of insulin sensitization with metformin to weight reduction by rimonabant on biochemical hyperandrogenaemia and insulin resistance in patients with PCOS.

Design.—A randomized, open-label parallel study.

Setting.—Endocrinology outpatient clinic in a referral centre.

Subjects.—Twenty patients with PCOS and biochemical hyperandrogenaemia with a body mass index (BMI) $\geq$ 30 kg/m^2 were recruited.

Intervention.—Patients were randomized to $1 \cdot 5$ g daily of metformin or 20 mg daily of rimonabant.

Main Outcome Measures.—The primary end-point of the study was a change in total testosterone.

Results.—After 12 weeks of rimonabant there was a significant reduction (mean ± SEM) in weight ($104 \cdot 6 \pm 4 \cdot 6$ *vs.* $98 \cdot 4 \pm 4 \cdot 7$ kg, $P < 0 \cdot 01$), waist circumference ($116 \cdot 0 \pm 3 \cdot 3$ *vs.* $109 \cdot 2 \pm 3 \cdot 7$ cm, $P < 0 \cdot 01$), hip circumference ($128 \cdot 5 \pm 4 \cdot 0$ *vs.* $124 \cdot 1 \pm 4 \cdot 2$ cm, $P < 0 \cdot 03$), waist-hip ratio ($0 \cdot 90 \pm 0 \cdot 02$ *vs.* $0 \cdot 88 \pm 0 \cdot 01$, $P < 0 \cdot 01$) free androgen index (FAI) ($26 \cdot 6 \pm 6 \cdot 1$ *vs.* $16 \cdot 6 \pm 4 \cdot 1$, $P < 0 \cdot 01$), testosterone [$4 \cdot 6 \pm 0 \cdot 4$ *vs.* $3 \cdot 1 \pm 0 \cdot 3$ nmol/l ($132 \cdot 7 \pm 11 \cdot 5$ *vs.* $89 \cdot 4 \pm 8 \cdot 65$ ng/dl), $P < 0 \cdot 01$] and insulin resistance as measured by the homeostasis model assessment (HOMA) method ($4 \cdot 4 \pm 0 \cdot 5$ *vs.* $3 \cdot 4 \pm 0 \cdot 4$, $P = 0 \cdot 05$). There was no change in any of these parameters in the metformin-treated group.

Conclusion.—This study suggests that the weight loss through rimonabant therapy may be of use in patients with PCOS and appears superior to insulin sensitization by metformin in reducing the FAI and insulin resistance in obese PCOS patients treated over a 12-week period.

▶ Polycystic ovary syndrome (PCOS) is a common disorder in women of reproductive age and is characterized by insulin resistance, the metabolic syndrome, oligomenorrhea, and androgen excess. Metformin is commonly used to improve insulin resistance, body weight, and hyperandrogenemia. Rimonabant, a cannabinoid receptor 1 blocker, has been reported to improve the metabolic syndrome, lipid parameters, and insulin resistance in obese persons. This study compared the effects of 12 weeks of treatment with metformin or rimonabant in women with PCOS. Rimonabant but not metformin significantly improved characteristics of the metabolic syndrome and free testosterone index and total testosterone during the therapy. Rimonabant treatment did not significantly affect triglycerides or high-density lipoprotein (HDL) cholesterol. The reduction in weight loss but not in insulin resistance correlated well with androgen reduction in the rimonabant-treated group. While the lack of benefit with metformin is not consistent with other studies, rimonabant has promise in the treatment of PCOS, and long-term studies are needed to determine safety and efficacy.

A. W. Meikle, MD

Effects of aromatase inhibition in hypogonadal older men: a randomized, double-blind, placebo-controlled trial

Burnett-Bowie S-AM, Roupenian KC, Dere ME, et al (Massachusetts General Hosp and Harvard Med School, Boston)
Clin Endocrinol 70:116-123, 2009

Objective.—To assess the effects of sustained aromatase inhibition in older hypogonadal men.

Design and Patients.—In a 1-year randomized, double-blind, placebo-controlled trial, 88 men, aged 60 years and older with testosterone levels between 5·2 and 10·4 nmol/l on a single measure or between 10·4 and 12·1 nmol/l on two consecutive measures, and with symptoms of hypogonadism were recruited. Subjects received either anastrozole 1 mg daily or placebo.

Measurements.—Changes in gonadal steroid hormone levels, body composition [by computerized tomography (CT) and dual X-ray absorptiometry (DXA)], strength, prostate specific antigen (PSA), symptoms of benign prostatic hypertrophy (BPH), haematocrit and lipid levels were assessed.

Results.—Testosterone levels increased from 11·2 ± 3·3 nmol/l at baseline to 18·2 ± 4·8 nmol/l at month 3 ($P < 0·0001$ *vs.* placebo) while bioavailable testosterone levels increased from 2·7 ± 0·8 nmol/l at

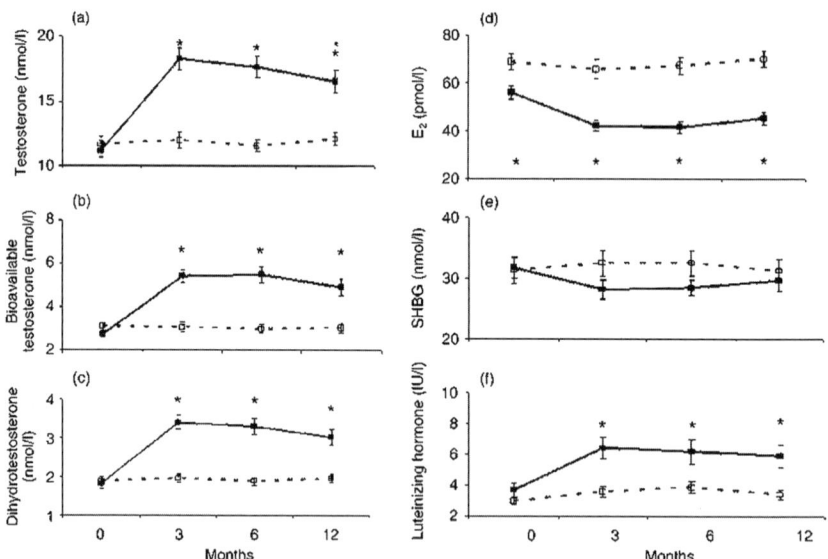

FIGURE 2.—Mean (± SE) (a) testosterone (b) bioavailable testosterone (c) dihydrotestosterone (d) E_2 (e) SHBG, and (f) LH with anastrozole (solid line) *vs.* placebo (dashed line). *$P < 0·05$ as compared to placebo. (Reprinted from Burnett-Bowie S-AM, Roupenian KC, Dere ME, et al. Effects of aromatase inhibition in hypogonadal older men: a randomized, double-blind, placebo-controlled trial. *Clin Endocrinol.* 2009;70:116-123, with permission from Blackwell Publishing Ltd.)

baseline to $5 \cdot 4 \pm 1 \cdot 7$ nmol/l at month 3 ($P < 0 \cdot 0001$ *vs.* placebo). Testosterone and biotestosterone levels peaked at month 3 and then declined by month 12 (though they remained significantly higher than baseline and greater than placebo). E_2 levels decreased from $55 \cdot 8 \pm 15 \cdot 4$ pmol/l at baseline to $42 \cdot 2 \pm 13 \cdot 6$ pmol/l at month 3 and then remained stable ($P < 0 \cdot 0001$). Body composition and strength did not change, nor did PSA, BPH symptoms, haematocrit or lipid levels.

Conclusions.—Anastrozole administration normalized androgen production in older hypogonadal men and decreased E_2 production modestly. These alterations did not improve body composition or strength (Fig 1).

▶ Aging men often have declining serum testosterone concentrations and clinical manifestations associated with testosterone deficiency in younger men, which includes decreased libido, increased fat mass, decreased lean body mass, depressed mood, erectile dysfunction, and reduced strength. There are many studies showing that testosterone administration to older men with testosterone deficiency can reverse the clinical features of testosterone deficiency. The long-term efficacy and safety have yet to be determined in older men replaced with testosterone therapy. Because the defects in gonadal function are in part from central dysfunction and diminished Leydig cell function, suppressing estrogen production, or action with aromatase inhibition or estrogen receptor blockade might reverse testosterone deficiency in older as well as younger men with testosterone deficiency. The study by Burnett-Bowie et al treated elderly men with relative testosterone deficiency, and established that an aromatase inhibitor compared with placebo increased serum testosterone and dihydrotestosterone and LH. They did not observe benefit in body composition and strength, but also did not observe adverse effects on prostate-specific antigen (PSA) or lipids. The use of aromatase inhibitors long-term are a concern with respect to bone health.

A. W. Meikle, MD

Diminished paternity and gonadal function with increasing obesity in men
Pauli EM, Legro RS, Demers LM, et al (The Pennsylvania State Univ College of Medicine, Hershey, PA)
Fertil Steril 90:346-351, 2008

Objective.—To examine the relationship of male obesity and reproductive function.

Design.—Observational study.

Setting.—Academic medical center.

Patient(s).—Eighty-seven adult men, body mass index (BMI) range from 16.1 to 47.0 kg/m^2 (mean = 29.3 kg/m^2; SD = 6.5 kg/m^2).

Intervention(s).—None

Main Outcome Measure(s).—Reproductive history, physical examination, inhibin B, FSH, LH, T, and unbound T levels, and semen analysis.

Result(s).—Body mass index was negatively correlated with testosterone ($r = -0.38$), FSH ($r = -0.22$), and inhibin B levels ($r = -0.21$) and was positively correlated with E_2 levels ($r = 0.34$). Testosterone also negatively correlated with skinfold thickness ($r = -0.30$). There was no correlation of BMI or skinfold thickness with semen analysis parameters

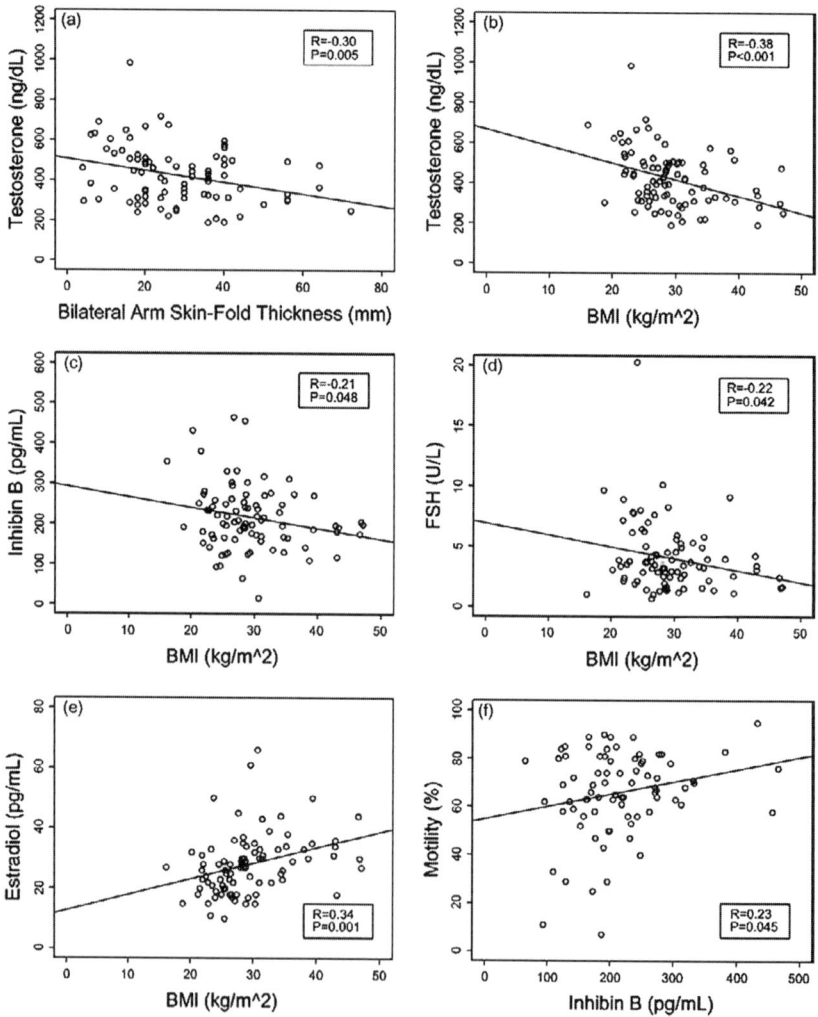

FIGURE 1.—(a) Testosterone level and bilateral arm skin fold thickness; (b) testosterone level and body mass index; (c) inhibin B level and body mass index; (d) FSH level and body mass index; (e) estrogen level and body mass index; (f) sperm motility and inhibin B level. (Reprinted from Pauli EM, Legro RS, Demers LM, et al. Diminished paternity and gonadal function with increasing obesity in men. *Fertil Steril.* 2008;90:346-351, with permission from the American Society for Reproductive Medicine.)

(sperm density, volume, motility, or morphology). Inhibin B level correlated significantly with sperm motility ($r = 0.23$). Men with paternity had lower BMIs (28.0 kg/m^2 vs. 31.6 kg/m^2) and lower skinfold thickness (24.7 mm vs. 34.1 mm) than men without.

Conclusion(s).—Obesity is an infertility factor in otherwise normal men. Obese men demonstrate a relative hypogonadotropic hypogonadism. Reduced inhibin B levels and diminished paternity suggest compromised reproductive capacity in this population (Fig 1).

▶ Obesity is associated with a reduction in serum testosterone concentrations, sex hormone binding globulin, inhibin B, follicle-stimulating hormone (FSH), and elevation of serum concentrations of estrogen. Fertility also appears to be diminished by obesity. Hammoud et al[1] observed that obesity resulted in low sperm counts and motility. Reduced paternity has been reported in obese men. There is limited information about inhibin B in obese men, but inhibin B has been found to be a marker of spermatogenesis. The study by Pauli et al confirmed that obesity is associated with a reduction in total serum testosterone, FSH, inhibin B, and an elevation of serum estradiol concentrations. The reduction in FSH could adversely affect Sertoli cell function and diminish inhibin and sperm production. Currently, there are no studies to confirm that these hormonal and spermatogenesis abnormalities are reversible with weight loss, and what degree of weight loss is needed to enhance fertility potential.

A. W. Meikle, MD

Reference

1. Hammoud AO, Wilde N, Gibson M, et al. Male obesity and alteration in sperm parameters. *Fertil Steril.* 2008;90:2222-2225.

59 Thyroid

Calcitonin Measurement in the Evaluation of Thyroid Nodules in the United States: A Cost-Effectiveness and Decision Analysis
Cheung K, Roman SA, Wang TS, et al (Yale Univ School of Medicine, New Haven, CT; Medical College of Wisconsin, Milwaukee; et al)
J Clin Endocrinol Metab 93:2173-2180, 2008

Context.—European studies have shown that the use of routine calcitonin screening for detection of medullary thyroid cancer (MTC) in patients with thyroid nodules increases the detection of occult MTC and may improve patient outcomes. Calcitonin screening for MTC has not been recommended in recent U.S. practice guidelines.

Objective.—Our objective was to determine the cost-effectiveness (C/E) of routine calcitonin screening in adult patients with thyroid nodules in the United States.

Settings/Subjects.—A decision model was developed for a hypothetical group of adult patients presenting for evaluation of thyroid nodules in the United States. Patients were screened using current American Thyroid Association guidelines only, or American Thyroid Association guidelines with routine serum calcitonin screening. Input data were obtained from the literature, the Surveillance Epidemiology and End Results and Healthcare Cost and Utilization Project's Nationwide Inpatient Sample databases, and the Medicare Reimbursement Schedule. Sensitivity analyses were performed for a number of input variables.

Main Outcome Measures.—C/E, measured in dollars per life years saved (LYS), was calculated.

Results.—Addition of calcitonin screening to current American Thyroid Association guidelines for the evaluation of thyroid nodules would cost $11,793 per LYS ($10,941–$12,646). When extrapolated to the national level, calcitonin screening for MTC in the United States would yield an additional 113,000 life years at a cost increase of 5.3%. Calcitonin screening C/E is sensitive to patient age and gender, and to changes in disease prevalence, specificity of fine needle aspiration and calcitonin testing, calcitonin screening level, costs of testing, and length of follow-up.

Conclusion.—Routine serum calcitonin screening in patients undergoing evaluation for thyroid nodules appears to be cost effective in the

United States, with C/E comparable to the measurement of thyroid stimulating hormone, colonoscopy, and mammography screening.

▶ Medullary thyroid carcinoma (MTC) arises from the C cells of the thyroid. There is a sporadic and a familial form consisting of familial MTC and the multiple endocrine neoplasia type 2. MTC is characterized by the overproduction of calcitonin, a 32 amino acid long polypeptide hormone. Because calcitonin is mainly produced by the C cells of the thyroid gland, it can be used for diagnosing clinically occult MTC, sometimes in connection with a pentagastrin test.[1-3] Therefore, MTC belongs to the group of rare cancers, which can be safely detected by measurement of a serum tumor marker. Importantly, it has also been demonstrated[4] that early detection of MTC is associated with an improvement in patient outcome. Based on that, there is a long-lasting debate on whether calcitonin screening should be generally recommended. In 2006, the European Thyroid Association and Cancer Research Network followed the lead of individual European countries and developed a European consensus report on the management of differentiated thyroid carcinoma, including the use of calcitonin screening in patients with thyroid nodules. These guidelines recommended the use of calcitonin measurement in the initial diagnostic evaluation of thyroid nodules.[5] In the United States, the American Thyroid Association management guidelines for patients with thyroid nodules could not "recommend either for or against the routine measurement of serum calcitonin" because of unresolved issues of sensitivity, specificity, assay performance, cost-effectiveness (C/E), and lack of pentagastrin availability in the United States. The article by Cheung et al presents for the first time a formal C/E analysis of the addition of routine serum calcitonin screening to current American Thyroid Association guidelines in the United States. The authors calculated additional costs of almost $12 000 per life years saved. These are almost the same costs as those for measurement of thyroid stimulating hormone, for colonoscopy and mammography screening. In my eyes and based on these clear data, the American Thyroid Association should follow the Europeans and should recommend a calcitonin screening in all patients presenting with 1 or more thyroid nodules.

M. Schott, MD, PhD

References

1. Vierhapper H, Niederle B, Bieglmayer C, Kaserer K, Baumgartner-Parzer S. Early diagnosis and curative therapy of medullary thyroid carcinoma by routine measurement of serum calcitonin in patients with thyroid disorders. *Thyroid.* 2005;15:1267-1272.
2. Costante G, Meringolo D, Durante C, et al. Predictive value of serum calcitonin levels for preoperative diagnosis of medullary thyroid carcinoma in a cohort of 5817 consecutive patients with thyroid nodules. *J Clin Endocrinol Metab.* 2007; 92:450-455.
3. Elisei R, Bottici V, Luchetti F, et al. Impact of routine measurement of serum calcitonin on the diagnosis and outcome of medullary thyroid cancer: experience in 10,864 patients with nodular thyroid disorders. *J Clin Endocrinol Metab.* 2004; 89:163-168.

4. Pacini F, Schlumberger M, Dralle H, Elisei R, Smit JW, Wiersinga W. European consensus for the management of patients with differentiated thyroid carcinoma of the follicular epithelium. *Eur J Endocrinol.* 2006;154:787-803.
5. Cooper DS, Doherty GM, Haugen BR, et al. Management guidelines for patients with thyroid nodules and differentiated thyroid cancer. *Thyroid.* 2006;16: 109-142.

Phase II Trial of Sorafenib in Advanced Thyroid Cancer

Gupta-Abramson V, Troxel AB, Nellore A, et al (Univ of Pennsylvania, Philadelphia)

J Clin Oncol 26:4714-4719, 2008

Purpose.—Given the molecular pathophysiology of thyroid cancer and the spectrum of kinases inhibited by sorafenib, including Raf kinase, vascular endothelial growth factor receptors, platelet-derived growth factor receptor, and RET tyrosine kinases, we conducted an open-label phase II trial to determine the efficacy of sorafenib in patients with advanced thyroid carcinoma.

Patients and Methods.—Eligible patients with metastatic, iodine-refractory thyroid carcinoma received sorafenib 400 mg orally twice daily. Responses were measured radiographically every 2 to 3 months. The study end points included response rate, progression-free survival (PFS), and best response by Response Evaluation Criteria in Solid Tumors.

Results.—Thirty patients were entered onto the study and treated for a minimum of 16 weeks. Seven patients (23%; 95% CI, 0.10 to 0.42) had a partial response lasting 18+ to 84 weeks. Sixteen patients (53%; 95% CI, 0.34 to 0.72) had stable disease lasting 14 to 89+ weeks. Seventeen (95%) of 19 patients for whom serial thyroglobulin levels were available showed a marked and rapid response in thyroglobulin levels with a mean decrease of 70%. The median PFS was 79 weeks. Toxicity was consistent with other sorafenib trials, although a single patient died of liver failure that was likely treatment related.

Conclusion.—Sorafenib has clinically relevant antitumor activity in patients with metastatic, iodine-refractory thyroid carcinoma, with an overall clinical benefit rate (partial response + stable disease) of 77%, median PFS of 79 weeks, and an overall acceptable safety profile. These results represent a significant advance over chemotherapy in both response rate and PFS and support further investigation of this agent in these patients (Figs 1-3).

▶ In line with the article by Sherman et al,[1] there was this highly interesting article from Gupta-Abramson et al dealing with the treatment of advanced iodine-refractory thyroid cancers with the multityrosine kinase inhibitor sorafenib with multiple targets, including B-type Raf kinase (BRAF) and vascular endothelial growth factor (VEGF) receptor.[1,2] It has already been demonstrated that thyroid tumors are highly vascular and overexpress VEGF.[2] Moreover, it is known that inhibition of VEGF receptor (VEGFR) signaling inhibits growth of

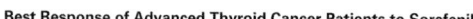

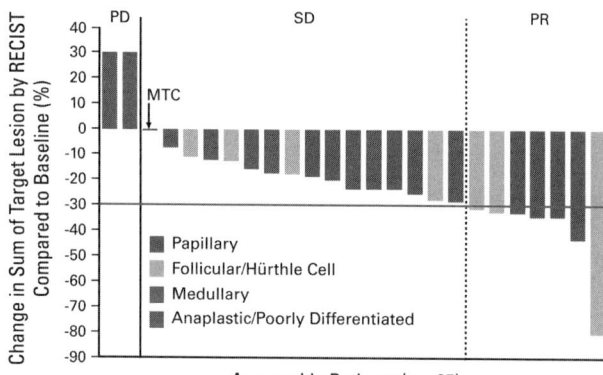

FIGURE 1.—Best overall percentage of change from baseline in target lesion measurement. Baseline radiographic measurements of target lesions were compared with measurements over the course of the study to determine the best change in target lesion size for each patient with data. RECIST, Response Evaluation Criteria in Solid Tumors; PD, progressive disease; SD, stable disease; PR, partial response; MTC, medullary thyroid cancer. (Reprinted from Gupta-Abramson V, Troxel AB, Nellore A, et al. Phase II trial of sorafenib in advanced thyroid cancer. *J Clin Oncol.* 2008;26:4714-4719, with permission from the American Society of Clinical Oncology. All rights reserved.)

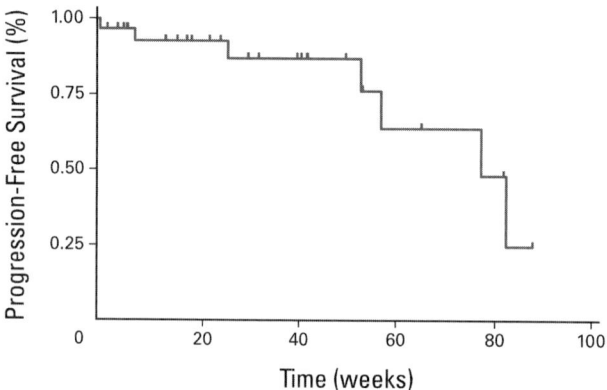

FIGURE 2.—Kaplan-Meier estimate of progression-free survival (PFS) for patients on study. Median PFS was 79.0 weeks. (Reprinted from Gupta-Abramson V, Troxel AB, Nellore A, et al. Phase II trial of sorafenib in advanced thyroid cancer. *J Clin Oncol.* 2008;26:4714-4719, with permission from the American Society of Clinical Oncology. All rights reserved.)

thyroid tumors in xenograft models,[3] thereby providing a strong rationale for targeting VEGFR in this disease. Besides, the BRAF in the mitogen-activated protein kinase signaling pathway also plays a key role in thyroid cancer, and an acidic substitution at a single amino acid residue, V600E, occurs frequently.[4] BRAF[V600E] is associated with substantially higher basal kinase activity compared with wild-type BRAF, and transfection experiments have shown that expression of BRAF[V600E] is associated with 70- to 138-fold greater

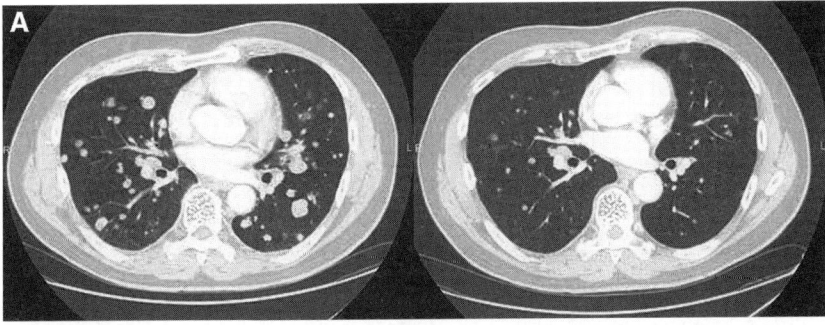

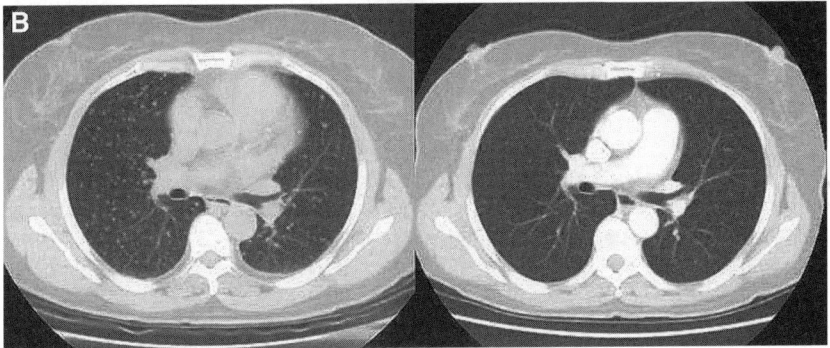

FIGURE 3.—(A) A 60-year-old man with follicular thyroid cancer had metastatic disease in the lung (left). Computed tomography (CT) scans confirm partial response in target lesions (right) after 16 weeks of treatment with sorafenib. (B) A 59-year-old woman with papillary thyroid cancer had widespread miliary lung metastases (left). CT scans show marked improvement in the burden of lung disease after 33 weeks of treatment with sorafenib (right). (Reprinted from Gupta-Abramson V, Troxel AB, Nellore A, et al. Phase II trial of sorafenib in advanced thyroid cancer. *J Clin Oncol.* 2008;26:4714-4719, with permission from the American Society of Clinical Oncology. All rights reserved.)

transformation efficacy.[4] In thyroid cancer, BRAF^{V600E} has been found in 29% to 69% of papillary thyroid cancers,[5] and has been associated with aggressive features, including extrathyroidal extension and advanced stage.[6] Based on these data, there was this rationale to test the multikinase inhibitor in humans. This study clearly demonstrates that this treatment approach has a clear benefit with regard to the response rate (Fig 1) and the progression-free survival (Fig 2) compared with the classical chemotherapy. Fig 3 shows an impressive result in a 60-year-old patient following treatment with sorafenib. Importantly, this study consisted mostly of patients with differentiated thyroid cancer; 27 of 30 patients had either papillary or follicular subtypes. Thus, the results demonstrated not being generalizable to other subtypes of thyroid cancer. Notably, the 2 patients who had progressive disease as their best response had poorly differentiated/anaplastic disease. Nonetheless, the results suggest that sorafenib warrants further investigation in the treatment of advanced thyroid cancer.

M. Schott, MD, PhD

References

1. Sherman SI, Wirth LJ, Droz JP, et al. Motesanib diphosphate in progressive differentiated thyroid cancer. *N Engl J Med.* 2008;359:31-42.
2. Tuttle RM, Fleisher M, Francis GL, Robbins RJ. Serum vascular endothelial growth factor levels are elevated in metastatic differentiated thyroid cancer but not increased by short-term TSH stimulation. *J Clin Endocrinol Metab.* 2002; 87:1737-1742.
3. Bauer AJ, Terrell R, Doniparthi NK, et al. Vascular endothelial growth factor monoclonal antibody inhibits growth of anaplastic thyroid cancer xenografts in nude mice. *Thyroid.* 2002;12:953-961.
4. Davies H, Bignell GR, Cox C, et al. Mutations of the BRAF gene in human cancer. *Nature.* 2002;417:949-954.
5. Namba H, Nakashima M, Hayashi T, et al. Clinical implication of hot spot BRAF mutation, V599E, in papillary thyroid cancers. *J Clin Endocrinol Metab.* 2003;88: 4393-4397.
6. Xing M, Westra WH, Tufano RP, et al. BRAF mutation predicts a poorer clinical prognosis for papillary thyroid cancer. *J Clin Endocrinol Metab.* 2005;90: 6373-6379.

Effects of T4 replacement therapy on glucose metabolism in subjects with subclinical (SH) and overt hypothyroidism (OH)

Handisurya A, Pacini G, Tura A, et al (Med Univ of Vienna, Austria; Natl Res Council, Padova, Italy)
Clin Endocrinol 69:963-969, 2008

Objective.—To evaluate β-cell function and insulin sensitivity in subjects with overt (OH) and subclinical hypothyroidism (SH) before and after T4 replacement therapy.

Background.—Disturbances in glucose metabolism have been observed in hypothyroid states. However, the clinical significance and potential reversibility of these alterations by T4 replacement therapy remain to be elucidated especially in patients with SH.

Design and Patients.—Parameters of glucose metabolism have been investigated in subjects with OH ($n = 12$) and SH ($n = 11$). Insulin sensitivity has been assessed by the euglycaemic–hyperinsulinaemic clamp technique and β-cell function by mathematical modelling of data derived from an oral glucose tolerance test.

Results.—Fasting and dynamic glycaemia as assessed by the $AUC_{Glucose}$ remained unaltered following substitution therapy ($P > 0\cdot05$). Insulin sensitivity significantly improved only in subjects with OH ($P < 0\cdot05$). Fasting insulin and proinsulin concentrations increased proportionally in both groups ($P < 0\cdot05$) with the proinsulin: insulin ratio remaining unchanged ($P > 0\cdot05$). Total insulin secretion was higher in OH before initiation of therapy ($P < 0\cdot05$). In both groups, dynamic parameters including total insulin secretion, hepatic insulin extraction and the adaptation index were significantly attenuated ($P < 0\cdot05$) after restoration of thyroid function, whereas the disposition index and the basal insulin secretion rate remained unaltered ($P > 0\cdot05$).

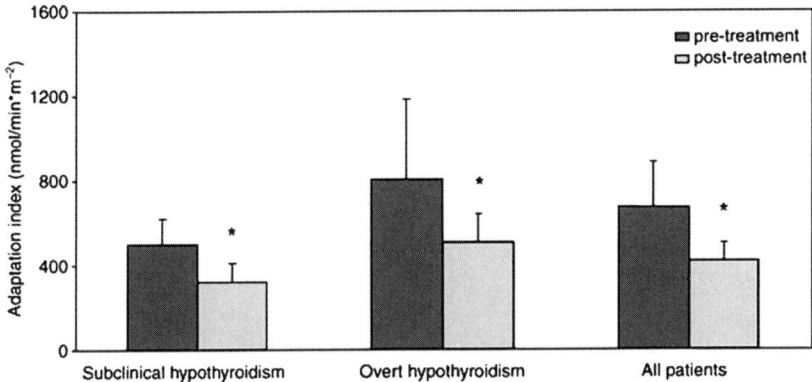

FIGURE 2.—Adaptation index in subjects with SH, OH and in all patients. *$P < 0.05$: pretreatment *vs.* posttreatment. (Reprinted from Handisurya A, Pacini G, Tura A, et al. Effects of T4 replacement therapy on glucose metabolism in subjects with subclinical (SH) and overt hypothyroidism (OH). *Clin Endocrinol.* 2008;69:963-969, with permission from Wiley-Blackwell.)

Conclusion.—In summary, SH and OH are characterized by attenuated basal plasma insulin levels and increased glucose-induced insulin secretion. T4 replacement therapy partially ameliorates the insulin secretion profile and reduces the demand on pancreatic β-cells after glucose challenge to an extent that exceeds any effect attributable to the improvement in insulin sensitivity (Fig 2, Table 2).

▶ Although thyroid dysfunction has been postulated to be associated with dyslipidaemia and increased risk of cardiovascular disease, the effects of overt hypothyroidism (OH), and especially of subclinical hypothyroidism (SH) on glucose metabolism as well as the associated pathophysiological significance and the benefits of a T4 replacement therapy, are a matter of debate. It is known that abnormal glucose metabolism is common in thyrotoxicosis, and triiodothyronine is known to increase splanchnic release and peripheral uptake of glucose in healthy men. Although the underlying mechanisms are not fully understood, several explanations such as β-cell dysfunction, insulin resistance, and increased gluconeogenesis with increased hepatic glucose production have been suggested.[1] To date, few studies have investigated the impact of thyroid deficiency and its reversal by T4 replacement therapy on glucose metabolism and results, especially in SH, have been controversial.[2,3] The data presented here indicate that not only OH, but also SH, is associated with a deterioration of glucose metabolism. Table 2 shows detailed results of fasting plasma hormone concentrations in subjects with SH and OH before and after T4 replacement therapy. Fig 2 shows the adaptation indices, which represent the products between insulin sensitivity and the β-cell function indices. These data suggest that OH is characterized by reduced plasma insulin and increased plasma glucagon concentrations in the basal state due to an attenuation of endogenous glucose production and increased glucose-stimulated insulin secretion in response to elevated whole-body insulin resistance. The increased

TABLE 2.—Fasting plasma hormone concentrations in subjects with SH or OH before and after L-T4 replacement therapy

	Subclinical Hypothyroidism		Overt Hypothyroidism		All Patients Before vs.
	Before Therapy	After Therapy	Before Therapy	After Therapy	After Therapy
Glucose (mmol/l)	$5·3 \pm 0·2$	$5·4 \pm 0·2$	$5·4 \pm 0·3$	$5·0 \pm 0·2$	NS
Insulin (pmol/l)	$44·8 \pm 5·2$	$\mathbf{64·4 \pm 11·7\dagger}$	$52·5 \pm 6·2$	$\mathbf{74·7 \pm 8·6\ddagger}$	0·0014
C-peptide (pmol/l)	$600·1 \pm 52·4$	$582·8 \pm 34·7$	$746·2 \pm 78·9$	$663·7 \pm 73·9$	NS
Proinsulin (pmol/l)	$9·2 \pm 0·9$	$\mathbf{12·0 \pm 1·4\dagger\dagger}$	$9·4 \pm 1·0$	$\mathbf{14·9 \pm 2·8\ddagger}$	0·0144
Proinsulin : Insulin ratio	$0·22 \pm 0·02$	$0·20 \pm 0·01$	$0·19 \pm 0·02$	$0·19 \pm 0·02$	NS
Leptin (µg/l)					
Basal	$13·4 \pm 1·9$	$13·9 \pm 1·7$	$16·9 \pm 3·4$	$22·1 \pm 6·1$	NS
Stimulated (OGTT: 120 min)	$12·1 \pm 1·8$	$12·6 \pm 1·3$	$15·7 \pm 3·2$	$20·0 \pm 5·1$	NS
Cortisol (nmol/l)					
Basal	$491·5 \pm 65·2$	$513·6 \pm 80·5$	$417·3 \pm 52·5$	$423·6 \pm 52·7$	NS
Stimulated (OGTT: 120 min)	$366·9 \pm 43·0$	$\mathbf{308·7 \pm 63·2\dagger}$	$325·5 \pm 58·4$	$247·8 \pm 38·6$	0·0495
Glucagon (pmol/l)					
Basal	$45·9 \pm 4·0$	$42·1 \pm 3·2$	$50·2 \pm 3·4$	$\mathbf{42·8 \pm 2·8\ddagger}$	0·0213
Stimulated (OGTT: 120 min)	$57·0 \pm 6·1$	$48·1 \pm 7·3$	$59·3 \pm 5·7$	$\mathbf{50·8 \pm 3·5\ddagger}$	0·0108
Human GH (µg/l)					
Basal	$5·51 \pm 2·9$	$5·56 \pm 2·17$	$3·89 \pm 0·82$	$5·04 \pm 2·26$	NS
Stimulated (OGTT: 120 min)	$0·98 \pm 0·24$	$1·28 \pm 0·25$	$0·75 \pm 0·08$	$0·78 \pm 0·15$	NS
Free fatty acids (µmol/l)					
Basal	$523·3 \pm 110·5$	$458·0 \pm 66·5$	$659·7 \pm 57·7$	$\mathbf{292·3 \pm 62·6\ddagger\ddagger}$	0·0107
Stimulated (OGTT: 120 min)	$46·7 \pm 11·6$	$18·0 \pm 4·6$	$33·3 \pm 6·8$	$28·8 \pm 13·7$	0·0482

Reference range: Glucose 4·2–6·1 mmol/l, Insulin 34·7–173·6 pmol/l, C-Peptide 298·0–2351·0 pmol/l; $\dagger P < 0·05$, $\dagger\dagger P < 0·01$: SH before vs. after therapy, $\ddagger P < 0·05$, $\ddagger\ddagger P < 0·01$: OH before vs. after therapy.

(Reprinted from Handisurya A, Pacini G, Tura A, et al. Effects of T4 replacement therapy on glucose metabolism in subjects with subclinical (SH) and overt hypothyroidism (OH). *Clin Endocrinol*. 2008;69:963-969, with permission from Wiley-Blackwell.)

demand on β-cells following glucose loading also appears to be present in SH. Thus, therapeutic intervention might be of relevance in this patient collective, especially with regard to the high progression rate of SH to OH, and if other predisposing factors for an impaired glucose metabolism are present.

M. Schott, MD, PhD

References

1. Dimitriadis GD, Raptis SA. Thyroid hormone excess and glucose intolerance. *Exp Clin Endocrinol Diabetes*. 2001;109:S225-S239.
2. Brenta G, Berg G, Arias P, et al. Lipoprotein alterations, hepatic lipase activity, and insulin sensitivity in subclinical hypothyroidism: response to L-T(4) treatment. *Thyroid*. 2007;17:453-460.
3. Owecki M, Nikisch E, Sowinski J. Hypothyroidism has no impact on insulin sensitivity assessed with HOMA-IR in totally thyroidectomized patients. *Acta Clin Belg*. 2006;61:69-73.

Amiodarone-Induced Thyrotoxicosis Is a Predictor of Adverse Cardiovascular Outcome

Yiu K-H, Jim M-H, Siu C-W, et al (Univ of Hong Kong; Grantham Hosp, Hong Kong)

J Clin Endocrinol Metab 94:109-114, 2009

Background.—Amiodarone-induced thyrotoxicosis (AIT) is a clinical condition that is notoriously difficult to manage; the relative risk of adverse cardiovascular events in these patients compared with euthyroid patients is largely unknown.

Objective.—We compared the clinical characteristics and major adverse cardiovascular events (MACE) in AIT and euthyroid patients.

Method.—Patients at a tertiary referral center who had been prescribed amiodarone for at least 3 months were retrospectively analyzed. Baseline clinical characteristics, laboratory parameters, and outcome events were evaluated. MACE was defined as cardiovascular mortality, myocardial infarction, stroke and heart failure, or ventricular arrhythmias that required hospitalization.

Results.—A total of 354 patients (61.8 ± 14.1 yr; 64.7% male) with a mean follow-up of 48.6 ± 26.7 months were studied. AIT, euthyroid status, and amiodarone-induced hypothyroidism were identified in 57 (16.1%), 224 (63.3%), and 73 (20.6%) patients, respectively. No differences in baseline clinical characteristics were observed between AIT and euthyroid patients. Nonetheless AIT patients demonstrated a higher MACE rate (31.6 *vs.* 10.7%, $P < 0.01$), mostly driven by a higher rate of ventricular arrhythmias that required admission (7.0 *vs.* 1.3%, $P = 0.03$). Cox-regression multivariate analysis revealed that AIT (hazard ratio 2.68; confidence interval 1.53–4.68; $P < 0.01$) and left ventricular ejection fraction less than 45% (hazard ratio 2.52; confidence interval 1.43–4.42; $P < 0.01$) were independent predictors of MACE.

Conclusion.—In patients prescribed long-term amiodarone therapy, occurrence of AIT is associated with a 2.7-fold increased risk of MACE. Regular and close biochemical surveillance is thus advisable to identify and treat this high-risk group of patients (Fig 1).

▶ It is known that chronic use of amiodarone can be associated with significant side effects. One common side effect is thyroid dysfunction. This includes subclinical derangement of serum T_4 and T_3 or, in the extreme, overt clinical hypothyroidism or hyperthyroidism. Amiodarone contains 39% iodine by weight; chronic treatment is associated with a 40-fold increase in plasma and urinary iodide levels that is responsible for the thyroid dysfunction. Whereas amiodarone-induced hypothyroidism (AIH) is easily controlled by T_4 replacement, treatment for the less common amiodarone-induced thyrotoxicosis (AIT) is more complex and challenging.[1] Previous retrospective studies showed that AIT was associated with a greater increased risk of death and adverse cardiovascular events than Graves' thyrotoxicosis and toxic multinodular goitre, especially in the presence of left ventricular dysfunction.[2] The clinical outcome

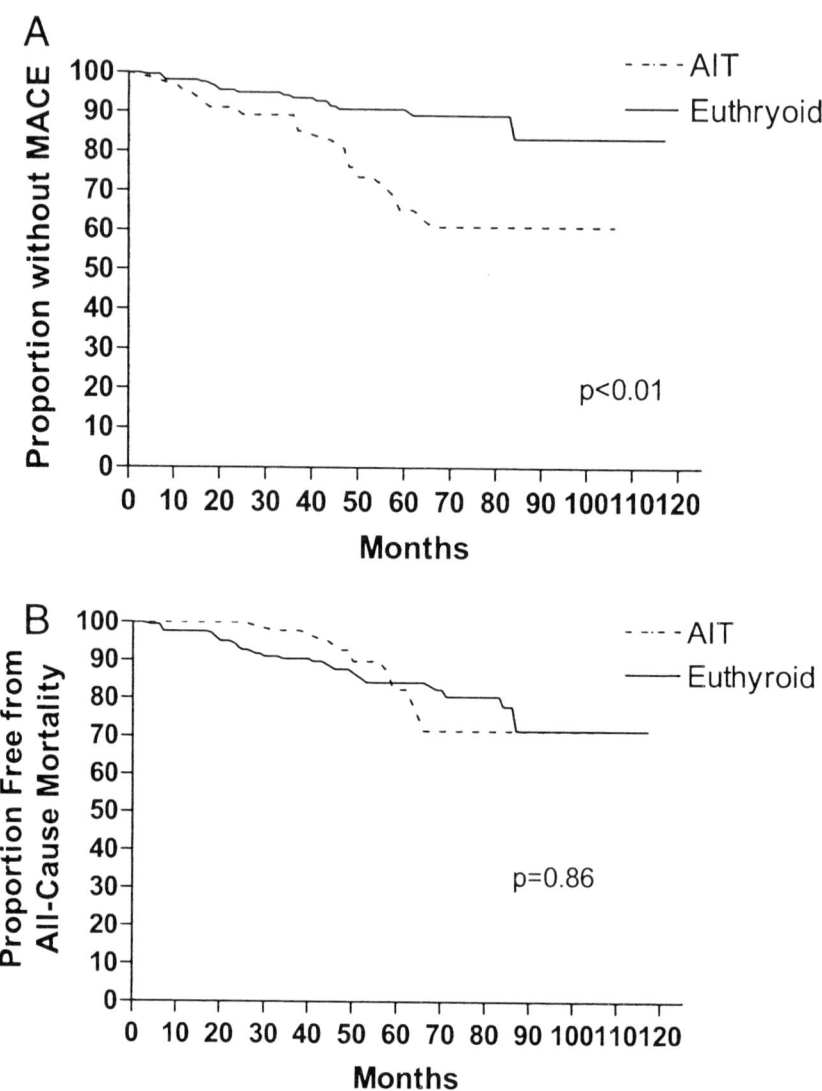

FIGURE 1.—A and B, Kaplan-Meier survival estimates of the development of MACE or all-cause mortality comparing patients with amiodarone induced thyrotoxicosis and euthyroid patients. (Reprinted from Yiu K-H, Jim M-H, Siu C-W, et al. Amiodarone-induced thyrotoxicosis is a predictor of adverse cardiovascular outcome. *J Clin Endocrinol Metab.* 2009;94:109-114, with permission from The Endocrine Society.)

for patients with AIT compared with those prescribed amiodarone but who remain euthyroid was unclear up to now. The aim of this study was to identify the frequency and clinical characteristics of patients prescribed amiodarone who develop thyroid dysfunction and determine whether the development of AIT or AIH can affect their clinical outcome. As shown in Fig 1, patients with

AIT have an increased risk of developing a major adverse cardiovascular event (MACE). There are several explanations for this. One is that AIT may destabilize any preexisting arrhythmia or provoke new arrhythmias under certain conditions. For that reason, it is recommended to look for antithyroperoxidase antibodies in patients receiving amiodarone. This author believes these patients should have regular 24-hour ECG monitoring studies to assess for arrhythmias.

M. Schott, MD, PhD

References

1. Bartalena L, Brogioni S, Grasso L, Bogazzi F, Burelli A, Martino E. Treatment of amiodarone-induced thyrotoxicosis, a difficult challenge: results of a prospective study. *J Clin Endocrinol Metab*. 1996;81:2930-2933.
2. Conen D, Melly L, Kaufmann C, et al. Amiodarone-induced thyrotoxicosis: clinical course and predictors of outcome. *J Am Coll Cardiol*. 2007;49:2350-2355.

Motesanib Diphosphate in Progressive Differentiated Thyroid Cancer
Sherman SI, Wirth LJ, Droz JP, et al (Univ of Texas M.D. Anderson Cancer Ctr, Houston; Dana–Farber Cancer Inst, Boston, MA; Centre Léon Bérard, Lyon, France; et al)
N Engl J Med 359:31-42, 2008

Background.—The expression of vascular endothelial growth factor (VEGF) is characteristic of differentiated thyroid cancer and is associated with aggressive tumor behavior and a poor clinical outcome. Motesanib diphosphate (AMG 706) is a novel oral inhibitor of VEGF receptors, platelet-derived growth-factor receptor, and KIT.

Methods.—In an open-label, single-group, phase 2 study, we treated 93 patients who had progressive, locally advanced or metastatic, radio-iodine-resistant differentiated thyroid cancer with 125 mg of motesanib diphosphate, administered orally once daily. The primary end point was an objective response as assessed by an independent radiographic review. Additional end points included the duration of the response, progression-free survival, safety, and changes in serum thyroglobulin concentration.

Results.—Of the 93 patients, 57 (61%) had papillary thyroid carcinoma. The objective response rate was 14%. Stable disease was achieved in 67% of the patients, and stable disease was maintained for 24 weeks or longer in 35%; 8% had progressive disease as the best response. The Kaplan–Meier estimate of the median duration of the response was 32 weeks (the lower limit of the 95% confidence interval [CI] was 24; the upper limit could not be estimated because of an insufficient number of events); the estimate of median progression-free survival was 40 weeks (95% CI, 32 to 50). Among the 75 patients in whom thyroglobulin analysis was performed, 81% had decreased serum thyroglobulin concentrations during treatment, as compared with baseline levels. The most common treatment-related adverse events were diarrhea (in 59% of the patients), hypertension (56%), fatigue (46%), and weight loss (40%).

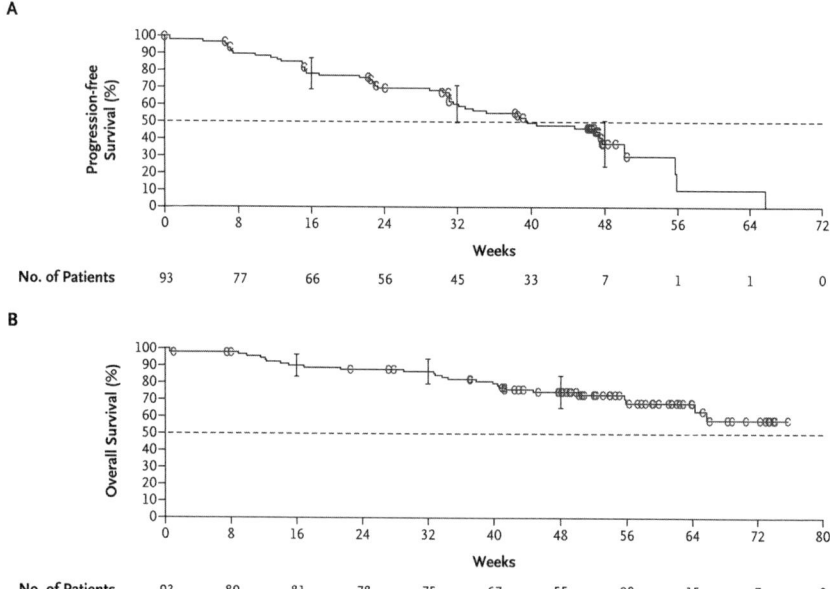

FIGURE 2.—Kaplan–Meier Analysis of Progression-free Survival and Overall Survival. Panel A shows progression-free survival among all 93 patients who received at least one dose of motesanib diphosphate. Panel B shows overall survival among the same patients. Eight patients died during the course of the study, within 30 days after the last administration of motesanib diphosphate; 19 additional patients died during long-term follow-up. The I bars indicate 95% confidence intervals. C denotes censored observation. (Reprinted from Sherman SI, Wirth LJ, Droz JP, et al. Motesanib diphosphate in progressive differentiated thyroid cancer. *N Engl J Med.* 2008;359:31-42, with permission from Massachusetts Medical Society. All rights reserved.)

Conclusions.—Motesanib diphosphate can induce partial responses in patients with advanced or metastatic differentiated thyroid cancer that is progressive (ClinicalTrials.gov number, NCT00121628.) (Fig 2).

▶ Thyroid cancer is the most common endocrine malignancy, with more than 30 000 new cases of thyroid cancers projected to be diagnosed in the United States in 2008. Differentiated thyroid carcinoma includes papillary and follicular subtypes and comprises 90% of all cases of thyroid cancer.[1] Once thyroid cancer metastasizes to distant sites and is no longer amenable to radioactive iodine therapy or surgery, expected survival declines rapidly. Chemotherapy with doxorubicin is still the first choice therapy (even though the protocol is quite old).[2] Low response rates, short duration of responses, and cardiotoxicity associated with prolonged treatment have, however, rendered doxorubicin a poor option.

A new therapy modality may represent a treatment with vascular endothelial growth factor (VEGF) inhibitors. VEGF is a potent angiogenesis stimulator. As prerequisite, an increased VEGF expression has already been demonstrated in differentiated thyroid cancers.[3] This was associated with increased growth, progression, and invasiveness of the tumor and with decreased recurrence-free survival.[4,5] For this reason, an inhibitor of angiogenesis may be effective when initial therapy fails. Motesanib diphosphate is an oral inhibitor of the tyrosine kinases of VEGF receptors 1, 2, and 3; platelet-derived growth factor receptor; and KIT. As demonstrated in Fig 1 in the original journal article, the oral treatment with motesanib diphosphate results in an objective response in 14% of patients. The progression-free survival and the overall survival are shown in Fig 2. The data clearly demonstrate that treatment with motesanib diphosphate can induce partial responses in a certain number of patients. The clear limitation of this trial is the lack of randomization with a control group. Because the study group specifically included patients with advanced differentiated thyroid cancer, traditional comparator therapies, such as cytotoxic chemotherapy, would have been inappropriate owing to their ineffectiveness and toxicity. I myself think that the large number of patients enrolled in this study still allow a reasonable estimate of clinical benefit of a treatment with motesanib diphosphate.

M. Schott, MD, PhD

References

1. Sherman SI. Thyroid carcinoma. *Lancet.* 2003;361:501-511.
2. Gottlieb JA, Hill CS Jr. Chemotherapy of thyroid cancer with adriamycin. Experience with 30 patients. *N Engl J Med.* 1974;290:193-197.
3. Bunone G, Vigneri P, Mariani L, et al. Expression of angiogenesis stimulators and inhibitors in human thyroid tumors and correlation with clinical pathological features. *Am J Pathol.* 1999;155:1967-1976.
4. Vieira JM, Santos SC, Espadinha C, et al. Expression of vascular endothelial growth factor (VEGF) and its receptors in thyroid carcinomas of follicular origin: a potential autocrine loop. *Eur J Endocrinol.* 2005;153:701-709.
5. Lennard CM, Patel A, Wilson J, et al. Intensity of vascular endothelial growth factor expression is associated with increased risk of recurrence and decreased disease-free survival in papillary thyroid cancer. *Surgery.* 2001;129:552-558.

Article Index

Chapter 1: Rheumatoid Arthritis

Chapter 2: Systemic Lupus Erythematosus

Chapter 3: Vasculitis

Chapter 4: Fibromyalgia

Chapter 5: Scleroderma

Chapter 6: Juvenile Idiopathic Arthritis

Chapter 7: Osteoporosis

Chapter 8: Spondyloarthropathies

Chapter 9: Toxicities of Antirheumatic Agents

Chapter 10: Pathogenesis of Infectious Diseases

Chapter 11: Infectious Disease Management

Chapter 12: Epidemiology and Management of Gram-Positive Infections

Chapter 13: Human Immunodeficiency Virus

Chapter 14: Tuberculosis

Chapter 15: Health Care Associated Infections

Chapter 16: Parasitic Infections

Chapter 17: Vaccines

Chapter 18: Influenza

Chapter 19: Cancer Prevention

Chapter 20: Cancer Screening

Chapter 21: Gynecologic Cancer

Chapter 22: Breast Cancer

Chapter 23: Prostate Cancer

Chapter 24: Lung Cancer

Chapter 25: Geriatric Oncology

Chapter 26: Supportive Care

Chapter 27: Miscellaneous Topics

Chapter 28: Metabolic Factors and Renal Disease Progression

Chapter 29: Hypertension

Chapter 30: Diabetes

Chapter 31: Acute Kidney Injury

Chapter 32: Chronic Renal Failure and Transplantation

Chapter 33: Lung Cancer

Chapter 34: Lung Transplantation

Chapter 35: Chronic Obstructive Pulmonary Disease

Chapter 36: Pleural, Interstitial Lung, and Pulmonary Vascular Disease

Chapter 37: Asthma and Cystic Fibrosis

Chapter 38: Sleep Disorders

Chapter 39: Critical Care Medicine

Chapter 40: Miscellaneous

Chapter 41: Cardiac Arrhythmias, Conduction Disturbances, and Electrophysiology

Chapter 42: Cardiac Surgery

Chapter 43: Coronary Heart Disease

Chapter 44: Hypertension

Chapter 45: Non-Coronary Heart Disease in Adults

Chapter 46: Pediatric Cardiovascular Disease

Chapter 47: Colon

Chapter 48: Pancreas

Chapter 49: Liver

Chapter 50: Miscellaneous

Chapter 51: Adrenal Cortex

Chapter 52: Calcium and Bone Metabolism

Chapter 53: Diabetes

Chapter 54: Lipoproteins and Atherosclerosis

Chapter 55: Neuroendocrinology

Chapter 56: Obesity

Chapter 57: Pediatric Endocrinology

Chapter 58: Reproductive Endocrinology

Chapter 59: Thyroid

Author Index

A

B

C

H

I

J

K

L

V

W

X

Y

Z